PATHOPHYSIOLOGY AND TREATMENT OF INHALATION INJURIES

LUNG BIOLOGY IN HEALTH AND DISEASE

Executive Editor: **Claude Lenfant**

Director, National Heart, Lung, and Blood Institute
National Institutes of Health
Bethesda, Maryland

PATHOPHYSIOLOGY AND TREATMENT OF INHALATION INJURIES

Edited by

Jacob Loke

Department of Medicine
Pulmonary Section
Yale University School of Medicine
New Haven, Connecticut

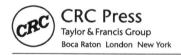

CRC Press
Taylor & Francis Group
Boca Raton London New York

CRC Press is an imprint of the
Taylor & Francis Group, an **informa** business

First published 1988 by Marcel Dekker, Inc.

Published 2019 by CRC Press
Taylor & Francis Group
6000 Broken Sound Parkway NW, Suite 300
Boca Raton, FL 33487-2742

© 1988 by Taylor & Francis Group, LLC
CRC Press is an imprint of Taylor & Francis Group, an Informa business

First issued in paperback 2019

No claim to original U.S. Government works

ISBN 13: 978-0-367-45136-3 (pbk)
ISBN 13: 978-0-8247-7795-1 (hbk)

**Visit the Taylor & Francis Web site at
http://www.taylorandfrancis.com**

**and the CRC Press Web site at
http://www.crcpress.com**

Pathophysiology and treatment of inhalation injuries.

(Lung biology in health and disease ; v. 34)
Includes bibliographies and indexes.
1. Gases, Asphyxiating and poisonous--Toxicology.
2. Lungs--Wounds and injuries. I. Loke, Jacob.
II. Series. [DNLM: 1. Air Pollutants, Environmental--
adverse effects. 2. Lung--injuries. 3. Lung--physio-
pathology. 4. Lung Diseases--therapy. 5. Respiratory
Tract Diseases--chemically induced. W1 LU62 v.34 /
WF 600 P2977]
RA1245.P38   1986   616.2'4   87-24553
ISBN 0-8247-7795-6

INTRODUCTION

Without question, Dr. Samuel S. Fitch (Fitch, 1853) of Philadelphia was no ordinary physician. He was, in fact, a visionary!

On October 17, 1844, R. R. Hinman, late Secretary of State of the State of Connecticut, wrote to Professor Kingsly of Yale College to introduce Dr. Fitch, who was about to visit New Haven. He said: "(Dr. Fitch) is not only a regularly educated physician, but he has been eminently successful in that branch of his profession which he has particularly pursued for many years past . . . You can rely on him as a gentleman . . . in every way worthy of the patronage of the public."

Dr. Fitch was a lung doctor whose specialty was what was then known as "consumption." The point of interest about him is that he believed that "it is utterly impossible to have pulmonary consumption so long as . . . the wall of the air cells (stay) free from engorgement or deposition of foreign matter." In one of his lectures Dr. Fitch explained the higher death rate from consumption in New York than in Philadelphia on supposition that the air in Philadelphia was devoid of (toxic) substances.

Whether the lungs can be impaired by a great variety of inert or active elements is no longer a question, but a fact of public health. Indeed, the lungs are our interface with an environment which in many ways is becoming more and more hostile as a consequence of industrial progress and societal evolution.

Until now, no volume of the series Lung Biology in Health and Disease has addressed the problem of inhalation injury. Although it is unclear to me whether Dr. Jacob Loke was inspired by knowledge of Dr. Fitch's visit to Yale College in 1844, it is fortunate that he contributed his expertise in pulmonary toxicology to edit *Pathophysiology and Treatment of Inhalation Injuries.* In toto, as well as in each individual chapter, this volume represents a new venture for this series of monographs. It covers many aspects of inhalation toxicology: dusts, vapors, heat, and radiation. All topics are addressed by authors whose recognized expertise is unchallenged. That this volume is at the forefront in facing today's problems is evidenced by the inclusion of a chapter concerning the inhalation of such drugs as cocaine. In reflecting on this type of self-imposed inhalation injury, its impact should be weighed against injuries to large populations, such as those resulting from the Bhopal and the Chernobyl catastrophes, or those that result from the industrial exploitation of the resources that provide us with comfort or enjoyment.

Inhalation toxicology is, and probably will remain, both a medical and a societal problem. This volume will undoubtedly serve as a reference, if not an inspiration, to potential students of this field. In one of his discourses, Dr. Fitch said "All may live to reach the utmost verge of longevity, provided accidents do not occur—diseases are obviated, and premature exhaustion of the system does not take place from our own war upon it."

Let this volume remind us of this prediction!

Reference

Fitch, Samuel Sheldon (1853). *Six Discourses on the Function of the Lungs.* S. S. Fitch & Co., New York.

Claude Lenfant, M.D.

PREFACE

In the world we live in, the potential toxic hazardous effects of gases, vapors, and particles in the environment on the lungs and other systems are always present. The toxic environment can develop due to natural disaster such as the release of clouds of toxic gases to the atmosphere from volcanic gas eruption in Cameroon, Africa, in 1986, or the manmade industrial pesticide plant accident due to the poison gas leak of methyl isocyanate in Bhopal, India, in 1984, which killed an estimated 1500 and 1600 people, respectively. The 1986 Chernobyl nuclear accident in Russia caused the release of radioactive material which not only produced death from excessive radiation, but will probably result in an increase in cancer deaths in the areas around Chernobyl related to the nuclear plant disaster for years to come. Closer to home, fires in homes and buildings claim the lives of 5000 people annually in the United States.

Inhalation toxicology covers a broad spectrum of multispecialty disciplines in science, namely, chemistry, pharmacology, toxicology, and medicine. In this volume, we have tried to cover several aspects of inhalation toxicology ranging from inhalation drug abuse (Chap. 9) to battlefield chemical inhalation lung injury, and emphasizing pathophysiology and therapy. Although cigarette smoking and asbestosis and silica also have deleterious effects on the lungs, these topics are not discussed here.

There is much to be learned from the pathophysiology of lung injury by toxic gases since Dr. Winternitz at Yale studied the effects of chemical war gas poisoning on the lungs and published his classical findings in 1920 (Chap. 8). So often with toxic inhalation lung injury, physicians merely treat the effect of the lung injury without identifying the toxicological characteristics of the gases, fumes, or particles. Animal studies have been done to correlate the exposure of specific toxic agents with lung injury in laboratory animals, and thus help us better understand the effects of these agents on the lungs of humans (Chap. 3). Using a specially designed exposure chamber for guinea pigs, obstructive patterns were demonstrated in these animals with methyl isocyanate exposure similar to the lung disease observed in surviving victims of Bhopal. Serial lung function tests and bronchoalveolar lavage in laboratory animals exposed to toxic materials or substances can provide us with a better understanding of the pathogenesis of inhalation lung injury and its therapy (Chap. 6).

Sampling of the gases in the toxic environment for toxicological analysis should be performed in addition to blood monitoring of fire victims, with smoke inhalation, for carboxyhemoglobin, methemoglobin, cyanide, benzene, and alcohol. Identification of the toxic gas exposure and analyses of blood samples for toxicological screening provide important clinical information for the rational management of inhalation lung injury.

Inhalation drug abuse is going to show an explosive growth, especially with progressive free-base cocaine abuse. While the pleasurable "rewards" of drug abuse are short-lived, it can lead to physical impairment, lung injury, life-threatening situations, and death. Detection of drug abuse in employees or patients has both medical and legal implications. Guidelines are given for identification of drug abuse screening in biological fluids with heroin, cocaine, marijuana, and phencyclidine.

Finally, there may be other "toxic" inhaled agents in the environment, radon, for example, or other substances yet to be identified that do not produce acute lung injury, but may be carcinogenic in nature, and produce lung cancer over an extended period of chronic exposure (Chap. 10).

Jacob Loke

CONTRIBUTORS

Yves Alarie, Ph.D. Professor and Chairman, Department of Industrial Environmental Health Sciences, University of Pittsburgh, Graduate School of Public Health, Pittsburgh, Pennsylvania

Caroline Chiles, M.D. Assistant Professor, Department of Radiology, Duke University Medical Center, Durham, North Carolina

Y. X. Du, M.D. Associate Professor and Chief, Department of Hygiene, Guangzhou Medical College, Director, Guangzhou Research Center for Lung Cancer, Guangzhou, China

Laurence W. Hedlund, Ph.D. Assistant Professor, Department of Radiology, Duke University Medical Center, Durham, North Carolina

William C. Hulbert, Ph.D. Assistant Research Professor, Department of Medicine, Division of Pulmonary Medicine, University of Alberta, Edmonton, Alberta, Canada

Peter Jatlow, M.D. Professor and Chairman, Laboratory Medicine and Professor Psychiatry, Yale University School of Medicine, and Director of Clinical Laboratories, Yale-New Haven Hospital, New Haven, Connecticut

Herbert D. Kleber, M.D. Professor, Department of Psychiatry, Yale University School of Medicine, and Director, Substance Abuse Treatment Unit, Connecticut Mental Health Center, New Haven, Connecticut

W. K. Lam, M.B., M.D., F.R.C.P. Senior Lecturer, Department of Medicine, University of Hong Kong and Queen Mary Hospital, Hong Kong

Jacob Loke, M.D. Associate Professor, Department of Medicine, Pulmonary Section, and Director of Pulmonary Function Laboratory, Yale University School of Medicine, New Haven, Connecticut

S. F. Paul Man, M.D. Professor, Department of Medicine, Division of Pulmonary Medicine, University of Alberta, Edmonton, Alberta, Canada

Richard A. Matthay, M.D. Professor, Department of Medicine, Pulmonary Section, Yale University School of Medicine, New Haven, Connecticut

Joseph A. Moylan, M.D. Professor and Director, Trauma Service, Department of Surgery, Duke University Medical Center, Durham, North Carolina

Basil A. Pruitt, Jr., M.D. Commander and Director, U. S. Army Institute of Surgical Research, Fort Sam Houston, San Antonio, Texas

Charles E. Putman, M.D. James B. Duke Professor of Radiology, Vice-Chancellor and Vice-Provost, Duke University Medical Center, Durham, North Carolina

Herbert Y. Reynolds, M.D. Professor and Head, Pulmonary Section, Department of Medicine, Yale University School of Medicine, New Haven, Connecticut

Richard Rowley, M.D. Chief Resident, Department of Medicine, Yale University School of Medicine, New Haven, Connecticut

Michelle Schaper, Ph.D. Research Associate, Department of Industrial Environmental Health Sciences, University of Pittsburgh, Graduate School of Public Health, Pittsburgh, Pennsylvania

Dean Sheppard, M.D. Assistant Professor, University of California, School of Medicine, San Francisco, California

Khan Z. Shirani, M.D. Chief, Surgical Study Branch, U. S. Army Institute of Surgical Research, Fort Sam Houston, San Antonio, Texas

William A. Skornik, M.S., Ph.D. Director, Laboratory for Inhalation Toxicology, Department of Environmental Science and Physiology, Respiratory Biology Program, Harvard University School of Public Health, Boston, Massachusetts

G. J. Walker Smith, M.D. Professor, Department of Pathology, Yale University School of Medicine, New Haven, Connecticut

John S. Urbanetti, M.D. Clinical Assistant, Professor, Yale University School of Medicine, New Haven, Connecticut, and Consultant of Toxic Inhalation to the U.S. Government

K. Randall Young, Jr., M.D. Medical Staff Fellow, Laboratory of Immunoregulation, National Institute of Allergy and Infectious Diseases, National Institutes of Health, Bethesda, Maryland

CONTENTS

1

Airway Repair and Adaptation to Inhalation Injury

S. F. PAUL MAN and WILLIAM C. HULBERT

University of Alberta
Edmonton, Alberta, Canada

There is a continuum of epithelial injuries due to the inhalation of noxious gases and fumes that exist in our environment today; the exposure extremes vary between acute massive and chronic low level. A massive exposure is usually the result of an accident, industrial or otherwise; often there are systemic effects in addition to severe injury to the lungs and eyes, and there is significant morbidity and mortality. Two recent examples of this level of exposure were the sodium cyanate exposure in Bhopal, India, where a large population was at risk, and the Lodgepole sour gas well blow out (of which hydrogen sulfide was a major component) in Alberta, Canada, where a few individuals were injured. These incidences are significant because they were industrial accidents, are potentially preventable, and invariably occur in or near populated areas.

At the other extreme of the spectrum is chronic low-level exposure to a large number of man-made noxious gases. Such low-level exposures, although unavoidable in our civilization, have only recently been recognized as serious health hazards. The total number of noxious gases in the environment and at the work site is increasing; the more common ones are the photochemical oxidants, oxygenated organic compounds such as the oxides of nitrogen and sulfur, ozone, and many others derived from fuel combustion. In contrast to the acute massive exposure, the pathologic changes in the airway following chronic low-level exposure are more subtle and at times difficult to assess. Whereas it is clear that massive acute exposures are life threatening, chronic low-level exposures are less so; indeed, the complex question regarding risk factors or a safety limit of exposure is only now being addressed and demands answers.

The epithelial repair processes following massive or low concentration exposures are different because the lesions caused by these different levels of exposure differ in severity. Adaptation to inhaled oxidant gases is, by definition, exclusively restricted to low-concentration, chronic exposures; as will be discussed later, the development of adaptation is not without a price. Unified concepts of the adaptative and repair processes are still evolving and, in most situations, the steps of these processes, though similar, are dependent upon a multitude of interacting factors.

In this chapter we will review data obtained primarily from animal experiments regarding the injury, repair, and adaptative processes following the inhalation of some of the more common oxidizing gases other than oxygen itself: sulfur dioxide (SO_2, an example of the sulfur oxides), nitrogen dioxide (NO_2, an example of the nitrogen oxides), and ozone (O_3).

I. Organization of the Airway Epithelium

In order to understand the processes of repair and adaptation, it is necessary to review briefly the structural organization of the airway epithelium and to define the function of the cellular constituents. The respiratory tract extends from the external nares to the respiratory bronchioles and at the level of the larynx is arbitrarily divided into the upper and lower tracts. The upper respiratory tract is connected to the paranasal sinuses, the eustachian tubes, and the mastoids. The lower tract is a series of conducting tubes whose branching pattern varies from species to species. The upper and the lower respiratory tracts are covered by a continuous layer of epithelium whose cellular composition changes in the transition from the nares to the peripheral respiratory bronchioles. As anticipated, functional changes of the airway epithelium are related to the cellular changes.

The morphology and population dynamics of the cells lining the nasal passages, the conducting airways, and the gas exchange units have been extensively studied and reviewed (Jeffery and Reid, 1977; Plopper, 1983; Plopper et al., 1980a,b,c, 1983; Gail and Lenfant, 1983). Although interspecies differences in the cellular composition of the respiratory tract epithelium are noted, some generalizations can be drawn. In the upper airway, except for parts of the anterior nares where it is squamous, the epithelium is mostly ciliated, columnar, and pseudostratified. On scanning electron microscopy (SEM), in the trachea and in the mainstem and lobar bronchi the epithelium appears as a dense ciliary mat because of the large surface area of the ciliated cells relative to the other superficial cell types. In the airways peripheral to the lobar bronchi, the epithelium becomes thinned to a single cell layer, the proportion of nonciliated to ciliated cells increases, and, in contrast to the ciliary mat seen in the trachea, on SEM the protruding apex of the nonciliated Clara cell is seen projecting into the bronchiolar lumen (Fig. 1).

Jeffery and Reid (1977) classified the cells in the airway epithelium into subgroups on the basis of their location within the mucosa, the presence of cilia, and the presence or type of secretory granules; a modification of their schema is shown in Figure 2. At least 10 cell types, 8 of them epithelial, are now recognized as resident mucosal cells although not all are present in every species. The distribution of these cells in the central airways has been found to vary between species although the number of ciliated vs. nonciliated cells that communicate with the airway lumen is fairly constant, comprising between 40 and 60% of the cell population (Plopper et al., 1980a,b,c). As shown in Figure 2, the nonciliated superficial cells (those that communicate with the airway lumen) are made up of two different populations: secretory and nonsecretory. Both cell classes have been studied extensively and it is well established that the ultrastructural characteristics of the two populations of nonciliated cells vary markedly between species, within an individual animal, and can change following exposure to irritant gases.

Several investigators (Spicer et al., 1971; Jones and Reid, 1973; Spicer et al., 1980; Plopper et al., 1984; St. George et al., 1985), using classic histochemical methods, lectins immunospecific for sugar residues on proteoglycans, and monoclonal antibodies, have examined the biochemical nature of secretory products within cells in the respiratory epithelium. As a result of these studies, three classes of secretory cells are generally recognized: mucous cells, serous cells, and Clara cells.

The Clara cell is perhaps the most extensively studied nonciliated superficial cell in the airway mucosa (Clara, 1937; Kuhn et al., 1974; Kuhn, 1976; Plopper et al., 1980a,b,c, 1983; Plopper, 1983; Young et al., 1986). This cell, as originally described by Max Clara, had unique ultrastructural characteristics. It was a cuboidal nonciliated cell in the bronchioles, the cellular apex of which projected into the airway lumen. Also, it was filled with dense granules. Recent studies (Plopper et al., 1980a,b,c; Plopper, 1983), however, showed that the ultrastructural features of this cell type vary considerably between species. For example, in the mouse, guinea pig, rat, hamster, and rabbit, there is an abundance of agranular endoplasmic reticulum (AER). The AER has been shown to have high levels of cytochrome p-450 monooxygenase activity and is postulated to be associated with the synthesis of secretory material and the detoxification of xenobiotic compounds. In other species, such as humans and primates,

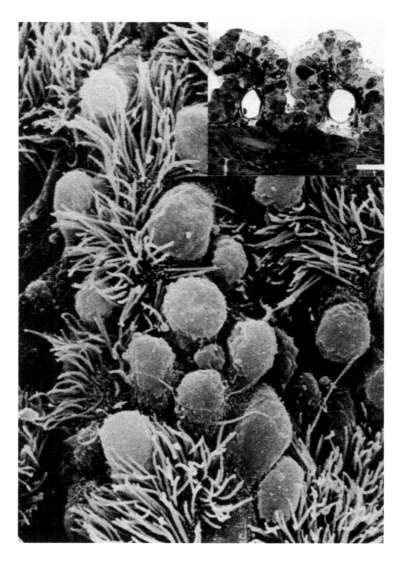

Figure 1 An SEM view of the surface of a bronchus from a guinea pig shows the protruding apices of the abundant nonciliated bronchiolar (Clara) cells and the ciliated cells. The marker bar represents 10 μm. The inset is a light micrograph of a bronchiolar cross-section showing the thick band of smooth muscle underlying the one-cell-layer-thick epithelium. In this view are examples of internalized bronchiolar circulation that causes the ridged appearance of the surface view. The marker bar represents 20 μm.

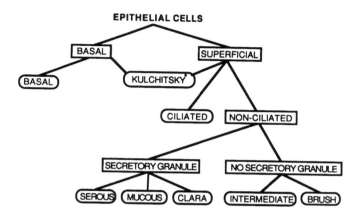

Figure 2 This schema is a modification of one published earlier (Jeffery and Reid, 1977) to illustrate the different residuent cell types in the tracheal mucosa. The Kulchitsky cell is also a superficial cell in the guinea pig.

the cells do not have abundant AER. The electron-dense granules in humans, the hamster, guinea pig, and rabbit stain positive for the vicinal hydroxyl group (or PAS-positive) whereas the granules in the mouse stain positive for phospholipid. The Clara cells in the cat do not contain granules. In addition, in most species examined, the Clara cells differ in their structural features depending upon the airway generation in which they are present, whereas in the mouse and rabbit they are the same throughout the airways.

A more recent study (Young et al., 1986) has shed some light on the heterogeneity of Clara cell structure. These investigators evaluated rat bronchus using three-dimensional reconstruction. Their findings suggest that some of the reported variability in Clara cell structure is due to the organelles not being randomly distributed throughout the cytoplasm. They found that within the same cell it was possible to obtain cross-sectional images characterized by a lack of mitochondria and numerous granules, or numerous mitochondria and no granules. Moreover, these same authors also found that the electron density of the granules varied from light to dense core within the same cell, had a polarized distribution, and yet exhibited cytochemical characteristics that were similar. Although these same investigators have perhaps identified a source of confusion over the variability in reports on Clara cell ultrastructure, they support previous findings (Plopper et al., 1980a,b,c) that considerable variability in the morphological characteristics exists between species. The role of the Clara cell in the detoxification of inhaled compounds and its contribution to the airway lining layer remains speculative and not well understood. However, it has been suggested that they are capable of synthesis and secretion of protein, carbohydrate, and possibly cholesterol (Widdicombe and Park, 1982). By contrast, the role of the Clara cell as a progenitor cell with an ability to redifferentiate into goblet or ciliated cells following exposure to inhaled irritants such as SO_2 (Lamb and Reid, 1968), NO_2 and O_3 (Evans et al., 1976; Lum et al., 1978), or cigarette smoke (Wells and Lamerton, 1975) has been well established.

The other two secretory cell types, the mucous or goblet and serous cells, are present in both the mucosal epithelium and the submucosal glands. The term goblet cell was originally applied to the mucous cells as a descriptive term to denote the cell shape when they are engorged with secretory granules. There are important differences between the mucous and serous cells in the structure of their granules, the secretory process, their stimulation by various neural and humoral factors, and their distribution in the submucosal gland (Borson et al., 1980; Reid and Jones, 1980; Coles and Reid, 1981; Leikauf et al., 1984).

Airway mucosal serous cells seem to be more cuboidal than mucous cells. Their granules are more apically oriented, smaller and more electron dense. Serous cell granules stain positive with PAS/Alcian blue (pH 2.6) and are not osmiophilic but contain lysozyme and protein, probably in the form of neutral glycoprotein. By contrast, the granules of the mucous cells are distributed throughout the apical/basal axis of the cells, are larger than those found in the serous cells, often have a dense core, stain positive with PAS due to the sialomucin or a mixture of sulfomucin and sialomucin, and do not contain lysozyme. The discharge of cellular contents also differs between the serous and mucous cells. In the serous cells, discharge is effected through numerous canaliculi extending throughout the cytoplasm in connection with the apical membrane; by contrast, mucous cell discharge is more classically epocrine and is followed by a decrease in cell height and width (Coles and Reid, 1981). Several investigators (Spicer et al., 1971; Jones and Reid, 1973; Plopper et al., 1984) have shown a high degree of variability in the nature of the mucins produced by the mucous and serous cells with the degree of sialiated and sulfated products differing between and within a species.

The control of secretion by the superficial serous and mucous cells may occur by direct cellular stimulation (Lamb and Reid, 1968); however, an electron micrograph of a mucous cell in the guinea pig trachea in juxtaposition to irritant receptors has been published (Hulbert et al., 1981). Whether this is a functional association is not known. On the other hand, the control of secretion by the serous and mucous cells in the submucosal glands has been shown to be sensitive to cholinergic, adrenergic, and peptidergic stimulation. It has been shown (Borson et al., 1980) that secretion from the tracheal glands of ferrets was increased by electrical stimulation, acetylcholine, and phenylephrine and that tetrodotoxin but not acetylcholine or phenylephrine blocked the effects of electrical stimulation. In addition, these same authors found that neither atropine nor phentolamine alone prevented the response to electrical stimulation, but together they did. They concluded that the adrenergic and cholinergic nerves mediate secretion by the glands via the respective receptors. Their data implied that the serous and mucous cells in the submucosal glands are differentially modulated by neural stimuli. This supposition was supported by the findings that adrenergic, but not muscarinic, stimulation produced secretions that differed from the control in viscoelastic properties, and that α-adrenergic stimulation caused serous cells to secrete whereas β-adrenergic stimulation caused mucous cells to do the same (Leikauf et al., 1984). The effects of vasoactive intestinal peptide (VIP) on submucosal gland secretion are mediated by its direct stimulation of both the mucous and serous cells and the smooth muscle in the collecting duct of the gland (Peatfield et al., 1983; Coles et al., 1984). Finally, others (Reid and Jones, 1980) have shown that the serous and mucous cells in the submucosal glands are organized in groups discrete from each other with the serous cells being distal to the mucous cells. The distribution of these cells presumably plays a role in the final constitution of the airway lining fluid.

The airway mucosa also has a resident population of nonciliated cells that cannot be classified as either serous, mucous, or Clara cells; however, it has been shown that in the Syrian hamster even these cells contain granules that stain positive for complex carbohydrates with lead-hematoxylin (Keenan et al., 1982a,b,c, 1983). These cells are further characterized by an extensive network of rough endoplasmic reticulum (RER), large numbers of mitochondria, and an electron-dense cytoplasm relative to that observed in ciliated cells. Variability in the ultrastructural characteristics of these cells is noted throughout the airway mucosa. It is possible that this variability is related to different stages of maturation or differentiation since it has been shown in rats that these cells are also progenitor cells and, following airway injury, have a mitotic activity level that at least equals that of the basal cells (Wells, 1970), and, in the Syrian hamster, a mitotic activity that exceeds that of the basal cells by an order of magnitude (Keenan et al., 1982b). We have extended these observations in our laboratory to show that superficial nonciliated cells also participate in the first stage of premitotic repair following inhalation injury; this is discussed below.

The other resident nonciliated nonsecretory cells in the airway mucosa are the basal cells, intermediate cells, brush cells, and the APUD, Helle-Zellen, or Kulchitsky cells (Jeffery and Reid, 1977). The basal cells, as indicated, are one of the other progenitor cells of the airway mucosa; however, because of the large numbers of hemidesmosomes on the basal surface, they may also serve to anchor the mucosa to the basement membrane. The intermediate cells are cells in the process of differentiation and migration to the airway lumen. The brush cells have been described in many species. They differ from nonciliated nonsecretory superficial cells because their apical membrane is organized into a profusion of microvillae similar to that observed in cells lining the gut. The role of these cells in health and disease is not known; however, based on their extensive brush border of microvillae, they may function in the transport of materials across the epithelium, possibly in absorbing fluid from the periciliary layer. The Kulchitsky or Helle-Zellen cell is another epithelial cell type whose functional role is subject to speculation. These cells are believed to be neuroendocrine cells derived from the neural crest and have been called APUD cells because of their ability to takeup and decarboxylate amines (Frohlich, 1949; Feyrter, 1954). The cells are either distributed singly throughout the airway mucosa or are observed aggregated to form neuroepithelial bodies (Palisano and Kleinerman, 1980).

The ciliated cell is by far the most prominent cell type, occupying the greatest surface area of the cells bordering the airway lumen. Although they constitute 40-60% of the superficial mucosal cells, they appear to be more prevalent than nonciliated cells. The reasons are that the apical diameter and therefore luminal surface area of the ciliated cells is significantly greater than that of the nonciliated cells (Man et al., 1984) and that the apices of the nonciliated cells (secretory and nonsecretory) usually form a crypt so that the cilia from adjacent ciliated cells extend across the crypt and obscure the presence of nonciliated cells (Fig. 3).

The prominent ultrastructural features of ciliated cells, in addition to the cilia, are a band of mitochondria adjacent to the ciliary basal bodies, perinuclear apical golgi complexes, extensive networks of rough endoplasmic reticulum, and a basal perinuclear glycogen body in some species such as the dog. The band of mitochondria is in close proximity to the primary energy-requiring organelle of these cells, the cilia whose structure, function, and beat frequency of between 10 and 13 Hz are well characterized (Satir, 1980). The synchronous wave-form movement of the ciliary beat is critical to maintaining the continuous and dynamic flow of the airway lining layer. Recently it has been documented (Jeffery and Reid, 1977) in humans, mice, and rats that there are small claw-like projections on the tips of the cilia; these may play a role in propelling the airway lining layer forward. Many structural and functional changes occur to the mucociliary apparatus following the inhalation of toxic gases.

The cells of the mucosa bordering the airway lumen are bonded at their apices by an anastomosis of membrane fusions that encircle the apex of each cell. These tight junctions or zonulae occludentes form a structural barrier to the paracellular movement of large-molecular-size substances, provide a strong mechanical bond between cells, and set up the necessary membrane constraints so that the cellular apical and basolateral membranes are polarized. For example, the Na^+-K^+ ATPase crucial to the maintenance of cell volume and low intracellular Na^+ activity is localized specifically on the basolateral membrane (Widdicombe and Welsh, 1980). The control of paracellular permeability is thought to be regulated through the structural configuration and continuity of the interconnecting

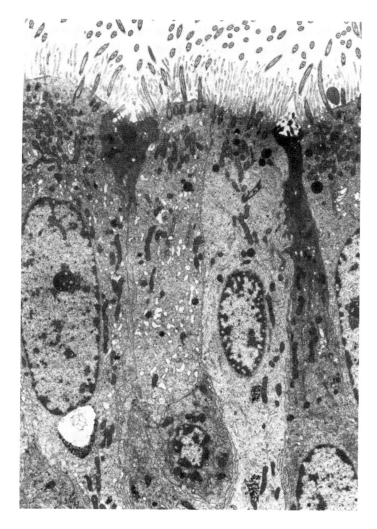

Figure 3 This TEM micrograph shows some of the characteristics of the ciliated and nonciliated nonsecretory cells from the canine tracheal mucosa. In the ciliated cell cytoplasm, directly below the ciliary basal bodies and immediately apical to the band of mitochondria, is a clear zone that is the terminal web of cytoskeletal elements. Other features include electron-dense granules and perinuclear Golgi distributed apically, and a glycogen body basally. Nonciliated, nonsecretory cells have an electron-dense cytoplasm and their apex usually forms a crypt. Mitochondria are distributed throughout the cell but the golgi complexes are primarily confined to the supranuclear portion of the cell. The marker bar represents 2.141 μm.

strands composing the tight junctions (Farquhar and Palade, 1963; Claude and Goodenough, 1973; Claude, 1978). However, others (Muller, 1980; Walker et al., 1984) have suggested that the corner pore formed by the apposition of three or more adjacent cells may also be a route of permeation.

Intracellularly, at the level of the tight junction, is a terminal web of cytoskeletal elements (actin, tubulin, and keratin fibers). This web further strengthens the apical bonds and forms membrane insertion points that act as organizing centers for the junctional units (Martinez-Palomo et al., 1980). Electrical communication between epithelial cells is via the well-described nexus or gap junction (Loewenstein, 1972; Inoue and Hogg, 1977; Loewenstein et al., 1978). Spot desmosomes with related intermediate filaments (keratin and prekeratin in mucosal cells) are found between all cells in the epithelium. The mucosal layer is anchored to the basement membrane by hemidesmosomes on the basal cells and cellular processes extending basally from the ciliated and nonciliated cells.

The control of junctional contacts has been studied extensively (Martinez-Palomo et al., 1980; Meza et al., 1980; Cereijido et al., 1981; Flagg-Newton et al., 1981; Flagg-Newton and Loewenstein, 1981; Azarnia et al., 1981; Radu et al., 1982). One feature of the regulatory properties shared by both the tight and gap junctions is up- and down-regulation by cellular levels of free Ca^{2+} ion. It has been suggested (Loewenstein, 1972) that closure, or down-regulation, of the communicating junction by increases in cellular Ca^{2+} is an important cellular defense mechanism. As is discussed below in more detail, a rise in cellular Ca^{2+} due to increased membrane permeability and/or inhibition of the Na^{+}-Ca^{2+} exchange mechanism is noted within minutes of cell injury.

The turnover rate of the airway mucosal cells has been found to be much longer than that observed in the gut, and it is dependent upon the sex, age, and airway generation, and the state of health of the animal. In a comprehensive study on the kinetics of cell proliferation in the tracheobronchial epithelium in rats (Wells, 1970), the labeling index of the basal and superficial cells gave a projected turnover time of between 24.3 and 41.6 days. In the same study, he reported that chronic airway disease significantly shortened the turnover time to between 11.2 and 22.4 days. In addition, it was also reported that young rats had a faster turnover rate, presumably due to the growth characteristics of the airway tissues. In the rat, the mitotic index of airway mucosal cells at five different levels in the airways decreased progressively from the trachea to the peripheral bronchioles (Bolduc and Reid, 1977). Moreover, these authors also found that the mitotic index in the trachea in males was higher than in females but was similar in the bronchus or peripheral bronchioles in both sexes. Evidently, the turnover rate is an important determinant of the repair process.

II. Function of Airway Epithelium and Morphologic Determinants

One of the recognized functions of the epithelium is that, similar to all other epithelia, it serves as a barrier separating two disparate milieus in juxtaposition. It separates the fluid and gas phases present within the airway lumen from the cellular and matrix components that lie beneath. This function depends on the presence of an intact layer of epithelial cells.

The airway lining layer, which is 95-98% water and rich in electrolytes, has several functions: it is a neutralizer for many toxins, and an important component of the mucociliary apparatus. Its role as a diffusion barrier under normal conditions is questionable since this layer is only approximately 5 μm thick. This contrasts with the situation in the gastrointestinal tract where the barrier properties of the mucous layer are well known. However, in the hypersecretory state, such as in acute inflammation, this layer may increase several-fold (Hulbert et al., 1982) and under these conditions, it may offer some resistance to diffusion. Various chemical and/or immune mediators have been demonstrated in the airway lining fluid (Boat and Cheng, 1980). These include all classes of immunoglobulins; complement and the associated fragments; secretory products of immunocytes, phagocytes, and lysozymes; and epithelial transfer component of IgA from serous epithelial cells. These compounds are postulated to be essential components of the epithelial defense mechanism(s) where they may function in the detoxification process of inhaled substances or as bactericidal agents.

Based on both in vivo and in vitro studies mainly in dogs, but also in other animal species, it is well established that the airway lining layer can be modulated by neural, humoral, and pharmacologic factors (Widdicombe and Welsh, 1980; Frizzell et al., 1981). Cholinergic α- and β-adrenergic stimultion can influence the rate and the biochemical nature of secretions from the airway epithelium. Also, it is evident that chemical mediators such as histamine, prostaglandins, vasoactive peptides, cyclic AMP and its analogues, and calcium may all alter the secretion of ions, movements of fluid, protein concentration, and mucous glycoproteins present in the airway lining layer. In the airway lining fluid, a number of breakdown products of arachidonic acid including LTD_4 have been identified (Johnson et al., 1983). However, the interplay between all the mechanisms that can influence airway secretion in controlling the characteristics of the airway lining layer under baseline and stimulated conditions is not well understood.

The central and peripheral airways are known to have different bioelectric properties (Boucher et al., 1980a), and the effects of autonomic agents on their ion transport have also been shown to be different (Boucher and Gatzy, 1982).

In the dog, the ionic composition of the airway lining fluid at the level of the trachea, bronchi, and subsegmental bronchi has been characterized (Man et al., 1979; Boucher et al., 1981a; Connolly et al., 1983), and the bioelectric and ionic flow measurements in excised canine bronchi have been reported (Boucher et al., 1981b). In the dog as well as in humans (Knowles et al., 1984) the central airway epithelium is involved in the reabsorption of airway lining fluid via Na^+ absorption. This supports a hypothesis previously put forward (Kilburn, 1968), which postulated that the airway lining fluid is regulated and absorption must occur in the central airways since the fluid produced in the large surface area of the alveoli and peripheral airways could not be accommodated as it is moved centrally by mucociliary clearance. In the trachea, a complex balance of active and passive flows is likely in operation and, in the dog at least, this results in a slightly hyperosmotic fluid bathing the mucosal surface (Man et al., 1979).

Mucociliary clearance is a complex process that depends on many variables, which can be grouped into ciliary and mucous factors. Among the ciliary factors are frequency and amplitude of the ciliary beating stroke, the generation of coordinated metachronal waves, the length of cilia, and the number of ciliated cells per unit of airway surface. In this regard, although no evidence for direct nervous control of ciliary function has been demonstrated, β-adrenergic agonists and digoxin have been demonstrated to enhance ciliary function (Verdugo et al., 1980; Wanner, 1977). Among the mucous factors are the nature of the periciliary fluid and its depth, and the viscoelastic properties of the mucus.

To help us understand fully the interrelationships controlling the production and movement of the airway lining layer and mucociliary clearance, measurements have been made on the viscoelastic properties of sputum collected from healthy and diseased individuals (Sturgess et al., 1971); however, few measurements have been made directly on the secretions that line the airway surface (King and Macklem, 1977).

Another function of the airway epithelium is to transport actively a variety of compounds from the air to the blood sides (Schanker, 1978; Brown and Shanker, 1983). It has been shown that the pulmonary epithelium in rats and other animal species actively transports a number of drugs and that these processes are metabolically dependent on the functional integrity of the epithelium. Recently, it has been demonstrated (Pitt et al., 1985) that in guinea pig lungs the pulmonary epithelial transfer of prostaglandin E_2 can occur via an energy-dependent, temperature-sensitive transport mechanism. Finally, biosynthesis of prostaglandins by isolated and cultured airway epithelial cells has been demonstrated (Xu et al., 1986). The exact role of these mechanisms in the overall function of the airway epithelium, and secondarily that of the lung, remains to be clarified.

III. Examples of Airway Epithelial Changes in Oxidant Gas Injury

It is beyond the scope of this chapter to include a detailed account of the changes to the respiratory tract due to the inhalation of all oxidizing gases. Specific examples are, however, discussed to illustrate generality of the findings and some of the points raised earlier.

Many of the problems related to a systematic study of inhalation injury due to oxidizing gases reside in the definition of the exposure parameters and these issues have been reviewed (Bils and Christie, 1980). The concentration of the gases and the time of exposure are important factors; however, other variables such as temperature, humidity, airflow, the presence of pathogens or other gases, pollutants, and particulates in the environment may also be important but often have received less attention. Moreover, another major shortcoming of studies on oxidant inhalation injury is the difficulty in obtaining a complete morphologic and physiological evaluation. This problem has been recognized (Dungworth et al., 1976) and in a review of morphologic methods for evaluation of pulmonary toxicity in animals it is suggested that the morphologic investigations combine the classic techniques of light microscopy with transmission electron microscopy and scanning electron microscopy. We suggest that their rationale be extended to include some physiological measures of the functional status of the epithelium so that the overall effects of the oxidant gases can be put into better perspective.

Epithelial cells have different turnover rates, different intrinsic functions, and different biochemical properties. Accordingly, it is important to question whether the inhalation of different gases, oxidants, and other irritants produce the same type of pathologic and physiological changes, and whether or not all epithelial cells are equally susceptible to injury. The answer to both questions may be that different forms of injuries are produced and that different cells have different susceptibilities to injury. On the other hand, once sustained, damage to an individual cell by whatever insult will likely produce a similar sequence of pathologic events. It is therefore to be expected that oxidant gases may produce cellular injuries and repair processes not too dissimilar from each other. Experimental data have shown that the physicochemical properties of gases, such as solubility, are among the principal determinants of the type of pathologic changes seen. Secondarily, determinants such as the species, age, the presence or absence of antioxidants such as vitamin E, and prior exposure to the gas in question or other gases, and presence of an infection may also be important. Table 1 summarizes some of the determinants of oxidizing gas injury.

For highly soluble gases such as SO_2 (Perry, 1950), the upper airways have been shown to be a very effective scrubber with much of the gas removed during

Table 1 Determinants of Oxidizing Gas Injury

Environmental conditions

    Physicochemical properties of gas

    Concentration of gas

    Duration of exposure

    Combination with other gases

Host factors

    Species

    Age

    Prior exposure

    Vitamin E and other antioxidants

    Presence of infection

a single passage through these structures. For example, it has been shown (Dalhamn and Strandberg, 1960) that in nose-breathing rabbits inhaling 400 ppm SO_2, less than 10 ppm reached the trachea. Because of this nasal scrubbing capacity, highly soluble gases only penetrate the lower respiratory tract when adsorbed on particulates or when the concentration is very high; accordingly, most of the changes caused by SO_2 are in the central airways and the peripheral airways tend to be much less affected. On the other hand, the lesser soluble gases such as O_3 (Perry, 1950) penetrate deeper into the lung and cause predominantly peripheral airway changes. Anatomically, among the animal species, rodents and dogs have short respiratory bronchioles whereas, similarly to humans, squirrel monkeys and subhuman primates have longer respiratory bronchioles (Bils and Christie, 1980). These anatomic differences may, in part, account for the observation that bronchiolitis and focal centroacinar pneumonitis are more often seen in primates and humans than in dogs and rodents.

    It has been shown that the age of the experimental animal can modify the response to an exposure of NO_2 (Cabral-Anderson et al., 1977; Evans et al., 1977). In these studies in which male rats ranging from 1 to 25 months old were exposed to NO_2 for up to 15 days, a proliferative response by the type II pneumocytes and Clara cells was observed in all animals. The proliferative response, however, differed between the animals of the two age groups. Although the injury was more severe and the proliferative response was greater in the old rats, there was a slower onset of repair; this finding suggests that the age of the animal was a major determinant of both the extent of tissue damage and the subsequent repair processes. These authors also showed that type 1 alveolar cells were more sensitive to injury in aging than in young rats and that the ciliated and type I pneumocytes sustained injury at these sublethal exposures whereas the nonciliated bronchiolar (Clara), type II and capillary endothelial cells did not. The authors noted, as a final comment, that it may well be the increased repair time of the older rats that caused an increase in their mortality since this would permit larger accumulations of edema in their alveoli.

The role of dietary interventions such as vitamin E and selenium against tissue injury by oxidizing gases has been addressed by several investigators (Goldstein et al., 1970; Menzel et al., 1972; Elsayed et al., 1983; McMillan and Boyd, 1982). It has been postulated that the antioxidant properties may be the result of vitamin E being preferentially oxidized by the oxidizing gas, thereby preventing the formation of lipid peroxides, or vitamin E may react with free radicals produced by lipid peroxidation (Tappel, 1982).

In a recent study, the respective roles of vitamin E and the age of the animals were examined (Stephens et al., 1983). In this study they evaluated the effects of O_3 and NO_2 on lung morphology in groups of pups, maturing animals, nursing maternal animals, and animals approximately 2 years old, which had been fed varying amounts of vitamin E. These authors also measured the levels of vitamin E in the lung tissue of the animals. They concluded that the age of the animal, not vitamin E levels, was the major determinant of the tissue responses, with the young pups showing less lung damage than those animals that were 2 years old. Selenium is important because it is a major component of glutathione peroxidase. Rats with selenium deficiency have shortened survival in hyperoxia (Cross et al., 1977).

It has been shown (Lamb and Reid, 1968) that SO_2 produces dose-related changes in airway cells in rats where levels as low as 25 ppm caused goblet cell hyperplasia (Fig. 4), and bronchial and tracheal gland hypertrophy. They also used exposures ranging from 400 ppm for 3 hr daily for 2-4 days, 5 days a week for 3-6 weeks, and examined the acute effects and changes during recovery over a period of 1, 4, 7, 14, and 21 days. They found that this exposure regimen produced changes that closely resemble human chronic bronchitis characterized by hypertrophy of tracheal glands and extension of goblet cells to peripheral airways. The recovery at 5 weeks postexposure was incomplete, since goblet cell and mucous gland hypertrophy as well as altered mucus composition had not returned to normal. Since plasma cells have been demonstrated in the airways of patients with chronic bronchitis but not in animals, this finding raises the possibility that the two disease states are different and that, in contrast to animal models, the immune system may play a vital role in the pathogenesis of the condition in humans.

In a recent study in dogs, it was demonstrated with SEM that in the trachea, and presumably in all central airways, ciliated cells are more susceptible

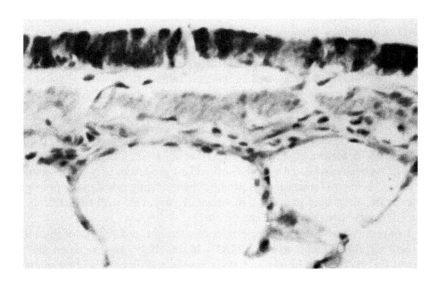

Figure 4 Bronchial epithelium from a rat exposed to sulfur dioxide for 6 weeks. Numerous goblet cells (black) are each larger than in the normal (buffered Formol-saline, PAS ×475; from Lamb and Reid, 1968 with permission).

to injury by SO_2 than nonciliated cells (Man et al., 1986); this has extended previous reports on the effects of O_3 on cat trachea (Boatman and Frank, 1974; Boatman et al., 1974) and on the effects of NO_2 on rat airway mucosa (Cabral-Anderson et al., 1977), where it was also demonstrated that ciliated cells are more sensitive than nonciliated cells to oxidizing gas injury. The inset in Figure 5 shows the surface appearance of the canine tracheal mucosa 1 hr after an acute exposure to SO_2 for 1 hr documenting the exfoliation of ciliated cells at this time. These observations on cell injury from experiments where three different irritant gases, with differing physiochemical properties were used, suggests that ciliated and nonciliated cells possess differing sensitivities to oxidant injury. The dog study (Man et al., 1986) has also extended the observations that inhalation injuries following exposure to O_3 are generally focal (Boatman et al., 1974). This canine study was of particular interest in this regard since the dogs inhaled 500 ppm SO_2 directly into the trachea via an endotracheal tube for a period of 1 hr and yet focal lesions were produced. The focal nature of these lesions from the SO_2 study is illustrated in Figure 5, which shows an SEM overview of the tracheal mucosa 6 hr following the acute exposure. The findings of both these studies raise the interesting question of the mechanisms of regional cytoprotection. This issue is of particular interest since both studies evaluated changes in

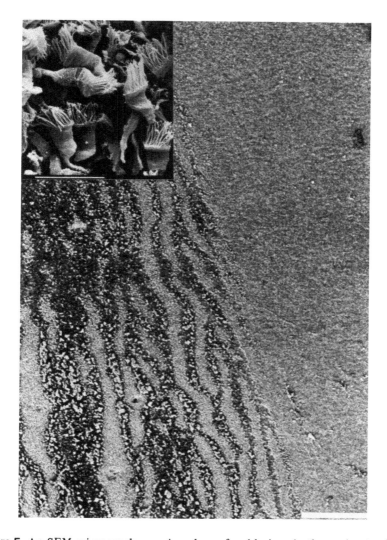

Figure 5 An SEM micrograph overview shows focal lesions in the canine tracheal epithelium 6 hr after exposure of the animal to 500 ppm SO_2 for 1 hr. On the left, the white-appearing spots and rows are cells still in the process of exfoliation and the adjacent dark areas are initial repair cells. The right portion shows normal tissue, as do the similar appearing bands between the exfoliating cells and repair areas on the left. The marker bar represents 500 μm. The inset shows exfoliating ciliated cells 1 hr after the acute exposure to 500 ppm SO_2. The marker bar represents 20 μm.

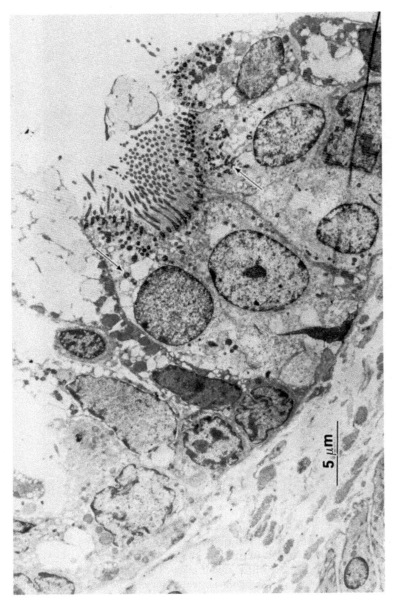

Figure 6 Portion of a medium airway (1.2 mm in diameter) from lung exposed to 0.26 ppm O_3. Cell lining is desquamated in two areas, and ciliated cells contain vacuoles and altered mitochondria (arrows) (X2,950; from Boatman et al., 1974, with permission).

the tracheal mucosa where one would expect that regional patterns of airflow will not be an important factor, and that all the epithelial cells are exposed to the irritant gases.

Ozone is less soluble than SO_2 (Perry, 1950) and it is a stronger oxidizing agent. Accordingly, the site and type of airway epithelial injury caused by ozone would be anticipated to be different from those caused by SO_2. Because of its presence in the atmosphere, it has received considerable attention (Castleman et al., 1973, 1980; Stephens et al., 1973, 1974; Boorman et al., 1980; Eustis et al., 1981; Last et al., 1984). Both long- and short-term studies have been carried out, in a number of animal species, and under different laboratory conditions. In general, while the upper airways are undoubtedly affected, the epithelium of the terminal bronchiole and alveoli shows the most profound morphologic damage. Further, the type I pneumocyte is the most sensitive alveolar cell to inhalation injury and the type II and cuboidal nonciliated bronchiolar cells act as the stem cells for repair (Castleman et al., 1980).

Short-term exposures (1/2 to 12 hr) to concentrations ranging between 0.2 and 3.0 ppm are sufficient to produce injuries at the terminal bronchiolar region characterized by a loss of cilia, swelling of the mitochondria, cytoplasmic vacuolization of the cell, and a loss of ciliated cells from the epithelium (Fig. 6). There is also proliferation of nonciliated secretory cells, desquamation of the epithelium, and development of squamous metaplasia. At the level of the alveoli the type I pneumocytes are replaced by cuboidal type II pneumocytes that demonstrate evidence of proliferation and hyperactivity.

At intermediate exposures using lower concentrations of ozone (0.1-1.3 ppm) for up to several weeks, there is a loss of cilia from ciliated cells, a replacement of the ciliated cells by nonciliated cells, and a replacement of degenerated and necrotic type I pneumocytes by type II cells. The nonciliated cells are presumably Clara cells, and it has been shown that they can transform into ciliated cells when the stress has ceased. In the primate, it has been shown (Castleman et al., 1977) that there is an accumulation of macrophages in the proximal alveoli at these exposure levels; however, the role played by these cells in the development of the pathologic sequelae is not clear. Severe superficial desquamative changes in the trachea and large bronchi that are seen in acute ozone exposure at high concentrations are unusual in the chronic long-term exposure at lower concentrations. Instead, severe peripheral airway and alveolar damage is seen. The end result of this damage is frequently chronic bronchiolitis and bronchiolar wall fibrosis.

Nitrogen dioxide is another gas that has been extensively studied because it is the major substance in oxidant smog (Freeman et al., 1966; Evans et al., 1971, 1975, 1976, 1977; Stephens et al., 1972; Cabral-Anderson, et al., 1977; Gordon et al., 1983). Although species differences were noted, short-term exposure to 30 ppm NO_2 for 3 hr produced significant pathologic changes in the lungs and airways of the study animals, which included rats, rabbits, and squirrel monkeys. The initial response was centroacinar hyperemia frequently associated with alveolar hemorrhage, an accumulation of pulmonary inflammatory exudates, airway epithelial necrosis with occasional sloughing of the epithelium, and an acute submucosal inflammatory response. These acute airway changes were followed by epithelial hyperplasia, particularly of Clara cells by the fourth day post-exposure. As a summary of these effects (Bils and Christie, 1980), it has been stated that the predominant pathologic finding was the slow mucosal repair with erosion, regeneration, and hyperplasia (particularly in the terminal bronchioles) all occurring coincidentally. The squirrel monkey was particularly susceptible to this form of oxidant injury. Following exposure to concentrations as low as 0.75 ppm for 4 hr daily for 4 days they not only demonstrated a greater acute inflammatory response than the rat or rabbit but also developed more extensive epithelial hyperplasia and metaplasia in the terminal bronchioles and alveolar wall thickening during the repair phase following the injury (Bils, 1974). Long-term continuous exposure to NO_2 in rats produced variable obstructive lesions, emphysema, and bronchiolar epithelial hypertrophy. Guinea pigs were susceptible than rats. Repair proceeded shortly after the injury was produced, indicating that inhibition of cell division was not a factor in the magnitude of the effect (Haydon et al., 1965, 1967; Freeman et al., 1966).

A common pathologic feature of oxidizing gas injury related to membrane structure and/or cell-cell interaction is an increase in paracellular permeability (Vai et al., 1980; Gordon et al., 1983). Currently however, there is controversy as to whether breaks in the junctional complex or separation of the corner pores represent the structural means by which this increase occurs (Walker et al., 1984). Nevertheless, although the structural mechanism of abnormal paracellular permeability is not resolved, it has been shown (Gordon et al., 1986) that breaks in the strands of tight junctions occur following exposure to NO_2 (Fig. 7) and that the return of the junctional complex to normal configuration in the bronchioles in hamsters was slower than that observed in the trachea.

The pathologic consequences of increased paracellular permeability due to oxidant gas injury are now better appreciated. Figure 8 illustrates the ease with which agonists or other larger molecules can gain access to the irritant nerve net when paracellular permeability is increased. This micrograph is from a guinea pig exposed to cigarette smoke, and horseradish peroxidase (40,000 Da) was used as the paracellular tracer (Boucher et al., 1980b). Hogg (1981) was the first investigator to draw attention to the possibility that increased paracellular permeability could cause bronchial hyperreactivity. A subsequent study (Hulbert et al., 1985) showed that this can happen when the increase in bronchial reactivity is mediated by the vagal reflex arc; however, others (Roum and Murlas, 1984)

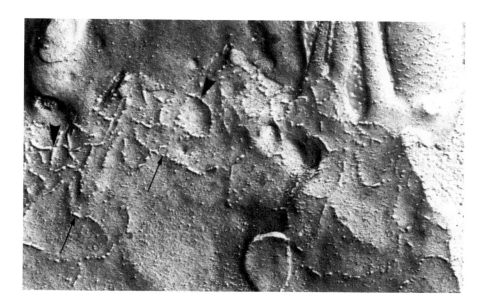

Figure 7 Micrograph of hamster exposed to NO_2 for 9 months shows a similar pattern of tight junction disruption in bronchiolar epithelium as compared to hamster exposed to NO_2 for 5 months (see Fig. 3). The disruption of tight junction fibrils (arrowheads) seen here is extensive. Individual tight junction particles and small fragments for the tight junction fibrils (arrows) (X6800; from Gordon et al., 1986, with permission).

have shown that increased permeability was not necessarily causally related to the bronchial hyperreactivity in guinea pigs exposed to ozone since the animals were also hyperreactive to intravenous acetylcholine. Two other consequences of increased paracellular permeability are the enhanced permeation of inert particles into the mucosa and/or submucosa, which may be coated with mutagenic and/or carcinogenic substances such as the benzopyrenes, or the offending agents themselves, and it has been suggested (Vai et al., 1980) that the persistent hyperpermeability following SO_2 exposure in rats leads to the development of chronic bronchopathy.

It is evident that while the central airways are more affected by SO_2, and the peripheral airways more by NO_2, the patchiness of the damage and the obvious susceptibility of the ciliated cells of the airway epithelium and type I alveolar epithelial cells seem to be common findings in all oxidizing gas injuries.

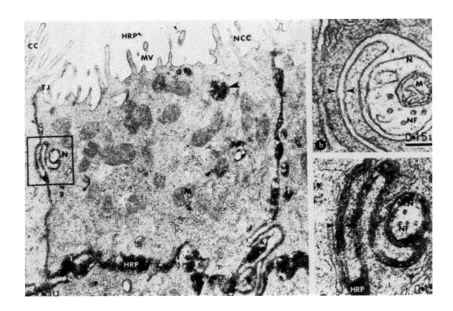

Figure 8 Smoke-exposed tracheal epithelium with HRP present in the intercellular space. Location of the nerve endings below the tight junction is outlined by a square and the inset shows higher magnification of the nerves from a normal (b) and smoke-exposed animal (c). HRP, horseradish peroxidase; MV, microvilli; TJ, tight junction (from Boucher et al., 1980b, with permission).

IV. Mechanisms of Epithelial Injury

The molecular mechanisms by which oxidizing gases cause cellular injury are not completely understood; however, the formation of free radicals by these agents is postulated to play a pivotal role. These mechanisms have been reviewed (Recknagel and Glende, 1977; Pryor, 1982; Menzel, 1984). The gases, O_3, NO_2, and SO_2 are strong oxidants that can react with many biochemical moieties to form free radicals. Free radicals formed by these interactions adversely affect the structure and function of cellular components such as proteins, especially enzymes containing sulfhydryl groups (SH), nucleic acids, and, more importantly, the cellular plasma membrane. The plasma membrane provides the containment of all cellular and organelle contents, and its permeability characteristics regulate the molecular species that enter and exit the cell and its organelles. The membrane is composed of lipoproteins rich in polyenoic long-chain fatty acids that are prone to undergo rancid or peroxidation decomposition under certain conditions. Free radicals, once formed, can react readily with molecular oxygen to form organic peroxy free radicals. When a peroxy free radical reacts with a phospholipid fatty acid side chain, it not only denatures the molecule but also produces another new organic free radical; this process is known as linear propagation of lipid hydroperoxide formation. Furthermore, new free radicals can be produced by the decomposition of organic peroxide via a number of cellular biochemical mechanisms (see Recknagel and Glende, 1977, for review).

The effects of lipid peroxidation on cell membrane permeability are well established. In red blood cells, there is a loss of water and electrolyte regulation, leakage of intracellular enzymes from the cells, and lysis. In other cells, there is inhibition of mitochondrial function, followed by their swelling and disintegration, disintegration of lysozomes, and fragmentation and swelling of the endoplasmic reticulum. Additional targets of lipid peroxidation are the phospholipids necessary for microsomal enzyme function; glucose-6-phosphatase and cytochrome P-450 are two of the better known examples. Thus, many pathologic changes result when there is peroxidation decomposition of structural lipids in cellular and subcellular membranes. While these have not been specifically studied in respiratory epithelial cells, the above mechanisms of action are believed to be common to all cell types.

Some of the biochemical changes following exposure to ozone have recently been outlined (Mustafa and Tierney, 1978). It has been demonstrated that oxygen consumption, monoamine oxidation, glucose utilization, NADPH formation, GSH reductase, disulfide reductase, nonprotein sulfhydryl content, GSH peroxidase, and superoxide dismutase all increase significantly. Also, a dose-related increase between ozone and cell titers of succinate oxidase, succinate cytochrome C reductase, NADPH-cytochrome C reductase, glucose-6-phosphate dehydrogenase (G6PDH), and glutathione peroxidase was found. In addition, the induction of the glutathione peroxidase has been demonstrated to occur in monkeys exposed to 0.2 ppm ozone for 8 hr/day (Mustafa and Lee, 1976).

While there seems to be good evidence that a group of enzymes, collectively referred to as antioxidant enzymes—superoxide dismutase, catalase (found in perixosomes), glutathione peroxidase (a cytoplasmic enzyme), glutathione reductase, and G6PDH—may play an important role in antioxidant defense, a recent study (Ospital et al., 1983) that examined the correlation between oxygen (another oxidizing gas) toxicity and the activity of glutathione peroxidase in rats failed to support the hypothesis.

In those experiments, the investigators compared the activity of these antioxidant enzymes and the degree of tolerance while the animals recovered in air following exposure to 85% oxygen. Although they found no correlation between activity levels of antioxidant enzymes and nonprotein sulfhydryl and oxygen tolerance, the authors were careful to point out that the glutathione peroxidase system may be only one of several mechanisms responsible for the protection. In a recent review (White and Repine, 1985), it has been concluded that the cause and effect relationship between increases in lung superoxide dismutase and/or other antioxidant enzymes and protection against lung injury from hyperoxia remains unproven. These authors considered that this is due to limitations in the ability to detect O_2 metabolites in vivo and to measure enzyme activities in anything but whole lung homogenates. Accordingly, local changes in antioxidant enzyme concentrations in specific cell types that may be essential to the development of tolerance can go undetected. Finally, though much needed, similar experiments have not been done on oxidizing gases other than oxygen to determine if the same conclusions would apply.

While it is evident that lipid peroxidation is the major biochemical mechanism in injuries due to oxidizing gases and there is a dose-response relationship between the duration and level of the exposure and the severity of the response, more research is needed to explain some observations noted following injury by a variety of gases. These include the focal nature of inhalation injuries, even though the exposure time may be hours in duration, and, the differential susceptibility of the epithelial cell types in cases when more ciliated than nonciliated cells are injured. If lipid peroxidation is the principal mechanism by which cell injury occurs, other undefined mechanisms may be in operation to explain the focal and selective nature of epithelial injury.

In addition to their obvious differences in function, three major molecular differences between ciliated and nonciliated cells have been documented, which may be related to their different susceptibilities to injury. These differences are their abilities to regulate cell volume, their tolerance to Na^+ loading, and their capacity for stem cell activity and redifferentiation.

When an osmotic load was placed on the submucosal side of an isolated canine tracheal tissue, the nonciliated and basal cell's volume was regulated but the ciliated cells shrunk; by contrast, when an osmotic load was placed on the mucosal side, all the cell types volume regulated (Man et al., 1986). This response is unique to the cells lining the airway epithelium (Spring and Ericson, 1983). When airway cells were incubated with amphotericin B, an Na^+ ionophore, ciliated but not nonciliated cells swelled and blebs formed on the apical membrane (Fig. 9) (Trump and Berezesky, 1983). Lastly, it is well established that only nonciliated airway cells are capable of mitotic activity and differentiation/redifferentiation. The exact role played by these differences in the susceptibility of the different cells types to oxidant injury is not certain.

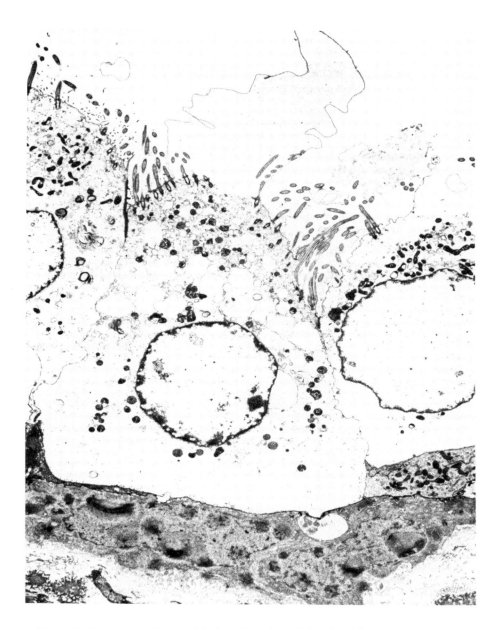

Figure 9 Hamster tracheal epithelium in culture following 2-hr exposure to
amphotericin B. Note the marked swelling of the cytosol and ER. Mitochondria are condensed, the nuclei show chromatin margination, and large blebs
occur at the apical surfaces. Note that the basal and mucous cells are not swollen
(from Trump and Berezesky, 1984, with permission).

V. Molecular and Morphologic Correlates in Cell Injury and Cell Death

Trump and associates (Trump and Berezesky, 1984; Trump et al., 1980, 1981) have examined the time course of the molecular events leading to cell injury and death and have related them to the ultrastructural features of cellular organelles and changes in cellular ionic compartmentalization. Although their work was conducted primarily on kidney cells, they have also examined some airway tissue. They have used anoxia, ischemia, metabolic poisons, membrane disrupters, and ionophores to induce cell injury and have conducted an elegant x-ray analysis of frozen tissues to evaluate the movements of ions during the different stages of cell death. They found that independent of the specific agent, the intracellular/extracellular ion gradients and ultrastructural changes to organelles were similar during what they have termed the reversible and irreversible phases of cell death.

During the reversible phase of cell death, the first key observable event was a rise in cellular Ca^{2+}, and this coincided with a dysfunction in Na^+ regulation by the cell. The rise in Ca^{2+} was speculated to result from either an increase in cell membrane permeability to Ca^{2+} or inhibition in the Na^+-Ca^{2+} exchange mechanism (Blaustein, 1977), or a combination of both. The associated ultrastructural features included the vacuolization of the cytoplasm resulting from dilation of the endoplasmic reticulum, condensation of the matrix proteins and dilation of cristae in mitochondria, the appearance of flocculent densities in the nuclei, and frequent formation of blebs on the apical membrane surface.

Initially, bleb formation was interpreted (Trump et al., 1980) as resulting from a rise in cellular Ca^{2+} causing either contraction of the actin-containing filaments and/or depolymerization of tubulin-containing cytoskeletal elements. Both elements are known to interact not only to stabilize the microvilli on the apical membrane surface, but to do so through interactive attachments at specific plasma membrane domains. This hypothesis was subsequently confirmed using Ca^{2+} ionophore that induced blebs like those observed in studies on the ultrastructural features of cell death.

In SO_2 injury (Hulbert et al., unpublished data), some ciliated airway cells also showed bleb formation whereas others did not (Fig. 10); however, although this finding was not universal, the other ultrastructural features of the reversible phase of cell death were. Figure 11 illustrates the mitochondrial abnormalities previously described (Boatman et al., 1974) and Figure 12 the dilation of the endoplasmic reticulum (ER), which results in a vacuolated appearance of the cytoplasm. In these figures, the causative agents were O_3 and SO_2, and they produce similar effects on the ultrastructural features of mitochondria from ciliated cells but have no effect, at this dose level, on nonciliated cells.

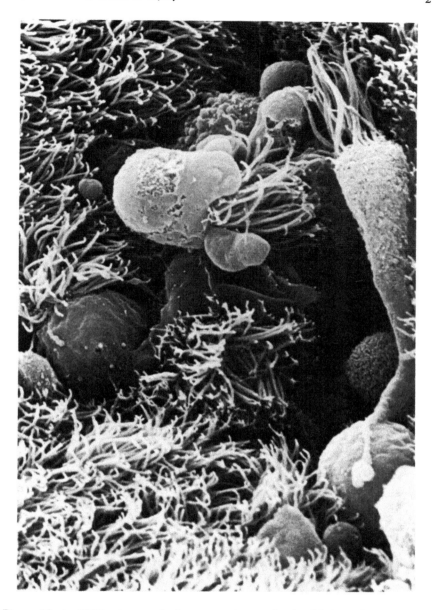

Figure 10 An SEM micrograph shows a canine tracheal epithelium from a dog exposed to 500 ppm SO_2 for 1 hr. This shows that not all exfoliating ciliated cells exhibited blebs, a feature characteristic of a disrupted cytoskeleton and abnormality in Ca^{2+} and volume regulation. The marker bar represents 10 μm.

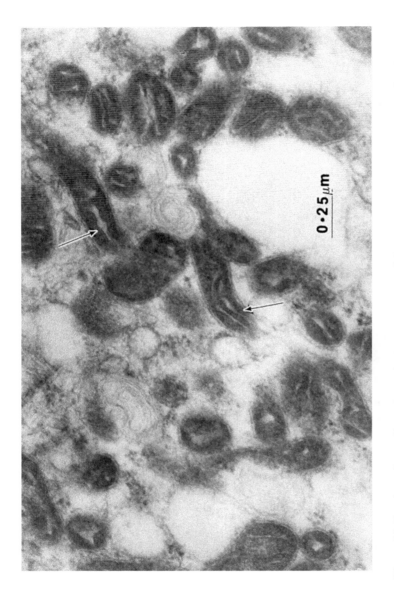

Figure 11 Portion of a medium airway (1.2 mm in diameter) from lung exposed to 0.26 ppm O_3 showing an area of ciliated cell cytoplasm. Note altered mitochondria with increased electron density of the matrix and abnormal cristae configuration (X34,320; from Boatman et al., 1974, with permission).

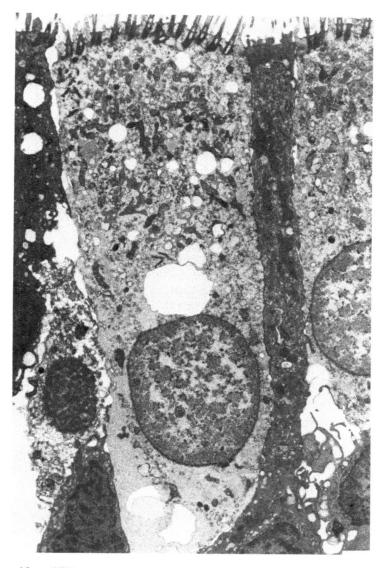

Figure 12 A TEM micrograph shows a canine tracheal epithelium from a dog exposed to 500 ppm SO_2 for 1 hr. It illustrates vacuolization of the cytoplasm in the ciliated cell centrally but a lack of vacuolization in the nonciliated cell. The vacuolated appearance of cells injured by oxidizing gases is due to dilation of the ER, which is a hallmark of cells in the reversible phase of cell death. The marker bar represents 1.28μm.

As implied by the term reversibility, the primary feature of the reversible phase of cell death is that if the cells are placed in an appropriate milieu and the inhaled agent(s) is removed, they will survive. This has been elegantly demonstrated by Trump and his associates in a variety of tissues (Trump and Berezesky, 1984) and in this laboratory on trachea from dogs acutely exposed to SO_2 (Fig. 5). In addition, using cultured MDCK cells exposed to hydrogen peroxide (H_2O_2), it has been shown that the effects of free radicals on membrane ion transport were reversible and, similar to our results on ciliated cell exfoliation following SO_2 injury, the cellular response was heterogeneous (Welsh et al., 1985).

Presently, we do not know the molecular events that enabled those ciliated cells with ultrastructural features of the reversible phase of cell death immediately following an acute exposure to SO_2 to remain intact within the mucosa and therefore result in focal lesions by 6 hr postexposure (Fig. 5). The definition of these mechanisms is important to complete our understanding of the processes of epithelial repair and the adaptive response. We can speculate that junctional formation and the reestablishment of the epithelial barrier against the passage of macromolecules occurs and that there is a return to normal ionic homeostasis at the cellular level. From recent work (Welsh et al., 1985), however, we can suggest that a major event in preventing the reversible phase of cell death to proceed to become irreversible is the inhibition or the blocking of membrane peroxidation. In oxidant gas injury in the whole animal, whether this is done through cellular antioxidant systems or other scavengers localized extracellularly remains the subject of speculation.

VI. Repair of Epithelial Injury

The repair sequence following inhalation injury has three stages: a premitotic stage, a mitotic stage, and a redifferentiation stage. Immediately following acute inhalation injury, when the damaged cells are exfoliating, the remaining viable superficial nonciliated cells expand laterally maintaining cellular contact and, as possible, the barrier properties of the epithelium. Concurrently, a wave of mitotic activity is initiated in the basal and superficial nonciliated cells. This mitotic activity is significantly increased above control levels by 12 hr and usually does not peak for approximately 48-72 hr (Lamb and Reid, 1968; Wells and Lamerton, 1975; Hulbert et al., 1981). The roles of these different stages in the overall defense strategy of the respiratory system are different. The premitotic repair stage is responsible for reestablishing the barrier function and confluent cellular layer (Gordon and Lane, 1976). By contrast, the mitotic repair stage is responsible for repopulating the epithelium and the redifferentiation stage ultimately reestablishes the proportion of ciliated to nonciliated cells lining the airway mucosa.

One would speculate that many factors could adversely affect the length and resolution of epithelial injuries induced by inhaling toxic gases. One major factor is the presence or absence of the oxidant gases. Another factor is the severity of the lesion itself. For example, damage caused by oxidant injury to the airway mucosa is dose-related to exposure and is present in three forms of severity: injury and exfoliation of individual, primarily ciliated cells leaving the superficial nonciliated and basal cells intact; damage to the mature differentiated layer causing desquamation of groups of cells but leaving the basal cells intact; and damage to the entire mature and undifferentiated mucosal cell layer leaving basement membrane exposed.

If we assume that the offending agent is removed, and the airway is allowed to recover, the following sequence usually occurs. If only the ciliated cells are damaged, the initial repair cells, which include the resident superficial nonciliated cells (Keenan et al., 1982a,b,c), can reseal the epithelium within a matter of hours. In fact, we have observed that following acute SO_2 exposure to the canine tracheal epithelium, the nonciliated superficial cells directly adjacent to a region of exfoliating cells undergo a change in shape from being approximately 20 μm high and 3 μm in apical diameter to being 20 μm in apical diameter and 3 μm high. The cells at this time are characterized by a very simple surface topography of microridges and the adjacent cell borders overlap extensively (Fig. 13). This initial repair phase is dynamic and resolution is generally complete within 6 hr. This is also the same time frame reported for the strands of the tight junction to form following mechanical injury to the airway mucosa (Marin et al., 1979) and for the increase in paracellular permeability following acute inhalation of cigarette smoke to also return to normal (Hulbert et al., 1981).

One very interesting feature of oxidant gas injury that causes selective cell exfoliation is that not all the injured ciliated cells are immediately cleared from the airway mucosa, some remain attached 6 hr after the exposure (Fig. 14). These cells are not yet necrotic so they can still undergo autodigestion. The process of autodigestion results in the metabolism of arachidonic acid and the production of various mediators with chemotactic activity (Trump et al., 1981). It may be that this is one phase of redundancy built into the defense processes that ensure that the appropriate chemical signals are present for a lengthy period of time after the insult for the recruitment of inflammatory cells.

The second level of epithelial injury due to the inhalation of oxidant gases, the loss of groups of mature surface cells leaving basal cells exposed, also resolves quickly in a sequence of events described earlier. That is, remaining cellular constituents are present to form contacts within a few hours. In both these examples of epithelial injury it is important to keep the perspective that repair is not complete with the establishment of barrier function and a cellular confluent layer because this is only the first step in the reciliation of an injured

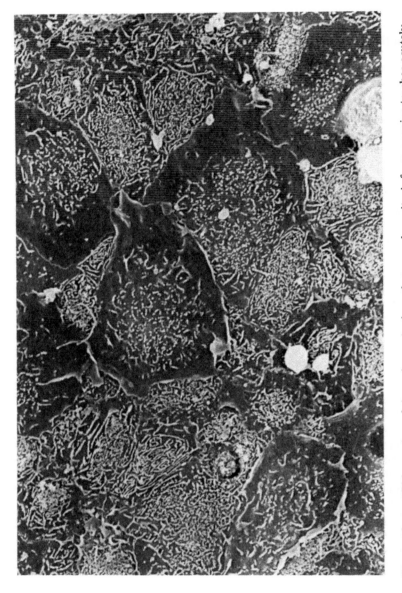

Figure 13 An SEM overview of the early repair phase that precedes mitosis from a canine trachea acutely exposed to 500 ppm SO_2 and examined 1 hr later. Unique to these cells is the simple surface topography indicating lateral migratory expansion. The marker bar represents 20 μm.

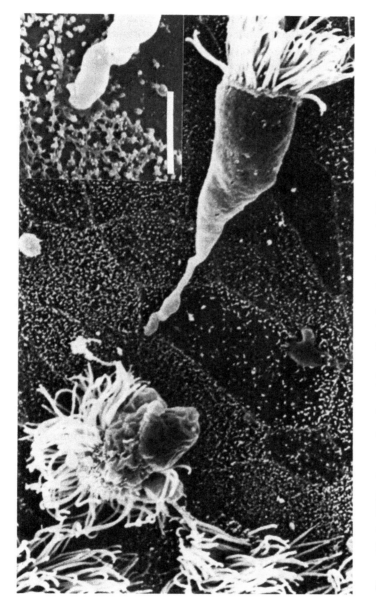

Figure 14 An SEM micrograph enlarged from the dark regions shown in Figure 5 to illustrate that 6 hr after acute inhalation injury by SO_2 some ciliated cells are not yet exfoliated and cleared from the airway surface. The marker bar represents 10 μm. The inset is a high-magnification enlargement of the attachment in the corner of three adjacent cells. The marker bar represents 4 μm.

area and the reestablishment of normal function for that area. Obviously, it is an important step since these injuries can potentially resolve at a faster rate than lesions where the entire mucosa is eroded and the basement membrane is exposed. This third level of injury has the greatest potential for life-threatening complications due to hemorrhage into the airway and subsequent development of significant pathologic sequelae. Injuries of this nature initially resolve at a rate dependent upon the lateral migration of cells at the wound margin; thus the larger the lesion, the more lengthy the resolution time. An additional factor influencing the initial repair phase of these lesions is whether the basement membrane remains intact, since both the migratory behavior and the differentiated cell phenotype is influenced by the substratum.

From this discussion, the concept can be developed that the three repair stages as well as the kind of lesion produced may be influenced by various host and environmentally derived factors. In addition to age and vitamin E in certain groups of animals, perhaps the most important host factor influencing the outcome of airway injuries is a cellular one involving the acute inflammatory response.

The inflammatory stimulus initiated by an acute injury to the airway epithelium causes an influx of polymorphonuclear leukocytes (PMN) within 4-6 hr (Metchnikoff, 1891; Hulbert et al., 1981). These cells, when actively phagocytosing, produce oxygen free radicals including superoxide anion, hydrogen peroxide, and hydroxy radicals (Fantone and Ward, 1982) that are effective bactericidal agents. However, these agents may also injure healthy tissues (Repine et al., 1982) by a mechanism similar to oxidizing gases. How this may affect the repair of epithelial injury is not determined; one would predict an attenuation of the repair process with a subsequent increase in repair time. Unfortunately, there have been no studies on the effects of activated PMNs on the repair of lesions caused by inhaling oxidizing gases nor have there been any studies on the sensitivity of repair cells to oxidants. However, if recent results (Sugahara et al., 1986) on the effects of phagocytosing PMNs on cultured epithelial monolayers can be extrapolated to the repair phase in situ following acute oxidizing gas injury, the increase in repair time postulated may indeed occur. In the lung, activated PMNs release proteases. These enzymes fragment fibronectin, which in turn may serve as one of the chemotactic stimuli for monocytes. It has been postulated (Henson et al., 1984) that the recruited monocytes then participate in the removal of cells and debris. Additionally, it has been suggested that these cells are capable of stimulating alveolar epithelial cell division and their differentiation into mature cells. Whether the role of the monocyte is similar in airway epithelial repair is unknown.

The focus of interest on the nonciliated superficial lining cell in the upper airways has expanded our knowledge as to their functional role during repair. Keenan and associates (1982a,b,c) have shown that following injury to the trachea in the Syrian hamster, the mitotic activity of the superficial nonciliated cells exceeds that of the basal cells by an order of magnitude. Their results confirm and extend earlier work (Evans et al., 1976) showing that the primary progenitor cell of the distal airways is the cuboidal nonciliated bronchiolar cell. Finally, others (Gordon and Lane, 1984) have also demonstrated that in the rat the nonciliated granular cells were a primary source of ciliated cells in the regenerating tracheal epithelium.

There is extensive evidence to suggest that epithelial cells other than basal cells are equally if not more important in the repair process following oxidant gas injury. For a teleologic point of view there may be good reason to have the capability of regeneration from two cell populations in the upper airways. One could speculate that the two progenitor cell populations in the upper airways are advantageous because many of the gaseous insults cause their most damage there. As a result, one would expect higher regenerative and repair capabilities of the tissues in the upper airways. This speculation is supported by the observations (Bolduc and Reid, 1977) that the turnover of tracheal cells is higher than observed in the peripheral airways.

VII. Epithelial Adaptation

In the context of this review, adaptation is defined as changes in airway morphology and physiological response following repeated exposure to nonlethal levels of oxidizing gases that confer an increase in tolerance to the inhaled agent. However, there is an important distinction between adaptation to inhaled irritant gases and adaptation of an organism to a new set of environmental conditions. In the classic description, the adaptation of an organism, a fish for example, to a new set of environmental conditions such as increase or decrease in water temperature, would result in the de novo production of the appropriate metabolic machinery necessary for the organism to sustain metabolism, and be sufficiently free of pathologic change to ensure reproduction and continual habitation in the new environment (Hochachka and Somero, 1973). Those species not capable of making the appropriate "changes" would not survive under the new conditions. The successful adaptation to irritant gases would result in the maintenance of normal function of the airway and lung epithelium despite repeated insults; however, this never occurs and this feature distinguishes "natural" adaptation from the development of "tolerance" and "adaptation" to inhaled gases. Because adaptation of the respiratory system to irritant gases is also accompanied by pathologic abnormalities and some loss in function, this has prompted Bromberg and Hazucha (1982) to question whether "adaptation" to an irritant gas, ozone for example, is really protective or advantageous.

The development of physiological adaptation to an irritating gas, ozone for example, is well documented (Hackney et al., 1977; Hazucha et al., 1977; Farrell et al., 1979; Folinsbee et al., 1980; Horvath et al., 1981). In fact, the continual exposure for only a few days is all that is required for the bronchial reactivity seen upon initial exposure to disappear. The mechanism(s) involved remain speculative. It has been suggested that the adaptive response or development of tolerance to ozone is due to a reduction in the sensitivity of airway receptors or possibly an increase in the production of mucus with decreased permeability of the airway lining layer (Gliner et al., 1983). Regardless of the precise mechanism for the physiological adaptation, a well defined pathologic appearance accompanies the adaptation to prolonged exposure to low levels of O_3 (Fujinaka et al., 1985). Because repeated exposure causes recurrent damage followed by repair, the changes seen in the airways following repeated exposure to sublethal concentrations of irritating gases closely resemble stages of repair that are incomplete.

Depending on the morphologic changes, aspects of epithelial function including mucociliary function and gas exchange can be affected. Following prolonged exposure to an oxidizing gas, the most common morphologic evidence of adaptation at the alveolar level is the replacement of type I alveolar cells by type II cells. Two factors have been postulated to relate this shift in cell populations. First, type II pneumocytes are progenitor cells in the alveoli and an increase in their numbers is necessitated by increased cell turnover. Second, type II pneumocytes are cuboidal and have a much smaller ratio of exposed membrane to cell volume. This translates to a higher ratio of antioxidant systems per unit surface membrane area, which may enable these cells to more efficiently handle free radicals. The increased number of type II cells lining the alveolar surface results in a decrease in gas exchange capacity, since the diffusion distances are increased from a few nanometers to several microns.

In the airways, the change in cell population is reflected by replacement of the ciliated by nonciliated cells with an increased proportion of secretory cells. In addition to these changes in the airway epithelium, in animals subchronically exposed to SO_2 there is an increase in the volume of submucosal mucous glands, an extension of the superficial secretory cells into the more peripheral airways, and a shift in the glycoconjugate from neutral and basic to more acidic residues in their contents (Lamb and Reid, 1968). Whether the Clara cells have a specific role in epithelial adaptation to oxidizing gases is not clear since their increase in numbers with prolonged exposure could simply be a reflection of increased cell turnover under these conditions. While biochemical and metabolic changes in the lungs following the development of tolerance have been demonstrated (Mustafa and Tierney, 1978), it is not certain whether these changes reflect a change in the cell population or actual change in cell biochemistry. Moreover, it is not known whether the same molecular changes have occurred in the airway epithelial cells.

Following these changes in the ratio of secretory to ciliated cells, one would anticipate an alteration in the composition of the airway lining secretions and the means to compensate mucociliary clearance due to reduced numbers of ciliated cells. With prolonged exposure to irritant gases the airway lining layer, like the secretory cells, has been shown to become more acidic (by staining with Alcian blue) and to contain a different group and proportion of protein species due to enhanced cell turnover and inflammation (Lamb and Reid, 1968; Boat and Cheng, 1980). This fundamental biochemical change in the number of free carboxyl and sulfhydryl residues may influence the degree of cross-linking, which may in turn change the viscoelastic properties of the lining layer. While this change in the viscoelastic properties may not be ideal for clearance by ciliary action, an increase in viscosity may be more suitable for clearance by cough (King, 1986). The changes in the mucus may be one adaptation to augment the function of the mucociliary apparatus by cough. The mucus layer covering the airway epithelium also has unique water retention capabilities (Negus, 1963); whether these changes in the composition of the layer have an effect on this property has not been studied. Similarly, the barrier property of the airway lining layer has not been addressed.

It is apparent that adaptation is a trade-off and complete and ideal adaptation of the airway epithelium to inhaled oxidants does not exist. Instead, the changes in the airway epithelium are more indicative of different stages of repair in response to recurrent injury. Until better techniques are available to study the different subpopulations of cells from the airway epithelium, it will not be certain if adaptation of the animal to oxidant gases is associated with true biochemical and metabolic changes of the cells.

VIII. Conclusion

Oxidizing gases are important contaminants of the environment, and their impact on human health is now better appreciated. The mechanisms, biochemical and morphologic, by which injuries to the pulmonary epithelium occur are becoming better known. What is unknown but is absolutely critical are the mechanism(s) responsible for cytoprotection that may explain the differential susceptibility of specific epithelial cell types and focal damages in oxidizing gas injury. Oxidizing gases can be used as a convenient tool to produce pathologic change and to assist in the study of different pulmonary diseases in which injury, repair, and adaptation are part of the pathogenesis of these conditions. Finally, true adaptation to the inhalation of oxidant gases does not exist.

Acknowledgments

The authors gratefully acknowledge grant support from the Medical Research Council of Canada, the Alberta Heritage Foundation for Medical Research, and the Alberta Lung Association. W. C. Hulbert is a Scholar of the Alberta Heritage Foundation for Medical Research. The support of Dr. J. Mehta in helping with the photography is also acknowledged.

References

Azarnia, R., Dahl, G., and Loewenstein, W. R. (1981). Cell junction and cyclic AMP: III. Promotion of junctional membrane permeability and junctional membrane particles in a junction-deficient cell type. *J. Membrane Biol.* **63**:133-146.

Bils, R. F. (1974). Effects of nitrogen dioxide and ozone on monkey lung ultrastructure. *Pneumonologie* **150**:99-111.

Bils, R. F., and Christie, B. R. (1980). The experimental pathology of oxidant and air pollutant inhalation. *Int. Rev. Exp. Pathol.* **21**:195-293.

Blaustein, M. P. (1977). Sodium ions, blood pressure regulation, and hypertension: a reassessment and a hypothesis. *Am. J. Physiol.* **232**:C165-C173.

Boat, R. F., and Cheng, P. W. (1980). Biochemistry of airway mucus secretions. *Fed. Proc.* **39**:3067-3074.

Boatman, E. S., and Frank, R. (1974). Morphologic and ultrastructural changes in the lungs of animals during acute exposure to ozone. *Chest* **65**:9S-11S.

Boatman, E. S., Sato, S., and Frank, R. (1974). Acute effects of ozone on cat lungs. II. Structural. *Am. Rev. Respir. Dis.* **110**:157-169.

Bolduc, P., and Reid, L. (1977). Mitotic index of the bronchial and alveolar lining of the normal rat lung. *Am. Rev. Respir. Dis.* **114**:1121-1122.

Boorman, G. A., Schwartz, L. W., and Dungworth, D. L. (1980). Pulmonary effects of prolonged ozone insult in rats. Morphometric evaluation of the central acinus. *Lab. Invest.* **43**:108-115.

Borson, D. B., Chinn, R. A., Davis, B., and Nadel, J. A. (1980). Adrenergic and cholinergic nerves mediate fluid secretion from tracheal glands of ferrets. *J. Appl. Physiol.* **49**:1027-1031.

Boucher, R. C., and Gatzy, J. T. (1982). Regional effects of autonomic agents on ion transport across excised canine airways. *J. Appl. Physiol.* **52**:893-901.

Boucher, R. C., Bromberg, P. A., Jr., and Gatzy, J. T. (1980a). Airway transepithelial electric potential *in vivo*: species and regional differences. *J. Appl. Physiol.* **48**:169-176.

Boucher, R. C., Johnson, J., Inoue, S., Hulbert, W., and Hogg, J. C. (1980b).

The effect of cigarette smoke on the permeability of guinea pig airways. *Lab. Invest.* **43**:94-100.

Boucher, R. C., Stutts, M. J., Bromberg, P. A., and Gatzy, J. T. (1981a). Regional differences in airway surface liquid composition. *J. Appl. Physiol.* **50**:613-620.

Boucher, R. C., Stutts, M. J., and Gatzy, J. T. (1981b). Regional differences in bioelectric properties and ion flow in excised canine airways. *J. Appl. Physiol.* **51**:706-714.

Bromberg, P. A., and Hazucha, M. J. (1982). Is "adaptation" to ozone protective? *Am. Rev. Respir. Dis.* **125**:489-490.

Brown, R. A., Jr., and Schanker, L. S. (1983). Absorption of aerosolized drugs from the rat lung. *Drug Metab. Disp.* **11**:355-360.

Cabral-Anderson, L. J., Evans, M. J., and Freeman, G. (1977). Effects of NO_2 on the lungs of aging rats I. Morphology. *Exp. Mol. Pathol.* **27**:353-365.

Castleman, W. L., Dungworth, D. L., and Tyler, W. S. (1973). Histochemically detected enzymatic alterations in rat lung exposed to ozone. *Exp. Mol. Pathol.* **19**:402-421.

Castleman, W. L., Tyler, W. S., and Dungworth, D. L. (1977). Lesions in respiratory bronchioles and conducting airways of monkeys exposed to ambient levels of ozone. *Exp. Mol. Pathol.* **26**:384-400.

Castleman, W. L., Dungworth, D. L., Schwartz, L. W., and Tyler, W. S. (1980). Acute respiratory bronchiolitis-An ultrastructural and autoradiographic study of epithelial cell injury and renewal in Rhesus monkeys exposed to ozone. *Am. J. Pathol.* **98**:811-840.

Cereijido, M., Meza, I., and Martinez-Palomo, A. (1981). Occluding junctions in cultured epithelial monolayers. *Am. J. Physiol.* **240**:C96-C102.

Clara, M. (1937). Sur histobiologie des bronchalepitels. *Z. Mikrosk. Anat. Forsch.* **41**:321-347.

Claude, P. (1978). Morphological factors influencing transepithelial permeability: a mode for the resistance of zonula occludents. *J. Membrane Biol.* **39**:219-232.

Claude, P., and Goodenough, D. A. (1973). Fracture faces of zonulae occludents from "tight" and "leaky" epithelia. *J. Cell Biol.* **58**:390-400.

Coles, S. J., and Reid, L. (1981). Inhibition of glycoconjugate secretion by colchicine and cytochalasin B. *Cell Tissue Res.* **214**:107-118.

Coles, S. J., Neill, K. H., and Reid, L. M. (1984). Potent stimulation of glycoprotein secretion in canine trachea by substance P. *J. Appl. Physiol.* **57**:1323-1327.

Connolly, T. P., Sproule, S. D., and Man, S. F. P. (1983). Regional ionic and albumin content of fluid in the tracheobronchial tree in dogs. *Clin. Invest. Med.* **6**:89-95.

Cross, C. E., Hasegawa, G., Reddy, K. A., and Omaye, S. T. (1977). Enhanced lung toxicity of O_2 in selenium-deficient rats. *Res. Commun. Chem. Pathol. Pharmacol.* **16**.695-706.

Dalhamn, T., and Strandberg, L. (1960). Acute effects on rate of ciliary beat in rabbit tracheal (*vivo* and *vitro*) and absorption capacity of nasal cavity. *Int. J. Air Water Pollution* **4**:154.

Dungworth, D. L., Schwartz, L. W., Tyler, W. S., and Phalen, R. F. (1976). Morphological methods for evaluation of pulmonary toxicity in animals. *Ann. Rev. Pharmacol. Toxicol.* **16**:381-399.

Elsayed, N. M., Hacker, A. D., Kuehn, K., Mustafa, M. G., and Schrauzer, G. N. (1983). Dietary antioxidants and the biochemical response to oxidant inhalation. II. Influence of dietary selenium on the biochemical effects of ozone exposure in mouse lung. *Toxicol. Appl. Pharmacol.* **71**:398-406.

Eustis, S. L., Schwartz, L. W., Kosch, P. C., and Dungworth, D. L. (1981). Chronic bronchiolitis in nonhuman primates after prolonged ozone exposure. *Am. J. Pathol.* **105**:121-137.

Evans, M. J., Stephens, R. J., and Freeman, G. (1971). Effects of nitrogen dioxide on cell renewal in the rat lung. *Arch. Intern. Med.* **128**:57-60.

Evans, M. J., Cabral, L. J., Stephens, R. J., and Freeman, G. (1975). Transformation of alveolar type 2 cells to type 1 cells following exposure to NO_2. *Exp. Mol. Pathol.* **22**:142-150.

Evans, M. J., Johnson, L. V., Stephens, R. J., and Freeman, G. (1976). Renewal of the terminal bronchiolar epithelium in the rat following exposure to NO_2 or O_3. *Lab. Invest.* **35**:246-257.

Evans, M. J., Cabral-Anderson, J., and Freeman, G. (1977). Effects of NO_2 on the lungs of aging rats II. Cell proliferation. *Exp. Mol. Pathol.* **27**:366-376.

Fantone, J. C., and Ward, P. A. (1982). Role of oxygen-derived free radicals and metabolites in leukocyte-dependent inflammatory reactions. *Am. J. Pathol.* **107**:397-418.

Farquhar, M. G., and Palade, G. E. (1963). Junctional complexes in various epithelia. *J. Cell Biol.* **17**:375-412.

Farrell, B. P., Kerr, H. D., Kulle, T. J., Sauder, L. R., and Young, J. L. (1979). Adaptation in human subjects to the effects of inhaled ozone after repeated exposure. *Am. Rev. Respir. Dis.* **119**:725-730.

Feyrter, F. (1954). Sur pathologie des argyrophilen helle-zellen-organes in bronchialbaum des menschen. *Virchows Arch.* **325**:723-732.

Flagg-Newton, J. L., and Loewenstein, W. R. (1981). Cell junction and cyclic AMP: II. Modulations of junctional membrane permeability, dependent on serum and cell density. *J. Membrane Biol.* **63**:123-131.

Flagg-Newton, J. L., Dahl, G., and Loewenstein, W. R. (1981). Cell junction and cyclic AMP: I. Upregulation of junctional membrane permeability and junctional membrane particles by administration of cyclic nucleotide or phosphodiesterase inhibitor. *J. Membrane Biol.* **63**:105-121.

Folinsbee, L. J., Bedi, J. F., and Horvath, S. M. (1980). Respiratory responses in humans repeatedly exposed to low concentrations of ozone. *Am. Rev. Respir. Dis.* **121**:431-439.

Freeman, G., Furiosi, N. J., and Hayden, G. B. (1966). Effects of continuous exposure of 0.8 ppm NO_2 on respiration of rats. *Arch. Environ. Health* **13**:454-456.

Frizzell, R. A., Welsh, M. J., and Smith, P. L. (1981). Hormonal control of chloride secretion by canine tracheal epithelium. An electrophysiological analysis. *Ann. N. Y. Acad. Sci.* **372**:558-570.

Frohlich, F. (1949). Die "Helle Zelle" der bronchialscheimhaut and ihre beziehungen zum problem der chemoreceptoren. *Frankfurt. Z. Pathol.* **60**:517-559.

Fujinaka, L. E., Hyde, D. M., Plopper, C. G., Typer, W. S., Dungworth, D. L., and Lollini, L. O. (1985). Respiratory bronchiolitis following long-term ozone exposure in Bonnet monkeys: a morphometric study. *Exp. Lung Res.* **8**:167-190.

Gail, D. B., and Lenfant, C. J. M. (1983). Cells of the lung:biology and clinical implications. *Am. Rev. Respir. Dis.* **127**:366-387.

Gliner, J. A., Horvath, S. M., and Folinsbee, L. J. (1983). Preexposure to low ozone concentrations does not diminish the pulmonary function response on exposure to higher ozone concentrations. *Am. Rev. Respir. Dis.* **127**: 51-55.

Goldstein, B. D., Buckley, R. D., Cardenas, R., and Balchum. O. J. (1970). Ozone and vitamin E. *Science* **1969**:605-606.

Gordon, R. E., and Lane, B. P. (1976). Regeneration of rat tracheal epithelium after mechanical injury. *Am. Rev. Respir. Dis.* **113**:799-807.

Gordon, R. E., and Lane, B. P. (1984). Ciliated cell differentiation in regenerating rat tracheal epithelium. *Lung* **162**:233-243.

Gordon, R. E., Case, B. W., and Kleinerman, J. (1983). Acute NO_2 effects on penetration and transport of horseradish peroxidase in hamster respiratory epithelium. *Am. Rev. Respir. Dis.* **128**:528-533.

Gordon, R. E., Solano, D., and Kleinerman, J. (1986). Tight junction alterations of respiratory epithelia following long term NO_2 exposure and recovery. *Exp. Lung Res.* **11**:179-193.

Hackney, J. D., Linn, W. S., Mohler, J. G., and Collier, C. R. (1977). Adaptation to short-term respiratory effects of ozone in men exposed repeatedly. *J. Appl. Physiol.* **43**:82-85.

Haydon, G. B., Freeman, G., and Furiosi, N. J. (1965). Covert pathogenesis of NO_2 induced emphysema in the rat. *Arch. Environ. Health* **11**:776-783.

Haydon, G. B., Davidson, J. T., Lillington, G. A., and Wasserman, K. (1967). Nitrogen dioxide induced emphysema in rabbits. *Am. Rev. Respir. Dis.* **95**: 797-805.

Hazucha, M., Parent, C., and Bates, D. V. (1977). Development of ozone tolerance in man. Research Triangle Park, N.C.: US EPA Publ. #EPA 600/3-
77-0001a, 527-541.

Henson, P. M., Larsen, G. L., Henson, J. E., Newman, S. L., Musson, R. A., and
Leslie, C. C. (1984). Resolution of pulmonary inflammation. *Fed. Proc.*
43:2799-2806.

Hochachka, P. W., and Somero, G. N. (1973). *Strategies of Biochemical Adaptation.* Philadelphia, W. B. Saunders, pp. 179-271.

Hogg, J. C. (1981). Bronchial mucosal permeability and its relationship to airways hyperreactivity. *J. Allergy Clin. Immunol.* **67**:421-425.

Horvath, S. M., Gliner, J. A., and Folinsbee, L. J. (1981). Adaptation to ozone:
duration of effect. *Am. Rev. Respir. Dis.* **123**:496-499.

Hulbert, W. C., Walker, D. C., Jackson, A., and Hogg, J. C. (1981). Airway permeability to horseradish peroxidase in guinea pigs: the repair phase after
injury by cigarette smoke. *Am. Rev. Respir. Dis.* **123**:320-326.

Hulbert, W. C., Forster, B. B., Laird, W., Phil, C. E., and Walker, D. C. (1982).
An improved method for fixation of the respiratory epithelial surface with
the mucous and surfactant layers. *Lab. Invest.* **47**:354-363.

Hulbert, W. C., McLean, T., and Hogg, J. C. (1985). The effect of acute inflammation on bronchial reactivity in guinea pigs. *Am. Rev. Respir. Dis.* **132**:
7-11.

Inoue, S., and Hogg, J. C. (1977). Freeze-etch study of the tracheal epithelium
of normal guinea pigs with particular reference to the intercellular junctions. *J. Ultrastruct. Res.* **61**:89-97.

Jeffery, P. K., and Reid, L. M. (1977). The respiratory mucous membrane in
Respiratory Defense Mechanisms, Part I. Edited by J. D. Brain, D. F.
Proctor, and L. M. Reid. New York, Marcel Dekker, pp. 193-238.

Jones, R., and Reid, L. (1973). The effect of pH on alcian blue staining of epithelial acid glycoproteins. I. Sialomucins and sulphomucins (singly or in
simple combinations). *Histochem. J.* **5**:9-18.

Johnson, H. G., Chinn, R. A., Chow, A. W., Bach, M. K., and Nadel, J. A. (1983).
Leukotriene-C_4 enhances mucus production from submucosal glands in
canine trachea in vivo. *Immunopharmacology* **5**:391-396.

Keenan, K. P., Combs, J. W., and McDowell, E. M. (1982a). Regeneration of
hamster tracheal epithelium after mechanical injury I. Focal lesions:
quantitative morphologic study of cell proliferation. *Virchows Arch.* **41**:
193-214.

Keenan, K. P., Combs, J. W., and McDowell, E. M. (1982b). Regeneration of
hamster tracheal epithelium after mechanical injury II. Multifocal lesions:
stathmokinetic and autoradiographic studies of cell proliferation. *Virchows
Arch.* **41**:215-229.

Keenan, K. P., Combs, J. W., and McDowell, E. M. (1982c). Regeneration of hamster tracheal epithelium after mechanical injury III. Large and small lesions: comparative stathmokinetic and single pulse and continuous thymidine labeling autoradiographic studies. *Virchows Arch.* **41**:231-252.

Keenan, K. P., Wilson, T. S., McDowell, E. M. (1983). Regeneration of hamster tracheal epithelium after mechanical injury IV. Histochemical, immunocytochemical and ultrastructural studies. *Virchows Arch.* **43**:213-240.

Kilburn, K. H. (1968). A hypothesis for pulmonary clearance and its implications. *Am. Rev. Respir. Dis.* **989**:449-463.

King, M. (1986). Role of mucus viscoelasticity in clearance by cough. *Eur. J. Respir. Dis.* in press.

King, M., and Macklem, P. T. (1977). The rheological properties of microliter quantities of normal mucus. *J. Appl. Physiol.* **42**:797-802.

Knowles, M., Murray, G., Shallal, J., Askin, F., Ranga, V., Gatzy, J., and Boucher, R. (1984). Bioelectric properties and ion flow across excised human bronchi. *J. Appl. Physiol.* **56**:868-877.

Kuhn, C. (1976). Ciliated and Clara cells. In *Lung Cells in Disease.* Edited by A. Bouhuys. New York, Elsevier/North-Holland, pp. 91-108.

Kuhn, C., Callaway, L. A., and Askin, F. B. (1974). The formation of granules in the bronchiolar Clara cells of the rat. I. Electron microscopy. *J. Ultrastruct. Res.* **49**:387-400.

Lamb, D., and Reid, L. (1968). Mitotic rates, goblet cell increase and histochemical changes in mucus in rat bronchial epithelium during exposure to sulphur dioxide. *J. Pathol. Bacteriol.* **96**:97-111.

Last, J. A., Reiser, K. M., Tyler, W. S., and Ruckler, R. B. (1984). Long-term consequences of exposure to ozone. I. Lung collagen content. *Toxicol. Appl. Pharmacol.* **72**:111-118.

Leikauf, G. D., Ueki, I. F., and Nadel, J. A. (1984). Autonomic regulation of viscoelasticity of cat tracheal gland secretions. *J. Appl. Physiol.* **56**:426-430.

Loewenstein, W. R. (1972). Cellular communication through membrane junctions. *Arch. Intern. Med.* **129**:299-305.

Loewenstein, W. R., Kanno, Y., and Socolar, S. J. (1978). The cell-to-cell channel. *Fed. Proc.* **37**:2645-2650.

Lum, H., Schwartz, L. W., Dungworth, D. L., and Tyler, W. S. (1978). A comparative study of cell renewal after exposure to ozone or oxygen. Response of terminal bronchiolar epithelium in the rat. *Am. Rev. Respir. Dis.* **118**:335-345.

Man, S. F. P., Adams, G. K. III, and Proctor, D. F. (1979). Effects of temperature, relative humidity, and mode of breathing on canine airway secretions. *J. Appl. Physiol.* **46**:205-210.

Man, S. F. P., Hulbert, W., Park, D. S. K., Thomson, A. B. R., and Hogg, J. C. (1984). Asymmetry of canine tracheal epithelium: osmotically induced changes. *J. Appl. Physiol.* **57**:1338-1346.

Man, S. F. P., Hulbert, W. C., Mok, K., Ryan, T., and Thomson, A. B. R. (1986). Effects of sulfur dioxide on pore populations of canine tracheal epithelium. *J. Appl. Physiol.* **60**:416-426.

Marin, M. L., Gordon, R. E., and Lane, B. P. (1979). Development of tight junctions in rat tracheal epithelium during the early hours after mechanical injury. *Am. Rev. Respir. Dis.* **119**:101-106.

Martinez-Palomo, A., Meza, I., Beaty, G., and Cereijido, M. (1980). Experimental modulation of occluding junctions in a cultured transporting epithelium. *J. Cell Biol.* **87**:736-745.

McMillan, D. D., and Boyd, G. N. (1982). The role of antioxidants and diet in the prevention or treatment of oxygen-induced lung microvascular injury. *Ann. N. Y. Acad. Sci.* **384**:535-543.

Menzel, D. B. (1984). Ozone: an overview of its toxicity in man and animals. *J. Toxicol. Environ. Health* **4**:183-204.

Menzel, D. B., Roehan, J. N., and Lee, S. D. (1972). Vitamin E: the biological and environmental antioxidant. *J. Agric. Food Chem.* **20**:481-486.

Metchnikoff, E. (1891). Lecture I. Delivered at the Pasteur Institute in 1891. *Lectures on the Comparative Pathology of Inflammation.* (Translated from the French by F. A. Starling and E. H. Starling). New York, Dover Publications, 1968, p. 10.

Meza, I., Ibarra, G., Sabanero, M., Martinez-Palomo, A., and Cereijido, M. (1980). Occluding junctions and cytoskeletal components in a cultured transporting epithelium. *J. Cell Biol.* **87**:746-754.

Muller, W. (1980). Cell junctions with funnels in the olfactory mucosa of frogs (*Rana temporia* L.). *Cell Tissue Res.* **207**:165-169.

Mustafa, M. G., and Lee, S. D. (1976). Pulmonary biochemical alterations resulting from ozone exposure. *Ann. Occup. Hygiene* **19**:17-26.

Mustafa, M. G., and Tierney, D. F. (1978). Biochemical and metabolic changes in the lung with oxygen, ozone, and nitrogen dioxide toxicity. *Am. Rev. Respir. Dis.* **118**:1061-1090.

Negus, V. E. (1963). The function of mucus. *Acta Otolaryngol.* **56**:204-214.

Ospital, J. J., Kasuyama, R. S., and Tierney, D. F. (1983). Poor correlation between oxygen toxicity and activity of glutathione peroxidase. *Exp. Lung Res.* **5**:193-199.

Palisano, J. R., and Kleinerman, J. (1980). APUD cells and neuroepithelial bodies in hamster lung: methods, quantitation, and response to injury. *Thorax* **35**: 363-370.

Peatfield, A. C., Barnes, P. J., Bratcher, C., Nadel, J. A., and Davis, B. (1983). Vasoactive intestinal peptide stimulates tracheal submucosal gland secretion in ferret. *Am. Rev. Respir. Dis.* **128**:89-93.

Perry, J. H. (1950). Physical characteristics. In *Chemical Engineers Handbook,* 3rd ed. Edited by J. H. Perry. New York, McGraw-Hill, pp. 668-693.

Pitt, B. R., Moalli, R., Man, S. F. P., and Gillis, N. C. (1985). Alveolar transfer of prostaglandin E_2 in isolated perfused guinea pig lungs. *J. Appl. Physiol.* **59**:691-697.

Plopper, C. G. (1983). Comparative morphologic features of bronchiolar epithelial cells. The Clara cell. *Am. Rev. Respir. Dis.* **128**:S37-S41.

Plopper, C. G., Mariassy, A. T., and Hill, L. H. (1980a). Ultrastructure of the nonciliated bronchiolar epithelial (Clara) cell of mammalian lung: I. A comparison of rabbit, guinea pig, rat, hamster, and mouse. *Exp. Lung. Res.* **1**:139-154.

Plopper, C. G., Mariassy, A. T., and Hill, L. H. (1980b). Ultrastructure of the nonciliated bronchiolar epithelial (Clara) cell of mammalian lung: II. A comparison of horse, steer, sheep, dog, and cat. *Exp. Lung Res.* **1**:155-169.

Plopper, C. G., Hill, L. H., and Mariassy, A. T. (1980c). Ultrastructure of the nonciliated bronchiolar epithelial (Clara) cell of mammalian lung. III. A study of man with comparison of 15 mammalian species. *Exp. Lung Res.* **1**:171-180.

Plopper, C. G., Mariassy, A. T., Wilson, D. W., Alley, J. L., Nishio, S. J., and Nettesheim, P. (1983). Comparison of nonciliated tracheal epithelial cells in six mammalian species: ultrastructure and population densities. *Exp. Lung Res.* **5**:281-294.

Plopper, C. G., St. George, J. J., Mishio, S. J., Etchision, J. R., and Nettesheim, P. (1984). Carbohydrate cytochemistry of tracheobronchial airway epithelium of the rabbit. *J. Histochem. Cytochem.* **32**:209-218.

Pryor, W. A. (1982). Free radical biology: xenobiotics, cancer and aging. *Ann. N. Y. Acad. Sci.* **393**:1-22.

Radu, A., Dahl, G., and Loewenstein, W. R. (1982). Hormonal regulation of cell junction permeability: upregulation by catecholamine and prostaglandin E_1. *J. Membrane Biol.* **70**:239-251.

Recknagel, R. O., and Glende, E. A., Jr. (1977). Lipid peroxidation: a specific form of cellular injury. In *Handbook of Physiology Reactions to Environmental Agents.* Edited by D. H. K. Lee, H. L. Falk, S. D. Murchy, and S. R. Geiger. Baltimore, Williams and Wilkins, pp. 591-601.

Reid, L., and Jones, R. (1980). Mucous membrane of respiratory epithelium. *Environ. Health Perspect.* **35**:113-120.

Repine, J. E., Bowman, C. M., and Tate, R. M. (1982). Neutrophils and lung edema. *Chest* **81**:47-50.

Roum, J., and Murlas, C. G. (1984). Ozone-induced bronchial hyperreactivity is not explained by airway mucosal hyperreactivity. *Fed. Proc.* **43**:883 (Abstr).

Satir, P. (1980). Structural basis of ciliary movement. *Environ. Health Perspect.* **35**:77-82.

Schanker, L. S. (1978). Drug absorption from the lung. *Biochem. Pharmacol.*
27:381-385.

Spicer, S. S., Chakrin, L. W., Wardell, J. R., Jr., and Kendrick, W. (1971). Histochemistry of mucosubstances in the canine and human respiratory tract. *Lab. Invest.* 25:483-490.

Spicer, S. S., Mochizuki, I., Setser, M. E., and Martinez, J. R. (1980). Complex carbohydrates of rat tracheobronchial surface epithelium visualized ultrastructurally. *Am. J. Anat.* 158:93-109.

Spring, K. R., and Ericson, A. C. (1983). Epithelial cell volume modulation and regulation. *J. Membrane. Biol.* 69:167-176.

Stephens, R. J., Freeman, G., and Evans, M. J. (1972). Early response of lungs to low levels of nitrogen dioxide. *Arch. Environ. Health* 24:160-179.

Stephens, R. J., Freeman, G., Satara, J. F., and Coffin, D. L. (1973). Cytologic changes in dog lungs induced by chronic exposure to ozone. *Am. J. Pathol.* 73:711-726.

Stephens, R. J., Sloan, M. F., Evans, M. J., and Freeman, G. (1974). Alveolar type I cell response to exposure to 0.5 ppm O_3 for short periods. *Exp. Mol. Pathol.* 20:11-23.

Stephens, R. J., Buntman, D. J., Negi, D. S., Parkhurst, R. M., and Thomas, D. W. (1983). Tissue levels of vitamin E in the lung and the cellular response to injury resulting from oxidant gas exposure. *Chest* May supplement:37S-39S.

St.George, J. A., Cranz, D. L., Zicker, S. C., Etchison, J. R., Dungworth, D. L., and Plopper, C. G. (1985). An immunohistochemical characterization of rhesus monkey respiratory secretions using monoclonal antibodies. *Am. Rev. Respir. Dis.* 132:556-563.

Sturgess, J., Palfrey, A. J., and Reid, L. (1971). Rheological properties of sputum. *Rheol. Acta* 10:36-43.

Sugahara, K., Cott, G. R., Parsons, P. E., Mason, R. J., Sandhaus, R. A., and Henson, P. M. (1986). Epithelial permeability produced by phagocytosing neutrophils *in vitro. Am. Rev. Respir. Dis.* 133:875-881.

Tappel, A. L. (1982). Vitamin E and free radical peroxidation of lipids. *Ann. N. Y. Acad. Sci.* 203:12-28.

Trump, B. F., and Berezesky, I. K. (1984). Role of sodium and calcium regulation in toxic cell injury. In *Drug Metabolism and Drug Toxicity.* Edited by J. R. Mitchell, and M. G. Horning. New York, Raven Press, pp. 261-300.

Trump, B. F., Berezesky, I. K., Laiho, K. U., Osornio, A. R., Mergner, W. J., and Smith, M. W. (1980). The role of calcium in cell injury. A review. *Scanning Electron Microscopy* 2:1437-1462.

Trump, B. F., Berezesky, I. K., and Phelps, P. C. (1981). Sodium and calcium regulation and the role of the cytoskeleton in the pathogenesis of disease: a review and hypothesis. *Scanning Electron Microscopy* 2:435-454.

Vai, F., Fournier, M. F., Lafuma, J. C., Touaty, E., and Pariente, R. (1980). SO$_2$-induced bronchopathy in the rat: Abnormal permeability of the bronchial epithelium *in vivo* and *in vitro* after anatomic recovery. *Am. Rev. Respir. Dis.* 121:851-858.

Verdugo, P., Johnson, N. T., and Tam, P. Y. (1980). β-adrenergic stimulation of existing ciliary activity. *J. Appl. Physiol.* 48:868-871.

Walker, D. C., MacKenzie, A., Wiggs, B. R., Hulbert, W. C., and Hogg, J. C. (1984). The structure of tight junctions in the tracheal epithelium may not correlate with permeability. *Cell Tissue Res.* 235:605-613.

Wanner, A. (1977). Clinical aspects of mucociliary transport. *Am. Rev. Respir. Dis.* 116:73-125.

Wells, A. B. (1970). The kinetics of cell proliferation in the tracheobronchial epithelia of rats with and without chronic respiratory disease. *Cell Tissue Kinetics* 3:185-206.

Wells, A. B., and Lamerton, L. F. (1975). Regenerative response of the rat tracheal epithelium after acute exposure to tobacco smoke: a quantitative study. *J. Natl. Cancer Inst.* 55:887-891.

Welsh, M. J., Shasby, M., and Husted, R. M. (1985). Oxidants increase paracellular permeability in a cultured epithelial cell line. *J. Clin. Invest.* 76:1155-1167.

White, C. W., and Repine, J. E. (1985). Pulmonary antioxidant defense mechanisms. *Exp. Lung Res.* 8:81-96.

Widdicombe, J. G., and Park, R. J. (1982). The Clara cell. *Eur. J. Respir. Dis.* 63:202-220.

Widdicombe, J. H., and Welsh, M. J. (1980). Ion transport by dog tracheal epithelium. *Fed. Proc.* 39:3062-3066.

Xu, G. L., Sivarajah, K., Wu, R., Nettesheim, P., and Eling, T. (1986). Biosynthesis of prostaglandins by isolated and cultured airway epithelial cells. *Exp. Lung Res.* 10:110-114.

Young, S. L., Fram, E. K., and Randell, S. H. (1986). Quantitative three-dimensional reconstruction and carbohydrate cytochemistry of rat nonciliated bronchiolar (Clara) cells. *Am. Rev. Respir. Dis.* 133:899-907.

2

Mechanisms of Airway Responses to Inhaled Sulfur Dioxide

DEAN SHEPPARD

University of California School of Medicine
San Francisco, California

Sulfur dioxide (SO_2) is the major air pollutant produced by combustion of sulfur-containing fossil fuels. Because these fuels are an important source of electrical power, approximately 70% of the SO_2 emitted into the atmosphere in the United States comes from power plants (Committee on Sulfur Oxides, 1978). Other major outdoor sources of SO_2 include oil refineries and metal smelters. Until recently SO_2 was not an important pollutant in indoor air. However, kerosene space heaters, a form of household heating that has gained worldwide popularity over the past several years, can produce large quantities of SO_2 leading to indoor concentrations that may exceed maximal outdoor concentrations by 10-fold or more (Leaderer, 1982). In addition to its importance as an air pollutant, sulfur dioxide is widely used in industry. In 1974, the National Institute for Occupational Safety and Health estimated that 500,000 workers in the United States are regularly exposed to SO_2 in industries ranging from smelters and paper pulp mills to wineries and food processing plants (NIOSH, 1974).

The first suggestion that sulfur dioxide might produce important adverse effects on human health came from observations of clear increases in mortality in association with several episodes of severe air pollution that occurred in the middle of this century (Shy et al., 1978). Although information about the specific pollutants present during these episodes is incomplete, the best estimates suggest that large concentrations of sulfur dioxide were present. The excess deaths attributable to pollution during these episodes were generally clustered among patients with preexisting cardiopulmonary disease, suggesting that the pollutants present might be exerting their adverse effects on the lung. Patients with asthma were found to be especially susceptible to these episodes of pollution; one report noted that 88% of patients with asthma experienced exacerbations of their disease during the pollution episode that occurred in Donora, Pennsylvania, in 1948 (Schrenk et al., 1949). In addition to effects attributed to sulfur dioxide in ambient air, several studies have suggested that occupational exposure to SO_2 can have adverse effects on the lung. The effects most commonly described are a modest reduction in maximal expiratory flow and an increase in the prevalence of cough and sputum production in workers chronically exposed to SO_2 (Smith et al., 1977, 1978; Skalpe, 1964). Over the past 30 years, these epidemiologic observations have stimulated a series of laboratory studies examining the effects of this ubiquitous pollutant on the airways of animals and of human subjects. The results of these studies form the basis of this chapter.

I. Effects of SO_2 on Animals

Investigators have examined the effects of SO_2 on several species of animals including mice, guinea pigs, rats, dogs, cats, donkeys, and monkeys. The two most important effects observed have been an increase in airflow resistance and an alteration in mucus secretion. Acute inhalation of SO_2 has been reported to increase airflow resistance rapidly in dogs, cats, and guinea pigs (Nadel et al., 1965; Frank and Speizer, 1965; Amdur, 1966). Generally, this effect has only occurred after inhalation of concentrations of SO_2 above 5 ppm, well in excess of the concentrations encountered in polluted outdoor air. The one exception is a report of a statistically significant increase in pulmonary resistance in guinea pigs exposed to concentrations of SO_2 less than 1 ppm (Amdur, 1966). These responses, though statistically significant, were quite small. The same investigator found that 46 ppm SO_2 was required to increase resistance by 50% above baseline. Thus, extrapolation from these experiments in animals would not predict an important acute effect of SO_2 in the concentrations encountered in polluted air (generally less than 1 ppm) on airflow resistance.

These observations did provide an experimental system in which to examine the mechanism(s) by which inhalation of sulfur dioxide causes an increase in airflow resistance. The most direct information about this mechanism comes from experiments in which the pulmonary resistance of cats was measured during brief exposures to a high concentration of SO_2. Pulmonary resistance increased after SO_2 was instilled either through a tracheostomy into the low airways or into an anatomically separated upper tracheal pouch. Both responses could be abolished by atropine and by vagal section (Nadel et al., 1965). These results suggested that SO$_2$ causes bronchoconstriction in the cat by activating a vagal reflex.

Several lines of evidence suggest that inhalation of SO$_2$ effects mucus secretion in animals. Alterations in measurements of mucociliary clearance have been reported after both acute and chronic exposures to SO$_2$ in a variety of species (Committee of Sulfur Oxides, 1978; Spiegelman et al., 1968). Because clearance can be affected by alterations in airway caliber and ciliary function as well as by alterations in secretory products contributed by glands and epithelial cells, we cannot infer the mechanisms of action of SO$_2$ from these experiments. The effect of SO$_2$ on the volume of secretion from submucosal glands has recently been examined more directly in a preparation in which a segment of dog trachea was coated with tantalum powder and photographed during exposure of the lower airways to air or to SO$_2$. In these experiments, SO$_2$ was shown to cause a dramatic increase in submucosal gland secretion. This response, similarly to the bronchomotor effect of SO$_2$ in cats, was abolished by vagal cooling, which suggests that it too is mediated by a vagal reflex (Hahn et al., 1983).

In general, SO$_2$ has not acutely caused direct lower respiratory injury in animals unless it was inhaled in high concentrations (in excess of 25 ppm). Repeated exposure to SO$_2$ has been shown to cause goblet cell hyperplasia and hypertrophy of submucosal glands in both rats and dogs (Reid, 1963; Seltzer et al., 1984). These changes in morphology were associated with an increase in basal mucus secretion and thus in some ways resembled chronic bronchitis in humans.

II. Effects of SO$_2$ on Human Subjects

Several studies have examined the effects of acute inhalation of SO$_2$ on normal human subjects. In most of these studies, inhalation of concentrations in excess of 5 ppm was shown to cause small but significant decrements in airway function (Nadel et al., 1965; Frank et al., 1962). Occasional "sensitive" subjects were found to respond in a similar fashion to concentrations as low as 1 ppm (Frank et al., 1962; Amdur, 1969). Because these effects were small, and usually required inhalation of concentrations of SO$_2$ well in excess of those encountered in polluted outdoor air these results were interpreted to imply that SO$_2$ itself was not likely to be responsible for the adverse health effects of air pollution.

However, studies from several different laboratories have recently shown that concentrations of SO$_2$ that have little or no effect on normal healthy subjects can produce marked symptomatic bronchoconstriction in subjects with asthma (Sheppard et al., 1980, 1981; Kirkpatrick et al., 1982; Bethel et al.

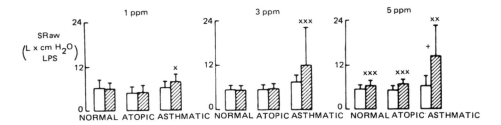

Figure 1 Specific airway resistance (SRaw) after 5 min of breathing filtered air (□) and during the last 5 min of exposure (▨) to 1, 3, and 5 ppm of SO_2 in normal, atopic, and asthmatic subjects. Data are mean ± SD; n = 7 except for asthmatic subjects breathing 5 ppm; in this group, n = 6. x, xx, xxx significantly different from value after exposure to air; $P < 0.05$, 0.025, and 0.01, respectively; + SRaw significantly different from SRaw for the other two groups; $p < 0.005$ (from Sheppard et al., 1980; reprinted with permission).

1983b, 1985; Koenig et al., 1981; Linn et al., 1983; Schacter et al., 1984). In one such study, 10 min of breathing 1 ppm SO_2 at rest caused a significant increase in specific airway resistance (SRaw) in seven subjects with mild asthma and a similar period of breathing 5 ppm SO_2 caused a mean doubling of SRaw and symptoms of an asthma attack in four of the seven (Fig. 1). In contrast, inhalation of 1 and 3 ppm SO_2 had no effect on SRaw in seven normal subjects or in seven atopic subjects without asthma, and inhalation of 5 ppm by these subjects caused an increase in SRaw that was statistically significant but quite small (approximately 15% above baseline) (Sheppard et al., 1980).

The bronchomotor effect of SO_2 in subjects with asthma is greatly potentiated if the pollutant is inhaled during exercise. Thus, when a group of seven subjects with mild asthma inhaled 0.25 and 0.5 ppm SO_2 during mild exercise (work rate 300 kilopond m/min (kpm)), both concentrations caused significant bronchoconstriction with significant symptoms in most subjects after inhalation of 0.5 ppm (Sheppard et al., 1981b). The two most sensitive subjects also developed bronchoconstriction after inhaling 0.1 ppm SO_2 (Fig. 2). Furthermore, the increase in SRaw caused by inhalation of 0.5 ppm during exercise was greater than that caused by resting inhalation of 5.0 ppm in the earlier study. This dramatic difference was not merely due to the increased dose of SO_2 delivered to the mouth during exercise, since minute ventilation during exercise exposures was only approximately three times higher than it was during resting exposures. These findings suggested that during exercise a greater percentage of inhaled SO_2 may have been reaching the relevant target sites within the airways. Such a result would be compatible with the results of studies with S^{35}-labeled SO_2 showing greater than 95% uptake of SO_2 in the oropharynx at low inspiratory flow rates but a progressive decrease in oropharyngeal uptake as inspira-

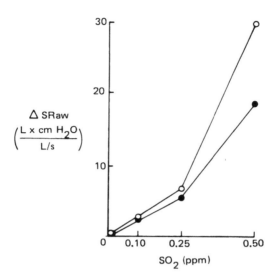

Figure 2 Dose-response to SO_2 inhaled during exercise in two subjects (● and ○). The Δ SRaw is the difference between baseline specific airway resistance and specific airway resistance after inhalation of SO_2. The subjects exercised on a bicycle ergometer for 10 min on separate days at a work rate of 300 kilopond m/min while they breathed partially humidified filtered air containing 0, 0.1, 0.25, or 0.5 ppm SO_2 through a mouthpiece (from Sheppard et al., 1981: reprinted with permission).

tory flow increased (Frank et al., 1969). That the increased effect of SO_2 inhaled during exercise were entirely due to the ventilatory response to exercise was confirmed by the finding that this effect was mimicked when the same subjects inhaled SO_2 during voluntary eucapnic hyperpnea at the same minute ventilation (Sheppard et al., 1981b) (Fig. 3).

At the same time that these experiments were demonstrating the bronchomotor effects of low concentrations of SO_2 on adult subjects with asthma, other investigators were finding similar effects of SO_2 administered with or without a sodium chloride aerosol to adolescent subjects with asthma (Koenig et al., 1981). These investigators subsequently extended their observations to include adolescent subjects with airway hyperresponsiveness but without a clinical history of asthma (Koenig et al., 1982).

These initial studies were performed by having subjects with asthma inhale SO_2 through a mouthpiece. Because of the previous observation that the human nose is an efficient filter for SO_2, it was suggested that mouthpiece studies might not be relevant to naturally occurring exposures to SO_2. More recent studies, per-

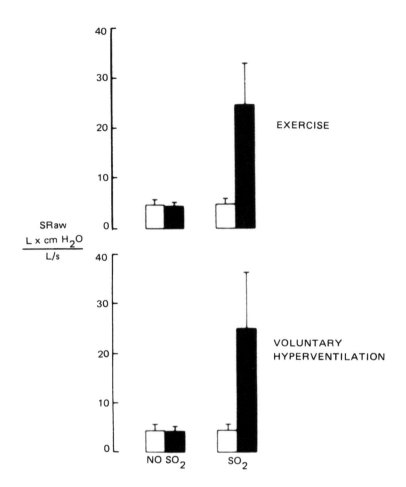

Figure 3 Effect of exercise (upper bars) and voluntary eucapnic hyperventilation (lower bars) on the response of specific airway resistance (SRaw) to inhaled SO_2 (1.00 ppm) in 6 asthmatic subjects. ($\square$ = control value during normal breathing at rest. $\square$ = value after intervention). Neither exercise alone nor hyperventilation alone (left columns) had any effect on SRaw. Exercise while breathing SO_2 and voluntary hyperventilation with SO_2 (right columns) both increased SRaw ($P < 0.005$) (from Sheppard et al., 1981; reprinted with permission).

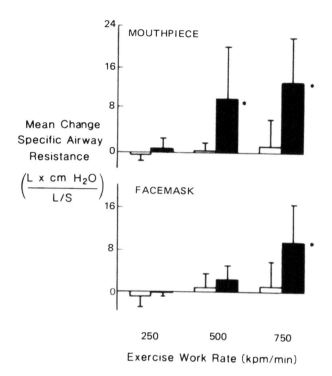

Figure 4 Mean change in specific airway resistance from before to after exercise in nine asthmatic subjects breathing SO_2-free air (□) or 0.5 ppm SO_2 (□) through a mouthpiece and through a face mask during exercise at 250, 500, and 750 kpm/min. The bar extensions are standard deviations; * = significant increase ($P < 0.001$) (from Bethel et al., 1983; reprinted with permission).

formed both through face masks and in whole body exposure chambers, have confirmed that a given concentration of SO_2 causes a somewhat smaller bronchomotor effect when it is inhaled during oronasal rather than purely oral breathing (Kirkpatrick et al., 1982; Bethel et al., 1983). However, in one study, 0.5 ppm SO_2 caused significant bronchoconstriction during exercise even when it was forced entirely through the nose by mouth occlusion (Kirkpatrick et al., 1982). Furthermore, the protective effects of oronasal breathing can be overcome by increasing the exercise work rate during SO_2 exposure (Bethel et al., 1983) (Fig. 4). Taken together, this series of experiments has shown that inhalation of concentrations of SO_2 as low as 0.25 ppm during exercise causes statistically significant bronchoconstriction even with unencumbered breathing in an exposure

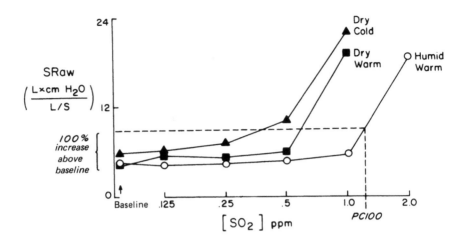

Figure 5 Specific airway resistance (SRaw) after inhalation of increasing concentrations of SO_2 in dry cold air (▲), dry warm air (■), and humid warm air (○) in one subject with asthma. The subject inhaled each concentration of SO_2 through a mouthpiece for 3 min at a minute ventilation of 40 liters/min. The concentration of SO_2 required to increase SRaw by 100% above baseline was more than 50% less when SO_2 was inhaled in dry air than when it was inhaled in humid air. Repeated inhalation of dry air alone at the same minute ventilation had no effect on SRaw (from Sheppard et al., 1984; reprinted with permission).

chamber (Bethel et al., 1985), and concentrations of 0.4 ppm or greater can cause symptomatic bronchoconstriction (Linn et al., 1983; Bethel et al., 1983a).

To avoid the potentially confounding effects of hyperpnea with cold or dry air on subjects with asthma, all of the studies discussed above administered SO_2 in warm partially humidified air. However, exposure to SO_2 in the environment often occurs when the outdoor air is cold or dry. Recently, two sets of studies have demonstrated that the bronchoconstrictor effects of SO_2 are potentiated if the gas is inhaled in dry air, even at a ventilatory rate at which dry air itself has no effect (Bethel et al., 1984; Sheppard et al., 1984) (Fig. 5). This potentiation is similar for cold dry air and warm dry air (Sheppard et al., 1984).

On the basis of early studies showing that SO_2 caused bronchoconstriction in cats entirely by activating a muscarinic reflex via the vagus nerves (Nadel et al., 1965), it has generally been assumed that SO_2-induced bronchoconstriction in humans is also mediated by a muscarinic reflex. This assumption fit well with the high aqueous solubility of SO_2 discussed above and its preferential deposition in the upper airways, a site of dense afferent innervation. Initial human studies, both in normal subjects and in subjects with asthma, provided further support for the viewpoint by demonstrating prevention of the bronchoconstriction induced by single concentrations of SO_2 by treatment with inhaled atropine (Sheppard et al., 1980). Recently, however, it has become clear that SO_2 induced bronchoconstriction in people with asthma is *not* solely mediated by a muscarinic reflex. By administering a wide range of doses of the muscarinic antagonist ipratroprium bromide and then performing dose-response curves to inhaled SO_2, it has been possible to study the role of the muscarinic pathway in more detail. In one study, sulfur dioxide continued to cause a marked increase in SRaw even after maximal inhibition of the muscarinic reflex pathway in every subject with asthma, if a high enough concentration of SO_2 was inhaled. This nonmuscarinically mediated increase in SRaw did appear to be due to contraction of airway smooth muscle, since it could be completely inhibited and/or reversed by the beta-adrenergic agonist metaproterenol (Tam et al., 1983).

The mechanism of this nonmuscarinic component of SO_2-induced bronchoconstriction has not been determined. Some evidence suggests that SO_2 may cause bronchoconstriction in part by an effect on airway mast cells. The major line of evidence supporting this hypothesis is the repeated observation that SO_2-induced bronchoconstriction can be inhibited by treatment with cromolyn (Harris et al., 1981; Sheppard et al., 1981a, Myers et al., 1986), a drug thought to work by stabilizing mast cell membranes. However, the significance of this observation is unclear, since cromolyn may prevent bronchoconstriction by other mechanisms, independent of an action on mast cells. In one recent study, SO_2 dose-response curves were obtained for nine subjects with asthma after treatment with either placebo, inhaled atropine (2.0 mg) alone, inhaled cromolyn (200 mg) alone, or the combination of atropine and cromolyn. Despite the fact that the dose of atropine had previously been shown to inhibit maximally the muscarinic component of SO_2-induced bronchoconstriction, treatment with atropine and cromolyn caused significantly greater inhalation of SO_2-induced bronchoconstriction than did atropine alone (Myers et al., 1986) (Fig. 6). These results suggest that the protective effects of cromolyn are not merely due to an inhibitory effect of this drug on the muscarinic reflex pathway, but that cromolyn is affecting the nonmuscarinic component of the response to SO_2.

A. Acute Massive Human Exposures

When SO_2 is inhaled in extremely high concentrations during industrial accidents, it has been reported to cause severe pulmonary injury and death from respiratory failure (Galea, 1964). Although most people who survive massive SO_2 inhalation probably recover normal lung function, some reports describe individuals who have persistent abnormalities in lung function for several years after a single massive exposure to SO_2 (Charan et al., 1978; Harkonen et al., 1983). In one such report, nine workers were presumably exposed to a concentration of SO_2 esti-

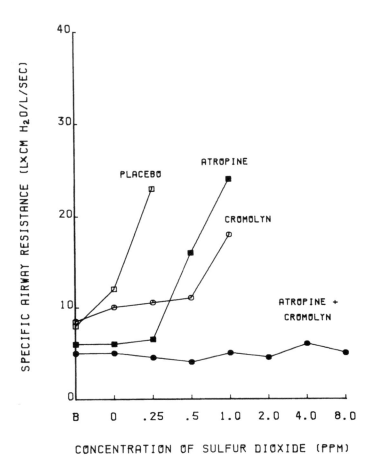

Figure 6 Effects of treatment with either inhaled atropine (2 mg), inhaled cromolyn (200 mg by spinhaler), the combination of atropine and cromolyn, or placebo on the increase in specific airway resistance caused by inhalation of doubling concentrations of SO_2 in one subject with asthma. The dose of atropine used was previously shown to cause maximal inhibition of the muscarinic component of SO_2-induced bronchoconstriction (data from Myers et al., 1986).

mated to be several hundred ppm as a result of a pyrite dust (FeS_2) explosion in an underground mine (Charan et al., 1979). One worker died and seven of eight survivors were evaluated over the next 4 years with serial measurements of lung function. In six of seven workers FEV_1, FVC, and maximal midexpiratory flow (**MMEF**) were markedly reduced from preexposure values within the first week after the accident and improved somewhat over the next 4 weeks. However, despite normal preexposure lung function, all six had persistent reductions in all three tests of lung function throughout the subsequent 4 years. The pattern of abnormality, with larger decreases in FEV_1 and MMEF than in FVC, suggested that the principal site of abnormality was in the airways. Four of these six were also found to have what the authors considered to be abnormally increased bronchomotor responsiveness to inhaled histamine 4 years after the explosion, although no preexposure data on histamine responsiveness was available. Although it is likely that SO_2 was the major chemical present in the mine air following this explosion, according to the authors such explosions can also produce nitrogen dioxide (NO_2) in concentrations of 2-25 ppm. It is therefore possible that the persistent airway dysfunction seen in these miners was due to NO_2 or to the combined effects of SO_2 and NO_2.

B. Chemical Mechanisms Underlying the Bronchomotor Effect of SO_2

Sulfur dioxide dissolves in water to form bisulfite ion, sulfite ion and hydrogen ion. These reactions are described by the following equilibrium relationships:

$$SO_2 + H_2O \xrightleftharpoons{\quad 1 \quad} HSO_3^- + H^+ \xrightleftharpoons{\quad 2 \quad} SO_3 = +2H^+$$

The pKa of reaction 1 is 1.86 (Huss and Eckert, 1977) and the pKa of reaction 2 is 7.2 (Hayon et al., 1972). The hydrolysis of SO_2 occurs very rapidly in aqueous environments, so that within fluid-filled structures such as cells, tissues, and blood vessels any effects of SO_2 exposure must be due to effects of bisulfite and/or sulfite anion. However, during inhalation of SO_2, SO_2 gas itself would be present at the air-liquid interface, so the initial effects of SO_2 on cells at the luminal surface of the airways could be due to direct chemical effects of SO_2 gas rather than to the effects of bisulfite or sulfite. Because of the difficulty in studying exposures of cells to SO_2 in the absence of water, nothing is known about such a direct effect of SO_2. The two major hydrolysis products, sulfite and bisulfite, are present in roughly equal concentrations at physiologic pH as determined by the pKa of their equilibrium reaction ($\sim$7.2). However, at the pH reported at the luminal surface of the airways, 6.6 (Boden et al., 1983), the ratio of bisulfite to sulfite is approximately 5:1. This may be unfortunate, since bisulfite is generally more chemically reactive than sulfite. Recent studies comparing the bronchoconstrictor effects of inhaled SO_2 and acidic and basic sulfite solutions in subjects with asthma suggest that sulfite ion is not likely to mediate SO_2-induced bronchoconstriction, whereas bisulfite ion might (unpublished observation). Although the hydrolysis of SO_2 also generates hydrogen ion, it is not likely that hydrogen ion generation causes SO_2-induced bronchoconstriction. The concentration of hydrogen ion generated by inhalation of the concentrations of SO_2 required to cause bronchoconstriction is trivial compared to the concentration of inhaled hydrogen ion required to cause bronchoconstriction in similar asthmatic subjects when they inhaled aerosols of a variety of acidic solutions (Fine et al., 1987).

Since bisulfite ion is a likely intermediary in the chemical effects of SO_2 on the airways, it is reasonable to review some of what is known about the biochemical reactivity of bisulfite. Bisulfite is a nucleophile that reacts with many biomolecules by substitution at electrophilic sites (Neta and Huie, 1985). One of these reactions leads to disruption of disulfide bonds and the production of thiosulfates by the following reaction (Petering and Shih, 1975):

$$R\text{-}S\text{-}S\text{-}R + HSO_3^- \rightleftharpoons RSSO_3^- + RSH$$

This reaction is probably the most important one for HSO_3^- absorbed into the bloodstream, since thiosulfates (RSH) are the major form of ^{35}S found in the bloodstream of animals after inhalation of $^{35}SO_2$ (Yokohama et al., 1971). Since disulfide bonds are widely found in tissue proteins, it is possible that bisulfite formed at the airway surface during SO_2 inhalation initiates bronchoconstriction by such an effect on surface proteins. However, there is no direct experimental evidence to confirm or refute such a mechanism of action of SO_2.

Most absorbed $^{35}SO_2$ is eventually excreted in the urine as sulfate (SO_4) (Yokohama et al., 1971), but the mechanism of bioconversion to sulfate is not determined (Neta and Huie, 1985; Petering and Shih, 1975). Bisulfite ion is converted to sulfate by sulfite oxidase, an enzyme found in lung, liver, and a variety of other tissues. Since thiosulfates, not bisulfite, are the principal chemical form of absorbed SO_2 in the bloodstream, the importance of sulfite oxidase in SO_2 clearance remains uncertain (Petering and Shih, 1975). Sulfite can also be converted to sulfate by nonenzymatic autooxidation that occurs in the presence of oxygen. Although this reaction is usually slow, it can be catalyzed by trace metal ions (Hoffmann and Boyce, 1983). This reaction is also a source of free radicals that could contribute to the tissue toxicity of SO_2 (Neta and Huie, 1985).

The intimate chemical relationship between SO_2, bisulfite, and sulfite ion has led to speculation that the bronchoconstriction that follows oral ingestion of sulfite-containing foods and beverages in some patients with asthma is mechanistically related to SO_2-induced bronchoconstriction (Stevenson and Simon, 1984). At least three different mechanisms may contribute to bronchoconstriction after sulfite ingestion. Since sulfite-sontaining foods, especially at acid pH, can off-gas significant concentrations of SO_2 (Freedman, 1980), some of the effects of sulfite ingestion may actually be due to inhalation of SO_2, either during ingestion or in association with eructation after the foods have been acidified in the stomach (Hoffmann and Boyce, 1983). This mechanism is the most likely explanation for the reported observation that some patients with presumed "sulfite sensitivity" develop bronchoconstriction after oral ingestion of acidified sulfite solutions but not after these solutions are instilled directly into the gastrointestinal tract via a nasogastric tube (Delohery et al., 1984). A second possible mechanism was suggested by a report that cultured fibroblasts from patients with bronchomotor sensitivity to ingested sulfite had a relative deficiency of the enzyme sulfite oxidase (Hoffman and Boyce, 1983). This observation suggested that sulfite sensitivity might be due to impaired clearance of HSO_3^- and SO_3^- leading to increases in the concentrations of these anions delivered to the lungs and perhaps increased off-gassing of SO_2 delivered to the lungs via the circulation. However, since, as noted above, the importance of sulfate oxidase in the overall clearance of ingested or inhaled sulfites is the subject of debate, this hypothesis requires further experimental validation. A third possible mechanism of sulfite-induced bronchoconstriction is immediate hypersensitivity. Although this mechanism does not seem to be important in most affected patients, it may play a role in the rare reports of systemic anaphylaxis from sulfites. The observation that dermal sensitivity to sulfite could be passively transferred via the serum of one affected patient is consistent with a humoral immune mechanism of response (Simon and Wasserman, 1986).

III. Summary

Sulfur dioxide is a ubiquitous air pollutant encountered in significant concentrations in outdoor air, in industry, and in homes heated by kerosene space heaters. The most important health effect of SO_2 is that it causes bronchoconstriction in people with asthma, especially when inhaled during exercise. Although the bronchoconstriction caused by high concentrations of SO_2 in animals is mediated primarily via a muscarinic reflex, there is an important nonmuscarinic component to the bronchoconstriction caused by low concentrations of SO_2 in people with asthma. In aqueous environments SO_2 is rapidly hydrolyzed to form sulfite, bisulfite, and hydrogen ions. Sulfite and hydrogen ions are not likely to cause SO_2-induced bronchoconstriction, but the relative importance of bisulfite and SO_2 gas itself remains to be determined, as does the initial cellular site of action of either of these forms of SO_2. Although it is intriguing to relate the bronchoconstrictor effects of inhaled SO_2 to those of ingested sulfites, the nature of the link between these events requires further investigation.

References

Amdur, M. O. (1966). Respiratory absorption data and SO_2 dose-response curves. *Arch. Environ. Health* **12**:729-736.

Amdur, M. O. (1969). Toxicologic appraisal of particulate matter, oxides of sulfur and sulfuric acid. *J. Air Pollut. Control Assoc.* **19**:638-644.

Bethel, R. A., Epstein, J., Sheppard, D., Nadel, J. A., and Boushey, H. A. (1983a). Sulfur dioxide-induced bronchoconstriction in freely breathing exercising asthmatic subjects. *Am. Rev. Respir. Dis.* **128**:987-990.

Bethel, R. A., Erle, D. J., Epstein, J., Sheppard, D., Nadel, J. A., and Boushey, H. A. (1983b). Effect of exercise rate and route of inhalation on sulfur dioxide-induced bronchoconstriction in asthmatic subjects. *Am. Rev. Respir. Dis.* **128**:592-596.

Bethel, R. A., Sheppard, D., Epstein, J., Tam, E., Nadel, J. A., and Boushey, H. A. (1984). Interaction of sulfur dioxide and airway cooling in causing bronchoconstriction in people who have asthma. *J. Appl. Physiol.* **57**: 419-423.

Bethel, R. A., Sheppard, D., Geffroy, B., Tam, E., Nadel, J. A., and Boushey, H. A. (1985). Effect of 0.25 ppm sulfur dioxide on airway resistance in freely breathing, heavily exercising, asthmatic subjects. *Am. Rev. Respir. Dis.* **131**:659-661.

Bodem, C. R., Lampton, L. M., Miller, D. P., Tarka, E. F., and Everett, E. D. (1983). Endobronchial pH. *Am. Rev. Respir. Dis.* **127**:39-41.

Charan, N. B., Myers, C. G., Lakshminarayan, S., and Spencer, T. M. (1979). Pulmonary injuries associated with acute sulfur dioxide inhalation. *Am. Rev. Respir. Dis.* **119**:555-560.

Committee on Sulfur Oxides (1978). *Sulfur Oxides.* Washington, D.C., National Academy of Sciences.

Delohery, Z. J., Simmul, R., Castle, W., and Allen, D. (1984). The relationship of inhaled sulfur dioxide reactivity to ingested metabisulfite sensitivity in patients with asthma. *Am. Rev. Respir. Dis.* **130**:1027-1032.

Fine, J. M., Gordon, T., Thompson, J., and Sheppard, D. (1987). Acid aerosol-induced bronchoconstriction in asthmatics. *Am. Rev. Respir. Dis.* **135**: 826-830.

Frank, N. R., and Speizer, F. E. (1965). SO_2 effects on the respiratory system in dogs: changes in mechanical behavior at different levels of the respiratory system during acute exposure to the gas. *Arch. Environ. Health* **11**: 624-634.

Frank, N. R., Amdur, M. O., Worcester, J., and Whittenberger, J. H. (1962). Effects of acute controlled exposure to SO_2 on respiratory mechanics in healthy male adults. *J. Appl. Physiol.* **17**:252-258.

Frank, N. R., Yoder, R. E., Brain, J. D., and Yokoyama, E. (1969). SO_2 (^{35}S-labeled) absorption by the nose and mouth under conditions of varying concentration and flow. *Arch. Environ. Health* **18**:315-322.

Freedman, B. J. (1980). Sulfur dioxide in foods and beverage: its use as a preservative and its effect on asthma. *Br. J. Dis. Chest* **74**:128-135.

Galea, M. (1964). Fatal sulfur dioxide inhalation. *Can. Med. Assoc. J.* **91**:345-347.

Hahn, H. L., Fabbri, L., Graf, P. D., and Nadel, J. A. (1983). Bronchokonstricktion und hypersekretion nack schwefeldioxid (SO$_2$)–ein laryngealer reflex? *Prax. Klin. Pneumol.* 37:666-669.

Harkonen, H., Nordman, H., Korhonen, O., and Winblad, I. (1983). Long-term effects of exposure to sulfur dioxide. Lung function four years after a pyrite dust explosion. *Am. Rev. Respir. Dis.* 128:890-893.

Harries, M. G., Parkes, P. E. G., and Lessof, M. H. (1981). Role of bronchial irritant receptors in asthma. *Lancet* 1:5-7.

Hayon, E., Treinin, A., and Wilf, J. (1972). Electronic spectra, photochemistry, and autoxidation mechanism of the sulfite-bisulfite-pyrosulfite systems, the SO_2^- SO_3^-, SO_4^-, and SO_5^- radicals. *J. Am. Chem. Soc.* 94:47-57.

Hoffmann, M. R., and Boyce, S. D. (1983). Catalytic autoxidation of aqueous sulfur dioxide in relationship to atmospheric systems. In *Trace Atmospheric Constituents: Properties, Transformations, and Fates.* Edited by S. E. Schwartz. New York, John Wiley, pp. 147-189.

Huss, A., and Eckert, C. A. (1977). Equilibria and ion activities in aqueous sulfur dioxide solutions. *J. Phys. Chem.* 81:2268-2270.

Kirkpatrick, M. B., Sheppard, D., Nadel, J. A., and Boushey, H. A. (1982). Effect of the oronasal breathing route on sulfur dioxide-induced bronchoconstriction in exercising asthmatic subjects. *Am. Rev. Respir. Dis.* 125:627-631.

Koenig, J. Q., Pierson, W. E., Horike, M., and Frank, R. (1981). Effects of SO$_2$ plus NaCl aerosol combined with moderate exercise on pulmonary function in asthmatic adolescents. *Environ. Res.* 25:340-348.

Koenig, J. Q., Pierson, W. E., Horike, M., and Frank, R. (1982). Bronchoconstrictor response to sulfur dioxide or sulfur dioxide plus sodium chloride droplets in allergic, nonasthmatic adolescents. *J. Allergy Clin. Immunol.* 69:339-344.

Leaderer, B. P. (1982). Air pollutant emission from kerosene space heaters. *Science* 218:1113-1115.

Linn, W. S., Venet, T. G., Shamoo, D. A., Valencia, L. M., Anzar, U. T., and Spier, C. E., and Hackney, J. D. (1983). Respiratory effects of sulfur dioxide in heavily exercising asthmatics: a dose-response study. *Am. Rev. Respir. Dis.* 127:278-283.

Myers, D. J., Bigby, B. G., Calvagrac, P., Sheppard, D., Boushey, H. A. (1986). The combination of cromolyn and atropine inhibits sulfur dioxide-induced bronchoconstriction more than either agent above. *Am. Rev. Respir. Dis.* 133:1154-1158.

Nadel, J. A., Salem, H., Tamplin, B., and Tokiwa, G. (1965). Mechanism of bronchoconstriction during inhalation of sulfur dioxide. *J. Appl. Physiol.* 20:164-167.

National Institute for Occupational Safety and Health (1974). Criteria for a recommended standard: Occupational exposure to sulfur dioxide. Washington, D.C. USDHEW p. 16.

Neta, P., and Huie, R. E. (1985). Free radical chemistry of sulfite. *Environ. Health Perspect.* **64**:209-217.

Petering, D. H., and Shih, N. T. (1975). Biochemistry of bisulfite-sulfur dioxide. *Environ. Res.* **9**:55-65.

Reid, L. An experimental study of hypersecretion of mucus in the bronchial tree. *Br. J. Exp. Pathol.* **44**:437-445.

Schachter, E. N., Witek, T. J., Beck, G. J., Hosein, H. R., Colice, G., Leaderer, B. P., and Cain, W. (1984). Airway effects of low concentrations of sulfur dioxide: dose-response characteristics. *Arch. Environ. Health* **39**:34-42.

Schrenk, H. H., Heiman, H., Clayton, G. D., Gafafen, W., and Wexler, H. (1949). Air pollution in Donora, Pennsylvania. Epidemiology of the unusual smog episode of October 1948). Public Health Bulletin 1949. Washington, D.C., U.S. Gov. Printing Office.

Seltzer, J., Scanlon, P. D., Drazen, J. M., Ingram, R. H., and Reid, L. (1984). Morphologic correlation of physiologic changes caused by SO_2-induced bronchitis in dogs. *Am. Rev. Respir. Dis.* **129**:790-797.

Sheppard, D., Wong, S. C., Uehara, C. F., Nadel, J. A., and Boushey, J. A. (1980). Lower threshold and greater bronchomotor responsiveness of asthmatic subjects to sulfur dioxide. *Am. Rev. Respir. Dis.* **122**:873-878.

Sheppard, D., Nadel, J. A., and Boushey, H. A. (1981a). Inhibition of sulfur dioxide-induced bronchoconstriction by disodium cromoglycate in asthmatic subjects. *Am. Rev. Respir. Dis.* **124**:257-259.

Sheppard, D., Saisho, A., Nadel, J. A., and Boushey, H. A. (1981b). Exercise increases sulfur dioxide-induced bronchoconstriction in asthmatic subjects. *Am. Rev. Respir. Dis.* **123**:486-491.

Sheppard, D., Eschenbacher, W. L., Boushey, H. A., and Bethel, R. A. (1984). Magnitude of the interaction between the bronchomotor effects of sulfur dioxide and those of dry (cold) air. *Am. Rev. Respir. Dis.* **130**:52-55.

Shy, C. M., Goldsmith, J. R., Hackney, J. D., Lebowitz, M. D., and Menzel, D. B. (1978). Health effects of air pollution. New York, American Lung Association.

Simon, R. A., and Wasserman, S. I. (1986). IgE mediated sulfite sensitive asthma. *J. Allergy Clin. Immunol.* **77**(suppl):157.

Skalpe, I. O. (1964). Long-term effects of sulfur dioxide exposure in pulp mills. *Br. J. Indust. Med.* **21**:69-73.

Smith, T. J., Peters, J. M., Reading, J. C., and Castle, C. H. (1977). Pulmonary impairment from chronic exposure to sulfur dioxide in a smelter. *Am. Rev. Respir. Dis.* **116**:31-39.

Smith, T. J., Wagner, W. L., and Moore, D. E. (1978). Chronic sulfur dioxide exposure in a smelter. *J. Occup. Med.* **20**:83-95.

Spiegelman, J. R., Hanson, G. D., Lazarus, A., Bennett, B. J., Lippman, M., and Albert, R. E. (1968). Effect of acute sulfur dioxide exposure on bronchial clearance in the donkey. *Arch. Environ. Health* **17**:321-326.

Stevenson, D. D., and Simon, R. A. (1984). Sulfites and asthma. *J. Allergy Clin. Immunol.* **74**:469-472.

Tam, E., Sheppard, D., Epstein, J., Bethel, R. A., and Boushey, H. A. (1983). Lack of dose dependency for ipratropium bromide's inhibitory effect on sulfur dioxide-induced bronchospasm in asthmatic subjects. *Am. Rev. Respir. Dis.* **127**:257.

Yokohama, E., Yoder, R. E., and Frank, N. R. (1971). Distribution of ^{35}S in the blood and excretion of dogs exposed to [35]SO_2. *Arch. Environ. Health* **22**:389-395.

3

Pulmonary Performance in Laboratory Animals Exposed to Toxic Agents and Correlations with Lung Disease in Humans

YVES ALARIE and MICHELLE SCHAPER

University of Pittsburgh
Graduate School of Public Health
Pittsburgh, Pennsylvania

Since the pioneering effort of Amdur and Mead (1955) to introduce an objective method for evaluation of the pulmonary toxicity of airborne chemicals, little progress has been made. Indeed, even this method has been found to be indicated primarily for recognition of acute effects (Costa, 1985). Other methods introduced since then (Costa, 1985; O'Neil and Raub, 1984) are difficult to use for toxicologic investigation because of one or more of the following drawbacks: invasive techniques, inability to perform measurements while animals are being exposed, need for anesthesia, too much restraint on animals, and time-consuming. The problems facing pulmonary toxicologists today are much broader than 30 years ago when the main interest was centered upon the effects of airborne chemicals. Now, a wide variety of drugs (primarily used as antineoplastic agents; Ginsberg and Comis, 1982), natural toxins in food, food additives, herbicides, etc., have been found to induce pulmonary toxicity (Boyd, 1980). Thus, the need is even greater to develop simple methods to detect whether or not pulmonary toxicity can be induced by inhaled chemicals or chemicals given by other routes. These detection methods can be viewed as "screening methods" and are not necessarily diagnostic. Once pulmonary toxicity is detected, a second level must be reached, that is, recognition of the type of effect induced, or discrimination. Finally, we must be able to predict what a "safe" level of exposure for humans is likely to be. Furthermore, simple methods are needed for several scenarios, including single exposures at different concentrations, multiple exposures at different concentrations, development of cumulative pulmonary toxicity, and recovery, if any, following pulmonary injury.

This chapter presents new methods to detect pneumotoxicity, describes how they can be used to detect both acute and chronic effects, and demonstrates the similarities between findings in animals and lung diseases in humans.

I. Statement of the Problem

Pulmonary toxicologists today are faced with evaluation of new chemicals being introduced on the market, as well as evaluation of a variety of pollutants found in urban atmospheres and indoors. Typically, when new chemicals are introduced, the first segment of the population exposed is the industrial workforce and the principal routes of exposure are inhalation and dermal. Thus, a rapid evaluation of each chemical is needed to establish the potential for acute pulmonary toxicity and to determine, when pulmonary toxicity is induced, whether or not recovery is likely. Let us assume that the method of choice is that involving measurement of airway resistance and pulmonary compliance, as developed by Amdur and Mead, (1955). Even with data reduction with a digital computer (Alarie et al., 1971a), how long would it take to evaluate a chemical? With 8-10 animals/group, and 6-8 exposure concentrations to obtain a concentration-response relationship from which the threshold or no effect level can be established, the entire study would take several months. It is very unlikely that a manufacturer would conduct such a study. It is more likely that animals will be acutely exposed, with some sacrificed 1 day later and some 14 days following exposure. Their lungs would then be examined grossly and at the light microscopic level. Functional tests have not been favored because of cost. Yet functional tests that can be used repeatedly on the same animals should be much more revealing and less costly than histopathologic evaluation to follow the development of pulmonary toxicity as well as recovery from it. A severe limitation of functional tests is the size of the animals involved. Typically, toxicity tests of new products are initiated using small rodents. Functional tests used in humans have been adapted to unanesthetized and restrained primates (Alarie et al., 1970, 1971a,b). However, cost is prohibitive and the use of nonhuman primates cannot be justified, at least in the initial screening of new products.

The situation is worse for chronic studies. Typically, a chronic study will involve a control group and at least three exposure groups with a large number of animals in each. Let us assume that 10-20 animals from each group would be selected for pulmonary function testing at least once a week. Thus, 40-80 animals would need to be evaluated every week. In recent studies on cotton dust, animals were evaluated daily, before and after exposure, to determine whether a pattern of response similar to that observed in humans could be obtained. The method(s) for evaluation had to be very rapid since 40 animals needed to be tested daily, prior to and following exposure (Ellakkani, 1985; Alarie et al., 1985).

The final problem confronting us is that we have no idea of the type of pulmonary toxicity likely to be induced by a new chemical, unless the agent is related to a previously studied one. The effect may be on the conducting airways or at the alveolar level, or on both, and it may be fast or slow in developing. Thus, the choice of a method becomes critical. In this chapter, we will defend the position that a method to detect pneumotoxicity should be as broad as possible.

II. Selection of a Method

Recent reviews by Costa (1985) and O'Neil and Raub (1984) present methods currently used by many investigators to evaluate pneumotoxicity. None are general enough to detect all possible types of pneumotoxicity. Only one general method has been proposed and that is based on the evaluation of control of ventilation, or ventilatory performance (Wong and Alarie, 1982). Ventilatory performance in lung disease is abnormal for a wide variety of reasons (Anthonisen and Cherniack, 1981). It is our intention to propose a test of ventilatory performance as an ideal screening method for pneumotoxicity.

Ventilatory pattern (tidal volume and respiratory frequency) may be normal during air breathing, but in the face of stimuli such as exercise or CO_2 (administered CO_2 or via rebreathing), abnormalities may be seen. This was reported long ago by Haldane et al. (1918a,b), who observed unusual ventilatory patterns in soldiers exposed to phosgene, a pulmonary irritant. These soldiers exhibited a rapid, shallow breathing pattern during air breathing that was even more exaggerated during exercise.

In laboratory animals, one method has been used in unrestrained and unanesthetized guinea pigs to produce higher tidal volume, respiratory frequency, and flow rates using a challenge with 10% CO_2 (Wong and Alarie, 1982). When the animal is breathing tidally, tidal volume, respiratory frequency, and airflow abnormalities may not be detected unless a relatively maximal maneuver is performed on inspiration and expiration, similar to the maximal expiratory flow-volume curves obtained in humans to detect obstructive and restrictive lung disease. In addition, the respiratory center can be evaluated with CO_2 challenge, although this will not be explored here.

III. Adaptation of the CO_2 Challenge Method for Toxicologic Screening

A. Apparatus and Respective Ventilatory Parameters Obtained

Whole-Body Plethysmograph: ΔP and f

In 1982, Wong and Alarie proposed that the barometric method could be adapted to measure volume (V), tidal volume (VT), respiratory frequency (f), and minute ventilation (VT·f) in unanesthetized, unrestrained guinea pigs. With their system, VT was actually measured as a change in whole-body plethysmograph pressure (ΔP), which was calibrated in ml rather than cm H_2O. The first practical application of the barometric method was by McCutcheon (1951) using rats. This was followed by Chapin (1954) using hamsters. Drobaugh and Fenn (1955) used it with newborn infants and the principles, and limitations, have been well-described (Bargeton and Barres, 1956; Epstein et al., 1980). The arrangement, as shown in Figure 1, permitted these measurements to be made rapidly with the animal first breathing room air, followed by 10% CO_2 challenge (10% CO_2, 20% O_2, 70% N_2). This CO_2 concentration was selected as optimal for increasing ΔP and f based on a series of experiments using from 3-20% CO_2 (Wong and Alarie, 1982) and arterial blood gas measurements (Alarie and Stock, 1986b).

It has been shown that for normal guinea pigs ΔP in the whole-body plethysmograph is proportional to VT during air breathing, as well as during CO_2 challenge (Wong and Alarie, 1982). A comparison of this system with other systems used in rabbits or humans and the limitations of such systems has been presented (Alarie et al., 1985).

Head Chamber Within Whole-Body Plethysmograph: $\dot{V}$, V, VT, ΔP, and f

The apparatus to measure $\dot{V}$, V, VT, f, and ΔP during air and CO_2 challenge is presented in Figure 2 (Matijak-Schaper et al., 1983). ΔP was measured as above, but VT (also designated VI or VE for inspiratory or expiratory volume) was measured directly by integration of airflow ($\dot{V}$) with time. Each animal was first fitted with a head chamber to which a pneumotachograph was attached, thus allowing the measurement of inspiratory ($\dot{V}I$) and expiratory airflows ($\dot{V}E$). This approach involves some restraint via the head chamber, although it is mild. As with the whole-body plethysmograph, continuous measurements can be made with the head chamber system while the animal is breathing air or a 10% CO_2 mixture. However, by using the head chamber system, it is possible to evaluate the relationship between two variables simultaneously (e.g., flow and volume, $\dot{V}$-V; pressure and volume, ΔP-V) during a given breath (Schaper et al., 1985). Since the volume measured during air is tidal volume (VT) and it is simply aug-

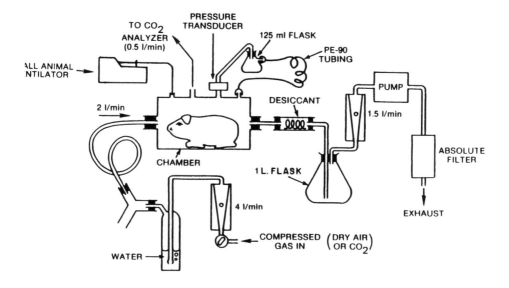

Figure 1 Lateral view of whole-body plethysmograph. This is a flow-through arrangement which permits continuous measurement of ΔP, proportional to VT, and f of an unrestrained, unanesthetized guinea pig while breathing air or a mixture containing 10% CO_2. A small animal ventilator is attached, which is used for calibration at frequencies from 60 to 220/min. (Modified from Wong and Alarie, 1982, reprinted with permission from Academic Press.)

mented during CO_2 challenge, the flow-volume ($\dot{V}$-V) or pressure volume (ΔP-V) relationships will be abbreviated $\dot{V}$-VT and ΔP-VT, respectively. The utility of such measurements will be demonstrated in a subsequent section. Several investigators have obtained flow-volume or pressure-volume relationships using a similar system with rabbits (Bargeton and Barres, 1956), rats (Johanson and Pierce, 1971), guinea pigs (Pennock et al., 1979), and humans (Bargeton and Barres, 1956; Jaeger and Otis, 1964). Their measurements, however, were obtained during air breathing only. A comparison of these systems has been presented (Alarie et al., 1985).

B. Response to CO_2 : ΔP, VT, and f

Whole-Body Plethysmograph

In guinea pigs, the ΔP and f responses to CO_2 are rapid and reach a plateau within a few minutes, as shown in Figure 3. In normal animals, ΔP increases

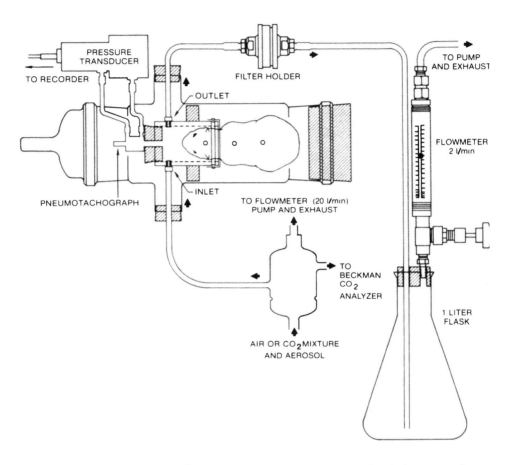

Figure 2 Overhead view of head chamber within a whole-body plethysmograph. This is a flow-through arrangement, which permits continuous measurement of ΔP, VT, and f of an unanesthetized but mildly restrained guinea pig. Attached to the head chamber is a pneumotachograph to measure $\dot{V}$ from which VT is obtained by integration with time. As illustrated, a Statham PM-15 differential pressure transducer was used to measure $\dot{V}$ (and ΔP as in Fig. 1, not shown). Because of their smaller size, Gaeltec 8T-2 transducers are now used and can be attached directly to the pneumotachograph within the whole-body plethysmograph. As shown, a filter holder is placed in line before the flowmeter. This is used to obtain the concentration of an aerosol when added to CO_2, as described in the text. The 1 liter flask is used to minimize the influence of the exhaust pump on the $\dot{V}$ signal. (From Matijak-Schaper et al., 1983, reprinted with permission from Academic Press.)

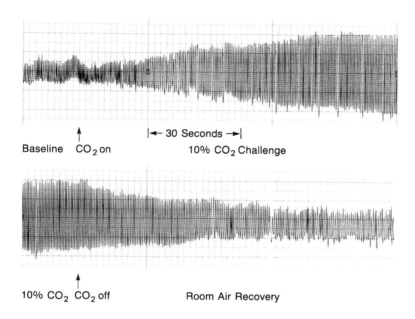

Figure 3 Normal ventilatory response of a guinea pig to 10% CO_2, in 20% O_2 and 70% N_2 as measured in the whole-body plethysmograph shown in Figure 1. The signal, ΔP, was calibrated in ml using a Harvard Apparatus small animal ventilator (see Schaper et al., 1985). The ΔP amplitude shown here during baseline was around 0.3 ml. (Modified from Wong and Alarie, 1982, reprinted with permission from Academic Press.)

by a factor of about 3 or higher, while the increase in f is 1.3-1.5 (Wong and Alarie, 1982). There is very little variation between animals and the ventilatory response to CO_2 is very reproducible. Over a period of 5 days, the coefficients of variation for ΔP were less than 12% of the average values for eight animals tested (Wong and Alarie, 1982). Also, over a 1 year period (as illustrated below), the ventilatory response to CO_2 was very stable. This permits the use of very few animals/group (even as few as four) and is of considerable importance for toxicologic evaluation. In comparison, there is wider interindividual variation in normal human subjects challenged with CO_2 (Read, 1967; Rebuck et al., 1974; Pengelly et al., 1979). However, the short-term and long-term reproducibility in the same subject is very good (Read, 1967; Irsigler, 1976). While ΔP is measured here, rather than VT, it has been shown that the two are well-correlated in normal guinea pigs during CO_2 challenge (Wong and Alarie, 1982).

Head Chamber Within Whole-Body Plethysmograph

The response of a guinea pig to CO_2 is even more rapid in the head chamber apparatus than in the whole-body plethysmograph. This is due to the small volume (head chamber, 152 ml, vs. whole-body plethysmograph, 2500 ml), which is quickly equilibrated with the CO_2 mixture. Respiratory frequency (f) increases during CO_2 challenge by a factor of 1.3-1.5 (Schaper et al., 1984), whereas VT and ΔP increase during CO_2 challenge by a factor of 2-3 (Matijak-Schaper et al., 1983). The difference in CO_2 response for VT and ΔP in the head chamber apparatus (two to three times) and the whole-body plethysmograph (three to four times) must be attributed to the mild restraint used at the neck of each animal. Similar effects are introduced in humans during CO_2 challenge with a face mask compared to mouth piece and nose clip (Hirsch and Bishop, 1982) or when comparing a canopy system with a neck seal to a mouthpiece plus nose clip (Weissman et al., 1984). As with the results obtained in the whole-body plethysmograph, little variation between CO_2 responses of different animals was found when using the head chamber (Matijak-Schaper et al., 1983; Schaper et al., 1984, 1985).

C. Use of the CO_2 Challenge Method, Acute Effects: Abnormal ΔP, VT, and f

To illustrate the use of the CO_2 method to detect pneumotoxicity, several examples are given here.

Pre-/Postexposure Measurements of the CO_2 Response
Sulfuric Acid Mist
Guinea pigs were exposed to sulfuric acid mist for 30 min at exposure concentrations between 23.5 and 72.7 mg/m^3 (Wong and Alarie, 1982). The particle size varied between 0.8 and 1.0 μm (mass median diameter). Prior to exposure, ΔP and f were obtained in the whole-body plethysmographs during air breathing and during CO_2 challenge. The same measurements were obtained at 0.5 and 3 hr postexposure, as well as every day during the following 5 days. The results presented in Figure 4 show that both ΔP and f during CO_2 decreased in a concentration-dependent fashion following exposure to sulfuric acid. Also, it can be seen that recovery occurred during the following 5 days. The effect was more pronounced on ΔP than on f and recovery was also slower for ΔP than for f.

Other agents producing similar effects are smoke from wood (Wong et al., 1984), smoke from polyvinylchloride (Wong et al., 1983), toluene diisocyanate (Wong et al., 1985), and hydrogen chloride (Burleigh-Flayer et al., 1985a). In each case, the effect on ΔP and f was easily recognized as that seen with sulfuric

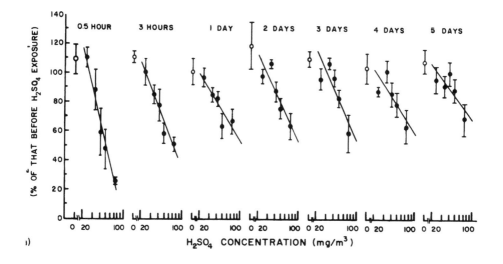

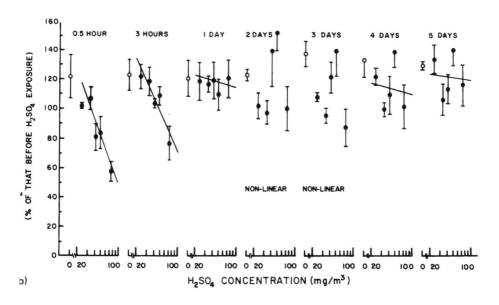

Figure 4 Decrease in VT (as measured by ΔP) and decreases in f, following a 30-min exposure to sulfuric acid mist at different concentrations. The measurements were made using the whole-body plethysmograph system. Each point represents the mean of four animals and the decrease in VT and f during CO_2 challenge were found to be concentration-dependent. Recovery was complete for f by day 5 and for VT by day 13 (data not shown). The data for a control group is shown at concentration = 0. (From Wong and Alarie, 1982, reprinted with permission from Academic Press.)

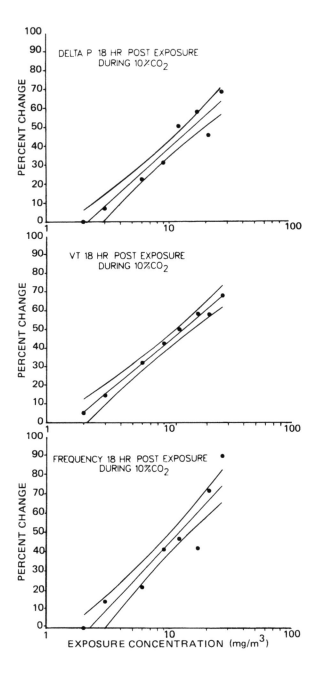

acid mist and recovery was easily followed by repeated CO_2 challenges as shown with sulfuric acid mist.

Cotton Dust

Groups of guinea pigs were exposed to respirable particles of cotton dust at concentrations of 2.0-27.0 mg/m^3 (Ellakkani et al., 1985a). Each exposure lasted 6 hr and the animals were challenged with CO_2 prior to exposure, following exposure and at 18 hr postexposure. In these experiments, the head chamber apparatus was utilized as described above and VT, ΔP, and f were measured. The maximal effect with exposure to cotton dust was observed at 18 hr postexposure and these results are shown in Figure 5. It can be seen that both ΔP and VT decreased in a concentration-dependent manner and it can also be seen that VT and ΔP were well-correlated ($r = 0.96$). The effect on f was opposite of the examples given above. As shown in Figure 5, there was a concentration-dependent increase in f. Thus, the pattern of breathing can be described as rapid and shallow. This same type of abnormal response to CO_2 challenge was also obtained following inhalation or intraperitoneal injections of paraquat (Burleigh-Flayer et al., 1985b; Burleigh-Flayer and Alarie, 1986) and following inhalation of hexamethylene diisocyanate (HDI) trimer aerosols (Ferguson et al., 1985).

Continuous Measurements of the CO_2 Response with the Addition of an Aerosol

Description of Protocol and Rationale

Using the exposure systems described above (Fig. 2), an alternative protocol may be employed that, as the pre/post exposure protocol, enables the recognition of acute effects of aerosols. Here, animals are also challenged with CO_2 but while they are breathing CO_2, an aerosol is added. Modifications in the normal CO_2 response can be easily detected. Most of the experiments following this approach have been conducted with the head chamber apparatus to obtain VT, ΔP, and f. The whole-body plethysmograph will also be suitable, using only ΔP and f.

Figure 5 Concentration–response relationships (with 95% confidence limits) for ΔP, VT, and f during CO_2 challenge performed at 18 hr following a 6 hr exposure to respirable particles from cotton dust. Measurements made using the head chamber added within the whole body plethysmograph as shown in Figure 2. Each point represents the mean of four exposed animals at each concentration. The % change, as labeled on the Y-axis, refers to the change in each variable during CO_2 postexposure from pre-exposure measurements. For ΔP and VT, it is a % decrease while for f, it is a % increase. (From Ellakkani et al., 1985a, reprinted with permission from Academic Press.)

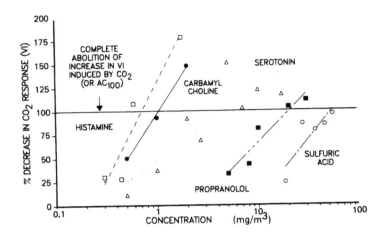

Figure 6 Concentration-response relationships for VT (or inspiratory volume, VI) for five aerosols during their addition to 10% CO_2 mixtures. Each point represents the mean of four exposed animals at each concentration. The percent decrease was calculated as follows. First, VI was measured during air breathing and during CO_2 challenge prior to addition of the aerosol. The increase in VI due to CO_2 was set equal to 100. Diminution in VI caused by the aerosol was then calculated from this level and thus a 100% decrease simply indicates that VI during CO_2 was reduced to the VI level during air breathing. A % decrease above 100% indicates that VI was lowered further than VI during air breathing. To compare the potency of various aerosols, a horizontal line was drawn at the 100% level to illustrate that concentration of each aerosol that abolishes the CO_2 response by 100% (AC_{100}). (From Schaper and Alarie, 1985, reprinted by permission from *Acta Pharmacologica et Toxicologica*.)

When guinea pigs are challenged with CO_2, their VT (or ΔP) and f increases (see Fig. 3) and this increase remains stable for 55 min (Matijak-Schaper et al., 1983) and for as long as 3 hr (unpublished) and probably longer. In rats, this increase has been shown to be stable for several days (Lai et al., 1981). Thus, if an aerosol or a gas is added while the animals are being challenged with CO_2, there should be a reduction in VT if the aerosol or gas induces constriction of the conducting airways or decreases the compliance of the lungs. Both effects increase the work of breathing and the ventilatory response to CO_2 should decrease.

Effects on VT or ΔP

By adding the following aerosols to CO_2: histamine, carbamylcholine, serotonin, propranolol, and sulfuric acid, a decrease in VT resulted. Furthermore, the magnitude of reduction of VT or ΔP during CO_2 was dependent upon the aerosol concentration (Schaper et al., 1984; Schaper and Alarie, 1985). VT was, however, a somewhat more sensitive indicator of acute responses to the aerosols than was ΔP. Accordingly, concentration-response relationships using only VT are presented in Figure 6. To compare the potency of these aerosols, we can calculate from each concentration-response relationship the concentration that completely abolishes the increase in VT due to CO_2, termed the AC100. This is, in effect, the aerosol concentration needed to reduce VT from its amplitude during CO_2 back to its amplitude during air breathing prior to CO_2 challenge. The AC100 values for the above aerosols showed histamine to be the most potent chemical and sulfuric acid the least potent. The effect of sulfuric acid was, however, longer lasting than that for histamine (Schaper et al., 1984), as also previously shown by Amdur (1958). It is of interest to compare the sensitivity of this method with the results of Amdur (1958, 1966), who used sulfuric acid and histamine aerosols of similar particle size. When we compare her concentration-response relationships based on increases in pulmonary airflow resistance with those given here based on reductions in VT during CO_2, these methods have an equal detection capability (Schaper et al., 1984).

Effects on f

Although the five agents given above decreased VT in a concentration-dependent manner, their effect on f was not the same. For histamine, sulfuric acid, and carbamyl choline, f decreased. f also decreased for serotonin at the beginning of a 30 min exposure. In contrast, f increased immediately for propranolol and for serotonin at the end of a 30 min exposure (Schaper et al., 1984; Schaper and Alarie, 1985).

D. Use of the CO_2 Challenge Method, Chronic Effects: Abnormal VT, ΔP, and f

Cotton Dust

This study was conducted using 20 control guinea pigs and 20 exposed animals (Ellakkani, 1985; Ellakkani et al., 1985b). The animals were exposed to 20 mg/m^3 respirable particles generated from cotton dust collected in a textile mill (Weyel et al., 1984). These animals were exposed for 6 hr/day, 5 days/week for 1 year. Prior to and following each daily exposure, each animal was placed in the whole-body plethysmograph shown in Figure 1 and ΔP and f during air breathing were obtained followed by the same measurements obtained during CO_2 challenge. A preliminary 6-week study demonstrated that the daily effect of cotton dust obtained by measuring ΔP was the same as that with a direct measurement of VT using the head chamber apparatus shown in Figure 2 (Ellakkani et al., 1984a).

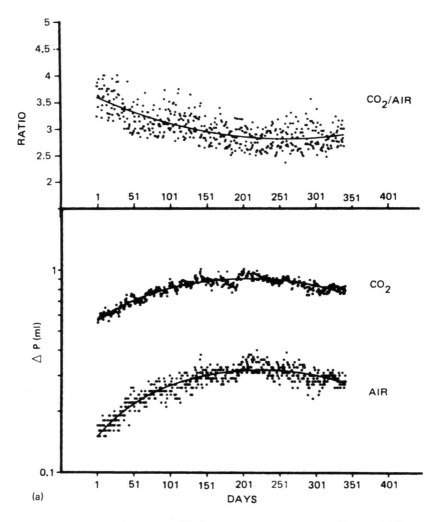

Figure 7 Trends for ΔP, f, and $\Delta P \cdot f$ obtained during air breathing and CO_2 challenge for a control group of guinea pigs. Measurements were obtained twice daily, before and after a 6 hr sham exposure. Each point represents the mean response of 20 animals. The solid line was obtained using a second degree polynomial to fit the data points. (From Ellakkani, 1985).

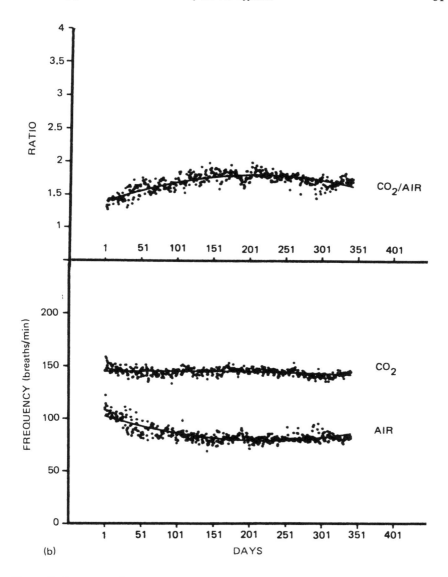

Figure 7 (continued)

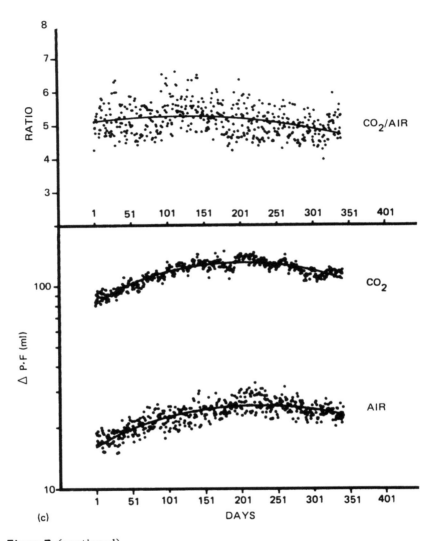

(c)

Figure 7 (continued)

The body weights of these animals were recorded daily and no difference between these two groups was observed until day 225 of exposure, when the control group had a slightly higher body weight than the exposed group.

Daily CO_2 Challenges for the Control Group

From Figure 7 it can be seen that the ventilatory response to CO_2 was very reproducible over a period of 1 year. For ΔP, f, and $\Delta P \cdot f$, there was less variation during CO_2 than during air. It is interesting to note that the ratios of CO_2/air for ΔP versus f displayed opposite trends with time. The ratio was higher for ΔP in young animals and decreased with age and increasing body weight. For f, the ratio was lower in young animals due to a higher f during air, which slowly decreased with age. Thus, the ratio of CO_2/air for $\Delta P \cdot f$ remained fairly stable for the entire year but f contributed more at the end of the year than at the beginning. A similar decrease in f with an increase in VT has also been observed in growing laboratory animals (Parot et al., 1984; Mortola, 1984). There is an indication from Figure 7 that $\Delta P \cdot f$ was beginning to decline toward the end of the year and that both ΔP during air and ΔP during CO_2 values were also declining after reaching a maximum. In humans, there is a decrease in the ventilatory response to CO_2 with age when young (22-37 years) subjects were compared to older (65-72 years) subjects (Brischetto et al., 1984).

Daily CO_2 Challenges for the Group Exposed to Cotton Dust

Cotton dust exposure changed the normal ΔP and f response to CO_2 challenge, as shown in Figure 8. Although CO_2 challenge was conducted daily, prior to and following exposure (Alarie et al., 1984; Ellakkani et al., 1984b, 1985b), only the results obtained on Mondays of each exposure week are shown to illustrate the utility of the technique.

First, f was much higher than normal following exposure to cotton dust. The pre-postexposure difference was larger at the beginning of exposure than at the end, due to an upward trend in preexposure values. Secondly, ΔP during CO_2 was altered in two major ways. There was a pre-postexposure difference during the entire year with the postexposure values always lower than preexposure. Also, the ΔP values for preexposure, although similar to the control group during the first 4 weeks of exposure, never reached the higher level of the control group during growth. Therefore, other airborne chemicals could be tested using the same protocol to investigate chronic pneumotoxic effects.

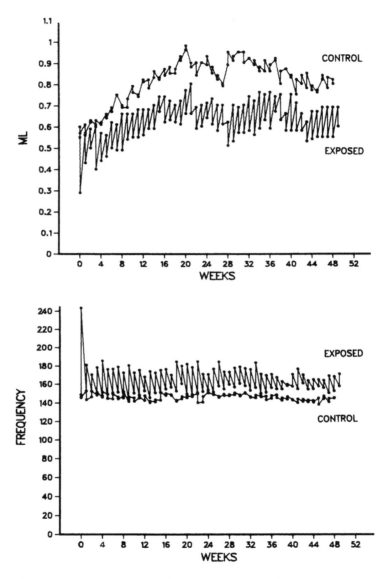

Figure 8 Average values for ΔP (ml) and f (breaths/min) of control animals and animals and animals exposed daily to cotton dust (20 mg/m^3). The values presented were obtained during CO_2 challenge and are shown for pre-exposure and postexposure on Mondays during the 1 year of exposure. For the exposed group, f values were always higher and ΔP values were always lower after exposure than prior to exposure. No such trend was observed for the control group. (From Ellakkani, 1985.)

IV. Types of Abnormal CO_2 Responses Observed Acutely or Chronically: VT (or ΔP) and f

A. Animal Studies

As shown above, all agents tested reduced VT (or ΔP) during CO_2 challenge, but one group also reduced f, while an increase in f was observed with the second group. The agents in the first group are listed under the type I abnormal response and the agents in the second group are listed under the type II abnormal response in Table 1. Because of the nature of the agents involved (i.e., known bronchoconstrictors usually associated with decreasing f with intense bronchoconstriction and the pattern of rapid, shallow breathing [increasing f] with the other group of agents), the two different types (type I and type II) of abnormal response were arbitrarily defined as "obstruction" and "restriction." This follows the findings of McIlroy et al. (1956) that in normal individuals added resistive loads reduce VT and reduce f, while with added elastic loads VT is restricted from increasing but f compensates for the reduced VT. Since only VT (or ΔP) and f were measured, this classification scheme is speculative. Lung volume measurement as well as other measurements are necessary to classify more clearly the obstruction or restriction pattern. Nevertheless, there were two different types of abnormal responses to CO_2 induced by these agents and with further measurements (described in a subsequent section) it appears that this proposed scheme is probably correct. Thus, at this point, the results presented above with measurements of VT (or ΔP) and f during CO_2 challenge provide the information needed to answer important toxicologic questions:

> At a given exposure concentration, do we observe a normal ventilatory response to CO_2 in terms of the expected increase in VT (or ΔP) and f observed in normal animals?

> Is there a concentration-response relationship in the change from the normal increase in VT (or ΔP) and f and can a threshold level be established?

> Is the change permanent or how long is the period of time for recovery?

> Can a chronic effect be detected?

The method is extremely simple and requires few animals. This is what a detection method should do. Next, an attempt must be made to determine if both types of abnormal ventilatory responses to CO_2 also exist in humans.

B. Are There Similarities Between the Normal and Abnormal Responses Observed in Guinea Pigs With Observations Obtained in Humans?

In the previous sections we have presented evidence that a wide variety of chemicals can modify the normal VT and f responses to CO_2 challenge. In all cases,

Table 1 Changes in VT and f During CO_2 Challenge in Laboratory Animals and Humans

A. Normal Response

The normal response to CO_2 challenge is an increase in VT and f where the percent increase in VT is larger than the percent increase in f.

I. Laboratory animals

Guinea pigs: Wong and Alarie, 1982; Matijak-Schaper et al., 1983; Blake and Banchero, 1985

Dogs: Lee et al., 1980

Rats: Wong and Alarie, 1982; Hayashi et al., 1982; Lai et al., 1981; Walker et al., 1985; Saeta and Mortola, 1985

Hamsters: Walker et al., 1985; Schlenker, 1984; Javaheri et al., 1980

Rabbits: Maskrey and Nicol, 1980; Richardson and Widdicombe, 1969; Russell et al., 1984

Mole rats: Arieli and Ar, 1979

Cats: Gautier, 1976

II. Humans

Askanazi et al., 1979

Cunningham and Gardner, 1977

Donald and Christie, 1949a,b

Fishman et al., 1955

Garrard and Lane, 1978

Guz et al., 1966

Haldane and Priestley, 1905

Haywood and Bloete, 1969

Hey et al., 1966

Irsigler, 1976

Kellog, 1964

Lambertsen, 1960

Lindhard, 1911

Maranetra and Pain, 1974

Pengelly et al., 1979

Read, 1967

Table 1 (continued)

II. Humans (continued)

Rebuck et al., 1974

Reynolds et al., 1972

Schaefer, 1958

Scott, 1920

Weissman et al., 1982, 1984

B. Type I: Obstruction

With CO_2 challenge, there is a failure to increase VT and f as in normal conditions and VT·f is always lower than in normal conditions.

I. Observed in guinea pigs with exposure to:

Sulfuric acid mist: Wong and Alarie, 1982; Matijak-Schaper et al., 1983; Schaper et al., 1984

Aerosols of histamine: Matijak-Schaper et al., 1983; Schaper et al., 1984

Smoke from wood: Wong et al., 1984

Smoke from polyvinylchloride: Wong et al., 1983

Toluene diisocyanate: Wong et al., 1985

Hydrogen chloride: Burleigh-Flayer et al., 1985a

Aerosols of serotonin: Schaper and Alarie, 1985[a]

Aerosols of carbamylcholine: Schaper and Alarie, 1985

Cotton dust exposure for 1 year: Alarie et al., 1985; Ellakkani et al., 1985b[a]

II. Observed in humans with emphysema and chronic obstructive lung diseases and in normal individuals with added resistive loads:

Brodovsky et al., 1960

Cherniack, 1965

Cherniack and Snidal, 1956

Clark, 1968

Clark and Cochrane, 1972

Clark and Godfrey, 1969

Donald and Christie, 1949a

Duara et al. (in infants), 1985

Eldridge and Davis, 1959

Fritts et al., 1957

Table 1 (continued)

II. Observed in humans with emphysema and chronic obstructive lung diseases and in normal individuals with added resistive loads: (continued)

Lopata et al., 1985

Lourenco and Miranda, 1968

Milic-Emili and Tyler, 1963a,b

Richards et al., 1958

Scott, 1920

Tenney, 1954

III. In humans with severe asthma and during their recovery:

Rebuck and Read, 1971

IV. In severely affected cotton workers:

Prausnitz, 1936

C. Type II: Restriction

With CO_2 challenge the increase in VT is less than in normal conditions while f increases higher than in normal conditions.

I. Observed in guinea pigs with exposure to:

Single exposure to cotton dust: Ellakkani et al., 1985a

During first 6 weeks of exposure to cotton dust: Alarie et al., 1984; Ellakkani et al., 1984

After exposure to cotton dust for 51 weeks: Alarie et al., 1985[a]

Aerosols of hexamethylene diisocyanate trimer: Ferguson et al., 1985

Aerosols of dichloroisoproterenol: Schaper and Alarie (unpublished)

Aerosols of propranolol: Schaper and Alarie, 1985

Aerosols of serotonin: Schaper and Alarie, 1985[a]

Aerosols of paraquat: Burleigh-Flayer and Alarie, 1986

Aerosols of endotoxin: Karol et al., 1985

II. Observed in rats following exposure to:

Paraquat injection: Burleigh-Flayer et al., 1985b

Chronic exposure to silica: Chavlova et al., 1974[a]

III. Observed in dogs

With exposure to ozone: Lee et al., 1979, 1980

With experimental pneumonitis: Phillipson et al., 1975

Aerosols of histamine: Bleecker et al., 1976

Table 1 (continued)

IV. Observed in humans

Following exposure to phosgene: Haldane et al., 1918a,b

Following exposure to ozone: Folinsbee et al., 1975; Beckett et al., 1985; Gibbons and Adams, 1984

With allergic alveolitis: Jones, 1981

With disease of pulmonary arteries: Nadel et al., 1966; Nadel et al., 1968

With mild pulmonary fibrosis and in cases of dyspnea of unknown origin: Fishman and Ledlie, 1979

Reduced lung compliance following pulmonary resection: Easton et al., 1983

External elastic loading: Lopata and Pearle, 1980; Shekleton et al., 1976; Freedman et al., 1972

With diffuse pulmonary fibrosis: Lourenco et al., 1965; Turino and Goldring, 1976

Expiratory nonelastic loading in normal individuals: Garrard and Lane, 1978, 1979

Proliferative stage of fibrosis: Cotes et al., 1970

Hyperinflation of the thorax: Grassino et al., 1973

Pulmonary fibrosis: West and Alexander, 1959

Inspiratory muscle fatigue: Gallagher et al., 1985; Gribbin et al., 1983

Interstitial lung disease: Burdon et al., 1983

[a]Both Type I and II abnormal response were observed; see text.

VT was prevented from increasing as in normal conditions. For one group, f was lower than normal and this was termed "obstruction." For the second group, f was higher than normal, and this was termed "restriction." We have searched the literature to determine what constitutes a normal CO_2 response in humans and to find as many examples of abnormal ventilatory responses (for VT or f) to CO_2 in humans.

Normal Ventilatory Response to CO_2 in Humans, Guinea Pigs, and Other Laboratory Animals

From this survey, we found that in normal individuals the ventilatory response to CO_2 is the same as in guinea pigs and is as follows: an increase in VT that is always higher than the increase in f. In fact, in two studies involving humans who inspired several air concentrations of CO_2 (Reynolds et al., 1972; Schaeffer, 1958), the results are very similar to those obtained in guinea pigs. All studies are listed in Table 1.

Abnormal Ventilatory Response to CO_2 in Humans, Guinea Pigs, and Other Laboratory Animals

Type I: Obstruction

The studies listed in Table 1 dealt with patients who had obstructive disease and/or emphysema as characterized by classic pulmonary function tests or clinical evaluation. Upon challenge with CO_2, these individuals failed to respond in a normal manner. Their minute ventilation was consistently below that of normal subjects. The same pattern was found in normal individuals breathing with added resistive loads. Again, this pattern was observed in asthmatics during a severe asthma attack and during recovery. Listed in Table 1 are the results obtained in guinea pigs with a variety of agents that induced a similar abnormal ventilatory response, (i.e., failure to increase VT and f upon CO_2 challenge to that level of control animals, resulting in lower than normal minute ventilation). Thus, as stated earlier, there is an increase in the work of breathing with obstruction causing a reduced ventilatory response to CO_2.

Type II: Restriction

The studies listed as type II in Table 1 are from a wider variety of sources than those listed under type I, but all share a common feature. When challenged with CO_2 (or mild to moderate exercise), the response was abnormal in that VT failed to increase as in normal conditions, while f increased much higher than normally. The causes of this abnormal type of ventilatory response may be numerous.

Reflex Restriction. The first report that an abnormal ventilatory response to mild exercise could be due to stimulation of vagal nerve endings was presented by Haldane et al. (1918a,b), who coined the term "reflex restriction" to describe the rapid and shallow breathing in soldiers recovering from phosgene poisoning. Lee et al. (1979, 1980) have demonstrated that ozone, another classic pulmonary irritant, induced the same type of abnormal ventilatory response in dogs during CO_2 challenge or exercise challenge. This abnormal response was abolished upon vagal nerve cooling, thus providing good evidence that the abnormal response is due to stimulation of vagal nerve endings. Indeed, a wide variety of pulmonary irritants, including phosgene and ozone, are known to induce rapid, shallow breathing in a wide variety of laboratory animals and in humans during normal air breathing (Alarie, 1981). Thus, as characterized by Lee et al. (1979, 1980), CO_2 challenge or exercise further exaggerated the effect. Paintal (1981) and Widdicombe (1982) have provided ample evidence that this pattern of breathing can be due to stimulation of a variety of vagal nerve endings, in particular, type J receptors. Thus, with CO_2 or mild to moderate exercise challenge, the rapid shallow breathing is further exaggerated. Further evidence for this mechanism was obtained with propranolol. The response was abolished by cervical vagal block-ade with cocaine infiltration but not by an aerosol of isoproterenol (Schaper and Alarie, 1986). Pulmonary edema and congestion are also adequate stimuli for type J vagal nerve endings (Paintal, 1981; Widdicombe, 1982; Trenchard et al., 1972) and can explain why this abnormal response to CO_2 can be observed during an in-flammatory reaction. The effect of ozone in humans was recently reported (Gib-bons and Adams, 1984) as similar to the effect of phosgene reported by Haldane et al., (1918a,b) and of ozone reported by Lee et al. (1979, 1980) in dogs. Further evidence of the involvement of vagal receptors in mediating the response following ozone treatment has been presented by Gertner et al. (1984) and Beckett et al. (1985). There are definite indications that vagal afferents play a major role in de-termining f during normal conditions and during CO_2 challenge or mild exercise (von Euler et al., 1970; Clark and von Euler, 1972; Guz et al., 1966; Richardson and Widdicombe, 1969; Phillipson et al., 1970; Russell et al., 1984; Gertner et al., 1984; Easton et al., 1985; Savoy et al., 1982; among others). The results of Rus-sell et al. (1984) and Green et al. (1984) suggest that nonmyelinated vagal endings and nonmyelinated vagal fibers are responsible. Therefore, it is not surprising that direct stimulation of vagal afferents or pathologic conditions resulting in their stimulation, will result in an exaggerated increase in f and a lower than normal increase in VT during CO_2 challenge or during mild or moderate exercise.

Restrictive Disease and Decreases in Lung Compliance. Another cause for this pattern of abnormal response to CO_2 is a decrease in lung compliance as ob-served with fibrosis and restrictive diseases. Here, there is a mechanical advantage in breathing shallowly and rapidly to minimize the work to overcome elastic re-sistance (Mead, 1960). However, the situation is more complex than simply minimizing work. Lourenco et al. (1965) presented an appraisal of the mechan-ism responsible for the augmented minute ventilation in patients with diffuse fibrosis. They tested the same patients with two ventilatory stimuli: exogenous CO_2 and exercise. Both induced the same abnormal response: VT increased less than in normals while f increased more than in normals, thus resulting in a higher than normal minute ventilation. They concluded that the higher work of breath-ing was not the limiting factor. This abnormal pattern of response could instead be due to an abnormally large number of afferent nervous impulses reaching the respiratory center from the lungs and/or respiratory muscles. However, as also noted by these authors, in patients with pulmonary fibrosis the fraction of the vital capacity used during CO_2 challenge (tidal volume/vital capacity $\times$ 100) is much higher than that used by normal individuals. Thus, this mechanical factor (limitation) must have also contributed in restricting VT from increasing as in normal conditions. Cotes et al. (1970) also reported a similar abnormal ventila-tory response during the proliferative stage of fibrosis and attributed it to activa-tion of vagal nerve endings. Renzi et al. (1982) concluded that, in diffuse lung fibrosis, the pattern of rapid shallow breathing is in proportion to the decrease in lung elastance and is qualitatively similar to that observed when external elastic loads are added to normal subjects. They concluded "hence high lung elastance seems to be the main determinant of their breathing pattern likely via chest wall receptors and reflexes via the vagus nerve from the lung parenchyma."

Inspiratory Muscle Fatigue. This has also been demonstrated to be a cause of a more rapid and shallower than normal breathing. Particularly in the case of an overinflated chest, the inspiratory muscles are no longer operating at their normal resting levels since they are in a stretched position. CO_2 or exercise challenge results in a lower than normal VT and a higher than normal f (Gallagher et al., 1985; Hannhart et al., 1979).

Thus, in humans and guinea pigs, types I and II abnormal ventilatory responses have been observed. Other investigative methods are needed to allow us to confirm and understand fully the elements of these abnormal responses measured during CO_2 challenge.

V. Flow-Volume Loops and Other Ventilatory Parameters

A. Normal CO_2 Response in the Guinea Pig

We begin by characterizing the normal CO_2 response in terms of other parameters besides VT (or ΔP) and f. This will then provide a basis for comparisons with responses obtained during and following exposure to airborne chemicals and further characterize the two types of abnormal responses described. As mentioned earlier, the measurements of $\dot{V}$, VT, ΔP, and f were conducted using the head chamber apparatus. By using this apparatus, two variables can be examined simultaneously for a given breath. Thus, it was possible to plot flow-volume ($\dot{V}$-VT) and pressure-volume loops (ΔP-VT) (Schaper et al., 1985). Results of such measurements are shown in Figure 9 for one control animal breathing air, then during CO_2 challenge. Also shown in Figure 9 is the relationship between ΔP and $\dot{V}$ at 0.5 VT, which can be used to obtain a measure of resistance (R) (Bargeton and Barres, 1955; Johanson and Pierce, 1971; Schaper et al., 1985). Table 2 gives the numerical results for numerous ventilatory parameters such as inspiratory/expiratory airflows ($\dot{V}I/\dot{V}E$), time of inspiration/expiration (TI/TE), area of ΔP-VT loops, and resistance (R) both during air and CO_2. Areas of ΔP-VT loops were examined since they are substantially proportional to flow-resistive work (Bargeton and Barres, 1955; Jaeger and Otis, 1964). The data in Table 2 for air breathing and CO_2 challenge were collected from 12 animals and each value in the table represents the mean of this group. The coefficient of variation is also given for each mean value.

As shown in the earlier illustration of CO_2 challenges (Fig. 3), it may be concluded that the overall effect of CO_2 is one of "magnification." This is clearly demonstrated by the results given in Table 2. The only variable that did not change during CO_2 was R, which implied that no bronchoconstriction was induced by CO_2 itself. The flow-resistive work, as indicated by increases in area of ΔP-VT loops from air to CO_2 challenge, was greater during CO_2. This can be explained by the higher $\dot{V}$ during CO_2 than during air. The additional work was necessary to maintain the higher airflows evoked by CO_2. Thus, while VT increased by 2.4 from air to CO_2, the ΔP-VT loop area increased by a factor of 6.6, or slightly more than the square of the increase in VT.

B. Abnormal CO_2 Response in the Guinea Pig

As we have stated above, two types of abnormal CO_2 responses have been observed in guinea pigs. To understand why, in both cases, there is a reduction in VT, while f changes in opposite directions, $\dot{V}$-VT loops, ΔP-VT loops, R, TI, and TE measurements can be extremely useful.

Type I: Obstruction
Carbamylcholine: Obstruction Induced Acutely

By adding an aerosol while an animal is breathing CO_2, it is possible to recognize its acute pulmonary effects via a reduction in VT. The aerosol concentration can be regulated so that it will reduce VT during CO_2 to that VT level obtained during air breathing prior to CO_2 challenge (i.e., the increase in VT due to CO_2 alone is completely abolished by the added aerosol: the concentration producing this effect is termed the AC_{100}). In this manner, all variables can be compared to the results obtained at the normal VT during air (i.e., 1.5 ml) in effect, normalizing on VT. The effect of carbamylcholine at the AC_{100} level can be seen for one animal in Figure 9. Table 2 presents the data on carbamylcholine, also from exposures at the AC_{100} level, where each value represents the mean response of four animals. These results can be compared with those from animals breathing air or 10% CO_2 mixtures (columns A and B).

From Figure 9, it can be seen that VT was reduced during exposure to carbamylcholine to that level seen during air breathing (1.5 ml). There are obvious airflow interruptions during expiration, the area of the ΔP-VT loop is increased, R is increased, and f is decreased due to a lengthening of the duration of expiration (TE). This effect can be reversed by adding an aerosol of isoproterenol but is not abolished by cervical vagal blockade with cocaine infiltration. Thus, the effect is indeed one of airway obstruction, increasing the work of breathing and reducing the CO_2 response. This pattern was obtained for carbamylcholine, histamine, sulfuric acid, and at the beginning of exposure to serotonin. The results for serotonin are shown in Table 2.

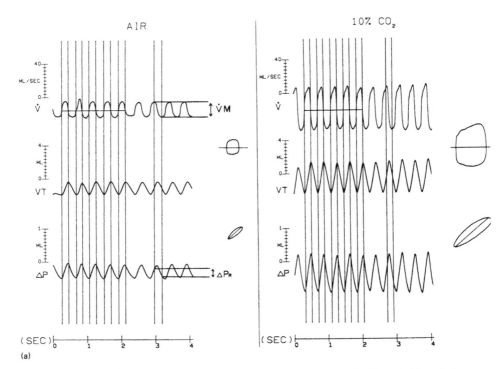

Figure 9 (a) $\dot{V}$, VT, and ΔP recorded during air breathing (left) and CO_2 challenge (right), as measured with the apparatus shown in Figure 2 for 300-400 g normal guinea pigs. The horizontal line passing through $\dot{V}$ indicates 0 flow with inspiration and expiration above and below this line, respectively. Vertical lines drawn through the points of zero flow on the first five breaths indicate the phase differences between VT and ΔP. For the seventh breath, vertical lines were drawn through the points at midtidal volume (0.5 VT of 0.5 VI and 0.5 VE). From these, 0.5 $\dot{V}I$ and 0.5 $\dot{V}E$ values were obtained. Also, 0.5 $\dot{V}I$ plus 0.5 $\dot{V}E$ was set equal to $\dot{V}M$. The ΔP amplitude between 0.5 VI and 0.5 VE was also obtained and termed ΔPr, as shown. Resistance (R) was obtained by the ratio of $\Delta Pr/\dot{V}M$ and was expressed in ml/ml/sec since ΔP was calibrated in ml. From one of the first five breaths, a $\dot{V}$-VT loop and a ΔP-VT loop are presented at the right of each group of tracings during air and CO_2. The line passing through the $\dot{V}$-VT loop separates inspiration (top) from expiration (bottom). Likewise, the line drawn through the ΔP-VT loop separates inspiration (right) from expiration (left), permitting the calculation of areas for inspiration (ΔP-VT, area I) and expiration (ΔP-VT, area E) representing flow-resistive work during each breath.

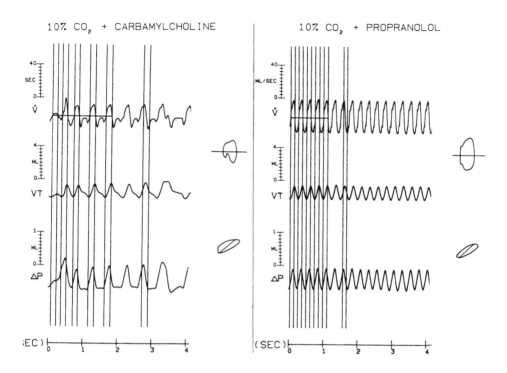

Figure 9 (b) V̇, VT, and ΔP signals and V̇-VT and ΔP-VT loops as described in
(a). These were obtained in two guinea pigs, with one inhaling an aerosol of
carbamylcholine (left side) and the other inhaling an aerosol of propranolol
(right side). Each aerosol was added to CO_2 only after VT was increased to a
level similar to that seen in the right panel of 9a (3.6 ml). The aerosol concentration used in both cases was adjusted to reduce the VT amplitude during CO_2
back to that VT amplitude during air (1.5 ml). Thus, the changes induced by
both aerosols can be compared for the same VT of a control animal (see left
panel of Fig. 9a). (From Schaper et al., 1985, reprinted with permission from
Academic Press.)

Table 2 Results Obtained in Normal Guinea Pigs Breathing Air or During 10% CO_2 and During 10% CO_2 Plus Aerosols of Carbamylcholine, Propranolol, or Serotonin

Variables measured[b]	A Air		B 10% CO_2			C 10% CO_2 + Carbamylcholine			D 10% CO_2 + Propranolol			E 10% CO_2 + Serotonin		
	X^a	C.V.[c]	X	C.V.	B/A	X	C.V.	C/A	X	C.V.	D/A	X	C.V.	E/A
VT (ml)	1.50	10.7	3.64	3.3	2.42	1.51	23.8	1.00	1.68	6.0	1.12	1.50	11.3	1.00
f (breaths/min)	120	3.6	140.4	6.3	1.16	97.0	72.6	0.80	245	4.4	2.04	119	7.4	0.99
VT·f (ml/min)	180	–	511	–	2.83	146	–	0.81	411	–	2.28	178	–	0.99
TI (sec)	0.23	6.1	0.20	9.0	0.87	0.23	18.8	1.00	0.12	8.3	0.52	0.20	5.4	0.87
TE (sec)	0.28	3.2	0.24	11.9	0.86	0.50	42.6	1.78	0.12	8.3	0.43	0.32	12	1.14
ΔP (ml)	0.38	13.8	1.00	5.8	2.63	0.58	7.6	1.52	0.56	8.9	1.47	0.53	6.6	1.39
VT-ΔP area I (ml²)	0.12	24.4	0.80	12.2	6.66	0.26	10.2	2.16	0.21	14.3	1.75	0.24	6.8	2.00
VT-ΔP area E (ml²)	0.12	22	0.79	9.1	6.58	0.26	21.8	2.16	0.21	14.3	1.75	0.23	18.4	1.92
VI at 0.5 VI (ml/sec)	8.70	10.7	23.30	4.2	2.68	10.12	44.6	1.16	18.87	4.7	2.16	10.54	1.4	1.21
VE at 0.5 VE (ml/sec)	6.59	17	19.21	12.5	2.91	3.59	67.6	0.54	19.31	8.3	2.93	4.22	23.8	0.64
VM (ml/sec)	15.47	12	42.37	8.8	2.73	13.55	45.1	0.87	38.18	4.7	2.47	14.76	5.9	0.95
ΔPr (ml)	0.19	10.5	0.49	6.4	2.57	0.41	6.8	2.15	0.29	20.7	1.52	0.38	5.5	2.00
R (ml/ml/sec)	0.013	7.7	0.012	16.7	0.92	0.037	35.1	3.08	0.008	25	0.6	0.026	15.4	2.00

[a] Average for 12 animals during air and CO_2 challenge. Four of these were then exposed to either carbamylcholine, propranolol, or serotonin and the average is for four animals for each agent. For carbamylcholine and propranolol, the variables were measured after 30 min addition of these agents to CO_2, while with serotonin they were measured after 10 min. The aerosol concentrations were 1.0 mg/m³ for carbamylcholine, 20.0 mg/m³ for propranolol and 4.5 mg/m³ for serotonin.

[b] Abbreviations and calculations of each variable as given in Figure 9.

[c] Coefficient of variation (standard deviation/average × 100).

From Schaper et al. (1985), reprinted with permission from Academic Press.

Type II: Restriction

Propranolol: Restriction Induced Acutely

As with the experiments where a carbamylcholine aerosol was added to CO_2, similar experiments were conducted using propranolol at its respective AC_{100} level. Again, the results are based on responses of four animals; mean values are given in Table 2. Representative $\dot{V}$-VT and ΔP-VT loops for one animal during exposure to a propranolol aerosol are seen in Figure 9. During propranolol added to CO_2, the $\dot{V}$-VT loop is more rectangular than square, due to a higher airflow during both inspiration and expiration than during air breathing at the same VT. The major effect is an increase in f, which was twice that f obtained during air breathing at a comparable VT. The flow-resistive work, as measured by the area of the ΔP-VT loops during inspiration and expiration, was also doubled. The increase in f occurred by an equal shortening of TI and TE. This effect was not reversible by an aerosol of isoproterenol, in contrast to that with carbamylcholine. However, the effect was prevented by cervical vagal blockade with cocaine infiltration. Thus, VT was restricted from increasing reflexively (reflex restriction). The same pattern was obtained with serotonin after 30 min of inhalation of this aerosol (Schaper and Alarie, 1985) and after a single 6 hr exposure to cotton dust (Ellakkani et al., 1985a).

Types I and II: Mixed Effects

Propranolol and Carbamylcholine: Mixed Effects Induced Acutely

To produce a mixed response, two agents producing opposite effects on f, carbamylcholine, and propranolol were used at different concentrations to explore the variety of $\dot{V}$-VT loop patterns. In Figure 10, a series of $\dot{V}$-VT loops is shown to illustrate the effect of propranolol alone and propranolol with the addition of carbamylcholine at two concentrations. First, A and B were loops obtained during air and CO_2 challenge, respectively. Then, propranolol aerosol (20 mg/m^3) was added to CO_2, resulting in a typical decrease in VT, an increase in f, and a rectangular $\dot{V}$-VT loop (loops C). All three features are characteristic of a restriction pattern. At 29 min, CO_2 and propranolol exposure was continued, but an aerosol of carbamylcholine (0.4 mg/m^3) was also added. There was a further decrease in VT but no major change in the shape of the loops (loops D), except that airflow was not maintained at a plateau during expiration. A noticeable drop occurred after reaching maximum expiratory flow, indicating airflow obstruction. Both propranolol and carbamylcholine were then removed, continuing with CO_2 exposure only and recovery (not complete) occurred by min 71. Then the series was repeated again, using a higher concentration (0.6 mg/m^3) of carbamylcholine. Again, the addition of propranolol diminished VT amplitude and increased f (loops C at 78 and 83 min) but a "check-valve" during expiratory flow was now apparent, perhaps indi-

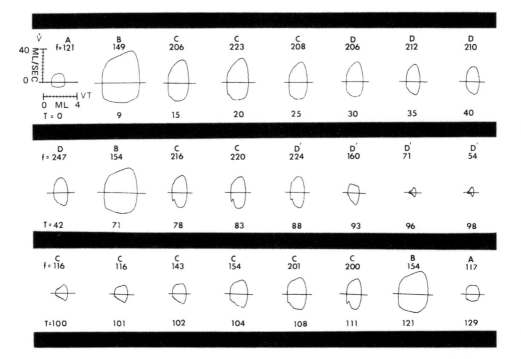

Figure 10 $\dot{V}$-VT loops obtained in one guinea pig using the apparatus described in Figure 2 to illustrate the variety of patterns that can be obtained using combination of different aerosols. Time (T) in minutes is noted under each loop as exposure conditions changed. Respiratory frequency (f) is noted above each loop and represents the average value for 12 breaths under each condition. The letter above each loop indicate the following conditions:

1. A = air.
2. B = 10% CO_2.
3. C = 20 mg/m^3 propranolol aerosol added to 10% CO_2, starting at min 10 and continuing until min 43.
4. D = 0.4 mg/m^3 carbamylcholine aerosol added to 20 mg/m^3 propranolol and 10% CO_2, starting at min 29.
5. At min 43, both propranolol and carbamylcholine were removed, leaving only 10% CO_2. Loop B at 71 min can be compared to loop B at 9 min, which indicates that recovery (although not complete) occurred.
6. At min 72, the same concentration of propranolol was added to 10% CO_2, resulting in loops C, which are slightly different than those during the first addition of propranolol (compare with loops C at min 15, 20, and 25).

cating a lingering effect of carbamylcholine. Addition of carbamylcholine drastically changed the appearance of the loops (loops D′) with a further decrease in VT and now a decrease in f occurred. At min 99, the carbamylcholine exposure was terminated and its action faded gradually, leaving the action of propranolol. Exposure to propranolol was terminated at min 112 and recovery was almost complete at min 121 with only CO_2 exposure and at min 129 during air breathing.

This series of experiments demonstrates the utility of this method to detect rapidly a change from control with introduction of aerosols. It also demonstrates that although two categories of change, obstruction, and restriction, have been proposed, a variety of mixed patterns exist that can be obtained. Furthermore, one agent, depending on the exposure concentration, can mask the effect of another. In the example given, carbamylcholine, at the higher concentration, induced such an intense obstruction that the rapid, shallow breathing first induced by propranolol could no longer be sustained. The masking of the propranolol effect by carbamylcholine is similar to the findings of Pack et al. (1982) with aerosols of histamine. When the increase in respiratory resistance was prevented from occurring by administration of isoproterenol and atropine, histamine aerosols increased phrenic nerve activity via a vagal reflex. Also, with intravenous injection of histamine, the rapid, shallow breathing is easily elicited from stimulation of type J vagal endings before bronchoconstriction occurs (Miserocchi et al., 1978). In guinea pigs, both histamine and carbamylcholine are capable of inducing rapid shallow breathing if the aerosol concentration is very low (or if bronchoconstriction is prevented by isoproterenol). However, the effect is difficult to obtain since, as the concentration increases slightly, bronchoconstriction occurs quickly with a decrease in both VT and f (Schaper and Alarie, 1985).

We have shown how the addition of V̇ measurement through use of the head chamber provided additional information and was very helpful in further characterizing the two types of abnormal response to CO_2 challenge.

Figure 10 (continued)

7. At minute 87, 0.6 mg/m³ carbamylcholine aerosol was added to propranolol and 10% CO_2, resulting in a drastic change with exposure time shown in loops D′. These can be compared with loops D at a lower carbamylcholine concentration.

8. At min 99, carbamylcholine was removed, leaving only 10% CO_2 and a propranolol aerosol (loops C, from min 100 to 111).

9. At minute 112, propranolol was removed, leaving only 10% CO_2. Air breathing was initiated at min 122. Loops A and B at min 121 and 129 can be compared with loops A and B at min 0 and 9 obtained under the same conditions prior to adding the aerosols.

Cotton Dust: Mixed Effects Induced Chronically

As stated earlier, responses to CO_2 were evaluated in a group of 20 animals prior to and following daily exposure to cotton dust over a 1-year period using the whole-body plethysmograph approach. This was also done for a group of controls. $\dot{V}$-VT loops and other ventilatory parameters were also examined in both groups, but on a weekly basis. In 17 exposed animals measured after 51 weeks of exposure to cotton dust, obvious changes from control were detected. Four animals presented a clear pattern of obstruction and three animals presented a clear pattern of restriction, as shown in Figure 11 where a control is also shown for comparison purposes. The other animals (10) had $\dot{V}$-VT loops in between the two extremes presented in Figure 11.

C. Similarities Between Flow-Volume Loops Obtained in the Guinea Pig and Humans

General

Since the introduction of the interrelations among pressure, flow, and volume (Fry et al., 1954), many researchers have used flow-volume loops (or curves) to investigate pulmonary diseases in humans. Abnormal flow-volume loops in patients with variable or fixed extra- or intrathoracic obstruction, interstitial fibrosis, emphysema, etc., have been well-described (Hyatt, 1986; Anthonisen, 1986). There is, however, one drawback when comparing $\dot{V}$-VT loops in guinea pigs with flow-volume loops obtained in humans. Those obtained in humans have the residual volume to total lung capacity relationship in addition to airflow rates, which greatly helps in diagnosing the types of abnormalities involved. This is not obtainable in guinea pigs, at least not with the system shown in Figure 2. Thus, once abnormal $\dot{V}$-VT loops are recognized in guinea pigs, other variables measured in humans can also be measured by appropriate techniques in the animals. The examples of abnormal flow-volume loops given by Hyatt (1986) and Anthonisen (1986) are nevertheless good starting points for evaluation of abnormal $\dot{V}$-VT loops obtained in guinea pigs.

Also to be noted, flow-volume curves in humans are obtained during maximal inspiratory and expiratory maneuvers. The $\dot{V}$-VT loops obtained in guinea pigs were obtained during normal breathing and when VT was increased by CO_2 challenge. These can be compared to flow-volume curves obtained in humans at less than maximal ventilatory effort, such as in humans during exercise, as shown in Figure 12, or in humans during partial maximal effort. There is, however, less information available for this category than for flow-volume curves obtained with maximal effort.

Specific: Methyl Isocyanate

Following the methyl isocyanate (MIC) release in Bhopal, India, on December 2-3, 1984, widespread morbidity and mortality occurred. Flow-volume patterns were studied in 35 cases by Kamat et al. (1985). These authors reported highly abnormal flow-volume patterns, including an inspiratory sawtooth pattern, expiratory concavity on the descending limb, and expiratory doming (Kamat et al., 1985). Examples of abnormal flow-volume curves were also provided by S. R. Kamat in a personal communication. In view of this, a study was undertaken with exposure of guinea pigs to MIC to possibly correlate the findings. Some results are presented in Figures 13 and 14. These results were obtained from one of two animals surviving a 3 hr exposure to MIC at 37 ppm, which was lethal for six of the eight exposed animals (Alarie et al., 1987). Thus, this exposure concentration was capable of inducing very severe pulmonary damage that was most likely the cause of death in the other six animals. It is also a concentration estimated to produce very severe eye, nose, and throat irritation in humans (Ferguson et al., 1986). The results shown in Figure 13 indicate highly abnormal $\dot{V}$-VT loops, during both air breathing and CO_2 challenge up to 35 days postexposure. The main effect was one of obstruction. This can be further observed from Figure 14. The low f values observed were from an increase in TE. The response to MIC was very severe immediately postexposure (3 hr) and worsened over the next 2 days. The $\dot{V}$-VT loops were highly abnormal and the animal failed to increase VT or f during CO_2 challenge. From days 5 to 14, there was some recovery but $\dot{V}$-VT loops were still highly abnormal and the response to CO_2 challenge was still much lower than normal. There was a worsening observed at day 21 but progression toward recovery at day 35. Nevertheless, the $\dot{V}$-VT loop on this day was still highly abnormal. Grossly, this animal appeared normal on this day and was gaining weight. The other surviving animal presented the same pattern. Both will be evaluated to assess whether recovery will be complete. At lower exposure concentrations (21 ppm), we also observed the predominant pattern to be obstruction but some animals also showed a pattern of restriction with evidence of obstruction during expiration as observed with the carbamylcholine-propranolol mixture (Fig. 10). Kamat et al. (1985) also reported flow-volume loop patterns indicating a predominant restrictive pattern in some individuals and some with mixed effects.

Histopathologic examination of the eyes and lungs of rats exposed to MIC revealed the potency of this agent as an irritant (Salmon et al., 1985; Nemery et al., 1985). It is particularly interesting to note that animals surviving high exposure concentrations exhibited acute signs of airway narrowing and develop-

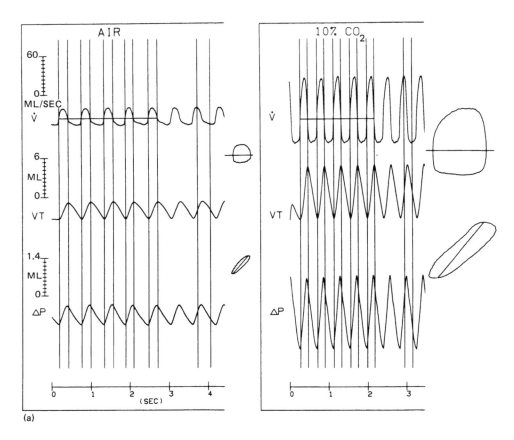

Figure 11 V̇, VT, ΔP, signals and V̇-VT and ΔP-VT loops, as recorded in Figure 9. (a) Taken from one guinea pig, with a body weight of 1200 g, representative of the control animals measured over 1 year. (b) Worst of the four animals presenting an obstruction pattern after 51 weeks of exposure to 20 mg/m³ cotton dust, similar body weight to the control animal shown in (a). (c) One of the three animals (all three had a very similar pattern) presenting a restriction pattern after 51 weeks of exposure to 20 mg/m³ cotton dust; although there is airflow limitation as indicated by the drop in airflow during expiration occurring after maximum airflow at the beginning of expiration; similar body weight to the control animal shown in (a). (From Alarie et al., 1985, with permission from the National Cotton Council of America.)

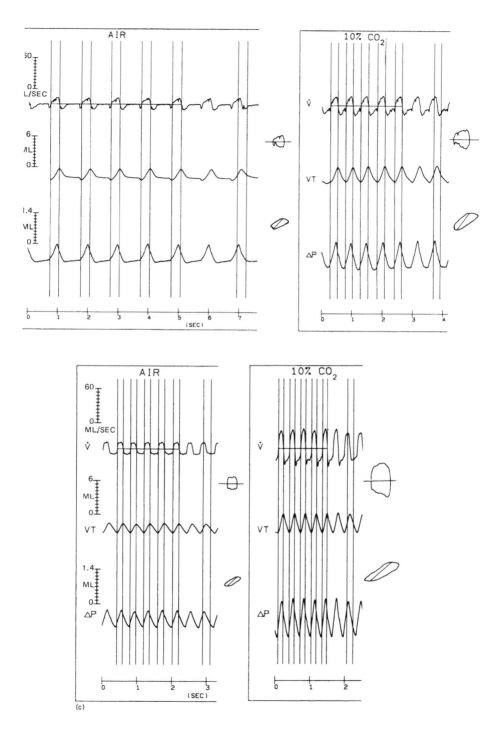

Figure 11 (continued)

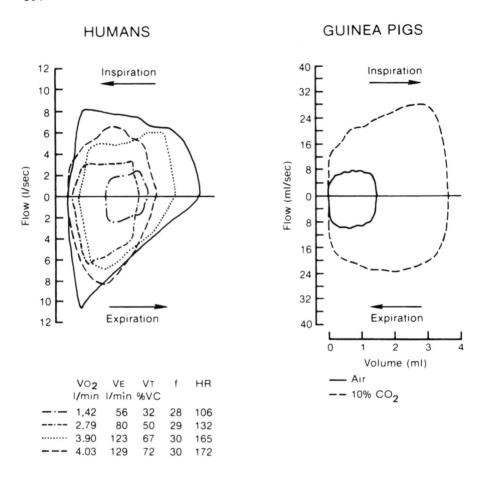

Figure 12 Maximal ventilatory effort flow-volume loop (solid line) obtained in a subject and V̇-VT loops obtained in the same subject at lower VT values during exercise as indicated. Inspiration and expiration phases were inverted from the original figure by Grimby et al. (1971) for an easier comparison with V̇-VT loops obtained in guinea pigs. (Reprinted by permission from *Bulletin Européen de Physiopathologie Respiratoire.*)

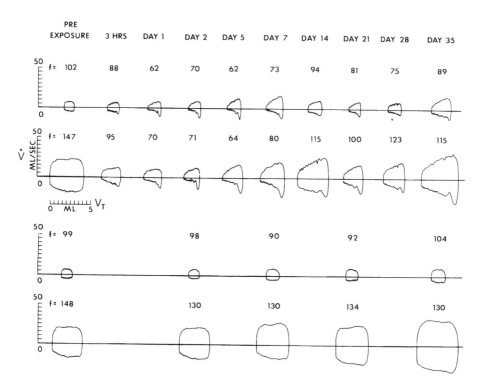

Figure 13 $\dot{V}$-VT loops during air and CO_2 challenge in one animal exposed to methyl isocyanate for 3 hr at 37 ppm (top two lines) and for one control animal (bottom two lines). Both had a body weight of 350 g prior to exposure. Each $\dot{V}$-VT loop is separated by a horizontal line with inspiration and expiration above and below the line, respectively. The scale for $\dot{V}$ and VT is the same for all the loops. Respiratory frequency (f) is given in breaths/min at the top of each loop and represents the average value of 12 breaths. The first measurement was performed immediately after exposure (3 hr) and at various times following exposure as indicated above each loop. (From Alarie et al., 1987, reprinted with permission from *Environmental Health Perspectives*.)

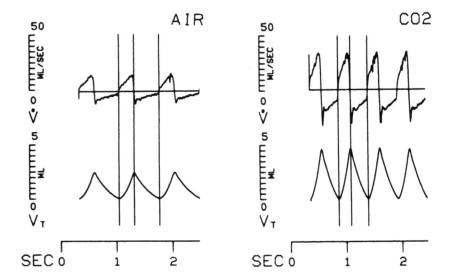

Figure 14 $\dot{V}$ and VT signals recorded during air and CO_2 challenge on day 35 after exposure to methyl isocyanate from which the $\dot{V}$-VT loops presented in Figure 13 were obtained. (From Alarie et al., 1987, reprinted with permission from *Environmental Health Perspectives.*)

ment of hemorrhagic pulmonary edema. This obviously can explain the highly abnormal $\dot{V}$-VT loops and poor response to CO_2 immediately following exposure and during the next few days. However, as reported by Nemery et al. (1985), epithelial lesions were repaired rapidly, which can explain the recovery (although not complete) by day 14. These researchers also noted residual peribronchial fibrosis and signs of renewed injury and inflammation after the first recovery phase. We also observed a worsening by day 21 and again recovery (although not complete) at day 35. Thus, the dynamics of recovery, uncovered by histopathologic examination and by pulmonary function testing, seem to be well-correlated.

VI. Other Conditions Capable of Increasing VT and f and Variations Between Species of Small Laboratory Animals in Their Response to CO_2

There is the possibility to stress further the ventilatory system by using both CO_2 and exercise simultaneously. In mild to moderate exercise, the increase in ventilation is also due to a larger increase in VT than f (Jones, 1981, 1984) but higher frequencies can be reached than with CO_2 challenge (Askanazi et al., 1979). When both CO_2 and exercise are used, there is a synergistic effect (Poon and Greene, 1985; Craig, 1955). However, it is not as easy to measure VT and f in small, exercising laboratory animals as in humans or larger animals. Nevertheless, such studies should be undertaken since CO_2 and exercise involve two different types of stimuli and both may test complementary functions (Askanazi et al., 1979; Menitove et al., 1984).

The possibility of using hypoxia to increase ventilation has been explored. However, small laboratory animals such as rats, hamsters, and guinea pigs are not responsive to hypoxia (Blake and Banchero, 1985; Schlenker, 1984; Walker et al., 1985). Furthermore, combining hypoxia (10% O_2) with 10% CO_2 and 80% N_2 did not modify the ventilatory response of guinea pigs from 10% CO_2 in 20% O_2 and 70% N_2 (Ellakkani et al., 1984a).

Of the small animal species listed in Table 1, the guinea pig seems to have the greatest ventilatory response to CO_2. This is perhaps due to the low $PaCO_2$ of these animals. During air breathing, their $PaCO_2$ was only around 28 mmHg, which increased to 35 mmHg during 10% CO_2 (Alarie and Stock, 1986). In contrast, Lucey et al. (1982), Javaheri et al. (1980), and Walker et al. (1985) reported $PaCO_2$ values around 50 mmHg in hamsters. In rats, Walker et al. (1985) reported values for $PaCO_2$ around 36 mmHg, breathing air and 46 mmHg breathing 5% CO_2.

VII. Advantages and Disadvantages of the CO_2 Challenge Method

A. Use of Whole-Body Plethysmograph for Measurement of Only ΔP and f

Clearly, the advantages of this system include (1) the rapidity with which CO_2 challenges can be performed, (2) the low variability in the response of a control group, and (3) the fact that CO_2 challenges can be performed repeatedly in the same animals. Because of this last feature, it is possible to detect acute pulmonary effects as well as the development of chronic pulmonary effects. Furthermore, recovery from induced pulmonary effects can be assessed by this method. One general disadvantage of CO_2 challenges themselves is that an abnormal response to CO_2 can occur because of toxicity within or outside the pulmonary system and, thus, the test is not diagnostic. Another disadvantage should be noted. While the amplitude of ΔP measured from minima to maxima is proportional to VT, this is not so during the entire breath (Bargeton and Barres, 1986). During the breath, not only are thermal and humidification effects contributing to ΔP but also added is the pressure to overcome airway resistance (Bargeton and Barres, 1956). If intense bronchoconstriction is present, the minima and maxima are shifted in time and no longer reflect VT amplitude, and, in fact, overestimate VT (Alarie et al., 1985; Wong et al., 1985; Schaper et al., 1985). This can be clearly seen in Figures 9 and 11. With intense bronchoconstriction, f decreases, particularly due to a longer expiratory phase (TE) and this will alert the investigator.

B.   Use of the Head Chamber Within the Whole-Body Plethysmograph for Measurement of $\dot{V}$, VT, ΔP, and f

The major advantage in using this system when conducting CO_2 challenges lies in the larger amount of data that can be collected. By combining variables (e.g., $\dot{V}$ and VT, VT and ΔP, ΔPr and $\dot{V}M$), more information can be obtained, which provides an indication of the probable cause(s) of the abnormal response to CO_2. Since this approach is noninvasive, the same animals can also be tested repeatedly. Thus, it would seem to be an ideal method for assessing pneumotoxicity. One drawback in using this system is the time involved in data collection and data analysis. It is undoubtedly much easier to measure ΔP and f in the whole-body plethysmograph. Which system should be used?

There are several alternatives in such a selection. First, in the chronic study of cotton dust, all animals were tested daily using the whole-body plethysmograph while only a fraction of them was challenged weekly using the head chamber apparatus. This is just one way that a study can be designed to obtain desired information, yet conserve valuable time. A second alternative to the problem is the construction of a new system. Based on the parameters that appeared most useful in evaluating pulmonary performance, this was done and a schematic diagram is shown in Figure 15. In essence, only the head chamber is being utilized since the outer chamber serves only to hold the animal in place. With this system, it is possible to measure $\dot{V}$, VT, and f and to obtain $\dot{V}$-VT loops, which have proven to be an extremely valuable tool. Since ΔP is not measured, R is not obtainable. However, airflow obstruction is easily detected from $\dot{V}$-VT loops. As with the whole-body plethysmographs, it is easy to challenge four animals at a time. With a four-channel recorder, $\dot{V}$ is measured and displayed for four animals during air and CO_2 challenge. Each $\dot{V}$ signal is digitized (250 samples/sec) for storage on floppy disk. A computer program integrates $\dot{V}$ with time to obtain VT and $\dot{V}$-VT loops are then displayed on a video terminal, as are the $\dot{V}$ and VT waves obtained from digital integration. From these, TI and TE are calculated and $\dot{V}$ at different VI and VE are also calculated. This system has been used successfully in evaluating responses of guinea pigs exposed to methyl isocyanate, as presented in Figures 13 and 14. Thus, if this system is used, obstruction and restriction patterns in guinea pigs during CO_2 challenge would be indicated as follows from the examples presented in this chapter:

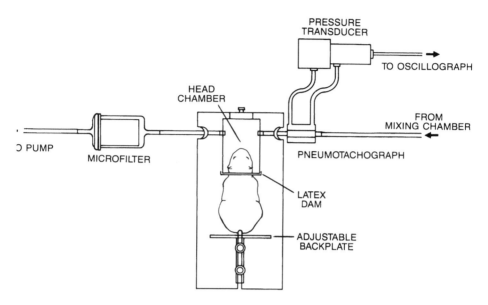

Figure 15 Overhead view of new system designed to measure $\dot{V}$, VT (through integration of $\dot{V}$ with time), and f. Similarly to the other systems described earlier, this is a flow-through arrangement that permits continuous monitoring of an unanesthetized guinea pig. Each animal is fitted with a head chamber (Plexiglas) that is positioned inside a cylinder (Plexiglas). This cylinder has an adjustable back plate, serving to restrain the animal. Since the cylinder is open (unsealed), it is not possible to obtain ΔP with the new system. Using a pump, air and other mixtures (e.g., 10% CO_2 or 10% CO_2 plus an aerosol to be studied) are pulled from a mixing chamber and through the head chamber at 2 liters/min. A pneumotachograph is attached to a differential pressure transducer (Statham or Gaeltec) and placed after the mixing chamber at the inlet of the head chamber. It will measure both flow ($\dot{V}$) of air passing through the head chamber and flow associated with inspiratory ($\dot{V}I$) and expiratory ($\dot{V}E$) efforts of the guinea pig. The changes in flow created by the guinea pig are simply superimposed on the continuous head chamber flow signal. Four chambers, as the one shown here, are attached to one mixing chamber, thus enabling the ventilatory measurements of four guinea pigs simultaneously. (From Alarie et al., 1987, reprinted with permission from *Environmental Health Perspectives.*)

Obstruction	Restriction
Lower than normal VT	Lower than normal VT
Lower than normal f	Higher than normal f
Lower $\dot{V}$ during inspiration and expiration as well as $\dot{V}$ fluctuations as seen with methyl isocyanate, sometimes described as "check-valve," "saw tooth," or "fluttering" patterns	Rectangular $\dot{V}$-VT loops compared to controls
Lengthening of TE	Shortening of TI and TE

Mixed patterns can also be recognized. From these, cause(s) of the abnormal CO_2 response can be investigated further.

VIII. Conclusions

For toxicologic evaluation, the following needs must be met:

1. Detection: is there a change from normal?
2. Discrimination: if there is a change from normal, how different is this change?
3. Scaling or concentration-response relationship: how large is the difference from normal and how is it related to exposure concentration?
4. Mechanism: how is this change caused?
5. Extrapolation: safe levels for humans?

From what we have presented, it is obvious that with these new approaches we can detect, discriminate, and scale. As far as explaining the mechanisms for the observed changes, it is also obvious that these methods provide some clues as to the possible causes of the abnormalities observed. This, however, must be followed by further investigations using a variety of approaches. The final and most important need is extrapolation of safe levels of exposure for humans. So far, we have concentration-response relationships for three agents: paraquat, H_2SO_4, and cotton dust, for which "safe" levels of exposure for industrial workers have been established by the American Conference of Governmental Industrial Hygienists (1984) to prevent their pulmonary toxicity. These are called threshold limit values (TLVs). The TLVs for paraquat, H_2SO_4, and cotton dust are 0.1, 1.0, and 0.2 mg/m^3, respectively. We found a concentration-response relationship for all three agents in preventing VT to increase to its normal level during CO_2 challenge following acute exposures (Wong and Alarie, 1982; Ellakkani et al., 1985a; Burleigh-Flayer and Alarie, 1986). The exposure concentrations that reduced VT during CO_2 by 50% from the normal response were found to be 1.5, 50, and 13 mg/m^3, respectively, for paraquat, sulfuric acid, and cotton dust. If we divide these concentrations by 60 we obtain 0.02, 0.83, and 0.21 mg/m^3 as a "best guess" for a "safe" level of exposure to each for humans. For both sulfuric acid and cotton dust, these values are very close to their TLVs (i.e., 0.83 vs. 1.0 for sulfuric acid and 0.21 vs. 0.2 for cotton dust). For paraquat, 0.02 is five times lower than the TLV: 0.1 mg/m^3. The number of agents tested is too few to attempt an empirical correlation for prediction of safe levels for humans, but increasing the number of agents tested could provide such data. Indeed, with another animal model, an excellent correlation ($r^2 = 0.85$) was found for 41 industrial chemicals by comparing their sensory irritation potency with their TLV values (Alarie and Luo, 1986).

The other obvious needs for toxicologic evaluation are low cost and minimum amount of time required for the test procedure. The methods we have described here meet these requirements.

Acknowledgments

We thank Mrs. Evon Nigro and Miss Kate Detwiler for their help in preparing this chapter. This work was prepared under Grant RO1-ESO2747 from the National Institute of Environmental Health Sciences.

References

Alarie, Y. (1981). Toxicologic evaluation of airborne chemical irritants and allergens using respiratory reflex reactions. In *Proceedings of Inhalation Toxicology and Technology Symposium.* Edited by B. K. J. Leong. Ann Arbor, Michigan, Ann Arbor Science Pub., pp. 207-231.

Alarie, Y., and Luo, J. E. (1986). Sensory irritation by airborne chemicals: A basis to establish acceptable levels of exposure. In *Toxicology of the Nasal Passages.* Edited by C. S. Barrow. Washington, D.C., Hemisphere Pub. Co., pp. 91-100.

Alarie, Y., and Stock, M. F. (1986). Appropriate level of inspired CO2 for evaluation of the performance of the respiratory system in guinea pigs. *Toxicologist* 6:53.

Alarie, Y., Ellakani, M., Weyel, D., Mazumdar, S., and Karol, M. (1984). Monday post-shift respiratory response in guinea pigs following inhalation of cotton dust. In *Proceedings of the Eighth Cotton Dust Research Conference.* Edited by P. J. Wakelyn and R. R. Jacobs. Raleigh, N.C., National Cotton Council and Cotton Inc., pp. 84-86.

Alarie, Y., Ellakkani, M., Weyel, D., and Karol. M. (1985). Respiratory parameters which characterize the response of guinea pigs to inhalation of cotton dust. In *Proceedings of the Ninth Cotton Dust Research Conference.* Edited by P. J. Wakelyn and R. R. Jacobs. Raleigh, N.C., National Cotton Council and Cotton Inc., pp. 171-177.

Alarie, Y., Ferguson, J. S., Stock, M. F., Weyel, D. A., and Schaper, M. (1987). Sensory and pulmonary irritation and possible cyanide-like effects of methyl isocyanate in guinea pigs. *Environ. Health Perspect.* (in press)

Alarie, Y., Ulrich, C. E., Haddock, R. H., Jennings, H. J., and Davis, E. F. (1970). Respiratory system flow resistance with digital computer techniques; measured in cynomolgus monkeys and guinea pigs. *Arch. Environ. Health* **21**: 283-291.

Alarie, Y., Ulrich, C. E., Krumm, A. A., Haddock, R. H., and Jennings, H. J. (1971a). Mechanical properties of the lung in cynomolgus monkeys; measurements with real-time digital computerization. *Arch. Environ. Health* **22**:643-654.

Alarie, Y., Krumm, A. A., Jennings, H. J., and Haddock, R. H. (1971b). Distribution of ventilation in cynomolgus monkeys; measurement with real-time digital computerization. *Arch. Environ. Health* **22**:633-642.

Amdur, M. O. (1958). The respiratory response of guinea pigs to sulfuric acid mist. *Arch. Ind. Health* **18**:407-414.

Amdur, M. W. (1966). The respiratory response of guinea pigs to histamine aerosols. *Arch. Environ. Health* **13**:29-37.

Amdur, M. O., and Mead, J. (1955). A method for studying the mechanical properties of the lungs of unanesthetized animals: application to the study of respiratory irritants. In *Proceedings of the Third National Air Pollution Symposium.* Pasadena, California, pp. 150-159.

American Conference of Governmental Industrial Hygienists (1984). Threshold limit values for chemical substances and physical agents in the work environment and biological exposure indices with intended changes for 1984-85. In *Ann. Am. Conf. Gov. Ind. Hygienists* **11**:271-312.

Anthonisen, N. R. (1986). Tests of mechanical function. In *Handbook of Physiology.* Section 3. *The Respiratory System.* Edited by P. T. Macklem and J. Mead. Bethesda, Maryland, American Physiological Society, Vol. III, pp. 753-784.

Anthonisen, N. R., and Cherniack, R. M. (1981). Ventilatory control in lung disease. In *Lung Biology in Health Disease. Regulation of Breathing.* Part II. Edited by T. Horbein, New York, Marcel Dekker, pp. 965-987.

Arieli, R., and Ar, A. (1979). Ventilation of a fossorial mammal (Spalax ehrenbergi) in hypoxic and hypercapnic conditions. *J. Appl. Physiol.* **47**:1011-1017.

Askanazi, J., Milic-Emili, J., Broell, J. R., Hyman, A. I., and Kinney, J. M. (1979). Influence of exercise and CO2 on breathing pattern of normal man. *J. Appl. Physiol.* **47**:192-196.

Bargeton, D., and Barres, G. (1956). Measure volumetrique de la perte de charge dans les voies aeriennes. *C. R. Soc. Biol.* **150**:1343-1347.

Beckett, W. S., McDonnell, W. F., Horstman, D. H., and House, D. E. (1985). Role of the parasympathetic nervous system in acute lung response to ozone. *J. Appl. Physiol.* **59**:1879-1885.

Blake, C. I., and Banchero, N. (1985). Effects of cold and hypoxia on ventilation and oxygen consumption in awake guinea pigs. *Respir. Physiol.* **61**:357-368.

Bleecker, E. R., Cotton, D. J., Fischer, S. P., Graf, P. D., Gold, W. M., and Nadel, J. A. (1976). The mechanism of rapid shallow breathing after inhaling histamine aerosol in exercising dogs. *Am. Rev. Respir. Dis.* **144**:909-916.

Boyd, M. R. (1980). Biochemical mechanisms in chemical-induced lung injury: Role of metabolic activation. *CRC Crit. Rev. Toxicol.* **7**:103-176.

Brischetto, M. J., Millman, R. P., Peterson, D. D., Silage, D. A., and Pack, A. I. (1984). Effect of aging on ventilatory response to exercise and CO2. *J. Appl. Physiol.* **56**:1143-1150.

Brodovsky, D., MacDonnell, J. A., and Cherniack, R. M. (1960). The respiratory response to carbon dioxide in health and emphysema. *J. Clin. Invest.* **39**:724-729.

Burdon, J. G. W., Killian, N. J., and Jones, N. L. (1983). Pattern of breathing during exercise in patients with interstitial lung disease. *Thorax* **38**:778-784.

Burleigh-Flayer, H., and Alarie, Y. (1986). Concentration-dependent respiratory response of guinea pigs to paraquat aerosol. *Toxicologist* **6**:53.

Burleigh-Flayer, H., Wong, K. L., and Alarie, Y. (1985a). Evaluation of the pulmonary effects of HCl using CO2 challenges in guinea pigs. *Fund. Appl. Toxicol.* **5**:978-985.

Burleigh-Flayer, H., Wong, K. L., and Alarie, Y. (1985b). Respiratory effects of repeated paraquat injections. *Toxicologist* **5**:219.

Chapin, J. L. (1954). Ventilatory response of the unrestrained and unanesthetized hamster to CO2. *Am. J. Physiol.* **179**:146-148.

Chavlova, M., Kuncova, M., Havrankova, J., and Palacek, F. (1974). Regulation of respiration in experimental silicosis. *Physiol. Bohemoslov.* **23**:539-547.

Cherniack, R. M. (1965). Work of breathing and the ventilatory response to CO2. In *Handbook of Physiology.* Section 3. *Respiration.* Vol. II. Edited by W. O. Fenn and H. Rahn. Washington, D.C., American Physiological Society, pp. 1469-1474.

Cherniack, R. M., and Snidal, D. P. (1956). The effect of obstruction to breathing on the ventilatory response to CO2. *J. Clin. Invest.* **35**:1286-1290.

Clark, F. J., and von Euler, C. (1972). On the regulation of depth and rate of breathing. *J. Physiol.* **222**:267-295.

Clark, T. J. H. (1968). The ventilatory response to CO2 in chronic airways obstruction measured by a rebreathing method. *Clin. Sci.* **34**:559-568.

Clark, T. J. H., and Cochrane, G. M. (1972). Effect of mechanical loading on ventilatory response to CO2 and CO2 excretion. *Br. Med. J.* **1**:351-353.

Clark, T. J. H., and Godfrey, S. (1969). The effect of CO2 on ventilation and breath-holding during exercise and while breathing through an added resistance. *J. Physiol.* **201**:551-566.

Costa, D. L. (1985). Interpretation of new techniques used in the determination of pulmonary function in rodents. *Fund. Appl. Toxicol.* **5**:423-434.

Cotes, J. E., Johnson, G. R., and McDonald, A. (1970). Breathing frequency and tidal volume: Relationships to breathlessness. In *Breathing. Hering-Breuer Centenary Symposium.* Edited by R. Porter. London, Churchill Livingstone, pp. 297-314.

Craig, F. N. (1955). Pulmonary ventilation during exercise and inhalation of carbon dioxide. *J. Appl. Physiol.* **7**:467-471.

Cunningham, D. J. C., and Gardner, W. N. (1977). A quantitative description of the pattern of breathing during steady-state CO2 inhalation in man, with special emphasis on expiration. *J. Physiol.* **272**:613-632.

Donald, K. W., and Christie, R. V. (1949a). The respiratory response to carbon dioxide and anoxia in emphysema. *Clin. Sci.* **8**:33-44.

Donald, K. W., and Christie, R. V. (1949b). A new method of clinical spirometry. *Clin. Sci.* **8**:21-30.

Drobaugh, J. E., and Fenn, W. O. (1955). A barometric method for measuring ventilation in newborn infants. *Pediatrics* **16**:81-87.

Duara, S., Abbasi, S., Shaffer, T. H., and Fox, W. W. (1985). Preterm infants: ventilation and P100 changes with CO2 and inspiratory resistive loading. *J. Appl. Physiol.* **58**:1982-1987.

Easton, P. A., Arnup, M. E., de la Rocha, A., Fleetham, J. A., and Anthonisen, N. R. (1983). Ventilatory control after pulmonary resection. *Am. Rev. Respir. Dis.* **128**:627-630.

Easton, P. A., Jadue, C., Arnup, M. E., Meatherall, R. C., and Anthonisen, N. R. (1985). Effects of upper or lower airway anesthesia on hypercapnia ventilation in humans. *J. Appl. Physiol.* **59**:1090-1097.

Eldridge, F., and Davis, J. M. (1959). Effect of mechanical factors on respiratory work and ventilatory responses to CO2. *J. Appl. Physiol.* **14**:721-726.

Ellakkani, M. A. (1985). An animal model for byssinosis. Doctoral thesis. University of Pittsbutgh, Pittsburgh, Pennsylvania.

Ellakkani, M. A., Alarie, Y. C., Weyel, D. A., Mazumdar, S., and Karol, M. H. (1984a). Pulmonary reactions to inhaled cotton dust: an animal model for byssinosis. *Toxicol. Appl. Pharmacol.* **74**:267-284.

Ellakkani, M. A., Alarie, Y., Weyel, D., and Karol, M. H. (1984b). Chronic effect of cotton dust inhalation in a guinea pig model. *Toxicologist* **5**:71.

Ellakkani, M. A., Alarie, Y., Weyel, D. A., and Karol, M. H. (1985a). Concentration-dependent respiratory response of guinea pigs to a single exposure of cotton dust. *Toxicol. Appl. Pharmacol.* **80**:357-366.

Ellakkani, M., Alarie, Y., Weyel, D., and Karol, M. (1985b). Effects of 12-month inhalation of cotton dust. In *Proceedings of the Ninth Cotton Dust Research Conference.* Edited by P. J. Wakelyn and R. R. Jacobs. Raleigh, N. C., National Cotton Council and Cotton Incorporated, pp. 167-170.

Epstein, R. A., Epstein, M. A., Haddad, G. G., and Mellins, R. B. (1980). Practical implementation of the barometric method for measurement of tidal volume. *J. Appl. Physiol.* **49**:1107-1115.

Ferguson, J. S., Schaper, M. M., and Alarie, Y. (1985). Evaluation of the pulmonary effects of hexamethylene diisocyanate (HDI) trimer aerosols. *Toxicologist* **5**:73.

Ferguson, J. S., Schaper, M., Stock, M. F., Weyel, D. A., and Alarie, Y. (1986). Sensory and pulmonary irritation with exposure to methyl isocyanate. *Toxicol. Appl. Pharmacol.* **82**:329-335.

Fishman, A. P., and Ledlie, J. F. (1979). Dyspnea. *Bull. Eur. Physiopathol. Respir.* **15**:789-804.

Fishman, A. P., Samet, P., and Cournand, A. (1955). Ventilatory drive in chronic pulmonary emphysema. *Am. J. Med.* **19**:533-548.

Folinsbee, L. J., Silverman, F., and Shephard, R. J. (1975). Exercise responses following ozone exposure. *J. Appl. Physiol.* **38**:966-1001.

Freedman, S., Dalton, K. J., Holland, D., and Patton, J. M. S. (1972). The effects of added elastic loads on the respiratory response to CO2 in man. *Respir. Physiol.* **14**:237-250.

Fritts, H. W., Fishman, A. P., and Cournand, A. (1957). Factors contributing to the diminished ventilatory response to CO2 of patients with obstructive emphysema. *Fed. Proc.* **16**:41-42.

Fry, D. L., Ebert, R. V., Stead, W. W., and Brown, C. C. (1954). The mechanics of pulmonary ventilation in normal subjects and in patients with emphysema. *Am. J. Med.* **16**:80-97.

Gallagher, C. G., Im Hof, V., and Younes, M. (1985). Effect of inspiratory muscle fatigue on breathing pattern. *J. Appl. Physiol.* **59**:1152-1158.

Garrard, C. S., and Lane, D. J. (1978). The pattern of stimulated breathing in man during nonelastic expiratory loading. *J. Physiol.* **279**:17-29.

Garrard, C. S., and Lane, D. J. (1979). The pattern of breathing in patients with chronic airflow obstruction. *Clin. Sci.* **56**:215-221.

Gautier, H. (1976). Pattern of breathing during hypoxia or hypercapnia of the awake or anesthetized cat. *Respir. Physiol.* **27**:193-206.

Gertner, A., Bromberger-Barnea, B., Kelly, L., Traystman, R., and Menkes, H. (1984). Local vagal responses in the lung periphery. *J. Appl. Physiol.* **57**: 1079-1088.

Gibbons, S. I., and Adams, W. C. (1984). Combined effects of ozone exposure and ambient heat on exercising females. *J. Appl. Physiol.* **57**:450-456.

Ginsberg, S. J., and Comis, R. L. (1982). The pulmonary toxicity of antineoplastic agents. *Semin. Oncol.* **9**:34-51.

Grassino, A. E., Lewinsohn, G. E., and Tyler, J. M. (1973). Effects of hyperinflation of the thorax on the mechanics of breathing. *J. Appl. Physiol.* **35**: 336-342.

Green, J. F., Schmidt, N. D., Schultz, H. D., Roberts, A. M., Coleridge, H. M., and Coleridge, J. C. G. (1984). Pulmonary C-fibers evoke both apnea and tachypnea of pulmonary chemoreflex. *J. Appl. Physiol.* **57**:562-567.

Gribbin, H. R., Gardiner, I. T., Heinz III, G. J., Gibson, G. J., and Pride, N. B. (1983). Role of impaired inspiratory muscle function in limiting the ventilatory response to carbon dioxide in chronic airflow obstruction. *Clin. Sci.* **64**:487-495.

Grimby, G., Saltin, B., and Wilhelmsen, L. (1971). Pulmonary flow-volume and pressure-volume relationship during submaximal and maximal exercise in young well-trained men. *Bull. Physiopathol. Respir.* **7**:157-168.

Guz, A., Noble, M. I. M., Widdicombe, J. G., Trenchard, D., and Mushin, W. W. (1966). The effect of bilateral block of vagus and glossopharyngeal nerves on the ventilatory response to CO_2 of conscious man. *Respir. Physiol.* **1**: 206-210.

Haldane, J. S., and Priestley, J. G. (1905). The regulation of the lung-ventilation. *J. Physiol.* **32**:225-266.

Haldane, J. S., Meakins, J. C., and Priestley, J. G. (1918a). The reflex restriction of respiration after gas poisoning. Report No. 5 of the Chemical Warfare Medical Committee, Canadian General Hospital, England, pp. 1-11.

Haldane, J. S., Meakins, J. C., and Priestley, J. G. (1918b). Investigations of chronic cases of gas poisoning. Report No. 11 of the Chemical Warfare Medical Committee, Canadian General Hospital, England, pp. 1-13.

Hannhart, B., Preslin, R., Bohadana, A., and Teculescu, D. (1979). Ventilatory limitation during exercise in patients with chronic obstructive lung disease. *Bull. Eur. Physiopathol. Respir.* **15**:75-87.

Hayashi, F., Yoshida, A., Fukuda, Y., and Honda, Y. (1982). CO_2-ventilatory response of the anesthetized rat by rebreathing technique. *Pflugers Arch.* **393**: 77-82.

Haywood, C., and Bloete, M. E. (1969). Respiratory responses of healthy young women to carbon dioxide inhalation. *J. Appl. Physiol.* **27**:32-35.

Hey, E. N., Lloyd, B. B., Cunningham, D. J. C., Jukes, M. G. M., and Bolton, D. P. G. (1966). Effects of various respiratory stimuli on the depth and frequency of breathing in man. *Respir. Physiol.* 1:193-205.

Hirsch, J. A., and Bishop, B. (1982). Human breathing patterns on mouthpiece or face mask during air, CO2, or low O2. *J. Appl. Physiol.* 53:1281-1290.

Hyatt, R. E. (1986). Forced expiration. In *Handbook of Physiology.* Section 3. *The Respiratory System.* Edited by P. T. Macklem and J. Mead. Bethesda, Maryland, American Physiological Society, Vol. III, pp. 295-314.

Irsigler, G. B. (1976). Carbon dioxide response lines in young adults: the limits of the normal response. *Am. Rev. Respir. Dis.* 114:529-536.

Jaeger, M. J., and Otis, A. B. (1964). Measurement of airway resistance with a volume displacement body plethysmograph. *J. Appl. Physiol.* 19:813-820.

Javaheri, S., Lucey, E. C., and Snider, G. L. (1980). Ventilatory response to carbon dioxide breathing in unanesthetized unrestrained hamsters. *Clin. Res.* 28:529.

Johanson, W. J. Jr., and Pierce, A. K. (1971). A noninvasive technique for measurement of airway conductance in small animals. *J. Appl. Physiol.* 30:146-150.

Jones, N. L. (1981). Exercise tests. In *Clinical Investigation of Respiratory Disease.* Edited by T. J. H. Clark. London, Chapman and Hall, pp. 93-115.

Jones, N. L. (1984). Dyspnea in exercise. *Med. Sci. Sports Exerc.* 16:14-19.

Kamat, S. R., Mahashur, A. A., Tiwari, A. K. B., Potdar, P. V., Gaur, M., Kolhatkar, V. P., Vaidya, P., Parmar, D., Rupwate, R., Chatterjee, T. S., Jain, K., Kelkar, M. D., and Kimare, S. G. (1985). Early observations on pulmonary changes and clinical morbidity due to isocyanate gas leak at Bhopal. *J. Postgrad. Med.* 31:63-72.

Karol, M., Ellakkani, M., Barnet, M., Alarie, Y., and Fischer, J. J. (1985). Comparison of the respiratory response of guinea pigs to cotton dust and endotoxin from enterobacter agglomerans. In *Proceedings of the Ninth Cotton Dust Research Conderence.* Edited by P. J. Wakelyn and R. R. Jacobs. Raleigh, N. C., National Cotton Council and Cotton Inc., pp. 146-147.

Kellog, R. H. (1964). Central chemical regulation of respiration. In *Handbook of Physiology.* Section 3. *Respiration.* Vol. I. Edited by W. O. Fenn and H. Rahn. Washington, D.C., American Physiological Society, pp. 507-534.

Lai, Y. L., Lamm, J. E., and Hildebrandt, J. (1981). Ventilation during prolonged hypercapnia in the rat. *J. Appl. Physiol.* 51:73-83.

Lambertsen, C. J. (1960). Carbon dioxide and respiration in acid-base homeostasis. *Anesthesiology* 21.642-651.

Lee, L. Y., Dumont, C., Djokie, T. D., Menzel, T. E., and Nadel, J. A. (1979).

Mechanism of rapid, shallow breathing after ozone exposure in conscious dogs. *J. Appl. Physiol.* **46**:1108-1109.

Lee, L. Y., Djokic, T. D., Dumont, C., Graf, P. D., and Nadel, J. A. (1980). Mechanism of ozone-induced tachypneic response to hypoxia and hypercapnia in conscious dogs. *J. Appl. Physiol.* **48**:163-168.

Lindhard, J. (1911). On the excitability of the respiratory centre. *J. Physiol.* **42**:337-358.

Lopata, M., and Pearle, J. L. (1980). Diaphragmatic EMG and occlusion pressure response to elastic loading during CO_2 rebreathing in humans. *J. Appl. Physiol.* **49**:669-675.

Lopata, M., Onal, E., and Cromydas, G. (1985). Respiratory load compensation in chronic airway obstruction. *J. Appl. Physiol.* **59**:1947-1954.

Lourenco, R. V., and Miranda, J. M. (1968). Drive and performance of the ventilatory apparatus in chronic obstructive lung disease. *N. Engl. J. Med.* **279**:53-59.

Lourenco, R. V., Turino, G. M., Davidson, L. A. G., and Fishman, A. P. (1965). The regulation of ventilation in diffuse pulmonary fibrosis. *Am. J. Med.* **38**:199-216.

Lucey, E. C., Snider, G. L., and Javaheri, S. (1982). Pulmonary ventilation and blood gas values in emphysematous hamsters. *Am. Rev. Respir. Dis.* **125**: 299-303.

Maranetra, N., and Pain, M. C. F. (1974). Ventilatory drive and ventilatory response during rebreathing. *Thorax* **29**:578-581.

Maskrey, M., and Nicol. S. C. (1980). The respiratory frequency response to carbon dioxide inhalation in conscious rabbits. *J. Physiol.* **301**:49-58.

Matijak-Schaper, M., Wong, K. L., and Alarie, Y. (1983). A method to rapidly evaluate the acute pulmonary effects of aerosols in unanesthetized guinea pigs. *Toxicol. Appl. Pharmacol.* **69**:451-460.

McCutcheon, F. H. (1951). The mammalian breathing mechanism. *J. Cell. Comp. Physiol.* **37**:447-476.

McIlroy, M. B., Eldridge, F. L., Thomas, J. P., and Christie, R. V. (1956). The effect of added elastic and non-elastic resistance on the pattern of breathing in normal subjects. *Clin. Sci.* **15**:337-344.

Mead, J. (1960). Control of respiratory frequency. *J. Appl. Physiol.* **15**:325-336.

Menitove, S. M., Rapoport, D. M., Epstein, H., Sorkin, B., and Goldring, R. M. (1984). CO_2 rebreathing and exercise ventilatory responses in humans. *J. Appl. Physiol.* **56**:1039-1044.

Milic-Emili, J., and Tyler, J. M. (1963a). Relationship between work output of respiratory muscle and end-tidal CO_2 tension. *J. Appl. Physiol.* **18**:497-504.

Milic-Emili, J., and Tyler, J. M. (1963b). Relationship between PACO2 and respiratory work during external resistance breathing in man. *Ann. N.Y. Acad. Sci.* **109**:908-914.

Miserocchi, G., Trippenbach, T., Mazzarelli, M., Jaspar, N., and Hazucha, M. (1978). The mechanism of rapid shallow breathing due to histamine and phenyldiguanide in cats and rabbits. *Respir. Physiol.* **32**:141-153.

Mortola, J. P. (1984). Breathing pattern in newborns. *J. Appl. Physiol.* **56**: 1533-1540.

Nadel, J. A., Gold, W. M., Jennings, D. B., Wright, R. R., and Fudenberg, H. H. (1966). Unusual disease of pulmonary arteries with dyspnea. *Am. J. Med.* **41**:440-447.

Nadel, J. A., Gold, W. M., and Burgess, J. H. (1968). Early diagnosis of chronic pulmonary vascular obstruction. Value of pulmonary function tests. *Am. J. Med.* **44**:16-25.

Nemery, B., Dinsdale, D., Sparrow, S., and Ray, D. E. (1985). Effects of methyl isocyanate on the respiratory tract of rats. *Br. J. Ind. Med.* **42**: 799-805.

O'Neil, J. J., and Raub, J. A. (1984). Pulmonary function testing in small laboratory mammals. *Environ. Health Perspect.* **56**:11-22.

Pack, A. I., Hertz, B. C., Ledlie, J. F., and Fishman, A. P. (1982). Reflex effects of aerosolized histamine on phrenic nerve activity. *J. Clin. Invest.* **70**:424-432.

Paintal, A. S. (1981). Effects of drugs on chemoreceptors, pulmonary and cardiovascular receptors. In *International Encyclopedia of Pharmacology and Therapeutics.* Section 104. Respiratory Pharmacology. Edited by J. Widdicombe, Oxford, Pergamon Press, pp. 217-239.

Parot, S., Bonora, M., Gautier, H., and Marlot, D. (1984). Developmental changes in ventilation and breathing pattern in unanesthetized kittens. *Respir. Physiol.* **58**:253-262.

Pengelly, L. D., Tarshis, A. M., and Rebuck, A. S. (1979). Contribution of rib cage and abdomen-diaphragm to tidal volume during CO2 rebreathing. *J. Appl. Physiol.* **46**:709-715.

Pennock, B. E., Cox, C. P., Rogers, R. M., Cain, W. A., and Wells, J. H. (1979). A noninvasive technique for measurement of changes in specific airway resistance. *J. Appl. Physiol.* **46**:399-406.

Phillipson, E. A., Hickey, R. F., Bainton, C. R., and Nadel, J. A. (1970). Effect of vagal blockade on regulation of breathing in conscious dogs. *J. Appl. Physiol.* **29**:475-479.

Phillipson, E. A., Murphy, E., Kozar, L. F., and Schultze, R. K. (1975). Role of vagal stimuli in exercise ventilation in dogs with experimental pneumonitis. *J. Appl. Physiol.* **39**:76-85.

Poon, C. S., and Greene, J. G. (1985). Control of exercise hyperpnea during hypercapnia in humans. *J. Appl. Physiol.* **59**:792-797.

Prausnitz, C. (1936). Investigations on respiratory dust disease in operatives in the cotton industry. *Med. Res. Council Rep.*, London, England, p. 72.

Read, D. J. C. (1967). A clinical method for assessing the ventilatory response to CO_2. *Aust. Ann. Med.* **16**:20-32.

Rebuck, A. S., and Read, J. (1971). Patterns of ventilatory response to carbon dioxide during recovery from severe asthma. *Clin. Sci.* **41**:13-21.

Rebuck, A. S., Rigg, J. R. A., Kangalee, M., and Pengelly, L. D. (1974). Control of tidal volume during rebreathing. *J. Appl. Physiol.* **37**:475-478.

Renzi, G., Milic-Emili, J., and Grassino, A. E. (1982). The pattern of breathing in diffuse lung fibrosis. *Bull. Eur. Physiopathol. Respir.* **18**:461-472.

Reynolds, W. J., Milhorn, H. T. Jr., and Holloman, G. H. Jr. (1972). Transient ventilatory response to graded hypercapnia in man. *J. Appl. Physiol.* **33**: 47-54.

Richards, D. W., Fritts, H. W., and Davis, A. L. (1958). Observations on the control of respiration in emphysema: The effects of oxygen on ventilatory response to CO_2 inhalation. *Trans. Assoc. Am. Physicians* **71**:142-151.

Richardson, P. S., and Widdicombe, J. G. (1969). The role of the vagus nerves in the ventilatory responses to hypercapnia and hypoxia in anesthetized and unanesthetized rabbits. *Respir. Physiol.* **7**:122-135.

Russell, N. J. W., Raybould, H. E., and Trenchard, D. (1984). Role of vagal C-fiber afferents in respiratory response to hypercapnia. *J. Appl. Physiol.* **56**: 1550-1558.

Saetta, M., and Mortola, J. P. (1985). Breathing pattern and CO_2 response in newborn rats before and during anesthesia. *J. Appl. Physiol.* **58**:1988-1996.

Salmon, A. G., Muir, M. K., and Anderson, N. (1985). Acute toxicity of methyl isocyanate: a preliminary study of the dose response for eye and other effects. *Br. J. Ind. Med.* **42**:795-798.

Savoy, J., Dhingra, S., and Anthonisen, N. R. (1982). Inhaled lidocaine aerosol changes resting human breathing pattern. *Respir. Physiol.* **50**:41-49.

Schaefer, K. E. (1958). Respiratory pattern and respiratory response to CO_2. *J. Appl. Physiol.* **13**:1-14.

Schaper, M., and Alarie, Y. (1985). The effects of aerosols of carbamylcholine, serotonin and propranolol on the ventilatory response to CO_2 in guinea pigs and comparison with the effects of histamine and sulfuric acid. *Acta Pharmacol. Toxicol.* **56**:244-249.

Schaper, M., and Alarie, Y. (1986). New approaches for evaluating the effectiveness of drugs administered to prevent or reverse acutely induced responses to aerosols. *Pharmacologist* **28**:141.

Schaper, M., Kegerize, J., and Alarie, Y. (1984). Evaluation of concentration-response relationships for histamine and sulfuric acid aerosols in unanesthetized guinea pigs for their effects on the ventilatory response to CO_2. *Toxicol. Appl. Pharmacol.* 73:533-542.

Schaper, M., Thompson, R. D., and Alarie, Y. (1985). A method to classify airborne chemicals which alter the normal ventilatory response induced by CO_2. *Toxicol. Appl. Pharmacol.* 79:332-341.

Schlenker, E. H. (1984). An evaluation of ventilation in dystrophic Syrian hamsters. *J. Appl. Physiol.* 56:914-921.

Scott, R. W. (1920). Observations on the pathologic physiology of chronic pulmonary emphysema. *Arch. Intern. Med.* 26:544-560.

Shekleton, M., Lopata, M., Evanich, M. J., and Lourenco, R. V. (1976). Effect of elastic loading on mouth occlusion pressure during CO_2 rebreathing in man. *Am. Rev. Respir. Dis.* 114:341-346.

Tenney, S. M. (1954). Ventilatory response to carbon dioxide in pulmonary emphysema. *J. Appl. Physiol.* 6:477-484.

Trenchard, D., Gardner, D., and Guz, A. (1972). Role of pulmonary vagal afferent nerve fibres in the development of rapid, shallow breathing in lung inflammation. *Clin. Sci.* 42:251-263.

Turino, G. M., and Goldring, R. M. (1976). Techniques for measuring the responsiveness of the ventilatory apparatus in man in disease. *Chest* 70: 180-185.

von Euler, C., Herrero, F., and Wexler, I. (1970). Control mechanisms determining rate and depth of respiratory movements. *Respir. Physiol.* 10: 93-108.

Walker, B. R., Adams, M. E., and Voelkel, N. F. (1985). Ventilatory responses of hamsters and rats to hypoxia and hypercapnia. *J. Appl. Physiol.* 59: 1955-1960.

Weissman, C., Abraham, B., Askanazi, J., Milic-Emili, J., Hyman, A. I., and Kinney, J. M. (1982). Effect of posture on the ventilatory response to CO_2. *J. Appl. Physiol.* 53:761-765.

Weissman, C., Askanazi, J., Milic-Emili, J., and Kinney, J. M. (1984). Effect of respiratory apparatus on respiration. *J. Appl. Physiol.* 57:475-580.

West, J. R., and Alexander, J. K. (1959). Studies on respiratory mechanics and the work of breathing in pulmonary fibrosis. *Am. J. Med.* 27:529-544.

Weyel, D. A., Ellakkani, M., Alarie, Y., and Karol, M. H. (1984). An aerosol generator for the resuspension of cotton dust. *Toxicol. Appl. Pharmacol.* 76:544-547.

Widdicombe, J. G. (1982). Pulmonary and respiratory receptors. *J. Exp. Biol.* 100:41-57.

Wong, K. L., and Alarie, Y. (1982). A method for repeated evaluation of pulmonary performance in unanesthetized, unrestrained guinea pigs and its application to detect effects of sulfuric acid mist inhalation. *Toxicol. Appl. Pharmacol.* **63**:72-90.

Wong, K. L., Stock, M. F., and Alarie, Y. (1983). Evaluation of the pulmonary toxicity of plasticized polyvinyl chloride thermal decomposition products in guinea pigs by repeated CO_2 challenges. *Toxicol. Appl. Pharmacol.* **70**:236-248.

Wong, K. L., Stock, M. F., Malek, D. E., and Alarie, Y. (1984). Evaluation of the pulmonary effects of wood smoke in guinea pigs by repeated CO2 challenges. *Toxicol. Appl. Pharmacol.* **75**:69-80.

Wong, K. L., Karol, M. H., and Alarie, Y. (1985). Use of repeated CO2 challenges to evaluate the pulmonary performance of guinea pigs exposed to toluene disocyanate. *J. Toxicol. Environ. Health* **15**:137-148.

4

Inhalation Toxicity of Metal Particles and Vapors

WILLIAM A. SKORNIK

Harvard University School of Public Health
Boston, Massachusetts

The toxicology of inhalable metals involves about 80 elements and their compounds that range from comparatively simple salts to complicated structures, such as complexes consisting of a metal atom and a set of ligands, and organometallic compounds. With the possible exception of certain transuranic elements, metals have always been an intrinsic component of the earth's crust and as such many have been incorporated into the biochemical processes essential for all life forms. It is not surprising, therefore, that the relative abundance of metals found in plants and animals generally follows their abundance in the earth's crust.

Environmental pollution and human exposure to airborne metallic elements may occur naturally (e.g., volcanic activity), but it is particularly common from human activities (e.g., mining, refining, the manufacture of paper, cement, brick or glass, and the combustion of fossil fuels, including automobile exhaust). Industrial and commercial uses of metals continues to increase. New applications have been found for some less familiar metallic elements, particularly the transition metals. A large number of metals are used in the production of alloys in plating and increasing amounts are being used as catalysts in the modern chemical industry. Considerable amounts are also used in the production of plastics, such as polyvinyl chloride, particularly as heat stabilizers. Pigments, biocides, lubricants, fertilizers, and pesticides are still other examples of industrial uses of metals. All of these activities increase the discharge of metals into the environment, exposing humans to increased concentrations of metals, and thereby increasing the potential for metallic poisoning.

Metallic elements are found in all living organisms, where they play a variety of roles. They may be structural elements, stabilizers of biological structures, components of control mechanisms (e.g., in nerves and muscles), and most importantly, catalysts or cofactors in enzymatic processes. Calcium, potassium, sodium, and magnesium are involved in maintaining the physiological milieu necessary for sustaining life. Some metals are therefore essential elements and their deficiency results in impairment of biological functions. Of equal importance are the so-called "essential trace elements." About nine trace elements are essential for life (Cr, Mn, Fe, Co, Cu, Zn, Mo, Se, I). Seven of these, all metals, are found in air. All essential trace metals are toxic in high enough doses. Thus, when present in excess, essential metal nutrients may become toxic. Similarly, some "toxic" metals may be essential nutrients when provided in low quantities.

The remaining metals are foreign to the body and most are toxic. The metals having the greatest disease potential are those that tend to accumulate in the body. In general, the total amount of metals present in the body tends to increase with age and is often used as a yardstick of low-level exposure, for example, cadmium is a useful indicator of the amount of cigarette smoking. These metals can be toxic through direct action of the metal and through their inorganic salts; particularly in the ionized state or via organic compounds from which the metal can be easily detached, or introduced into cells.

In this chapter, the toxicity of inhalable metals is presented systemically. The toxicity of metals and their salts forms the main focus; radioactive metals are excluded. The toxicity of each nonradioactive metal is discussed in three parts: (1) general uses of the metal and its compounds; (2) metabolism of the metal, including absorption from the respiratory tract, distribution to various tissues, storage, excretion, and homeostasis; (3) toxicity, that is, its specific adverse effects in humans and animals at the whole organism, cellular, and molecular levels, carcinogenesis, and other pathologic conditions.

I. Historical Reports

Several metals have been known for centuries to be toxic to humans. The well-documented effects of lead in smelting and storage battery production include heompoietic alterations, lead paralysis, and colic. Inhalation of mercury vapor in mercury mining and in the felt hat industry has frequently given rise to severe symptoms from the central nervous system with a pronounced tremor as the dominant sign. Inhalation of manganese has long been recognized as causing central nervous system effects similar to those seen in Parkinson's disease.

At present, most of our information on metal toxicity to humans is derived from industrial health experience. Beginning in the 1960s, particular attention has been focused on mercury and cadmium, primarily because evidence of their effects is abundant in both industrial environments and contaminated general environments. However, at least 20 metals or metal-like elements can give rise to rather well-defined toxic effects in humans. In addition to mercury and cadmium, lead, manganese, and arsenic have been studied most thoroughly, but other metals are also of concern. Antimony and cobalt may have effects on the cardiovascular system, some organometallic tin compounds give rise to effects on the central nervous system, and molybdenum brings about gout-like signs. Effects on the lungs in the form of pneumoconioses can arise after exposure to such metals (or their compounds) as aluminum, antimony, barium, beryllium, cobalt, iron, tin, and tungsten.

A comprehensive summary of the toxicity of metals is available (*Handbook on the Toxicology of Metals*, Friberg, Nordberg, and Vouk, eds.).

II. Environmental Levels and Exposure by Inhalation

The sources of environmental contamination can be natural or man-made. Man-made sources deliver large amounts of potentially toxic materials to both the occupational and the residential environments. The distance from the source of emission of metals to their sink can be considerable. Atmospheric discharges from industrial centers are carried by the long distance transport of air masses, which often contain multielement particulates along with oxides of sulfur and nitrogen. These contaminants may travel hundreds of miles before returning to the land.

In the general environment, exposures always involve a spectrum of metals in combination with a variety of other environmental factors. Also, when considering occupational metal exposures, combinations of a number of metals often occur.

Metal ores invariably contain "guest" elements, amd as a result, there can be little doubt that metals in contaminated environments never occur singly but in association with other metals. For example, it is impossible to mine and move zinc without moving cadmium and to a lesser extent lead, antimony, arsenic, and indium. Similarly, nickel is commonly associated with cobalt and often copper, and uranium ores are associated with selenium and vanadium. Accurate evaluation of such situations, therefore, needs to take into account the possible interactions among metals and other environmental factors.

Urban air contains potentially toxic salts of metals such as cadmium, lead, antimony, selenium, thallium, vanadium, nickel, and zinc. Often these compounds are "enriched" in polluted urban air up to 1000-fold above the average levels at which these metals occur in the earth's crust (Natusch et al., 1975). Most toxic components of air pollution emanate from automobile exhausts, coal-fired power plants, incinerators, metallurgical and refinery operations, and aerosol cans of cosmetics, pesticides, paints, varnishes, and propellants. Humans and animals are exposed to these pollutants more through inhalation than through other modes of intake. Most metal compounds, while exerting some transient or secondary toxic effects in the lung, also produce toxic effects at primary sites elsewhere in the body.

Metals in air may occur as either vapors or particulates, called aerosols. In the industrial environment, human exposures to metals in vapor form may occur, for example, exposure to mercury vapor in chlor-alkali plants or in mercury mines, and to nickel carbonyl in some nickel refineries. However, in industry, metal aerosols occur much more commonly than metal vapors. When vapors given off by molten metals condense upon cooling, they form a fine aerosol or metal oxide fumes. These particles are often small, usually 1.0 μm in diameter or less, always form complex chains, and can be dispersed throughout the working environment. A number of metals are thus found, for example, in the fly ash from coal-fired power plants. Depending on the source of the coal, such fly ash may contain different concentrations of Pb, Cd, Zn, As, to name a few (Natusch et al., 1974, 1975; Coffin and Stokinger, 1977). With oil combustion, the dominant metal in the emitted aerosols is vanadium contained in oil. During the manufacture and use of steel, exposures to all types of metals contained in the various forms of steel (Fe, Mn, Mo, Cr, Ni) may occur.

Leaded gasoline (tetraethyl lead) gives rise to air pollution by lead-containing aerosols, particularly in cities and along highways. For smokers, inhalation exposure to metal compounds occurring in tobacco smoke is of great interest. Cigarette smoke contributes nickel, chromium, cadmium, lead, and aluminum compounds to the inhaled air. In this case there is a combined exposure to various metal compounds in aerosol form and a number of nonmetal gases and vapors, resulting in the potentiation of one harmful material by another (Bates, 1972). In addition, passive exposure of the nonsmoker to the contaminants in tobacco smoke occurs repeatedly.

In the home environment, exposure is a consequence principally of soldering, welding, use of organometals, or occasionally hobby-type activities. In all exposures, a major factor is the presence of high local concentrations which usually result from working in an inadequately ventilated enclosed space.

By way of introduction, before entering the area of inhalation toxicity of metals, it is likely that a brief summary of certain aspects of pulmonary physiology with special attention to particulates in the respiratory system will be helpful to some. Readers who feel the need for additional material are referred to the works of West (1974, 1977) and Doull et al. (1980).

III. The Respiratory Tract

The respiratory tract has three main regions: the nasopharyngeal; tracheobronchial; and (pulmonary) alveolar; each of which has distinctly different functions. The first section, the upper respiratory tract, consists of nose, paranasal sinuses, pharynx, and larynx. Its major functions are to warm and humidify inhaled air and to remove large particles and bacteria. Particle removal is accomplished partly through the sievelike action of coarse hairs in the anterior nares and partly by impaction on the respiratory mucosa. The second section, the major conducting airways, consist of the trachea, two main bronchi, numerous generations of cartilagenous bronchi, and multiple bronchioles ending in alveolar ducts. These airways carry the air to the periphery of the lung, while at the same time continuing to warm and humidify the air. More importantly, this part of the respiratory tract is highly developed as a defense against particles as will be discussed later. The third section consists of the respiratory airway, respiratory bronchioles, and alveoli, which are specially constructed to allow rapid gas exchange between alveoli and blood through the thin Type I epithelial cells and the capillary endothelium. During respiration, distention of the alveoli is made possible by the secretion of surfactant from Type II epithelial cells which lowers the surface tension in each alveolus. Without surfactant, expansion of the lung would be severely impaired. This structural division of the respiratory tract is of practical importance because the manifestations of toxic injury are different in the three sections.

Certain functional peculiarities make the lung vulnerable to toxic injury. Although situated deep within the body, the lung is in immediate contact with the external environment during each breath. During strenuous exercise or labor, the frequency and depth of respiratory effort, and as a result air intake, is markedly increased, leading to potentially greater toxic exposure. Secondly, the alveolar lining cells have a large surface area and thin cytoplasm with few organelles. This combination of large absorbing surface and modest defensive ability renders Type I cells vulnerable to toxic injury. Thirdly, the alveolar surface is extremely large, an area of approximately 140 m^2 in the adult human (Weibel, 1984) (as compared with a skin area of about 2 m^2), and its abundant thin-walled capillaries lie in intimate contact with epithelium. The alveolar surface represents the largest area in the body at which the blood comes into virtually direct contact with the external environment. Consequently, toxic particles and vapors are capable not only of injuring extensive areas of alveolar tissue and adjacent structures but also of initiating rapid absorption and distribution throughout the body to injure specific (target) organs, or the body as a whole.

IV. Particulate Deposition

The deposition, retention, and distribution pattern of inhaled metal particles and vapors are influenced by many anatomic features of the respiratory tract, including, for example, lung volume, alveolar surface area, and spatial relationships of conducting airways as well as particle shape, size, and solubility. Representative tidal volumes, respiratory frequencies, and minute volumes for different species are given in Table 1.

Although inhaled particles, theoretically, can be distributed uniformly throughout the respiratory tract, this is not normally the case. The actual distribution is governed by at least three distinct, interrelated factors: air flow velocity and deposition mechanisms, particle size, and physical characteristics. Ultimately, the amount deposited, absorbed, or exhaled depends on the total dosage and the physical characteristics of the aerosol particle or the chemical

Table 1 Comparison of Tidal Volume, Respiratory Frequency, and Minute Volume for Various Species at Rest

Species	Body weight (kg)	Tidal volume (ml)	Respiratory frequency (breaths/min)	Minute volume (liters/min)
Man	70	750	12	7.43
Horse	500	7500	10	200
Cow	400	3400	27	92
Sheep	60	362	20	7.1
Dog	20	320	18	5.21
Cat	4	34	30	0.96
Monkey (rhesus)	3	21	40	0.86
Guinea pig	0.47	1.8	90	0.16
Rat	0.11	0.86	86	0.073
Hamster	0.1	0.8	74	0.06
Mouse	0.02	0.15	163	0.024

Source: From Altman and Dittmer (1974).

form of the metal, and in conjunction with the health of the individual, will determine the toxicity of the inhaled particles.

A. Air Flow Velocity

The aerodynamics of the respiratory tract (Davies, 1961; Hatch and Gross, 1964), including air velocity and its directional change greatly influence the flow of vapors and as a result the deposition of particles.

During inhalation the air velocity is high in the nasopharyngeal region, where the cross-sectional area of the airways is low. The directional change of inhaled air is very abrupt in the nasopharyngeal region, and progressively less abrupt in the trachea and bronchi. Inspired air flows down to about the terminal bronchioles by bulk flow like water in a hose. Beyond that point, the combined cross-sectional area of the airways is so enormous, because of the large number of branches, that the forward velocity of the gas becomes very small. The cross-sectional area at the alveolar duct level is approximately 8000 cm^2 as compared with a value of less than 5 cm^2 at the mouth. The expansion of the airway lumen together with the termination of the respiratory efforts result in abrupt slowing of air flow at the level of distal air spaces.

B. Deposition Mechanisms

There are five physical processes involved in the deposition of particles. They have been reviewed by Brain and Valberg (1979) and are as follows: electrostatic precipitation; interception; inertial impaction; sedimentation; and diffusion (Brownian movement). In the respiratory tract, the last three are the most important in the removal of particles from the inhaled air.

Material inhaled through the nose enters a wind tunnel labyrinth in which the high velocity of the inspiratory air, with its rapid and abrupt change in direction, forces particulate material against mucus-covered turbinates. The settling velocity due to centrifugal force is high for large particles (5-30 μm), and most are trapped in the nasopharyngeal region by inertial impaction. The effectiveness of impaction increases with air velocity. Consequently, as total cross-sectional area increases, air velocity falls and inertial impaction decreases with depth into the respiratory tract. Thus, breathing patterns characterized by increased flows tend to lead to greater inertial impaction, especially for larger particles. Turbulent impaction is more important as a cause of particle deposition in the larger airways and primarily affects particles greater than 1 μm.

In the distal airways, where the airways are small and the velocity of the airflow is low, particles sediment under the influence of gravity, each falling at a constant speed which depends on Stokes' law. The speed at which a particle settles is known as the terminal velocity and is directly proportional to its density and the square of its diameter. Removal by sedimentation is favored by relatively still air and, thus, it increases with depth into the respiratory tract. Large particles settle more rapidly and sedimentation is no longer effective when the aerodynamic diameter reaches about 0.5 μm.

Submicron particles (<0.5 μm) are deposited on the walls of the smallest airways and within the alveolar region by diffusion, the result of bombardment of the particles by the constantly vibrating gas molecules of the surrounding air. This Brownian motion increases with decreasing particle size.

Particles 20 μm in diameter settle at a rate of about 1 cm/sec. This rate, plus their large size, would rarely allow them to penetrate the nasal labyrinth at normal respiration rates, 6-12 breaths/min. Particles 2-10 μm in diameter settle at about 0.05-0.3 cm/sec and are virtually all deposited in the nose, pharynx, and trachea. Particles less than 0.1 μm in diameter show virtually no deposition in the respiratory tract and resemble gases in this respect. Some metals, such as cadmium, accumulate in the lungs with age. During a lifetime, the accumulation of residual particulate matter is considerable (see p. 150).

C. Particle Size

In addition to chemical form, evaluation of the effects of airborne metal particles is complicated by the fact that these particles vary considerably with respect to size, shape, and density. These physical characteristics as well as inhalation pattern determine the extent to which deposition and retention of the particles will occur. Generally speaking, particles 10 μm in diameter and greater are removed in the upper respiratory tract, particularly in the nose. As particles become smaller, the removal efficiency falls until most particles below 3 μm in diameter pass through the upper respiratory tract and enter the lung. In the lung, the retention is maximal with particle size between 1 and 3 μm in diameter, then it falls sharply at sizes below 1 μm. Interestingly, very small particles, those 0.1 μm and less, are governed by diffusion forces and so retention may be significant.

It is important to distinguish two definitions when considering aerosol particles: *particle size* refers to the size of an individual particle, whereas *particulate size* refers to the mean characteristics of aggregated particles. Airway deposition is directly related to particulate size. In practice it is usual to refer to two broad divisions of aerosol: monodisperse aerosols, in which particles are all the same size, and polydisperse aerosols, where particle size is heterogenous. Except under controlled experimental conditions, monodispersed aerosols do not occur. Thus, a given metal aerosol can be expected to contain particles of many different sizes and shapes.

The deposition of irregular airborne particles is frequently described in terms of its equivalent aerodynamic diameter, which depends on the shape, size, and density of the particle. The aerodynamic diameter is equal to the diameter of a spherical particle of unit density (1 g/cc) with the same settling velocity in air as the particle under study. Between two particles of the same dimensions, that with higher density is considered to be a larger particle on an aerodynamic basis. It must also be remembered that particle size may not remain constant as the aerosol moves along the respiratory tract. Hygroscopic particles grow markedly on entry into the warm, water vapor-saturated respiratory tract, and volatile aerosols become smaller through evaporation.

The distribution of aerodynamic diameters of a particular aerosol can be measured experimentally and the frequency distribution can be determined. The size distribution of particles in a heterodispersed aerosol is usually log-normal. The count mean and median diameters are measures of the frequency at which particles of various sizes occur in the population. The count mean diameter is thus the mean of the diameters of all particles in the aerosol, and the count median diameter is the diameter above which there are as many larger particles as there are smaller ones below it. The mass mean diameter is the diameter of a particle with a mass equal to the mass of all the particles in the aerosol divided by the number of particles, and the mass median diameter is the diameter of a particle with the median mass. The mass mean and median diameters are measures of the mass distribution of the aerosol. Note that the mass (or volume) median diameter is often much larger than the count median diameter, because the larger particles make a greater contribution to the total mass of the aerosol. The mass median diameter and especially the mass median aerodynamic diameter are important in determining pulmonary deposition of particles. For a more detailed discussion of aerosol properties, generation, and measurement, see Raabe (1970), Mercer (1973), and Willeke (1980).

Physiologic Effect of Particle Size

In inhalation toxicity, the size of the particulate matter is a most important feature. Reactivity and surface area increase tremendously as particle size decreases. Metals are absorbed on the surfaces of particles, where they can readily react with tissues on which the particles deposit. Implications for differential toxicity of the same quantity of a metal absorbed onto a fine or a coarse microscopic particulate are evident. The former is deposited farther down the respiratory tract, and is much more harmful than the latter even when the same quantity of metal is involved. Furthermore, metal compounds are usually concentrated or adsorbed on the surfaces of colloidal particles; in some cases, they are distributed throughout the aerosol. The concentration of such toxicants increases with decreasing size of the metal particle and of the aerosol colloid to which it is attached. Flinn et al. (1940) noted that inhalation of a coarse dust of manganese oxide was asymptomatic, while pneumonitis resulted when a fine dust was inhaled. Dygert et al. (1949) found that the toxic action of uranium oxide was not evident until particles less than 3 μm in diameter were used. The larger particles were inactive; the small particles provided enough surface area to be highly active colloidal particles. High-temperature combustion sources emit a proportionally large number of extremely small toxic particles, especially the metal oxides; the higher the temperature, the smaller the particles and the greater their adsorptive surfaces (Hatch and Hemeon, 1948).

If the particle size becomes very small, the aerosol is readily exhaled, and absorption depends on the water solubility of gases and fine particulates. Except for physical blockage of airways, particulates greater than 10 μm in diameter are largely ignored in physiologic and public health considerations. Only 1-2% of the total dusts, the small particulates, accounts for most of the damage.

Some knowledge is thus available on how the size and surface properties of aerosols are related to the development of pathological processes following their inhalation. Further investigation of these relationships would be of interest.

D. Particle Clearance and Retention

Deposition and clearance must be considered together when assessing dosage. Of prime importance is the amount of a substance present in the respiratory tract at any time; this is called the retention. If exposure is continuous, then the concentration at equilibrium (achieved when the clearance rate equals the deposition rate) is also the retention. Thus, the relative rate constants of deposition and clearance determine the equilibrium levels. Presumably, it is this equilibrium level, or retention integrated over time, and the intrinsic properties of the metal particle that are related to the magnitude of the toxic response.

Particle size distribution as well as breathing pattern (e.g., deep or shallow) help specify the sites of deposition (Brain and Valberg, 1979; Sweeney et al., 1983), and hence affects clearance rates since various parts of the respiratory tract clear particles at different rates. This results in markedly different rates of retention.

A variety of mechanisms help facilitate the clearance of particles from the respiratory tract. Clearance mechanisms include solubilization, absorption, sneeze, cough, mucociliary transport, and alveolar clearance involving pulmonary macrophages among other mechanisms. Although these mechanisms are of considerable importance and must be taken into account in estimating retention, this review will focus on the three primary mechanisms by which particulate material is removed from the pulmonary region once it has been deposited: (1) particles may be phagocytized and cleared up the tracheobronchial tree via the mucociliary escalator; (2) particles may be phagocytized and removed via the lymphatic drainage; and (3) material may dissolve from the surface of particles and be removed via the bloodstream or lymphatics.

Removal of fine particles has been observed to occur in distinct phases (Hatch and Gross, 1964; Lourenco et al., 1971; Casarett, 1972; Gamsu et al., 1973; Doull et al., 1980). The rapid phase has a half-life of about 2 hours (Albert et al., 1967). This phase is completed within 6-24 hours. Particles are removed from the upper respiratory tract by colloidal movement of the mucous blanket at a rate of 1 cm/min. Tracheal material is completely removed within 20 hr by healthy respiratory cilia, according to tantalum insufflation studies by Gamsu et al. (1973). Much of the insoluble metal oxides that have been used to explore this phenomenon is excreted unabsorbed in the feces. A variety of irritants increase the secretion, flow, and discharge of this moving blanket. Allergies and certain disease states cause conditions considerably different from normal. Lourenco et al. (1971) found that smokers retain considerably more of the 2 μm particles than do nonsmokers during the first 3 hr; 24 hr following inhalation, retention was comparable in the two groups.

Material that is not rapidly cleared from the lungs has very different clearance characteristics. Much is usually deposited in the terminal bronchioles and the alveoli, where removal is slow. Gamsu et al. (1973) found that clearance time increased dramatically with decrease in size of bronchi. Microscopic particles deposited in the alveoli are mostly cleared from the pulmonary parenchyma by alveolar macrophages through phagocytosis. Most of this deposited material can be phagocytized in healthy lung tissue, as long as it is not overwhelmed with too much material. Macrophage clearance at a slow, constant rate characterizes this phase. The half-life of this intermediate clearance may extend from 1 month to several months, depending on the quantity and characteristics of the particles. Some metals are toxic to these cells (Waters et al., 1975). Skornik and Brain examined in hamsters the effect of metal sulfate aerosols on the ability of pulmonary macrophages to clear particles from the lung. Based on the concentration causing a 50% reduction in phagocytosis, the sulfates were ranked $Cu > Zn > Fe^{3+} > Zn - NH_4$. Since effects on pulmonary macrophages would be closely related to bacterial clearance, it is not surprising that their ranking is in general agreement with data studying susceptibility to respiratory infections in animals (Ehrlich et al., 1978; Ehrlich, 1980).

The material deposited in deep pulmonary regions is mostly less than 0.1 μm in diameter and becomes more readily soluble or moved by virtue of its colloidal properties. The lymph drainage of this area of the lung is effective. Macrophages readily transport fine particulates during the first few days following exposure. It is assumed that few particulates penetrate bronchioles or alveolar tissue prior to being phagocytized. Thus, only a small number of particles travel in the lymphatics or through tissues as naked particles.

The third phase of removal involves material that has been effectively sequestered from normal metabolic activities. Gamsu et al. (1973) found no movement for 15 months from tantalum in alveoli. Insoluble metal compounds and colloids with heavy metals combine with macromolecules to form a stable, nonreactive material (i.e., a denatured protein). This long-term clearance predominates when large quantities of particulates less than 1 μm in diameter are inhaled.

In addition to the clearance mechanisms described above, the very slow dissolution of "insoluble" materials, such as silicates, continues as long as there is an effective interface between the particulate material and living cells. Here they may be transformed into soluble ionic forms by very slow biochemical reactions and cell erosions. This action decreases if an effective tubercle is formed around the particulate. This slow clearance may continue for years.

In the discussion of particulate deposition, uptake, and removal, it is assumed that the respiratory system is normal. Drugs, infections, lung diseases, presence of irritants, and desquamation may dramatically change these clearance patterns.

E. Absorption

The Task Group on Metal Accumulation (1973) considered pulmonary absorption of metals to be the most important route for toxic metals to enter the human body and discussed general principles responsible for absorption by the lung. Metals are absorbed 10 times more effectively by the lungs than by the intestines. In humans, the total surface area of the lungs is about 70 times greater than that of the skin.

Gaseous and microparticulate (<0.2 μm diameter) absorption occurs primarily in the 300 million alveoli in man; this constantly moving surface of approximately 140 m² (Gehr et al., 1978; Weibel, 1984) equilibrates with 10,000 liters of air daily.

About 70% of each breath reaches the alveoli, where histologic structures and the slow movement of respiratory gas and alveolar capillary bed provide effective contact for gaseous exchange. Inhaled metallic vapors and particulates of submicroscopic size may be absorbed into the blood to the extent of their solubility; the major portion of insoluble microscopic particles will be retained or exhaled as shown in Table 2. Thus, inhalation may result in the direct transfer of soluble metal compounds, such as thallium, from the pulmonary tissues to the blood.

Natusch et al. (1974) estimated the absorption of lead from their data (Table 3). Assuming that 70% of the lead in the pulmonary region is absorbed and that only 10% of the lead from the upper respiratory tract is absorbed after it is swallowed, 22% of inhaled lead is absorbed from the lungs while 10% is absorbed from the alimentary tract. They suggest that the average city dweller obtains about 33% of his total lead intake each day (30 μg) by inhalation.

Similarly, the lung is an effective excretory organ for volatile metals such as selenium oxide. Although small concentrations may be involved, the continuous movement of air through the lung enhances contact with a vast capillary bed and makes exhalation an effective homeostatic mechanism for volatile metal salts. It can also provide a circuitous route for the transport of the metal to the

Table 2 Retention of Inhaled Particles in Different Regions of the Respiratory Tract[a]

	Retention (%)				
Region	0.2 μm[b]	0.6 μm	2 μm	6 μm	20 μm
Mouth	0	0	0	0	15
Pharynx	0	0	0	0	8
Trachea	0	0	0	1	10
Pulmonary bronchi	0	0	0	2	12
Secondary bronchi	0	0	1	4	19
Tertiary bronchi	0	0	2	9	17
Quarternary bronchi	1	1	2	7	6
Terminal bronchioles	6	4	6	19	6
Respiratory bronchioles	4	3	5	11	0
Alveolar ducts	11	8	25	25	0
Alveolar sacs	0	0	0	5	0
Totals	22	16	41	83	93

[a]Estimates of Hatch and Gross (1964) based on 450 cm^3 tidal volume and 4-sec cycle with 300 cm^3 air/sec.
[b]Particle size.

Table 3 Deposition of Metals in the Respiratory System

		% Deposited by region		
Metal	Diameter (μm)	Nasopharyngeal	Tracheobronchial	Pulmonary
Lead	0.56	17	6	32
Iron	2.7	48	7	22

Source: From Natusch et al. (1974).

tissues. Cilia of epithelial cells can carry insoluble metal particulates or compounds from the lungs into the gastrointestinal tract via the pharynx. Macrophages can transfer the metal directly to regional lymph nodes, blood, and other tissues or to the gastrointestinal tract.

The release of metal ions to tissues determines the dose-response sequence, with time as an important factor. Following inhalation, absorption results in the gradual exposure of tissues, in contrast with intravenous administration which delivers a high initial dosage to tissues.

Obvious differences in responses to metal toxicants following different routes of administration relate to how the material is absorbed, metabolized, sequestered, and excreted. Oral administration evokes a series of protective mechanisms: a physiologic response, such as vomiting; metal interactions; chemical action of hydrochloric acid in the stomach; enzyme action in the small intestine; and metabolism by intestinal microbes (10^{14} in humans). Inhalation processes are probably no less complex, since particulates may be carried by macrophages from lung tissues to other tissues, including the alimentary tract.

The species, time of day, and condition of the organism also modify the absorption, homeostasis, and toxicity. A variety of diseases alter the amount of toxicants absorbed and the response of the organism to a given dosage.

Prolonged inhalation of fine dust may considerably decrease the total absorptive capacity of the lungs. When industrial dusts accumulate in the bronchioles, the irritation reaction may include formation of fibrosis with subsequent dysfunction of that portion of the lung. This fibrosis may result in increased toxicity. Partial blockage tends to decrease pulmonary circulation, making the bronchial circulation important in absorption. Material absorbed in the bronchial arteries and veins goes directly from the arterial blood to tissues without benefit of the slow filtration through the reticuloendothelial components of lymphatic or pulmonary capillaries. The pulmonary blood is therefore a potentially dangerous pathway for absorption of metals in persons with lung dysfunction.

Any discussion of the deposition of inhaled metal particles and vapors would, however, be incomplete without considering the effect of other airborne contaminants. Irritating factors in the respiratory system can affect the fate and toxicity of inhaled particles by altering airway diameter, lung clearance mechanisms, or the function of the cells that line the airways.

In this connection, the potential effects of sulfur dioxide and of cigarette smoke have been discussed more than those of any other ambient air pollutant. The constriction of major airways can result in increased flow velocities and consequently increased particle deposition by impaction. Sulfur dioxide may also affect the clearance of particles deposited in the alveoli of animals or influence the vascular and lymphatic drainage.

V. Toxicity of Metals

The toxicity of a metal depends on its inherent capacity to adversely affect biological activity. Toxicity is a relative term used to compare one chemical or metallic compound with another. Some metals are essential for life because of the key role they play in maintaining biological processes. Toxic metals (including excessive levels of essential metals) tend to change biological structures and systems into irreversible and inflexible conformations leading ultimately to death. The generalized response of an organism to a toxicant is biphasic, a phase of biological effects being followed by a phase of pharmacotoxic actions.

Toxicity is only a single component in the complete activity spectrum or dose-response curve of a chemical in a living biological system. Depending on its characteristics and dose, a metal may be innocuous, essential as a nutrient, stimulatory, therapeutic, toxic, or lethal. The response varies according to the environment, diet, and condition of the animal as well as the form, dosage, and mode of administration of the metal or its salt. Synergisms and antagonisms among metals are included in these factors. Therefore, a broad overview is necessary for a thorough understanding of the complex spectrum of metals and their compounds. For example, cadmium, selenium, arsenic, and tin have long been known as toxic elements, but recently each has been proposed as an essential nutrient for animals. Alternatively many essential metals are being investigated for their toxicity in excessive amounts. This understanding is also needed to help counteract the simplistic labeling of a given metal as "good" or "bad," and to enable society to make enlightened decisions on a metal's biologic functions and limitations.

The toxicity of each metal or its compounds is influenced by a number of factors: (1) the dose; (2) the intrinsic or inherent toxicity; (3) the combining capacity; (4) the action of the biologic system to absorb and transport the metal to the target organ most susceptible to the metal; (5) the capacity to undergo biotransformation to a less toxic or more toxic form at the target organ or during transfer; (6) the ability to bind to essential macromolecules; and (7) the presence or absence of a mechanism for homeostasis (i.e., inactivation, transport, or excretory mechanisms).

Some of the more sensitive and susceptible biologic activities and systems affected by metals are: permeability of cell membranes and subcellular organelles, structure and function of nucleic acids and proteins; release of potent substances such as histamine; and biosynthetic formation of hormones. On the other hand, the defensive homeostatic mechanisms of the cells and tissues defend against metal toxicity either by sequestering the metal in a harmless form or by enhanced and rapid excretion of the toxic metal.

Acute toxicity is caused by a relatively large dose of a metal toxicant. The onset of symptoms is sudden, and the intensity of effects rises rapidly and if adequate procedures are not performed to neutralize or remove the toxicant, irreversible damage to tissues and systems may cause death. Chronic poisoning develops gradually following long and continued exposure to relatively small doses. Initially, no symptoms manifest, then there is a gradual onset of symptoms. There may be frequent remissions and recurrences of the symptoms. Many metals act as short-term poisons or toxicants in high doses and as long-term systemic poisons in low doses. Chronic poisoning also represents cumulative effects. A metallic toxicant can develop two different sets of symptoms, one for acute and one for chronic toxicity. Chronic toxicity can be reversed by removal of the toxicant, provided no irreversible damage has been done to vital systems. Groth (1972) found that metal interactions were effective in chronic experiments, with mercury toxicity being alleviated by selenium. Delayed, or latent, toxicity is the condition in which clinical effects are observable only months following exposure to the toxicant. Latent toxicity is exemplified by beryllium and chromium. Cumulative effects may or may not be associated with a build up of the toxicant. For example, there is no cumulative concentration of beryllium in pulmonary tissues in the pulmonary granuloma caused by chronic beryllium toxicity.

The study of the physicochemical properties of a metal and its interaction with biological macromolecules helps to explain its inherent toxicity and its overall toxicity in biological systems. Metal toxicity is associated with the physical and chemical properties of the metals, which differ according to their position in the periodic table (Pierre-Bienvenu et al., 1963). Although it is difficult to associate toxicity of a given metal with its group in the periodic table, toxicity can be related to its position in the horizontal period of the table. The physicochemical properties involved in metal toxicity are: (1) the electrochemical character and the oxidation state of the metal; (2) the particle size of the metal or compound, especially important in inhalation toxicity; (3) the stability and solubility of the metal compounds in body fluids and tissues and the degree of hydration of the ions formed; (4) the extent of hydrolysis of metal salts and the solubility and reactivity of these products; (5) the tendency of the metal compounds to exist in radiocolloidal (also designated microcolloidal), colloidal, and particulate forms in the tissues; and (6) the susceptibility of these metal compounds to be sequestered, metabolized, detoxified, and excreted.

The electrochemical character of a metal is directly involved in the capacity of the metal and its ions and compounds to coordinate or chelate with electron-donating oxygen, nitrogen, and sulfur atoms of biological ligands or macromolecules, cellular membranes, subcellular particulates, and tissue components. The stability of these bondings influences the toxicity of the metal involved in the chemical bond.

For example, essential metals, such as iron, copper, and vanadium, are involved in the oxygen and electron transport systems. These systems bind oxygen securely under certain environmental conditions, but release the oxygen under different conditions, thus, maintaining a dynamic continuity of function and turnover characteristic of all living cells. Other metals bind oxygen in an irreversible and stable condition. Toxic metals, therefore, are those which fix biological systems and structures into irreversible and inflexible conformation.

The bond strength of a metal and a ligand can be explained by the theory of hard and soft acids and bases of Pearson (1963, 1967, 1968) which is essentially based on electropositivity, electron mobility, or polarizability of the metal ion. A metal is a hard acid (electron acceptor) if it is characterized by low polarizability, high electropositivity, large positive charge or oxidation, small size, and electrostatic bond; the converse is true for the soft acid. The bond between soft Hg^{2+} and soft SH^{1-} is strong; similarly a strong bond is formed between hard acid and hard base (e.g., trivalent lanthanons and phosphates) but not between a soft acid and a hard base (e.g., Zn^{2+} and SO_4^{2-}). The strength of the bonding influences the metal toxicity in biological systems.

The retention of metal ions in mammalian systems depends on the affinity between the metal and the specific tissues where they are retained, the stability of the bonding involved, and the efficiency of any homeostatic mechanisms that control either the absorption or excretion of the metals. Other metals and anions may influence either retention or absorption, for example, the involvement of Cu^{2+} and SO_4^{2-} in Mo metabolism. Metal ions may either potentiate or reduce the toxicity of other metals.

VI. Inhalation Toxicity of Specific Metals

A. Group IA (Li, Na, K, Rb, and Cs)

Alkaline earth metals are elements which are essentially nontoxic. The body's homeostatic mechanisms are so efficient for these elements that excretion, chiefly in urine, or in sweat, prevents toxicity. However, excess intake of their salts, particularly in the presence of disease, can result in toxicity. The toxicity of rubidium and cesium results from their competition with and displacement of sodium and potassium in cell reactions (Browning 1969; Stokinger, 1981).

B. Group IB (Cu, Ag, and Au)

These metals are basically nontoxic. Copper, an essential element, is controlled by efficient homeostasis, whereas silver and gold salts are insoluble and have no effective homeostatic mechanism. Following entry into the body, removal occurs only by cell death. Silver can induce iron deficiency and as a consequence result in anemia. The side effects of therapy with gold salts are fibrosis of the lung and kidney damage, apparently because of hypersensitivity effects.

Copper

Copper is an essential element and is distributed widely in plant and animal tissues. The adult human body contains about 100 mg Cu, approximately 30% in muscle tissues. Copper has been used in tool making for 6000 years. The introduction of bronze (copper hardened by alloying with tin) heralded the end of the Stone Age. It is used extensively in industry because of its conductivity, malleability, and durability. It is an essential part of several of the most vital enzymes, such as tyrosinase, which is necessary for the formation of melanin, cytochrome oxidase, superoxide dismutase, peroxidase, and catalase. Copper is also essential for the incorporation of iron into hemoglobin (Piscator, 1977).

Inhalation Exposure and Limits

Except for a few areas of occupational exposure, inhalation of airborne copper, even near copper smelters or other major emitters, is negligible compared to oral ingestion (USEPA, 1980b).

The threshold limit value (TLV) as a time-weighted average for an 8 hr day is 1 mg/m^3 for copper dusts and mists, with a short-term exposure limit of 2 mg Cu/m^3 for 15 min. The TLV for copper fume is 0.2 mg/m^3 (ACGIH, 1983). The OSHA permissible exposure limit is 1 mg/m^3 for dusts and mists and 0.1 mg/m^3 for copper fumes (OSHA, 1981).

Toxicity

Metallic copper is toxic only when inhaled as a fume or fine dust (Gleason, 1969). Inhalation may cause "brass chills," a form of metal fume fecre (see Zinc, toxicity, p. 148 for general description of metal fume fever) that resembles influenza, but does not last as long. Symptoms generally disappear after 24 hours (Muir, 1972; Doull et al., 1980). An unusual characteristic of this condition is that immunity is built up as long as one is continually exposed to the metal oxide. However, this immunity is lost during short absences from work (in as few as 1 or 2 days) with symptoms recurring upon re-exposure (Muir, 1972).

Industrial exposure to copper dust or fumes has been common, but health surveys of workers engaged in processing copper have not revealed any other acute or chronic toxic reaction (Cohen, 1974). Lung changes have been reported in vineyard workers spraying vines with copper sulfate solutions (Villar, 1974). Since other compounds may contribute, the role of copper in these cases has not been fully elucidated.

Silver

Silver is used in electrical applications because of its excellent properties of conduction. Jewelry, coins, and eating utensils are some of the principal uses of this metal. Silver halides are used in photography; silver nitrate is used for making indelible inks and for medicinal purposes.

Inhalation Exposure and Limits

Ambient air concentrations of 10.5 ng/m³ have been reported in Kellog, Idaho, near where silver-lead ores were mined and smelted (USEPA, 1980f).

The threshold limit value as a time-weighted average in workroom air for an 8 hr day is 0.1 mg Ag/m³ for silver metal (ACGIH, 1983). The OSHA permissable exposure limit is 0.01 mg/m³ for silver metal and soluble compounds (OSHA, 1981).

Absorption, Excretion, and Toxicity

Silver and its salts are not industrial hazards and cases of poisoning are rare. Silver compounds may be absorbed via inhalation, but there are no quantitative data concerning the extent of this phenomenon. The deposition fraction of 0.5 μm spherical silver particles in the lung of dogs has been found to be about 17% (Phalen and Morrow, 1973). Dogs exposed to silver by inhalation accumulated most of the administered dosage in the liver, with lower concentrations in the lung, brain, and muscle (Phalen and Morrow, 1973). In an accidental exposure of a human being to radioactive silver, most of the inhaled dose had a biological half-life of one day, probably due to mucociliary clearance, swallowing, and fecal excretion. However, significant activity was found in the liver 16 days and later after exposure (Newton and Holmes, 1966).

Gold

Gold is used in jewelry, for other ornamental purposes, and for special industrial purposes where its properties of electrical and heat conductivity, malleability, and ductility outweigh its expense. Gold has also been used in the coating of space satellites and space suits, where it serves as a reflector of radiation. While gold and its salts have been used for a wide variety of medicinal purposes, their present uses are limited to the treatment of rheumatoid arthritis and rare skin diseases such as discoid lupus.

Absorption, Excretion, and Toxicity

The majority of information we have concerning the distribution of gold salts originates from its therapeutic use or through experimental studies. After injection of most of the soluble salts, gold is excreted via the urine, while the feces account for the major portion of insoluble compounds. Gold seems to have a long biologic half-life, and detectable blood levels can be demonstrated for ten months after the cessation of treatments. The skeleton permanently retains approximately half of the absorbed gold. There are no reports on inhalation of gold compounds, but it is presumed that clearance from the lungs would be similar to that from parenteral administration.

The toxicity of gold and its salts seems to be largely associated with its therapeutic use rather than its industrial use.

C. Group IIA (Be, Mg, Ca, Sr, and Ba)

These agents are essentially nontoxic except for beryllium, which is used to make durable steel, and in the nuclear and electronic industries. In the past, it was used widely in the manufacture of fluorescent lights and neon signs. Beryllium is highly toxic if inhaled and causes fever and progressive lung fibrosis. Beryllium inhibits enzyme activity, particularly that of alkaline phosphatase, but acts mainly by inducing a hypersensitivity response. Its toxicity is enhanced by its small molecular size which results in greater tissue penetration, its high charge to mass ratio, and the absence of a homeostatic control mechanism. Lung fibrosis is known to be associated with lung cancer. Magnesium and calcium are metals of major importance in normal body function and only cause toxicity at high dosage, usually because of existing internal disease rather than from excessive intake.

Beryllium

The industrial uses of beryllium include its function as a hardening agent in alloys, especially with Cu, the manufacture of nonsparking alloys for tools, and the manufacture of lightweight alloys and nuclear reactors. Formerly, it was used in the manufacture of fluorescent lamps (discontinued because of the dangers from the dust of broken lamps) and neon signs. The aerospace industry uses finely powdered beryllium compounds as propellants, providing a possible source of environmental exposure.

Inhalation Exposure and Limits

There is some airborne beryllium due to coal combustion, cigarette smoke, and, in some areas, beryllium processing plants (Reeves, 1977a; IARC, 1980a). The threshold limit value as time-weighted average in workroom air for an 8 hr day is 0.002 mg/m^3 for beryllium and its compounds (ACGIH, 1983). The OSHA permissible exposure limit is 0.002 mg/m^3, with a peak limit of 0.025 mg/m^3 over 30 min (OSHA, 1981).

Absorption and Excretion

The primary route of entry of beryllium into the body is through the lungs, where it binds with some proteins and is subsequently carried into the liver, spleen, and bone, with varying amounts remaining in the lungs (Doull et al., 1980). Beryllium particles are slowly cleared from the lungs (Stokinger, 1981). Sanders et al. (1975) measured the deposition, clearance, and retention of inhaled BeO in hamsters and rats, as well as the effect of BeO exposure on the clearance of a radioactive aerosol ($^{239}PuO_2$). Considerable variation was observed, however, females of both species had slower beryllium clearance than males. Reeves and Vorwald (1967) showed similar sex-related differences in the rate of clearance of beryllium sulfate. In both sexes the half-life of beryllium was greater than 9 weeks. The experiments with PuO_2 showed that exposure to beryllium also reduces the ability of the lungs to clear other particles. Exposures to beryllium are much less hazardous by the ingestion route than by the inhalation route. Compounds of beryllium are not well absorbed when given by any route: they tend to form insoluble precipitates at physiological pH. Experimental animals may absorb only 1% as a maximum. Beryllium excretion via urine and feces is extremely slow. Beryllium in the urine may reflect a recent exposure, but increased beryllium in the urine can be detected for years after exposure (Lauwerys, 1983).

Toxicity

Beryllium production commenced in quantity in the 1930s, and because of the early ignorance regarding its toxicity, no environmental controls were practiced until the late 1940s. Few measurements exist regarding the levels of beryllium to which workers were exposed in these early years, but, retrospectively, they must have been very high. In these early cases of acute pulmonary beryllium disease, frequently all segments of the respiratory tract were involved, resulting in rhinitis, pharyngitis, tracheobronchitis, and pneumonitis. These disorders were partially reversible if exposure to beryllium ceased. The acidity of beryllium salt solution probably played a major role in the etiology of the disease. There appeared to be a definite dose-response relationship both with respect to onset, severity, and duration of inflammation (Van Ordstrand et al., 1943). Acute beryllium disease is no longer common in the United States due to improved industrial hygiene.

Chronic beryllium toxicity in humans, caused by exposure to microgram quantities of airborne dusts of Be or its salts, develops into a granulomatous disease with primary manifestations in the lung. Chronic pulmonary beryllium disease has features of a systemic intoxication. Hardy and Tabershaw (1946) described a chronic pulmonary condition (berylliosis) among fluorescent light workers. The characteristics of this syndrome were quite different from that of the acute cases, with dyspnea being the leading symptom. Progressive pulmonary insufficiency, anorexia, weight loss, weakness, fatigue, chest pain, and constant hacking cough characterized the advanced disease. Cyanosis and clubbing of fingers were seen in about a third of cases, and cor pulmonale was another frequent sequela. Pulmonary x-rays showed miliary mottling (ground glass appearance), and histopathology of lung tissue showed interstitial granulomatosis.

Insoluble beryllium compounds, particularly low-fired oxide (approximately 500°C), appeared to be most often involved in the causation of this condition. There was no dose-response relationship evident between extent of exposure and severity of disease. Workers from the cleanest plants and family members of workers sometimes contracted the most severe clinical forms (DeNardi et al., 1949; Eisenbud et al., 1949; Sterner and Eisenbud, 1951; Hardy and Tepper, 1959; Lieben and Metzner, 1959). The onset of berylliosis was extremely variable, sometimes only a slight cough and fatigue which occurred as early as 1 year or as late as 25 years after exposure.

Two mechanisms were proposed to explain the toxicity of beryllium: a typical primary irritant reaction, and an immunologic reaction in which beryllium was the specific antigen (Sterner and Eisenbud, 1951). It is now clear that beryllium can trigger a cell-mediated immune response, as well as being directly cytotoxic (Cullen et al., 1986; Daniele et al., 1985).

Epidemiologic and experimental evidence have established the carcinogenicity of Be in mammals; the prolonged retention of Be in tissues enhances this involvement. Primary lung tumors develop in rats and monkeys following prolonged inhalation of Be compounds such as the sulfate or oxide (28 $\mu g/m^3$ for 10 months) (Vorwald, 1959; Schepers et al., 1957; Vorwald et al., 1966).

The presently available evidence on the carcinogenicity of beryllium in humans is incomplete and often contradictory. Notwithstanding, health authorities in Germany, Sweden, and the United States view beryllium as a potential human carcinogen.

Mancuso (1970) found that the incidence of respiratory cancers was significantly increased among beryllium workers who had been employed in beryllium plants for more than 15 months. The cancer risk was especially great in beryllium workers with prior respiratory illnesses (e.g., bronchitis and pneumonitis). Hasan and Kazemi (1974) reported a slight increase in the incidence of respiratory cancers in patients with chronic pulmonary berylliosis. On the other hand, Bayliss investigated the causes of deaths in 3900 men who had worked in beryllium factories, and he found no increase in mortality from respiratory cancers.

Magnesium

Magnesium metal is used extensively as a lightweight structural material in airplanes, cars, and boats. It is used in alloys, particularly those requiring light weight or resistance to corrosion. Magnesium is the second most abundant intracellular cation, after potassium (Stokinger, 1981). A normal adult body contains 21-28 g Mg, about 60% of it present in the skeleton, 29% in muscle tissues, 10% in soft tissues, and the rest in extracellular fluids. It is used in wire and ribbon for radios as well as for incendiary materials such as flares and incendiary bombs. Magnesium is an essential nutrient for living organisms because it forms part of the structure of the body and plays a critical role in cell metabolism. Magnesium is a cofactor of many enzymes and is contained in metalloenzymes; it is apparently associated with phosphate in these functions.

Absorption, Excretion, and Toxicity

Inhalation of soluble Mg salts results in transient retention of Mg in the lung before final absorption into the blood. Insoluble compounds such as MgO are retained for a longer period, causing local irritation and a temporary fall in body temperature. Freshly generated magnesium oxide can cause metal fume fever if inhaled in sufficient amounts. This is analogous to the effect caused by zinc oxide. Both zinc and magnesium exposure of animals produced similar effects (Hammond and Beliles, 1980; Stokinger, 1981).

Conjunctivitis, nasal catarrh, and coughing up discolored sputum results from industrial inhalation exposure. With industrial exposures increases in serum magnesium up to twice the normal levels failed to produce ill effects.

Calcium

Calcium is present in all plant and animal tissues and is a major essential constituent of bones, teeth, and soft tissues. A 70 kg adult human contains about 1200 g Ca, about 1.7% of the body weight; the skeleton contains 99% of the total body Ca.

Calcium metal and its compounds are used extensively in industry, medicine, and veterinary medicine. Metallic Ca is used as a deoxidizer in the purification of such metals as Cu and Be, and alloys such as steel (with Si). Some of the uses of Ca salts are: as a fixer in photography; dyeing, tanning, and curing of skins; insecticides; pesticides; and in the manufacture of melamine resin used in making plastic products. Slaked lime, with numerous uses, is a most inexpensive base used in the chemical industry.

Absorption, Excretion, and Toxicity

Calcium is an essential macroelement. It performs essential functions in bone structure, muscle contractility, nerve impulses, membrane permeability, blood coagulation, intracellular cement, and enzyme catalysis.

Calcium salts are considered nontoxic except at very high doses. Inhalation of moderately caustic calcium oxide or hydroxide causes chemical pneumonia and severe irritation of the upper respiratory tract. In humans, inhalation of calcium cyanamide causes transient vasomotor disturbances of the upper portion of the body; higher doses cause dermatitis, permanent vasomotor changes, and dyspnea (DeLarrad and Lazarini, 1954).

Strontium

The metallurgic uses are limited to the addition of small amounts in alloys of tin and lead. Strontium is also used as a deoxidizer in copper and bronze. Various strontium salts are used in paints and rubber, in the refinement of sugar from beets, and in freezing mixtures and refrigerators. Strontium is used in pyrotechnical devices such as tracer bullets and distress signal flares for its characteristic red color.

Absorption, Excretion, and Toxicity

The biologic action and physiologic function of strontium resemble those of calcium, especially with regard to bone. There is some evidence that strontium is essential for growth of animals and especially for the calcification of bones and teeth. Apparently a homeostatic balance between calcium and strontium exists that favors the absorption of calcium and the preferential excretion of strontium.

The concern over adverse effects of strontium intake is based on the radiation damage, since strontium-90, present in nuclear fallout, is a potent environmental health hazard. Chemically, toxicity from strontium is almost nil. No adverse effects from industrial use have been reported.

Barium

Barium and its salts are used extensively in the manufacture of various alloys, in paints, soap, paper, and rubber, and in the manufacture of ceramics and glass. Barium hydroxide is used in sugar refining. Barium fluorosilicate and carbonate have been used as insecticides and rodenticides. Barium sulfate, an insoluble compound, is used as a radiopaque material to aid in x-ray diagnosis.

Inhalation, Exposure and Limits

Barium may be a common pollutant of urban air. Barium organometallic compounds have been used in reducing black smoke emission from diesel engines (Smith et al., 1975). The threshold limit value as a time-weighted average in workroom air for an 8 hr day is 0.5 mg Ba/m^3 for soluble barium compounds (ACGIH, 1983). The OSHA permissible exposure limit is 0.5 mg/m^3 (OSHA, 1981).

Absorption, Excretion, and Toxicity

The toxicity of barium compounds depends on their solubility (Cuddihy et al., 1974). In man, the free ion is readily absorbed from all segments of the respiratory tract, but insoluble barium sulfate remains essentially unabsorbed and its accumulation in lung tissues increases with age. The soluble compounds once absorbed are transported by the plasma. The biologic half-life is short (less than 24 hours) (Stokinger, 1981). The major excretory route of absorbed barium appears to be the feces, although some is lost through the kidneys, sweat, and other routes (Reeves, 1977). The renal tubules reabsorb barium in the filtrate. Inhalation of barium sulfate (barite) dust causes a pulmonary reaction with mobilization of polymorphonuclear leukocytes and macrophages, and characteristic radiographic changes with dense, discrete, small opacities distributed throughout the lung fields ("baritosis"). However, the shadows appear to be due to the radiopacity of the barium sulfate itself rather than to any tissue lesions, and the condition is symptomless with no changes in pulmonary function (Wende, 1956; Stokinger, 1963; Levi-Vallensi et al., 1966). The radiologic changes are reversible if exposure to barium salt is stopped (Browning, 1969).

D. Group IIB (Zn, Cd, and Hg)

Zinc, cadmium, and mercury form strong covalent bonds resulting in stable chelates. This particularly affects thiol groups, which are frequently an active component of the structure of enzymes and so act as a major focus for the toxic action of these metals. The relative affinity for thiol groups is $Hg > Cd > Zn$. Zn is least toxic, being an essential trace element for which the body has homeostatic control. There is no homeostatic control for either Hg or Cd. Mercury toxicity is higher than that of cadmium because of its greater electropositivity, solubility, absorbability, and tissue penetration. Both have a cumulative effect which is eventually toxic.

Zinc

The principal uses of zinc are in the manufacture of galvanized iron, bronze, paint, rubber, pigments, glazes, enamel, glass, and paper and as a wood preservative, $ZnCl_2$, because of its fungicidal action. Zinc is one of the most abundant of the essential trace metals in the human body; after K, Ca, and Mg, it is the metal with the highest intracellular concentration. The human body contains about 2300 mg of zinc, 65% of it in muscles, 20% in bone, 6% in plasma, 2.8% in erythrocytes, and about 3% in the liver. Zinc appears to be essential for the proper functioning of several enzymes. Zinc is normally present in a number of metalloenzymes, peptidases (carbonic anhydrase, alkaline phosphatase, and alcohol dehydogenase), or as cofactors (arginase and histamine diaminase) used in the synthesis of DNA, RNA, protein, and insulin (Vallee, 1959). It is represented in every chemical pathway in the body so that toxicity can be widespread and serious if homeostatic clearance is exceeded.

Inhalation Exposure and Limits

The threshold limit value as a time-weighted average in workroom air for an 8 hr day is 1 mg/m^3 for zinc chloride fume and 5 mg/m^3 for zinc oxide fume, with a short-term exposure limit of 2 mg/m^3 and 10 mg/m^3, respectively (ACGIH, 1983). OSHA has adopted the TLVs for fumes of zinc chloride and zinc oxide (OSHA, 1981).

Absorption and Excretion

Inhalation of aerosols leads to rapid uptake with widespread, nonselective distribution. Excretion is mainly in the feces, only about 10% being voided in urine. Some zinc excreted into the bile is reabsorbed in the intestine. Considerable zinc may be lost in sweat during periods of extreme heat or exercise.

Toxicity

With regard to industrial exposure, the metal fume fever resulting from inhalation of freshly formed fumes of zinc oxide presents the most significant effect. Zinc oxide is a product or byproduct in zinc smelting, the manufacture of zinc oxide and powder, the production of brass, and the melting of galvanized iron. These processes yield an aerosol of zinc oxide particles of about 1 μm (Athanassiadis, 1969). It has been suggested that only the freshly formed material is potent. However, it is most likely that particle size is the most important factor (Johnson and Stonehill, 1961). The disease has an acute onset, and although there is no form of chronic metal fume fever, repeated bouts are common (Doig and Challen, 1964). It appears that following the initial response resulting in "chills," resistance to the condition develops after a few days of exposure, but also wears off quickly, hence the term Monday morning fever. Metal fume fever may occur on the first day a new worker is exposed, and there appears to be no latent period for sensitization to occur. Since metal fume fever occurs in the absence of prior exposure, it has been suggested that the fever and other symptoms are most likely due to chemotaxis of polymorphs and not to an immunologic reaction. While zinc oxide fumes ate the most common cause of metal fume fever, inhalation of other metal oxides (i.e., copper, magnesium, cadmium, iron, manganese, nickel, selenium, tin, and antimony) may induce this reaction.

By inhalation, the characteristic metal fume fever occurs at concentrations between 1 and 35 mg/m^3. Workers develop fever, chills, muscular aches and pains, fatigue, and cough. Exposure to high concentrations of zinc may be lethal, or may cause acute damage to the mucous membranes of the nasopharynx and respiratory tract along with pneumonitis and pulmonary edema. Chronic exposure leads to anemia with lowered serum levels of iron, ferritin, and hemoglobin, plus depressed reduced cytochrome C and catalase enzyme activities. It is not certain whether these effects are secondary to decreased Cu absorption.

Short term exposure to zinc sulfate and zinc ammonium sulfate of about 1-2 mg/m^3 produced increased pulmonary air flow resistance in guinea pigs. However, the sulfate had the main responsibility for this effect (Amdur et al., 1978).

Long-term exposure of rats to zinc oxide (ZnO) at concentrations of 15 mg/m^3 for 8 hr daily up to 84 days gave rise to minor microscopical changes with signs of chronic inflammation and slight changes in two of the ten pulmonary function tests studied. Histological examination of the lungs from rats exposed to zinc stearate at 5 mg/m^3 for 3-5 months did not show any signs of fibrosis (Weber et al., 1976).

Cadmium

Industrial uses of cadmium include electroplating other metals (iron, steel, and copper) to inhibit corrosion, in alloys (e.g., Ni-Cd rechargeable batteries, Cu-Cd telephone wires), in pigments for glass and paint, in nuclear reactors as a neutron absorber, and in insecticides. The manufacture of aluminum solder, dental amalgams, incandescent lamps, smoke bombs, small-arms ammunition, and storage batteries provides additional opportunity for industrial exposure. Cadmium from industrial effluents as well as from motor vehicle exhausts contributes to air pollution.

Inhalation Exposure and Limits

A recent European study noted that atmospheric cadmium comes from the steel industry and incineration of waste, followed by volcanic activity and zinc production. In the United States an air sampling study showed that most samples were < 10 ng/m^3, the limit of detection. Tobacco smoke contains considerable cadmium, up to 0.1 μg in the mainstream smoke and 0.4-0.7 μg in the sidestream smoke per cigarette (Nandi et al., 1969; NIOSH, 1976a).

The threshold limit value as a time-weighted average in workroom air for an 8 hr day is 0.05 mg/m^3 for cadmium dust and salts; the short-term exposure limit is 0.2 mg/m^3 (ACGIH, 1983). The OSHA permissible exposure limit is 0.2 mg/m^3 for cadmium fumes (OSHA, 1981).

Absorption and Excretion

Cadmium fumes or salt aerosols are readily absorbed in the lung. Animal data, both from single and chronic exposure studies, indicate high absorption of cadmium, between 10 and 60% of the inhaled cadmium, depending on its chemical form, particle size, and where in the lung it is deposited. For finely dispersed cadmium aerosols, for example, exposure via cigarette smoking, it can be calculated, based on cadmium concentration in cigarette smoke and autopsy data from people smoking different quantities of cigarettes, that absorption is between 25 and 50% (Lewis et al., 1972; Friberg et al., 1974; Elinder et al., 1976).

Following chronic low-level exposure, cadmium is absorbed and transported to the liver where it stimulates the synthesis of metallothionein. Bound to this carrier molecule, cadmium is then transported via the blood throughout the body. Inhaled cadmium eventually accumulates in the liver, kidneys, and testes because of the inability of the renal system to clear itself of the metal. Approximately one third of the cadmium in the body will be found in the kidneys, and most of the rest of the body burden is contained in the liver and muscles. The accumulation in the kidneys is explained by the fact that cadmium metallothionein in plasma is filtered via the glomeruli and then reabsorbed in the tubuli as are other low molecular weight plasma proteins. Catabolism of the cadmium metallothionein takes place after reabsorption and the "free" cadmium stimulates synthesis of metallothionein in the kidney tubular cells and is bound again. It is thought that kidney damage is prevented by this binding. However, when a sufficient amount of kidney cadmium can no longer be bound by metallothionein, renal tubular damage occurs. The exact mechanisms by which renal tubular damage results still remain to be determined. Regardless of the mechanisms, there is sufficient evidence that after long-term exposure renal damage occurs when the cadmium concentration in the renal cortex exceeds a certain critical concentration. This concentration varies among animal species and among individuals. Excretion is slow, but constant, and occurs mainly via the feces and urine.

With industrial exposure to levels of 0.1 to 0.5 $\mu g/m^3$, as much as 2 to 10 μg/day may be retained in the lungs. It has been estimated that occupational exposure to 13 $\mu g/m^3$ for 25 years, is sufficient for the critical concentration of cadmium to be reached in the kidney cortex, assuming a biologic half-life of 19 years and a pulmonary absorption of 25% (Friberg et al., 1974).

Smoking tobacco may be an important route of exposure for the general population. Smoking one cigarette, generally containing 1-2 μg cadmium, results in the inhalation of about 0.1-0.2 μg of the metal. In addition, cigarettes may be easily contaminated by cadmium-containing dust in the workplace (Piscator et al., 1976). Thus, smokers always have an additional exposure to cadmium compared with nonsmokers in the same working environment. It is estimated that the body burden is about doubled for a smoker compared to a nonsmoker (50 mg Cd) (Lewis et al., 1972; Lauwerys, 1983). The normal clearance of inhaled and deposited particles is impaired in smokers (Camner and Philipson, 1972), and this too may predispose smokers to respiratory disease as a consequence of occupational exposure to cadmium.

Toxicity

Cadmium is highly toxic because there is no homeostatic control and Cd has a propensity for binding with thiol groups. The basic action is enzyme inactivation but it may also bind to DNA and RNA. The major nonindustrial exposure results from smoking. Inhalation of cadmium compounds can give rise to both acute and chronic effects in the respiratory system. The severe acute effects from inhalation of cadmium fumes, mainly cadmium oxide, are well established and have been known for a long time (Bulmer et al., 1938). Symptoms may not appear until 24 hours after exposure has terminated, which may cause difficulties in obtaining the proper diagnosis (Friberg et al., 1974). The predominant symptoms and signs are shortness of breath, general weakness, fever, and in some cases respiratory insufficiency with shock and death (Lucas et al., 1980). The initial symptoms are similar to metal fume fever, a benign condition which may result from exposure to zinc fumes (Stokinger, 1963). The cadmium-induced acute pulmonary disorder that develops later is a chemical pneumonitis or sometimes a pulmonary edema. Death may occur several days after exposures. If survival occurs, delayed lung effects such as perivascular and peribronchial fibrosis accompanied by emphysema may remain.

This type of effect may most frequently result from the inhalation of fumes generated by welding cadmium-containing materials or by smelting or soldering such materials, both under conditions of poor ventilation. Lethal exposure has been estimated at 50 mg Cd/m^3 for one hour with regard to cadmium oxide dust and about one-half that for the fume (Friberg et al., 1971). Particles of larger size and particles with very low solubility will probably be in the lower part of this range, while particles with high solubility and smaller diameter will be in the upper part.

Chronic low-dose inhalation exposure to cadmium leads to severe lung disease with emphysema and chronic inflammatory change in the respiratory system. There is a high frequency of lung and prostatic cancer among workers occupationally exposed to cadmium (Potts, 1965; Kipling and Waterhouse, 1967; Kazantzis and Armstrong, 1983; Sorahan and Waterhouse, 1983, 1985).

In rats and mice, there is a marked increase in susceptibility to bacterial infections shortly after exposure to cadmium oxides and cadmium chlorides (Gardner et al., 1977). The authors pointed out that enhanced mortality after bacterial infections occurred even at exposure levels in the order of 0.1 mg $CdCl_2/m^3$, which is considerably lower than the levels which give rise to edema.

Recently, Takenaka et al. (1983) have shown that inhalation of cadmium aerosol may cause lung cancer in Wistar rats. This is the first report of its kind, in which animals were chronically exposed to a respirable cadmium aerosol. The exposure levels used in this experiment were comparably low, and in fact were at or below the threshold limit value (TLV) for cadmium ($50 \mu g/m^3$) still in use in most countries. As a result of these data, cadmium in the form of a cadmium chloride aerosol must definitely be regarded as a highly carcinogenic agent in animals.

Mercury

Mercury has widespread use in the scientific and electronic industries, chlorine-alkali-acid manufacture, as a catalyst in polyurethane foams, industrial and control instruments, and explosives. The chemical form of mercury to which exposure occurs is a very significant factor. Occupational exposure to mercury vapor is the most common inorganic form of mercury exposure. This type of exposure was first reported in connection with mining and historically was associated with the fur and felt hat industry, although other types of workers may suffer significant exposure. Although similar to Cd in toxicity, Hg is more important because it is used in greater bulk, in more varied industrial settings and has four metallic forms with differing toxic potential: metallic (Hg^0), mercurous (Hg^{1+}), mercuric (Hg^{2+}), and alkyl mercury.

Inhalation Exposure and Limits

Airborne mercury is predominantly elemental. The average concentration is about 20 ng/m^3, with variations from 0.5 to 50 ng/m^3. Much higher concentrations, up to 0.8 mg/m^3, have been observed near mercury mines (Berlin, 1977).

The threshold limit value as a time-weighted average in workroom air for an 8 hr day is 0.1 mg/m^3 for aryl and inorganic mercury compounds; 0.05 mg/m^3 for mercury vapor (all forms except alkyl); and 0.01 mg/m^3 for alkyl mercury; the short-term exposure limit for alkyl mercury is 0.03 mg/m^3/15 min (ACGIH, 1983). The OSHA permissible exposure limit is 0.01 mg/m^3 for alkyl mercury (OSHA, 1981).

Absorption and Excretion

The metal (Hg^0) vaporizes at room temperature and exposure to mercury vapor results in absorption via the lungs, but some mercury may also be absorbed through the skin. Elemental mercury vapor undergoes almost complete absorption from the inhaled air (Doull et al., 1980). In contrast, absorption of elemental mercury after oral ingestion is minimal. It is possible that inhaling mercury is more harmful than ingesting it. After absorption from the lungs, it exists physically dissolved in blood for a short time, in part as the oxide, and in this form, it easily crosses the blood-brain barrier and placenta (Stahl, 1969). Of the salts, mercurous (Hg^{1+}) salts are poorly soluble, whereas mercuric (Hg^{2+}) salts are absorbed. Organic mercury compounds (i.e., methylmercury salts) can also be readily absorbed through the lung. The amount of alkyl mercury salts absorbed depends upon particle size and their deposition in the respiratory tract.

All forms are distributed throughout the body with concentration in the liver and kidneys. Inorganic Hg has greater affinity toward thiol groups of soft tissue proteins, whereas alkyl Hg is preferentially concentrated in nervous tissue and red blood cells (Iverson et al., 1973). Alkyl Hg is approximately 100 times more soluble in lipid than water. Excretion is predominantly fecal with a significant proportion in the urine.

Toxicity

The toxicity of Hg salts has been known since 1500 B.C. Mercury binds with a variety of terminal groups and has a particularly high affinity for sulfhydryl groups in proteins and progressively less for other groups: $SH > CONH_2 > NH_2 > COOH > PO_4$. The mechanisms are not understood, but mercury salts are almost general-purpose enzyme inhibitors (USEPA, 1980a; Berlin, 1977). In particular, glucose-6-phosphatase, alkaline phosphatase, adenosine triphosphatase, succinic dehydrogenase, and Δ-amino-levulinic acid dehydrogenase are inactivated. This leads to blocking of active glucose transport into cells and to altered membrane permeability.

Although rare, metallic Hg can produce acute toxicity with severe vomiting, dehydration, coma, and death. Acute poisoning in humans has resulted from exposure to 1.2 to 8.5 mg Hg/m^3. Acute symptoms are related to pulmonary effects but are relatively rare. Experimentally, a massive single exposure causes severe hemorrhage of the kidneys, brain, heart, and colon, as well as the lungs.

High levels of mercury vapor are extremely irritating to the lung and cause erosive bronchitis and bronchiolitis with interstitial pneumonia (Berlin, 1977; Gerstner and Huff, 1977).

Chronic low-level exposure by elemental mercury vapor leads to neurotoxicity (mercurialism) which is often of delayed onset. The classic syndrome is characterized by psychic and emotional disturbances. There may be increased irritability, combativeness, defective patterns, ocular disturbances, and muscular tremors. These symptoms tend to regress very slowly, if at all, when the exposure ceases.

Inorganic Hg produces similar effects acutely, in addition, excessive salivation and diarrhea. The more common chronic inorganic poisoning has its main effect on the central nervous system. Symptoms relating to psychological and emotional dysfunction include irritability, combativeness, and varied types of nervous anxiety termed erythism.

Organic mercurials cause selective brain damage, especially the cerebellum and some parts of the cerebral cortex, resulting in impaired sensation, particularly of vision, with later paralysis and coma.

E. Group IIIA (Al, Ga, In, and Tl)

These metals rarely cause intoxication. Aluminum, the most common metal in the earth's crust (8.13%) is virtually nontoxic, whereas indium and thallium exposure are rare because of limited usage. Thallium compounds are extremely toxic. Total production, however, is unlikely to exceed a few thousand tons per year.

Aluminum

The use of metallic aluminum and its compounds is very extensive. Aluminum is widely used as a building material and for other uses where light weight and corrosion resistance are important. Aluminum oxide has industrial uses as an abrasive and catalyst. Medically, various soluble salts of aluminum have been used as astringents, styptics, and antiseptics. The insoluble salts are used as antacids and as antidiarrheal agents.

Inhalation Exposure and Limits

Inhalation of aluminum compounds has been used in the prevention and treatment of silicosis. Nonurban air usually contains < 0.5 μg Al/m^3, while urban air contains up to 10 μg/m^3 (Norseth, 1977).

The threshold limit value (TLV) as a time-weighted average in workroom air for an 8 hr day is 10 mg/m^3 for aluminum metal and oxide; the short-term exposure limit is 20 mg/m^3 for 15 min. The TLV is 2 mg/m^3 for aluminum soluble salts and alkyls, 5 mg/m^3 for aluminum pyro powders and welding fumes (ACGIH, 1983).

Absorption and Excretion

Aluminum has been demonstrated in all human organs analyzed, but the lungs invariably show the highest concentration, about 200-300 mg/kg. Most other organs are reported to contain 1/10 or less of the aluminum concentration of lung tissue. Aluminum in the lung is presumably the result of local deposition from inhaled air. Following inhalation, most of the insoluble Al salts are retained in the lung for a long time; soluble compounds are slowly absorbed into the blood. The Al in the lung tissues of industrial workers in Al refineries increases with duration of exposure. Aluminum is not absorbed readily through the skin.

Toxicity

Occupational exposure to aluminum and aluminum compounds is widespread, but the exposure has only to a limited degree turned out to be of toxicological importance.

Following inhalation, dusts of Al, Al$_2$O$_3$, and other Al compounds are retained in the lungs. In rats, the initial response to this deposit was the proliferation of macrophages within the alveolar spaces, resulting in lipoid pneumonia (Christie et al., 1963); prolonged exposure caused focal deposits of hyaline material in alveolar walls. Chronic inhalation of extremely fine dusts of Al compounds by humans caused a toxic pulmonary reaction; an interstitial fibrosis of a nonnodular type called Shaver's disease developed in the lungs (Shaver and Riddell, (1947).

Shaver's disease is the only aluminum-induced industrial disease. It may be the result of bauxite (the principal ore of aluminum) fume and the use of abrasive wheels containing aluminum. Exposure to the fume may produce weakness, fatigue, and chest x-rays may reveal extensive fibrosis with large blebs. Spontaneous pneumothorax is a frequent complication. Silicon may also play a contributing role in the disease because it is frequently inhaled along with aluminum in workers exposed to bentonite (an aluminosilicate clay). Fibrosis has also been noted after aluminum dust inhalation, but the mean exposure level recorded was 95 mg/m^3 respirable dust.

Gross et al. (1973) could not demonstrate fibrosis following inhalation of metallic aluminum powders in hamsters, guinea pigs, or rats, but fibrosis was demonstrated after intratracheal injections of high doses.

The main health hazard in primary aluminum production appears to be related to fluoride exposure, not exposure to aluminum or aluminum oxide. Both gaseous and particulate fluorides are found in the working atmosphere as well as in the emissions.

Gallium

Gallium is obtained as a byproduct of copper, zinc, lead, and aluminum. It is used in high-temperature thermometers, as a substitute for mercury in arc lamps, in the manufacture of alloys, and as a liquid sealant for glass joints and vacuum equipment. Gallium arsenide and phosphide are used in light-emitting diodes (LEDs).

Absorption, Excretion, and Toxicity

There are no reported adverse effects of gallium following industrial exposure.

Indium

Indium is recovered as a byproduct in the manufacture of other metals, chiefly zinc, but also tin, copper, and lead. Its industrial uses are in electroplating of nontarnishing silver and copper plate, corrosion-resistant alloys, glass manufacture, in nuclear energy processes, and in the manufacture of containers for foodstuffs.

Inhalation Exposure and Limits

Indium's ubiquitous presence in urban air, although at levels much lower than other industrial metals, probably reflects the fact that indium is a common contaminant of zinc. Elevated indium levels in ambient air might also be expected in areas near lead, copper, and tin smelters. In fact, concentrations up to 43 ng/m^3 have been reported, as compared to 0.04 to 0.2 ng/m^3 in rural and urban air (Smith et al., 1978).

The threshold limit value as a time-weighted average in workroom air for an 8 hr day is 0.1 mg In/m^3 for indium compounds; the short-term exposure limit is 0.3 mg In/m^3 (ACGIH, 1983).

Absorption, Excretion, and Toxicity

Indium compounds are moderately absorbed after inhalation. After one-time inhalation or intratracheal intubation of $In(OH)_3$ or indium citrate complex, at least 30% is absorbed within 8 days. The biological half-life for $InCl_3$ in the lungs is less than 1 hr, but InO_3 is absorbed much more slowly. The biological half-life for most indium compounds is about 2 months (Smith et al., 1978). Rats exposed 4 hr daily for 3 months to 64 mg $In_2 O_3/m^3$ showed marked growth depression; increased lung weight, enlargement of the tracheobronchial lymph nodes, and marked alteration of the alveolar walls.

No industrial injury has been reported in workers exposed to indium or its compounds that could be attributed solely to them. However, since other very toxic elements such as lead and arsenic are present in greater concentration (Smith et al., 1978), exposure to indium during its refining, while electroplating and while soldering must be considered hazardous.

Thallium

Thallium is used to make stainless steel alloys with Ag, corrosion-resistant alloys with Pb, and Hg-Tl alloy for subzero operating switches and low-temperature thermometers. Thallium salts are used as catalysts in organic reactions and firecrackers. Thallium oxide, with its high coefficient of refraction, is used in optical lenses and artificial gems. $Tl_2 SO_4$ is a rodenticide and $Tl_2 CO_3$ is a fungicide.

Thallium and its salts are considered to be industrial health hazards in coal, from its smoke as well as in the mining and refining of coal; Pb, Cd and As contaminants potentiate Tl toxicity.

Inhalation Exposure and Limits

In a review of environmental exposure to trace metals, Smith and Carson (1977) reported ambient air concentrations of thallium, 0.04 to 0.48 ng Tl/m^3, for Chadron, Nebraska, only

The OSHA permissible exposure limit and the threshold limit value (TLV) for thallium compounds as a time-weighted average in workroom air for an 8 hr day is 0.1 mg/m^3 (with a skin exposure warning) (ACGIH, 1983).

Absorption, Excretion, and Toxicity

Following inhalation of thallium oxides and salts, Tl is rapidly absorbed from mucous membranes of the respiratory tract, mouth, and lungs. After absorption into the blood, Tl^+ is rapidly distributed to the tissues; part of the Tl^+ is absorbed into the erythrocytes (Lauwerys, 1983). The transport of Tl in the blood appears to be in the ionic form; it has been shown that Tl^+ does not combine in vitro with the serum albumin or other proteins. Thallium easily passes through the blood-brain and placental barriers. In mammals, Tl^+ excretion is slow and prolonged, although Tl^+ appears in the urine a few hours after absorption. The amount of Tl^+ excreted in the urine is about three times that excreted fecally (Smith and Carson, 1977).

Although the specific effects resulting from the inhalation of Tl have yet to be determined, many reviews of the physiology and toxicology of Tl following other routes of administration in both humans and animals are available (Prick et al., 1955; Arena, 1974; Cavanagh et al., 1974; Smith and Carson, 1977; Stokinger, 1981).

F. Group IIIB (Sc, Y, Lanthanides, and Actinides)

Based on few reports, these metals are considered to be only slightly toxic because of their low solubility and rarity of exposure. A major exception is thorium because of its radioactivity.

Inhalation exposures in humans, while infrequent, have caused sensitivity to heat, itching, and an increased awareness of odor and taste. In animals, intratracheal administration or inhalation exposure to fluorides or oxides, or a combination thereof, resulted in transient pneumonitis, subacute bronchiolitis, and regional bronchiolar stricturing (Stokinger, 1981). Cancers of the blood vessels, kidney, liver, and other organs have occurred after exposure to thorium used as a radiopaque medium (Stokinger, 1981). For example, Verhaack et al. (1974) reported 45 cases of tumors of the renal pelvis related to Thorotrast pyelography. The severity of the neoplastic effect, however, did not appear to be dose related.

Lanthanum oxide fume and dust generated from carbon-arc lighting used to produce intense white illuminations in the lithographic industry may be responsible for worker's frequent complaints of headache and nausea (Stokinger, 1981).

G. Group IVA (Ge, Sn, and Pb)

Germanium and tin are of low solubility and toxicity except as organic compounds when they cause neurotoxicity.

Germanium

Germanium is produced as a byproduct of the production of electrolytic zinc. It finds use as a semiconductor in the manufacture of electronic components (transistors, diodes). Because of its high refractive index, germanium glass is used in wide-angle camera lens, microscope objectives, and infrared lenses. Germanium is used as a low-temperature catalyst in the hydrogenation of coal.

Inhalation Exposure and Limits

Because of the relatively high (1.6 to 7.5%) germanium concentration in coal, one would expect significant amounts of germanium to be present in urban air. The threshold limit value as a time-weighted average in workroom air for an 8 hr day is 0.6 mg/m^3 for germanium tetrahydride; the short-term exposure limit is 1.8 mg/m^3 (ACGIH, 1983).

Absorption, Excretion, and Toxicity

Animal experiments show that germanium compounds, both inorganic and organic, are rapidly and almost completely absorbed from the lungs. The distribution among organs to tissues is fairly uniform and there is no evidence of preferential uptake or accumulation. Germanium is rapidly excreted, mostly in the urine. In rabbits and dogs, over 75% was excreted within 72 hr (Browning, 1969).

Germanium tetrachloride is a strong irritant of the respiratory system, possibly because of easy hydrolysis producing HCl. In mice, the inhalation of high concentrations of GeCl$_4$ produced changes in the respiratory system, including necrosis of the tracheal mucosa, bronchitis, and interstitial pneumonia. There is no information on local effects of germanium compounds in the respiratory system in man. Exposure to germanium is not considered an industrial hazard, nor has it been implicated in any chronic diseases of humans.

Tin

Most tin is used as the metal in the manufacture of tin plate (a protective coating). Most of the rest is used in alloys, including solder, pewter, bronze, and brass. Stannous and stannic chlorides are used in dyeing textiles. Stannous fluoride is used in tooth pastes. Organic tin compounds have been used as antimicrobials, in antifouling paints, and as heat stabilizers in plastics (e.g., polyvinyl).

Inhalation Exposure and Limits

It has been estimated that the general population may inhale up to 7 μg Sn/day from ambient air (Snyder et al., 1975).

The threshold limit value (TLV) as a time-weighted average in workroom air for an 8 hr day is 2 mg Sn/m^3 for tin metal and inorganic compounds; the short-term exposure limit is 4 mg/m^3 for 15 min. For organotin compounds, the values are 0.1 and 0.2 mg Sn/m^3, respectively. The OSHA permissible exposure limit is 2 mg/m^3 for inorganic tin compounds except oxides (OSHA, 1981). NIOSH (1976b) has recommended a level of 0.1 mg Sn/m^2 for organotin compounds.

Absorption, Excretion, and Toxicity

The toxicity of tin after inhalation is low. In exposed workers, chronic inhalation of tin oxide dust or fumes leads to "stannosis," a benign pneumoconiosis without tissue reaction or pulmonary dysfunction (Barnes and Stoner, 1959). There are no data from animal experiments or from studies on human beings on deposition or absorption of inhaled inorganic tin or organotin compounds. The majority of inhaled tin or its salts remains in the lungs, most extracellularly, with some in the macrophages, in the form of SnO_2. The organic tins, particularly triethyltin, may be somewhat better absorbed and are considerably more toxic when taken orally (Piscator, 1977). Stannic hydride, an unstable gas, is more toxic than arsine and primarily affects the central nervous system.

Lead

Lead has been known to man since 2500 B.C. Lead toxicity, saturnism, was recorded by ancient Greek and Arab physicians. This metal has numerous commercial applications due to its physical properties and relative chemical inertness. Metallic lead is used in the manufacture of pipes, cisterns, lead shots, bullets, and linotype metal, and in alloys with antimony, tin, and copper for manufacture of accumulator plates in storage batteries. Unfortunately, inorganic and organic lead compounds are highly toxic.

Inhalation Exposure and Limits

The average atmospheric lead concentration in cities lies between 0.02 to 10 μg Pb/m^3, due to automobile exhausts and various industrial sources. Mid-ocean, baseline concentrations are about 0.001 $\mu g/m^3$ (Tsuchiya, 1977; USEPA, 1980d).

In the Northern Hemisphere, over 5 million tons of Pb have been used from 1920 through 1970 in automobile engines as tetraethyl lead. This widespread contamination of the environment amounts, over the 50-year period, to 120 pounds of Pb per square mile. Historically, the eccentric behavior of famous painters (e.g., Francisco Goya) has been attributed to their accidental ingestion and inhalation of lead pigments in the paints (Stoll, 1972). Today, however, the use of many lead compounds, such as inorganic pigments and tetraethyl lead for gasoline, is decreasing.

In the workplace, lead smelting and refining are probably the most hazardous operations with respect to exposure to lead. Mean concentrations of lead in air may reach 80-4000 $\mu g/m^3$ (WHO, 1977).

The threshold limit value as a time-weighted average in workroom air for an 8 hr day is 0.15 mg/m^3 for lead, inorganic dusts, and fumes; the short-term exposure limit is 0.45 mg/m^3 for 15 min (ACGIH, 1983). The OSHA permissible exposure limit is 0.2 mg/m^3 (OSHA, 1981), but NIOSH (1978a) has recommended <0.1 mg/m^3.

Absorption and Excretion

Since solubility conditions for deposited lead particles are very good in the alveolar region, exposure to the dust of the metal or $PbCl_2$, $PbBr_2$, or PbO_2 leads to high absorption—possibly as much as 90% if particles are less than 0.1 μm in diameter (Lauwerys, 1983). Tetraethyl lead (TEL) is readily absorbed through the lungs owing to the solubility of TEL in lipids and to its diffusibility. With a lead concentration of 2 μg/m^3 in the air and an inhaled volume of 15 m^3, the daily absorption of lead by an adult through inhalation is approximately 10 μg.

Urinary excretion is significant when there is an elevated level of blood Pb (Goyer, 1971).

Toxicity

The toxicology of lead is well known and documented. At low doses, Pb has a generalized stimulatory effect with increased DNA and protein synthesis, cell replication and production of red blood cells. The toxic effects of lead are mainly due to the inactivation of certain enzymes (Tsuchiya, 1977; Cullen et al., 1983). This inactivation is effected through the binding to the sulfhydryl groups of the protein components of the enzyme through a replacement of the other metal ions necessary for certain metabolic processes. Toxicity is associated with its divalent form and resembles the action of group IIB metals which is related to stable ligand formation with thiol, carboxylic, and phosphate groups. Most of these are membrane bound, particularly the phosphate ligands such as Na/K ATPase. There is little binding with amino and imidazole groups. The toxic action is directly related to the ready diffusibility of lead compounds and the lead content of individual tissues, particularly their level in the circulating blood. Total body content has little relation to toxicity because the bulk of Pb is fixed and inactive in bone. Thus, 90-95% of the total lead content in the body is an inactive store of lead in the adult skeleton. However, in children up to the age of 6, the intensive bone metabolism causes a low rate of lead deposition in the bone tissue. It is estimated that only about 64% of the total lead in the body of children is deposited in the bones. Therefore, children react in a particularly sensitive way to lead pollution and represent a high-risk group. A third important point is that toxicity has a cumulative effect.

Acute Toxicity

Acute toxicity is uncommon except for exposure to high concentrations of Pb dusts. Most symptoms relate to general malaise, gastrointestinal upset, and central nervous system symptoms, particularly convulsions and stupor. This progression usually ends in death.

There is no evidence that inhaled lead has local effects on the respiratory system in man, but inhalation of lead (10 μg/m^3 for 3-12 months) by rats reduced the number of macrophages that could be washed from the lungs (Bingham, 1970). Damage of alveolar macrophages by lead has been demonstrated in vitro (Beck et al., 1973).

Lead compounds are not considered carcinogenic to man, although there are reports in which benign and malignant tumors were produced in experimental animals (Tsuchiya, 1977; Stokinger, 1981).

H. Group IVB (Ti, Zr, and Hf)

Titanium

Most titanium is used, as the dioxide, in pigments. The metal is used structurally where its high strength and light weight outweigh its high cost (e.g., in military aircraft and missiles.) It is also used as a deoxidizer, in permanent magnets, in heat-resistant alloys, in pigments, in welding rods, in electrodes, in lamp filaments, and in surgical appliances.

Inhalation Exposure and Limits

Titanium is a contaminant of urban air with concentrations up to 1.1 μg Ti/m^3 (Snyder et al., 1975). Titanium dioxide is classified as a "nuisance particulate" in the workplace (ACGIH, 1983).

Absorption and Excretion

Titanium compounds that are common in the environment are thought to be poorly absorbed upon inhalation, but no quantitative information is available. The estimated soft tissue body burden of titanium is 9 mg. Most of it is in the lungs and lymph nodes, probably as a result of inhalation exposure (Snyder et al., 1975). Inhaled titanium tends to remain in the lungs for long periods. It has been estimated that about one third of the inhaled titanium is retained in the lungs. Newborns have little titanium reserves. Titanium can be absorbed and concentrated from the environment, and lung burdens tend to increase with age.

Toxicity

Titanium dioxide has been considered physiologically inert by all routes (ingestion, inhalation, dermal, and subcutaneous). Previous reports of pulmonary injury following exposure to titanium dioxide are now thought to be due to contamination (e.g., alumina, silica) (Stokinger, 1981). The metal and other salts are also relatively nontoxic except for titanic acid, which, as might be expected, will produce irritation. Inhalation of TiCl$_4$ by dogs caused severe bronchitis, edema, and death, but the toxicity was ascribed to the HCl released following hydrolysis (Lawson, 1961).

Zirconium

Zirconium is used in nuclear reactors as a shielding material for fuel rods, in metal alloys, as a catalyst in organic reactions, in the manufacture of water-repellent textiles, in dyes, in pigments on glass and ceramics, in abrasives, and cigarette lighter flints. Zirconium carbonate and oxide are used therapeutically for dermatitis from poison ivy. Zirconium oxychloride (ZrOCl$_2$) has been used as an antiperspirant; their use in aerosols was banned in 1974.

Inhalation Exposure and Limits

Few data are available on zirconium in ambient air, but it is expected to be present because of its high natural background concentration in soils. For zirconium compounds, the threshold limit value (TLV) as a time-weighted average in workroom air for an 8 hr day is 5 mg Zr/m^3; the short-term exposure limit is 10 mg Zr/m^3 for 15 min (ACGIH, 1983). The OSHA permissible exposure limit is 5 mg Zr/m^3 (OSHA, 1981).

Absorption, Excretion, and Toxicity

Although of low toxicity due to low solubility because of inactivation to protein, zirconium produces hypersensitivity reactions in the lung from use of deodorants and hair sprays. Retention in rat lungs is high following intratracheal instillation (Morishige, 1968). In guinea pigs exposed by nose only to ^{95}Zr oxalate in air for 0.5 hr, 12.1% of the total dose was found in the blood immediately following exposure while 17.8% was in other internal organs (Smith and Carson, 1978). Inhalation exposure of $ZrCl_4$ (6 mg Zr/m^3) for 60 days produced slight decrease in hemoglobin and red blood cell count in dogs and increased mortality in rats and guinea pigs. Zirconium oxide at 75 mg/m^3 caused no effect (Spiegl et al., 1956). Pulmonary granulomas developed in rabbits inhaling zirconium lactate aerosol (Prior et al., 1960).

Hafnium

Hafnium does not occur free in nature and does not form any of its own mineral ores; it occurs as up to 1-3% of the total Zr in zirconium minerals. Hafnium is used extensively as shielding material and as control rods in thermal nuclear reactors. Hafnium can absorb and give up heat twice as fast as Zr and Ti and thus has also been used as a construction material in space technology and in jet engines.

Inhalation Exposure and Limits

The threshold limit value (TLV) as a time-weighted average in workroom air for an 8 hr day is 0.5 mg/m^3 for hafnium; the short-term exposure limit is 0.5 mg/m^3 (OSHA, 1981).

Absorption, Excretion, and Toxicity

Hafnium is not essential to man or animals, and it is not reported to be involved in any biochemical systems; there are very few published reports about Hf metabolism. Toxicology studies on Hf are also rare. Lack of toxicology data on Hf leads to speculation on Hf toxicity. Owing to its similarity with Zr and Ti in chemical properties, one may assume that its metabolism in living tissues is similar but less traumatic because of the increased stability of the oxides formed. The higher electropositivity of Hf may render the chelation complexes of Hf with

OH-containing ligands very stable, and thereby confer somewhat higher toxicity to Hf than Ti or Zr.

I. Group VA (As, Sb, and Bi)

Arsenic

The major use of arsenic has been in the form of its compounds whose toxicity makes them valuable as insecticides, rodenticides, weed killers, and wood preservatives. Lead-arsenic alloys are also used because they are more rigid than pure lead. Antifouling paints and materials to control sludge formation in lubricating oils also contain arsenic.

Arsenic has been used therapeutically for more than 2000 years (Frost, 1967). Medicinal uses of arsenic have ranged from treatment of syphilis to use as a tonic. Arsenicals act locally and are slow corrosives; they have been used in the treatment of skin cancer. In the United States there has been a decline in the use of arsenicals in human medicine but the decrease has not been as great in veterinarian or agricultural use (e.g., sodium arsenite as a weed killer).

Inhalation Exposure and Limits

Arsenic is released into air by the combustion of coal, and by the smelting of ores or the use of pesticides containing it. The average level in the United States is $0.2 \mu g/m^3$, but near a copper smelter it has been much higher, $2.5 \mu g/m^3$ (Tsuchiya et al., 1977).

The threshold limit value (TLV) as a time-weighted average in workroom air for an 8 hr day is 0.2 mg As/m^3 for the metal and soluble compounds (ACGIH, 1983). The OSHA permissible exposure limit is 0.5 mg As/m^3 for organic arsenic and 0.01 mg/m^3 for inorganic arsenic (OSHA, 1981). NIOSH (1975) has recommended 0.002 mg/m^3 as the permissible exposure limit for inorganic arsenic.

Absorption, Excretion, and Toxicity

Although absorption is highly dependent on the chemical and physical form of the inhaled arsenic compounds, the common forms (particularly arsenic trioxide, the most prevalent) are fully absorbed from the lungs and mucous surfaces of the respiratory tract. It is generally true that trivalent arsenic compounds (arsenites) are more toxic than pentavalent compounds and that natural oxidation factors the conversion of trivalent arsenic to the pentavalent form.

Arsenites bind to tissue proteins and are concentrated in the leukocytes. They accumulate in the body primarily in the liver, muscles, hair, nails, and skin perhaps because of combination with sulfhydryl groups. Arsenic is excreted in the urine, the feces, and by the dermis as shed skin, hairs and nails (Tsuchiya et al., 1977; USEPA, 1980c).

While there has been some controversy, the epidemiologic evidence indicates that industrial and environmental exposure to inorganic arsenic compounds is implicated in cancer of the skin and respiratory tract (IARC, 1980b). Workers who have been exposed to inhalation of inorganic arsenic compounds in copper smelters, in gold mines, in agricultural operations (e.g., sheep-dip workers; vintners), and in manufacture of pesticides have increased incidences of lung cancers. Konetzke (1974) has tabulated 312 cases of lung cancer in workers who were occupationally exposed to arsenic compounds. Blejer and Wagner (1976) have reviewed 11 epidemiological studies from 1948 to 1975. Nine of the 11 studies showed, initially or upon review, significant excess mortality from respiratory cancer. In two studies, there appeared to be a dose-response relationship between arsenic exposure and lung cancer mortality. Blot and Fraumeni (1975) have reported increased mortality rates from lung cancer during 1950 to 1969 among men and women who resided in counties of the United States where copper, lead, or zinc refineries were located. Blot and Fraumeni have suggested that arsenic pollution of air in neighborhoods of the refineries may have been responsible for the increased mortality from lung cancer.

Arsine (AsH_3), the hydride of arsenic, is one of the more toxic arsenic compounds. Arsine may be generated when acids are combined with arsenic-containing metals. Poisoning by arsine is the principal source of industrial arsenic poisoning today and has been reported in connection with the refining or processing of tin, lead, and zinc. Poisonings from this source have dire consequences because arsine causes severe and extensive hemolysis, and the inadequacy of available therapy. Exposures as low as 10 ppm have produced delirium, coma, and death. If the exposure is not fatal, the signs of chronic arsenic poisoning may appear. Chronic inhalation of AsH_3 at subtoxic levels by laboratory animals leads to hemolysis of erythrocytes, leading to death from chemical asphyxia. Irritation from arsine also results in pulmonary edema.

Antimony

Antimony is alloyed with lead, copper, and other metals. Certain Sb compounds are used for flameproof textiles and for ceramics and glassware, pigments, and antiparasitic drugs. Uses of alloys include solder, ammunition, bearing metals, and lead storage batteries.

Inhalation Exposure and Limits

Tobacco contains 0.1 mg Sb/kg dry wt, about 20% of which is inhaled while smoking (Elinder and Friberg, 1977).

The threshold limit value as a time-weighted average in workroom air for an 8 hr day is 0.5 mg/m^3 for antimony and compounds and Sb_2O_3. Although no exposure is recommended in Sb_2O_3 production based on its carcinogenic potential in humans. The TLV for stibine (SbH_3), the volatile hydride, is also 0.5 mg/m³. Its short-term exposure limit is 1.5 m/m³ (ACGIH, 1983). Stibine gas exposure is a serious exposure risk when lead-acid storage batteries are charged in a closed area. The OSHA permissible limit for antimony and compounds is 0.5 Sb/m³ (OSHA, 1981).

Absorption, Excretion, and Toxicity

Inhalation studies with dogs suggest rapid absorption from the lungs and enhanced urinary excretion (Brieger et al., 1954). Urinary excretion is apparently higher for Sb(V) than for Sb(III) compounds. Workers exposed to ~3 mg Sb/m³ have 0.8 to 9.6 mg Sb/liter in their urine, much higher than normal (~0.5 to 2.6 μg/liter (Elinder and Friberg, 1977).

Acute effects in humans from inhalation exposure to $SbCl_3$ at 73 mg/m³ were irritation and soreness of the upper respiratory tract. After exposure to unknown high concentrations of $SbCl_5$, three workers developed severe pulmonary edema, and two died. Workers with heavy exposure to antimony fumes developed abdominal cramps, diarrhea, and vomiting (Elinder and Friberg, 1977).

Guinea pigs inhaling Sb_2O_3 at 45 mg/m³ for 33 to 609 hr showed signs of interstitial pneumonia. Rats and rabbits inhaling 3.1 and 5.6 mg Sb/m³ as Sb_2S_3 for 6 weeks developed parenchymatous degeneration of the myocardium (Elinder and Friberg, 1977).

Pneumoconiosis and obstructive lung diseases have been observed after longterm occupational exposure. Among antimony trioxide workers, the incidences of pneumoconiosis and emphysema were 21% and 42%, respectively. Rats exposed to unknown concentrations of Sb_2O_3 for up to 14 months developed pneumonitis, lipoid pneumonia, fibrous thickening of alveolar walls, and focal fibrosis (Elinder and Friberg, 1977).

In a study of about 1000 workers, between 1925 and 1971, at an antimony and zircon works, 15 workers died, a death rate about twice as high as the local death rate for lung cancer (Stokinger, 1981).

Bismuth

The primary U.S. source of bismuth is as a byproduct of the refining of lead and copper ores. Bismuth is used to produce low-melting alloys for use in fusible elements of specialized products such as sprinklers. It is also added to steel and iron to produce castings that can be machined more easily. The oxide and nitrate forms are used in glass and ceramics manufacture.

Inhalation Exposure and Limits

Ambient air in the United States contains <0.002 to 0.03 μg Bi/m³ (Snyder et al., 1975). The threshold limit value for bismuth telluride, Bi_2Te_3, as a time-weighted average in workroom air for an 8 hr day is 10 mg/m^3 and 20 mg/m^3 for the short-term exposure limit (ACGIH, 1983). The corresponding values for the Se-doped compounds are 5 and 10 mg/m^3.

Absorption, Excretion, and Toxicity

Humans exposed to $Bi_2 Te_3$ have foul breath, but no adverse health effects. Mild and reversible granulomatous lesions but no fibrosis were seen in laboratory animals exposed to daily inhalations of a mixture of $Bi_2 Te_3$ doped with $Bi_2 Se_3$, SnTe, and Te for 1 year. When exposed to $Bi_2 Te_3$ alone, only "inert" dust responses were seen in the lungs (Stokinger, 1981).

J. Group VB (V and Ta)

Vanadium

Vanadium is used extensively in the steel industry to increase hardness, malleability, and resistance to fatigue. Vanadium oxide is used as a catalyst in sulfuric and nitric acid manufacture. Vanadium compounds are also used as mordants in dyeing and printing cotton and for fixing aniline black on silk. Ammonium metavanadate, $NH_4 VO_3$, may be present in quick-drying inks.

Inhalation Exposure and Limits

Sources of vanadium in ambient air are combustion of coal, crude oils, and undersulfurized heavy fuel oils. Twice as much V appears in the air during the heating season as during spring and summer. In cities of northeast United States, ambient air concentrations have averaged up to 1320 ng V/m^3. Average concentrations in the west and midwest range up to 22 ng V/m^3 (NAS, 1974b).

The threshold limit value as a time-weighted average in workroom air for an 8 hr day is 0.05 mg $V_2 O_5$/m^3 for vanadium respirable dust and fume (ACGIH, 1983). The OSHA permissible exposure limit is 0.1 mg $V_2 O_5$/m^3 for vanadium dust, 0.5 mg $V_2 O_5$/m^3 for vanadium fume (OSHA, 1981).

Absorption, Excretion, and Toxicity

After inhalation or intratracheal instillation, V absorption from the lungs into the blood is more rapid than either intestinal absorption or absorption from parenteral sites. After rabbits were exposed to $V_2 O_5$ dust, V was found almost immediately in the urine (Massman, 1956), confirming the quick absorption of V compounds. Excretion of V is mostly in the urine, with smaller amounts in feces (Stokinger, 1981).

Industrial exposures are generally described as acute episodes with relapses and sometimes chronic coughing and chronic bronchitis as sequelae. Symptoms, generally upper and lower respiratory tract irritation, do not appear until after repeated exposure to vanadium compounds for a few days or a week, which may indicate development of delayed hypersensitivity. Respiratory symptoms are disabling (Stokinger, 1981).

Irritation of the human respiratory tract occurs with concentrations of $V_2 O_5$ and $NH_4 VO_3$ as low as 0.04 mg V/m^3 and 5-min exposure to 0.6 mg V/m^3 as $V_2 O_5$ is sufficient to produce coughing and rales. Acute exposure to the oxides and vanadates cause wheezing, rales, rhonchi, and chest pain. Ferro-vanadium exposure does not cause such severe symptoms. Chest pain, asthma-like bronchitis, and emphysema (although not conclusive) have been reported in workers exposed to vanadium compounds for longer than 6 months (NIOSH, 1977b).

Tantalum

Tantalum is used in the manufacture of capacitors and other electronic components, corrosion-resistant alloys for use in acid-proof chemical equipment, steel alloys, and in surgical and prosthetic appliances.

Inhalation Exposure and Limits
The threshold limit value as a time-weighted average in workroom air for an 8 hr day is 5 mg/m^3 for tantalum; the short-term exposure limit is 10 mg/m^3 for 15 min (ACGIH, 1983). The OSHA permissible exposure limit is 5 mg/m^3 (OSHA, 1981).

Absorption, Excretion, and Toxicity
Little has been reported about the absorption of tantalum. There appears to be early, rapid tracheobronchial clearance with inhaled tantalum, but prolonged (> 12 months) time is required for alveolar clearance (Stokinger, 1981).

Tantalum appears to be nontoxic in chronic studies. A study of workers exposed to tantalum carbide dust in the hard-metal cutting tool industry combined with a histological study of the lungs of rats similarly exposed found that tantalum carbide dust acted as a physiologically inert substance (Stokinger, 1981).

K. Group VIA (Se and Te)

Selenium

Selenium is used in the electronic industries for the manufacture of rectifiers, photocells (especially those involved in photocopying), in glass and ceramics, in pigments, in some metal alloys, and in rubber production. It was formerly used in insecticide sprays.

Inhalation Exposure and Limits

Urban regions have particulate selenium concentrations of 0.1 to 10 ng/m^3 (USEPA, 1980). Areas near metallurgical industries might even be higher (Snyder et al., 1975).

The threshold limit value as a time-weighted average in workroom air for an 8 hr day is 0.2 mg/m^3 for selenium and its compounds (ACGIH, 1983). The OSHA permissible exposure limit is 0.2 mg/m^3 (OSHA, 1981).

Absorption, Excretion, and Toxicity

Absorption through the lungs is rapid (Lauwerys, 1983). Extensive metabolism of selenium takes place, principally in the liver. Especially noteworthy is the reduction of selenite (SeO$_3$$^{-2}$) or selenate (SeO$_4$$^{-2}$) to hydrogen selenide (H$_2$Se), which is then methylated to dimethyl selenide and exhaled or to the trimethylselenonium ion and excreted in the urine. Excretion is predominantly in urine and is rapid. However, some fecal excretion (via the bile) occurs and significant amounts are exhaled, primarily as dimethyl selenide.

In humans exposed occupationally, acute toxicity is primarily due to the irritative and allergenic properties of selenious acid (H$_2$SeO$_3$), formed from water and selenium dioxide. SeO$_2$ is formed whenever selenium is heated in air. Symptoms are nonspecific, and include sneezing, coughing, dyspnea.

Tellurium

Tellurium is used in the steel industry in Cu and Pb alloys to provide increased resistance to corrosion and stress, in the glass industry as a coloring agent, and as an additive in rubber. Bismuth telluride is used as a thermocouple material in refrigeration equipment.

Inhalation Exposure and Limits

There is no significant tellurium intake from ambient air. The threshold limit value as a time-weighted average in workroom air for an 8 hr day is 0.1 mg Te/m^3 for tellurium (ACGIH, 1983). The OSHA permissible exposure limit is 0.1 mg/m^3 (OSHA, 1981).

Absorption, Excretion, and Toxicity

There is no information regarding absorption of tellurium by the lung. However, once tellurium is absorbed, metabolically active tissues evidently methylate it to volatile dimethyl telluride (Me$_2$Te), which has an unpleasant garlic-like odor, and which is exhaled (Stokinger, 1981).

Occupational exposure to tellurium has resulted in odor on the breath and drowsiness at levels of 0.1 to 1.0 mg Te/m^3. In other industrial exposures, additional symptoms reported were nausea, anorexia, suppression of sweat, dry itching skin, and constipation or diarrhea (Browning, 1969).

L. Group VIB (Cr, Mo, and W)

Chromium

Chromium is essential for most forms of animal life, as an essential component of the "glucose tolerance factor;" a low-molecular-weight cofactor for insulin activity. Chromium involvement in normal carbohydrate and lipid metabolism and its influence on glucose tolerance and lipogenesis have been extensively studied and reviewed (O'Dell and Campbell, 1971; NAS, 1974a; Langard and Norseth, 1977). Chromium does not serve as an essential component of any metalloenzyme nor as a specific enzyme activator.

Chromium compounds are used in tanning, pigments, and electroplating and as catalysts, corrosion inhibitors, and wood preservatives. Chromium metal is an essential ingredient of stainless steel, superalloys for jet engines, and other alloys.

Inhalation Exposure and Limits

Ambient air generally contains < 10 to 50 ng Cr/m^3 (Langard and Norseth, 1977). Chromium accumulates in the lungs with age, but the levels are usually harmless.

The threshold limit value as a time-weighted average in workroom air for an 8 hr day is 0.5 mg Cr/m^3 for chromium metal and Cr(II) and Cr(III) compounds. The TLV for certain water-insoluble chromium (VI) compounds is 0.05 mg Cr/m^3 (ACGIH, 1983). The OSHA permissible exposure limit is 0.5 mg Cr/m^3 for soluble compounds (OSHA, 1981). However, NIOSH (1975) has recommended 0.025 mg/m^3 as the limit (0.001 mg/m^3 for carcinogenic Cr(VI)).

Absorption, Excretion, and Toxicity

Chromium may be absorbed from the lungs, although some is deposited in an insoluble form (Langard and Norseth, 1977). Except for chromates, all chemical forms of chromium are rapidly cleared from the blood. The major excretory route for absorbed chromium is in the urine. Workers exposed to Cr(VI) at 0.05 mg/m^3 for 8 hr excrete 30 μg Cr/g creatinine, more than six times greater than normal values (Lauwerys, 1983).

Long-term inhalation of Cr(III) compounds reveal no adverse health effects, but long-term inhalation exposure to insoluble Cr(VI) compounds is associated with lesions of the mucosa and submucosa of the respiratory tract and other toxic effects. Workers exposed to chromates and chromic acid mist may develop contact dermatitis, skin ulcers, nasal membrane inflammation and ulceration, nasal septum perforation, rhinitis, liver damage, and pulmonary congestion and edema. Chronic rhinitis, laryngitis, and pharyngitis are also common (Stokinger, 1981). Progressive pulmonary fibrosis in a small number of workers was reported in 1962, but no subsequent reports have appeared (Stokinger, 1981). Pneumoconiosis has also been reported. Bronchial asthma is common among chromate workers.

An excessive incidence of lung cancer occurs in workers of the chromate producing industry and possibly of the pigment producing industry. Cr(II) has also been implicated in lung cancer cases (Stokinger, 1981; NIOSH, 1975).

Chromium complexes and precipitates proteins, which probably explains its cancer induction by combination with RNA and DNA. Observed/expected ratios of 5-40:1 have been reported for incidences of lung cancer in workers exposed to Cr(VI) compounds. Lung cancer is highest among heavy cigarette smokers. Cancer is also sometimes reported at other sites (Langard and Norseth, 1977).

Molybdenum

Molybdenum, an essential trace metal in mammals, is involved in flavin-dependent metalloenzymes. Most molybdenum is used as the oxide to alloy steel. Other uses include as a lubricant (MoS_2), as catalysts, as pigments (especially molybdates), and in ceramics.

Inhalation Exposure and Limits

The threshold limit value (TLV) as a time-weighted average in workroom air for an 8 hr day is 10 mg Mo/m^3 for insoluble molybdenum; the short-term exposure limit is 20 mg/m^3 for 15 min. The TLV for soluble molybdenum compounds is 5 mg/m^3; the short-term exposure limit is 10 mg/m^3 for 15 min (ACGIH, 1983). The OSHA permissible exposure limit is 15 mg/m^3 for insoluble molybdenum compounds and 5 mg/m^3 for soluble compounds (OSHA, 1981).

Absorption, Excretion, and Toxicity

Most inhaled molybdenum is absorbed by the lungs and distributed to other tissues, although some compounds, such as MoS_2, are poorly absorbed. Excretion of soluble Mo salts is rapid, mainly in the urine and partly in feces. Molybdenum salts are also excreted into bile and into intestines in the enterohepatic circulation (Friberg, 1977).

Inhalation of dusts of $CaMoO_4$ and MoS_2 is not toxic to rabbits, whereas the readily soluble MoO_3 is highly toxic (Fairhill et al., 1945). Exposure to MoO_3 dust at 164 mg Mo/m^3 for 1 hr/day was extremely irritating to guinea pigs; half died by the 10th exposure (Stokinger, 1981).

Tungsten

The largest use of tungsten is conversion to tungsten carbide (WC) for use in cutting and wear-resistant materials. Other uses include alloys, especially for high-strength alloys, incandescent lamp filaments, and compounds used as pigments and catalysts.

Inhalation Exposure and Limits

The threshold limit value (TLV) as a time-weighted average in workroom air for an 8 hr day is 1 mg W/m^3 for soluble tungsten compounds; the short-term exposure limit (STEL) is 3 mg/m^3 for 15 min. For insoluble tungsten compounds, the TLV is 5 mg W/m^3 and the STEL, 10 mg W/m^3 for 15 min (ACGIH, 1983).

Absorption, Excretion, and Toxicity

In one study in rats, inhaled tungstic acid (WO_3) was poorly absorbed (Stokinger, 1981). Urine appears to be the main excretory route (Kazantzis, 1977). Worker exposure, primarily to WC in grinding wheels, produces what is called "hard metal disease." The main symptoms are cough, dyspnea, and wheezing with minor radiological abnormalities. Hypersensitivity, asthma and marked radiological abnormalities are seen in some. This progresses to diffuse interstitial pulmonary fibrosis, which can cause (or contribute to) deaths from cor pulmonale, cardiac failure, and emphysema. Although the disease was formerly attributed to tungsten toxicity, later studies revealed that the cobalt present in tungsten carbide was probably the causative agent (Kazantzis, 1977; Stokinger, 1981).

M. Group VIIB (Mn)

Manganese

Manganese, an essential trace metal for animals, is also the least toxic of the essential metals. Manganese, primarily divalent, is widely distributed in the body. It is part of several enzymes (e.g., pyruvate carboxylase) and can substitute for magnesium in many. Enzyme systems in which manganese is essential are involved in protein and energy metabolism and in mucopolysaccharide formation.

The major use of manganese is in iron alloys. It is also used in nonferrous alloys (e.g., manganese-bronze), in dry cells as a depolarizer, and in matches and fireworks, in glass and ceramics as a pigment, and in various chemicals, especially potassium permanganate ($KMnO_4$) and other oxidizers. Manganese salts are used in paints, varnishes, inks, and dyes.

Inhalation Exposure and Limits

Exposure to manganese metal and salts occurs primarily through inhalation in industrial plants which make steel, alloys, glass, ceramics, etc. In industry, manganese salts in the air oxidize the toxic SO_2 to the even more toxic SO_3.

The threshold limit value (TLV) as a ceiling value in workroom air is 5 mg Mn/m^3 for manganese dusts and compounds. For manganese fumes, the TLV is 1 mg/m^3 as a time-weighted average with a short-term exposure limit of 3 mg/m^3 for 15 min (ACGIH, 1983).

Absorption, Excretion, and Toxicity

Inhaled manganese salts are deposited in the lungs where slow but continuous absorption takes place, the rate depends on the body's manganese reserves. Some of the manganese absorbed from the lung is transferred to the gastrointestinal tract, where it is absorbed again. Excretion of absorbed manganese is virtually entirely through the bile. However, occupational exposure has been correlated with manganese concentrations in the urine. Toxicity occurs when urinary Mn concentration exceeded 40-50 μg Mn/liter (normal: <3 μg/liter) (Lauwerys, 1983).

Inhalation of Mn compounds in aerosols or fine dusts produces "metal fume fever." Chronic inhalation of manganese oxides (dust particles: 3 μm) for a few months causes pulmonary pneumonitis in Mn workers. This pathologic condition is characterized by the onset of pneumonia, intense dyspnea, elevated body temperature, acute radiologic signs of lobar pneumonia, and hemorrhage in the lung with little expectoration. "Manganese pneumonia" has a high mortality rate. Fibrosis of the lung tissue has also been reported (Stokinger, 1983).

Chronic manganese toxicity ("manganism") is well known in miners, millworkers, and others exposed to dust and fumes. The usual signs and symptoms involve the central nervous system. This disease is reversible if recognized very early and if exposure to dust of Mn oxides is eliminated. However, after the onset of the disease, the neurological symptoms remain, even after the exposure to Mn is removed and the tissue Mn levels revert to normal. A peculiar slapping gait, cramps or tremors of the body and extremities, slurred speech, hallucinations, insomnia, mental confusion are some of the symptoms. At this stage, the symptoms resemble those of Parkinson's disease (Cotzias, 1958). In spite of the severity of the symptoms, manganism is not fatal, although it causes premanent disability.

N. Group VIII (Fe, Co, Ni, and Os)

Iron

Iron is the fourth most abundant element in the earth's crust, 5%. The industrial uses of iron are many, mainly in the fabrication of steel. The total production of steel exceeds that of all other metals combined. In addition to its structural uses, iron and its compounds are used in pigments, magnetic tapes, catalysts, feeds, and fuel additives.

Inhalation Exposure and Limits

Urban air may contain significant amounts of iron from industrial or geologic sources. Snyder et al. (1975) estimate that inhalation of iron in urban air may contribute about 27 μg/day.

The threshold limit value (TLV) as a time-weighted average in workroom air for an 8 hr day is 1 mg Fe/m^3 for soluble iron salts; the short-term exposure limit is 2 mg/m^3 (ACGIH, 1983).

Absorption, Excretion, and Toxicity

Iron is an essential nutrient for mammals, since Fe is involved in a number of physiologic reactions. Iron is involved in oxygen transport from the lungs to tissues by hemoglobin and in oxygen storage in myoglobin; divalent Fe is a cofactor in heme enzymes such as catalase and cytochrome c, and in nonheme enzymes such as aldolase and tryptophan oxygenase. Iron absorption by mammals has been studied extensively and excellent reviews are available (Forth and Rummel, 1971, 1973).

Absorption of Fe from the lungs depends upon the solubility of the compound. The lungs retain inhaled insoluble Fe compounds, while soluble compounds are readily absorbed into the blood. Absorbed iron is transported by transferrin, a β_1-globulin. Iron is stored intracellularly as ferritin and hemosiderin in the liver, bone marrow, and spleen. Iron is excreted mostly in feces, and smaller amounts in urine, sweat, and sloughed cells. Bleeding is another form of Fe excretion (Hammond and Beliles, 1980).

Long-term inhalation exposure to iron, particularly to iron oxide, leads to mottling of the lungs, a condition referred to as siderosis. This is considered a benign pneumoconiosis and does not ordinarily cause significant physiologic impairment (Stokinger, 1963). However, inhalation of iron oxides with silica produces the usual silicosis, and hematite inhalation has been reported to produce progressive, massive fibrosis (Stokinger, 1981).

Hematite miners have been reported in certain areas to have from 50 to 70% higher death rates attributable to lung cancer. It has been suggested that at least part of the increased incidence may be due to exposure to radon (Boyd et al., 1970).

Some Fe compounds are reported to be carcinogens. Iron oxides enhance the carcinogenic action of organic carcinogens such as benzpyrene by acting as an inert carrier to transport the carcinogen in high concentration to healthy cells (Stokinger and Coffin, 1968; Saffiotti et al., 1968).

Cobalt

It is used in high-temperature alloys and in permanent magnets. Its salts are useful in paint driers, as catalysts, and in the production of numerous pigments for use in glass and porcelain. Cemented carbide (hard metal) tools, used in metal-cutting operations, are produced primarily from tungsten carbide and 2-25% cobalt powders. Cobalt is an essential element in that 1 μg of vitamin B_{12} contains 0.0434 μg of cobalt. Vitamin B_{12} is essential in the prevention of pernicious anemia.

Inhalation Exposure and Limits

Major sources of cobalt in the atmosphere are probably the result of burning coal and residual fuel oil. The breakdown due to use of superalloys, hard-facing alloys, and cemented tungsten carbides also contributes. The predominant form of cobalt entering the air is probably CoO.

The threshold limit value (TLV) as a time-weighted average in workroom air for an 8 hr day is 0.1 mg/m^3 for cobalt metal, dust, and fumes (ACGIH, 1983), which is also the OSHA permissible exposure limit (OSHA, 1981).

Absorption, Excretion, and Toxicity

Industrial exposure to cobalt salts leads to respiratory effects, although there is some question as to whether cobalt is the sole agent responsible for these effects. Most industrial exposures come from cemented carbide industry where workers exposed to 0.1 to 0.2 mg Co/m^3 have shown mild to fibrotic pulmonary changes; (Coates and Watson, 1971). Sensitization may be an important part of this effect. Experimental studies in animals, however, confirm the lung-irritant effect of the metal as used in this industry but not of other cobalt compounds. NIOSH (1978b) considered it reasonable to consider all cobalt compounds as being capable of causing lung fibrosis. Although current data are not conclusive, it appears that cobalt metal, cobalt salts, and cobalt carbonyl do not cause human cancer. Industrial cases where malignancy has been associated with metals have usually involved exposure to a mixture (for example, tungsten or titanium carbide and cobalt cementing metal), thereby preventing assignment of causation to one specific metal such as cobalt.

Nickel

Nickel is extensively used in electroplating, in the manufacture of steel and other alloys, and in the manufacture of Ni-Cd batteries. Colored glass and ceramic industries use large quantities of Ni. It is not profitable to recover Ni; hence coal-fired power plants release Ni compounds into the atmosphere. The toxicity of nickel is considerably less serious than its carcinogenicity; nickel toxicity for mammals is low and is similar to chromium.

Inhalation Exposure and Limits

Airborne nickel is primarily the result of the combustion of coal and petroleum products. Recently, nickel levels in air have been decreasing, with levels averaging about 9 ng/m^3 in urban air and 2 ng/m^3 in nonurban air (USEPA, 1980e).

The threshold limit value (TLV) as a time-weighted average in workroom air for an 8 hr day is 0.1 mg/m^3, as nickel, for soluble nickel compounds; the short-term exposure limit is 0.3 mg/m^3 for 15 min. The TLV for nickel metal is 1 mg/m^3 (ACGIH, 1983). The OSHA permissible exposure limit is 1 mg Ni/m^3 (OSHA, 1981). However, NIOSH (1977a) has recommended 0.015 mg Ni/m^3 as the limit. The TLV for Ni(CO$_4$) is 0.35 mg/m^3 (ACGIH, 1983) and the OSHA permissible exposure level is 0.007 mg/m^3 (OSHA, 1981).

Absorption, Excretion, and Toxicity

The lungs retain inhaled Ni salts, especially those from cigarette smoke, and their removal from the pulmonary tissues is low. Approximately 50% of inhaled Ni dust is deposited on the bronchial mucosa and swept upward in mucous to be swallowed, about 25% is exhaled, and the rest deposited in the pulmonary parenchyma. Gaseous nickel compounds, such as nickel carbonyl, are deposited in much larger proportions. Excretion of absorbed Ni and Ni compounds is primarily urinary (60%) and the rest fecal. Inhaled nickel carbonyl is excreted primarily in urine (Sunderman and Selin, 1968).

Except for inhalation of nickel carbonyl, nickel is relatively nontoxic, ranking with iron, cobalt, copper, chromium, and zinc. Nickel metal is less toxic than its soluble salts. Inhalation of nickel carbonyl causes respiratory tract neoplasia and myocardial infarction; intra-alveolar hemorrhage, edema, and exudates are noticed prior to neoplasia. Perivascular leukocytosis and neuronal degeneration occur in the brain (NAS, 1975; USEPA, 1980e; Stokinger, 1981).

Nickel carbonyl causes the same toxic symptoms whether administered by inhalation, intravenously or parenterally. Immediate lethal toxicity occurs at 30 ppm in the air. An 8 hr exposure to 0.001 ppm Ni(CO)$_4$ in air is also toxic, producing severe pneumonitis. Inhalation of the less toxic nickel oxides and chlorides produces pneumonitis and increases the number of alveolar macrophages and the viscosity of pulmonary washings (Bingham et al., 1972).

The only effect of chronic exposure to nickel, which has been studied, is carcinogenesis. Chronic exposure to very low levels of Ni(CO)$_4$ produces squamous metaplasia of the bronchial epithelium and carcinoma of the upper respiratory tract and lungs (Sunderman et al., 1959). Nickel carcinogenicity from tobacco smoke is attributed to Ni(CO)$_4$ (Sunderman and Sunderman, 1961).

Epidemiologic studies among nickel refinery workers (NAS, 1975) and experimental studies in laboratory rodents have established Ni carcinogenesis in man and animals. Respirable particles of Ni, Ni subsulfide, nickel oxide, and vapors of nickel carbonyl are primarily responsible for Ni carcinogenicity. The highest risk of mortality from cancer of the respiratory tract is found among nickel mine workers involved in roasting, smelting, and electrolysis. Pulmonary carcinomas have been induced in rodents following the inhalation of nickel dust (particle size 4 μm) (Heuper, 1958) and following nickel carbonyl inhalation (Sunderman et al., 1959). Carcinogenic synergism between Ni compounds and polycyclic aromatic hydrocarbons, such as benzpyrene, has been established in rats (Maenza et al., 1971).

The latent period for induction of lung cancer in laboratory animals by inhalation of nickel carbonyl is about two years. Nickel carbonyl is able to cross cell membranes without hydrolysis because it is lipid soluble; this ability to penetrate cell barriers and to release Ni ions is responsible for its high toxicity and carcinogenicity. Other Ni compounds form complexes with serum proteins or ultrafiltrable molecules, such as histidine or other amino acids. These metal-protein (nickelocene) or amino acid complexes adsorb to the surface of a cell and enter the cell by endocytosis. Within the cell, lysosomal proteinases hydrolyze the carrier protein to release the electrophilic metal ion. Nickel ions then bind with nucleic acids and other cellular constituents (Hatem-Champy, 1961).

Osmium

Osmium, the most dense metal, is used in metal alloys with iridium in instrument pivots, compass needles, electrical contacts, and engraving tools. Until 1969, two osmium alloys were used as fountain pen tips. Academic and research laboratories are the major users of osmium. Osmium tetroxide is used as a tissue stain for histological preparations.

Inhalation Exposure and Limits

Since most osmium is recovered as a byproduct of copper refining, environmental exposures would be expected to occur in the vicinity of sites roasting and smelting copper concentrates. The threshold limit value (TLV) as a time-weighted average in workroom air for an 8 hr day is 0.002 mg Os/m^3 for OsO$_4$ (ACGIH, 1983). The short-term exposure limit is 0.006 mg Os/m^3. The OSHA permissible exposure limit is 0.002 mg Os/m^3 (OSHA, 1981).

Absorption, Excretion, and Toxicity

Osmium poisoning occurs through inhalation of OsO$_4$ which readily vaporizes from aqueous solutions even at room temperature; even Os-Ir alloy readily releases OsO$_4$ vapors at the heat required for annealing. The lungs and the respiratory tract retain most of the inhaled OsO$_4$ vapors. Severe irritation and black discoloration occur in the mucous membranes of the lungs, when OsO$_4$ comes in contact with tissues. OsO$_4$ is reduced to lower oxides and metallic Os by organic matter (McLaughlin et al., 1946). Inhalation of OsO_4 vapor produces acutely toxic symptoms; a concentration of 400 mg Os/m^3 is lethal to most laboratory animals (Brunot, 1933). Rabbits which survived four days after exposure to 250 mg Os/m^3 showed degenerative changes in the lungs in the form of a purulent bronchopneumonia. Chronic toxicity through inhalation of small doses of OsO_4 for a prolonged time reduced erythrocyte and leukocyte counts in the blood of guinea pigs (Mazturzo, 1951). The toxic action of Os seems to be in the bone marrow, affecting the maturation of reticulocytes.

References

ACGIH (1983). TLVs threshold limit values for chemical substances and physical agents in the work environment with intended changes for 1983-84. Cincinnati, OH: American Conference of Governmental Industrial Hygienists.

Albert, R. E., Lippmann, M., Spiegelman, J., Liuzz, A., and Nelson, N. (1967). The deposition and clearance of radioactive particles in the human lung. *Arch. Environ. Health* 14:10-15.

Altman, P. L., and Dittmer, D. S. (1974). *Biology Data Book,* Vol. III. Bethesda, MD, American Societies for Experimental Biology.

Arena, J. M. (1974). *Poisoning: Toxicology, Symptoms, Treatments,* 3rd edition. American Lecture Series, No. 903, American Lectures in Living Chemistry. Springfield, Charles C Thomas.

Athanassiadis, Y. C. (1969). Preliminary air pollution survey of zinc and its compounds. APTD 69. U.S. Department of Health, Education and Welfare, Raleigh, NC.

Barnes, J. M., and Stoner, H. B. (1959). The toxicology of tin compounds. *Pharmacol. Rev.* 11:211-231.

Bates, D. V. (1972). Air pollutants and the human lung. *Am. Rev. Respir. Dis.* 105:1-13.

Berlin, M. (1977). In *Toxicology of Metals,* Volume II. Springfield, VA, National Technical Information Service, pp. 301-344, PB 268-324.

Bingham, E., Barkley, W., Zerwas, M., Stemmer, K., and Taylor, P. (1972). Responses of alveolar macrophages to metals. I. Inhalation of lead and nickel. *Arch. Environ. Health* 25:406-414.

Blejer, H. P., and Wagner, W. (1976). Case study 4: Inorganic arsenic-ambient level approach to the control of occupational cancerigenic exposures. *Ann. N. Y. Acad. Sci.* 271:179-186.

Blot, W. J., and Fraumeni, J. F. Jr. (1975). Arsenical air pollution and lung cancer. *Lancet* **2**(7926):142-144.

Boyd, E. M. (1972). *Respiratory Tract Fluid.* Springfield, IL, Charles C Thomas.

Boyd, J. T., Doll, R., Faulds, J. S., and Leiper, J. (1970). Cancer of the lung in iron ore (hemitite) miners. *Br. J. Ind. Med.* **27**:97-105.

Brain, J. D., and Valberg, P. A. (1979). Deposition of aerosol in the respiratory tract. *Am. Rev. Respir. Dis.* **120**:1325-1373.

Brieger, H., Semisch, C. W., Stasney, J., and Piatneck, D. A. (1954). Industrial antimony poisoning. *Ind. Med. Surg.* **23**:521.

Browning, E. (1969). *Toxicity of Industrial Metals,* 2nd edition. London, Butterworths.

Brunot, F. R. (1933). The toxicity of osmium tetroxide (osmic acid). *J. Ind. Hyg.* **15**:136-143.

Bulmer, F. M. R., Rothwell, H. E., and Frankish, E. R. (1938). Industrial cadmium poisoning. *J. Can. Public Health* **29**:19-26.

Camner, P., and Philipson, K. (1972). Tracheobronchial clearance in smoking-discordant twins. *Arch. Environ. Health* **25**:60-63.

Casarett, L. J. (1972). The vital sacs: alveolar clearance mechanisms in inhalation toxicology. In *Essays in Toxicology,* Volume III. Edited by W. J. Hayes, Jr. New York, Academic Press, pp. 1-36.

Cavanagh, J. B., Fuller, N. H., Johnson, H. R. M., and Rudge, P. (1974). The effects of thallium salts, with particular reference to the nervous system. *Q. J. Med.* **43**:293-319.

Christie, H., Mackay, R. J., and Fischer, A. M. (1963). Pulmonary effects of inhalation of aluminum by rats. *Am. Ind. Hyg. Assoc. J.* **24**:47-56.

Coffin, D. L., and Stokinger, H. E. (1977). In *Air Pollution,* Volume 11. Edited by A. C. Stern. New York, Academic Press, 3rd ed., pp. 231-345.

Cotzias, G. C. (1958). Manganese in health and disease. *Physiol. Rev.* **38**:503-532.

Cullen, M. R., Robins, J. M., and Eskenazi, B. (1983). Adult inorganic lead intoxication: presentation of 31 new cases and a review of recent advances in the literature. *Medicine* **62**:221-247.

Cullen, M. R., Cherniack, M. G., and Kominsky, J. R. (1986). Chronic beryllium disease in the United States. *Sem. Resp. Med.* **7**:203-209.

Daniele, R. P., Elias, J. A., Epstein, P. E., and Rossman, M. D. (1985). Bronchoalveolar lavage: role in the pathogenesis, diagnosis and management of interstitial lung disease. *Ann. Int. Med.* **102**:93-108.

Davies, C. N. (1961). *Inhaled Particles and Vapors.* New York, Pergamon Press.

DeLarrad, J., and Lazarini, H-J. (1954). Intoxication par la cyanamide calcique, *Arch. Maladies Prof.* 15:282-287.

Doig, A. T., and Challen, P. J. R. (1964). Respiratory hazards in welding. *Ann. Occup. Hyg.* 7:223-231.

Doull, J., Klaassen, C. D., and Amdur, M. O. (Eds.). (1980). *Casarett and Doull's Toxicology, the Basic Science of Poisons,* 2nd ed. New York, Macmillan.

Dygert, H. P., LaBelle, C. W., Roberts, E., et al., (1949). Toxicity following inhalation. In *Pharmacology and Toxicology of Uranium Compounds.* Edited by C. F. Voegtlin and H. C. Hodge. New York, McGraw-Hill, pp. 423-700.

Eisenbud, M., Wanta, R. C., Dustan, C., Steadman, L. T., Harris, W. B., and Wolf, B. S. (1949). Non-occupational berylliosis. *J. Ind. Hyg. Toxicol.* 31:282-294.

Elinder, C-G., Kjellstroöm, T., Friberg, L., Lind, B., and Linnman, L. (1976). Cadmium in kidney cortex, liver, and pancreas from Swedish autopsies. *Arch. Environ. Health* 31:292-302.

Fairhill, L. T., Dunn, R. D., Sharpless, N. E., and Pritchard, E. A. (1945). Toxicity of Molybdenum, *U.S. Public Health Serv. Bull.* **293**

Flinn, R. H., Neal, P. A., Rhinehart, W. H., and Dallavilk, J. M. (1940). Chronic manganese poisoning in an ore-crushing mill, *U.S. Publ. Bull. No. 247,* Washington, D.C., U.S. Govt. Printing Office.

Forth, W., and Rummel, W. (1973). Iron absorption. *Physiol. Rev.* 53:724-793.

Forth, W., and Rummel, W. (1971). Absorption of iron and chemically related metals *in vitro* and *in vivo*: Specificity of the iron binding system in the mucosa of the jejunum. In *Intestinal Absorption of Metal Ions, Trace Elements and Radionuclides.* Edited by S. C. Skoryana and D. Waldron-Edward. New York, Pergamon Press, pp. 173-191.

Friberg, L. (1977). Molybdenum. In *Toxicology of Metals,* Volume II. Springfield, VA, National Technical Information Service, pp. 345-457, PB 268-324.

Friberg, L., Nordberg, F., and Vouk, V. B. (1979). *Handbook on the Toxicology of Metals.* New York, Elsevier/North Holland.

Friberg, L., Piscator, M., Nordberg, G. F., and Kjellstrom, T. (1974). *Cadmium in the Environment.* Cleveland, CRC Press.

Friberg, L., Piscator, M., and Nordberg, G. F. (1971). *Cadmium in the Environment.* Cleveland, Chemical Rubber Co. Press.

Frost, D. V. (1967). Arsenicals in biology: Retrospect and prospect. *Fed. Proc.* **26**:194-208.

Gamsu, G., Weintraub, R. M., and Nadel, J. A. (1973). Clearance of tantalum from airways of different caliber in man evaluated by a roentgenographic method. *Am. Rev. Respir. Dis.* **107**:214-224.

Gardner, D. E., Miller, F. J., Illing, J. W., and Kirtz, J. M. (1977). Alterations in bacterial defense mechanisms of the lung induced by inhalation of cadmium. *Bull. Eur. Physiopathol. Respir.* **13**:157-174.

Gerstner, H. B., and Huff, J. E. (1977). Clinical toxicology of mercury. *J. Toxicol. Environ. Health* **2**:491-526.

Gleason, M. N., Gosselin, R. E., Hodge, H. C., and Smith, R. P. (1969). *Clinical Toxicology of Commercial Products,* 3rd edition. Baltimore, Williams and Wilkins, Sect. II, p. 131.

Goyer, R. A. (1971). Lead and the kidney. *Curr. Top. Pathol.* **55**:147.

Groth, D. V. (1972). Mercury salts in chronic experiments. In *Trace Substances in Environmental Health,* Volume 6. Edited by D. D. Hemphill. Columbia, University of Missouri, p. 187-192.

Hammond, P. B., and Beliles, R. P. (1980). Metals. In *Casarett and Doull's Toxicology, the Basic Science of Poisons.* Edited by J. Doull, C. d. Klaassen, and M. O. Amdur. New York, Macmillan, pp. 409-467.

Hardy, H. L., and Tabershaw, I. R. (1946). Delayed chemical pneumonitis occurring in workers exposed to beryllium compounds. *J. Ind. Hyg. Toxicol.* **28**:197-211.

Hasan, F. M., and Kazemi, H. (1974). Chronic beryllium disease: a continuing epidemiologic hazard. *Chest* **65**:289-293.

Hatch, T., and Hemeon, W. C. L. (1948). Influence of particle size in dust exposure. *J. Ind. Hyg. Toxicol.* **30**:175-180.

Hatch, T. F., and Gross, P. (1964). *Pulmonary Deposition and Retention of Inhaled Aerosols.* New York, Academic Press.

Hatem-Champy, S. (1961). Cancers du nickel et complexe nickel-imidazole. *C. R. Acad. Sci.* **253**:2791-2792.

Heuper, W. C. (1958). Experimental studies in metal cancerigenesis IX. Pulmonary lesions in guinea pigs and rats exposed to prolonged inhalation of powdered nickel. *Arch. Pathol.* **64**:600-607.

IARC (1980a). Beryllium and beryllium compounds. International Agency for Research on Cancer Monograph, *Evaluation of Carcinogenic Risk of Chemicals to Humans* **23**:204.

IARC (1980b). Some metals and metallic compounds, arsenic and arsenic compounds. International Agency for Research on Cancer monograph, *Evaluation of Carcinogenic Risk of Chemicals to Humans* 23:39-141.

Iverson, F., Downie, R. H., Paul, C., and Trenholm, H. L. (1973). Methyl mercury-acute toxicity, tissue distribution and decay profiles in the guinea pig. *Toxicol. Appl. Pharmacol.* 24:545-554.

Johnson, F. A., and Stonehill, R. B. (1961). Chemical pneumonites from inhalation of zinc chloride. *Dis. Chest* 40:619-624.

Kazantzis, G. (1977). Tungsten. In *Toxicology of Metals,* Volume II. Springfield, VA, National Technical Information Service, pp. 442-453, PB 268-324.

Kazantzis, G., and Armstrong, B. G. (1983). A mortality study of cadmium workers from seventeen plants in England. In *Edited Proc. Fourth Int. Cadmium Conf.*, Munich, March 2-4, 1983, pp. 39-142.

Kipling, M. D., and Waterhouse, J. A. H. (1967). Cadmium and prostatic carcinoma (letter). *Lancet* 1(7492):730-731.

Konetzke, G. W. (1974). Die kanzerogene wirkung von arsen und nickel. *Arch. Geschwulstforsch.* 44:16-22.

Langard, S., and Norseth, T. (1977). Chromium. In *Toxicology of Metals,* Volume II. Springfield, VA, National Technical Information Service, pp. 164-187, PB-268-324.

Lauwerys, R. R. (1983). Biological monitoring of exposure to inorganic and organometallic substances. In *Industrial Chemical Exposure: Guidelines for Biological Monitoring.* Davis, CA, Biomedical Publications, pp. 9-50.

Lawson, J. J. (1961). Toxicity of titanium tetrachloride. *J. Occup. Med.* 3:7-12.

Lee, A. M., and Fraumeni, J. F. (1969). Arsenic and respiratory cancer in man: an occupational study. *J. Natl. Cancer Inst.* 42:1045-1052.

Lewis, G. P., Coughlin, L., Jusko, W., and Hartz, S. (1972). Contribution of cigarette smoking to cadmium accumulation in man. *Lancet* 1:291-292.

Lieben, J., and Metzner, F. (1959). Epidemiological findings associated with beryllium extraction. *Am. Ind. Hyg. Assoc. J.* 20:494-499.

Lourenco, R. V., Klimek, M. F., and Borowski, C. J. (1971). Deposition and clearance of 2μ particles in the tracheobronchial tree of normal subjects—smokers and non-somkers. *J. Clin. Invest.* 50:1411-1420.

Lucas, P. A., Jarivalla, A. G., Jones, J. H., Gough, J., and Vale, P. T. (1980). Fatal cadmium fume inhalation. *Lancet* 26:205.

Maenza, R. M., Pradhan, A. M., and Sunderman, Jr., F. W. (1971). Rapid induction of sarcomas in rats by a combination of nickel sulfide and 3,4 benz-pyrene. *Cancer Res.* 31:2067-2071.

Mancuso, T. F. (1970). Relation of duration of employment and prior respiratory illness to respiratory cancer among beryllium workers. *Environ. Res.* 3:251-275.

Massman, W. (1956). Experimentelle untersuchungen über die biologische wirkung von vanadinverbindungen. *Arch. Toxicol.* 16:182-186.

Mazturzo, A. (1951). Sangue periferico e mielogramma nella intossicazione sperimentalle da osmio. *Folia Med., Napoli* 34:27.

McLaughlin, A. I. G., Milton, R., and Perry, K. M. A. (1946). Toxic manifestations of osmium tetroxide. *Br. J. Ind. Med.* 3:183-186.

Mercer, T. (1973). *Aerosol Technology in Hazard Evaluation.* New York, Academic Press.

Morishige, T. (1968). Experimental studies on the effect of Sr^{95}-Nb^{95} on albino rats: distribution of Zr-Nb among the organs—microautoradiography of lungs on intratracheally incubated albino rats. *Jap. J. Hyg.* 23:404.

Nandi, M., Jick, H., Slone, D., Shapiro, S., and Lewis, G. P. (1969). Cadmium content of cigarettes. *Lancet* 2(7634):1329-1333.

NAS (1974a). Chromium. Committee on biological effects of atmospheric pollutants. National Academy of Sciences, Washington, D. C. 155 pp.

NAS (1974b). Vanadium. Committee on biological effects of atmospheric pollutants. National Academy of Sciences, Washington, D.C. 117 pp.

NAS (1975). Nickel. Committee on biological effects of atmospheric pollutants. National Academy of Sciences.

Natusch, D. F. S., Wallace, J. R., and Evans, C. A. (1974). Toxic trace elements: preferential concentration in respiratory particles. *Science* 183:202-204.

NIOSH (1975). Criteria for a recommended standard: occupational exposure to chromium (VI), Washington, D.C., U.S. Government Printing Office, DHEW (National Institute Occupational Safety and Health) Publication No. 76-129.

NIOSH (1976a). Criteria for a recommended standard: occupational exposure to cadmium. Washington, D.C., U.S. Government Printing Office, DHEW (National Institute Occupational Safety and Health) Publication No. 76-192.

NIOSH (1976b). Criteria for a recommended standard: occupational exposure to organotin compounds, Washington, D.C., U.S. Government Printing Office, DHEW (National Institute Occupational Safety and Health) Publication No. 77-115.

NIOSH (1977a). Criteria for a recommended standard: occupational exposure to inorganic nickel. Washington, D.C., U.S. Government Printing Office, DHEW(National Institute Occupational Safety and Health) Publication No. 77-164.

NIOSH (1977b). Criteria for a recommended standard: occupational exposure to vanadium, Washington, D.C., U.S. Government Printing Office, DHEW (National Institute Occupational Safety and Health) Publication No. 77-222.

NIOSH (1978a). Criteria for a recommended standard: occupational exposure to inorganic lead, Washington, D.C., U.S. Government Printing Office, DHEW (National Institute Occupational Safety and Health) Publication No. 78-158.

NIOSH (1978b). Environmental exposure to airborne contaminants in the nickel industry. Washington, D.C., U.S. Government Printing Office, DHEW (National Institute Occupational Safety and Health) Publication No. 78-178.

Norseth, T. (1977). Aluminum. In *Toxicology of Metals,* Volume II. Springfield, VA, National Technical Information Service, pp. 4-14, PB 268-324.

O'Dell, B. L., and Campbell, B. J. (1971). Trace elements: metabolism and metabolic function. In *Comprehensive Biochemistry,* Volume 21. Edited by M. Florkin and E. H. Stotz. Amsterdam, Elsevier Publishing Co., pp. 179-266.

OSHA (1981). Occupational Safety and Health Standards. Subpart 2—Toxic and hazardous substances. Code of federal regulations 29 (Part 1910.1000), Occupational Safety and Health Administration, pp. 673-679.

Pearson, R. G. (1968). Hard and soft acids and bases—HSAB, Part I. Fundamental principles. *J. Chem. Ed.* **45**:581-587; Part II. Underlying theories. *J. Chem. Ed.* **45**:643-648.

Pearson, R. G. (1967). Hard and soft acids and bases. *Chem. Br.* **3**:103-107.

Pearson, R. G. (1963). Hard and soft acids and bases. *J. Am. Chem. Soc.* **85**: 3533-3539.

Pierre-Bienvenu, M. M., Notre, C., and Cier, A. (1963). Comparative general toxicity of metallic ions: relation with periodic system. *C.R. Acad. Sci.* **256**:1043-1044.

Piscator, M. (1977). Copper. In *Toxicology of Metals,* Volume II. Springfield, VA, National Technical Information Service, pp. 206-221, PB 268-324.

Piscator, M., Kjellström, T., and Lind, B. (1976). Contamination of cigarettes and pipe tobacco by cadmium-oxide dust (letter). *Lancet* **2**(7985):587.

Potts, C. L. (1965). Cadmium proteinuria—the health of battery workers exposed to cadmium oxide dust. *Ann. Occup. Hyg.* **8**:55-61.

Prick, J. J. G., Smitt, W. G. S., and Muller, L. (1955). *Thallium Poisoning.* Amsterdam, Elsevier.

Prior, J. T., Cronk, G. A., and Ziegler, D. D. (1960). Pathological changes associated with the inhalation of sodium zirconium lactate. *Arch. Environ. Health* **1**:297-300.

Reeves, A. L., and Vorwald, A. J. (1967). Beryllium carcinogenesis II. Pulmonary deposition and clearance of inhaled beryllium sulfate in the rat. *Cancer Res.* 27:446-451.

Reeves, A. L. (1977a). In *Toxicology of Metals*, Volume II. Springfield, VA, National Technical Information Service, pp. 85-109, PB 268-324.

Reeves, A. L. (1977b). Barium. In *Toxicology of Metals*, Volume II. Springfield, VA, National Technical Information Service, pp. 71-84, PB 268-324.

Saffiotti, U., Cefis, F., and Kolb, L. H. (1968). A method for the experimental induction of bronchogenic carcinoma. *Cancer Res.* 28:104-124.

Sanders, C. L., Cannon, W. C., Powers, G. J., Adee, R. R., and Meier, D. M. (1975). Toxicology of high-fired beryllium oxide inhaled by rodents. *Arch. Environ. Health* 30:546-551.

Schepers, G. W. H., Durkan, T. M., Delahant, A. B., and Creedon, F. T. (1957). The biological action of inhaled beryllium sulfate. *Arch. Ind. Health* 15: 32-58.

Shaver, C. G., and Riddell, A. R. (1947). Lung changes associated with the manufacture of alumina abrasives. *J. Ind. Hyg. Toxicol.* 29:145-147.

Smith, I. C., and Carson, B. L. (1977). *Trace Metals in the Environment*, Volume I, *Thallium.* Ann Arbor, MI, Ann Arbor Science Publishers, Inc., pp. 394.

Smith, I. C., and Carson, B. L. (1978). *Trace Metals in the Environment,* Volume III, *Zirconium.* Ann Arbor, MI, Ann Arbor Science Publishers, Inc., pp. 405.

Smith, I. C., Carson, B. L., and Hoffmeister, F. (1978). *Trace Metals in the Environment,* Volume V, *Indium.* Ann Arbor, MI, Ann Arbor Science Publishers, Inc., pp. 552.

Smith, I. C., Ferguson, T. L., and Carson, B. L. (1975). Metals in new and used petroleum products: quantities and consequences. In *The Role of Trace Metals in Petroleum.* Edited by T. F. Yen. Ann Arbor, MI, Ann Arbor Science Publishers, pp. 123-148.

Snyder, W. S., Cook, M. J., Nasset, E. S., Karhausen, L. R., Howells, G. P., and Tipton, I. H. (1975). International Commission on Radiological Protection. Report of the task group on reference man. New York, ICRP Publication 23.

Sorahan, T., and Waterhouse, J. A. H. (1985). Cancer of prostate among nickel-cadmium battery workers (letter). *Lancet* 1(8426):459.

Sorahan, T., and Waterhouse, J. A. H. (1983). Mortality study of nickel-cadmium battery workers by the method of regression models in life tables. *Br. J. Ind. Med.* 40:293-300.

Sterner, J. H., and Eisenbud, M. (1951). Epidemiology of beryllium intoxication. *Arch. Ind. Hyg. Occ. Med.* 4:123-151.

Stokinger, H. E. (1963). The metals (excluding lead). In *Industrial Hygiene and Toxicology*, Volume II. Edited by D. W. Fasset and D. D. Irish. New York, Interscience, pp. 987-1188.

Stokinger, H. E. (1981). The metals. In *Patty's Industrial Hygiene and Toxicology*, 3rd edition, Volume IIA, *Toxicology*. Edited by G. D. Clayton and F. E. Clayton. New York, Wiley-Interscience, John Wiley & Sons, pp. 1493-2060.

Stokinger, H. E., and Coffin, D. L. (1968). Biological effects of air pollutants. In *Air Pollution*. Edited by A. C. Stern. New York, Academic Press, pp. 446-546.

Stoll, E. (1972). Medical portraits: Goya and Van Gogh. *The Sciences* 12(4): 16-21.

Sunderman, F. W., Jr., and Selin, C. E. (1968). The metabolism of nickel carbonyl. *Toxicol. Appl. Pharmacol.* 12:207-218.

Sunderman, F. W., and Sunderman, Jr., F. W. (1961). Nickel poisoning indication of nickel as a pulmonary carcinogen in tobacco smoke. *Am. J. Clin. Pathol.* 35:203-209.

Sunderman, F. W., Donnelly, A. J., West, B., and Kincaid, J. F. (1959). Nickel poisoning. II-IX. Carcinogenesis in rats exposed to nickel carbonyl. *AMA Arch. Ind. Health* 20:36-41.

Sweeney, T. D., Brain, J. D., and LeMott, S. (1983). Anesthesia alters the pattern of aerosol retention in hamsters. *J. Appl. Physiol. : Respirat. Environ. Exercise Physiol.* 54:37-44.

Takenaka, S., Oldiges, H., König, H., Hochrainer, D., and Oberdörster, G. Carcinogenicity of cadmium chloride aerosols in Wistar rats. *J. Natl. Cancer Inst.* 70:367-373.

Task Group on Metal Accumulation. (1973). Accumulation of toxic metals with special reference to their absorption, excretion and biological half-times. *Environ. Physiol. Biochem.* 3:65-107.

Tsuchiya, K. (1977). In *Toxicology of Metals*, Volume II. Springfield, VA, National Technical Information Service, pp. 242-300, PB 268-324.

USEPA (a980a). Ambient water quality criteria for mercury. Springfield, VA, National Technical Information Service, No. PB 81-117699, U.S. EPA.

USEPA (1980b). Ambient water quality criteria for copper, Springfield, VA, National Technical Information Service. PB 81-117475, U.S. Environmental

Protection Agency.

USEPA (1980c). Ambient water quality criteria for arsenic. Springfield, VA, National Technical Information Service, No. PB 81-117327, U.S. Environmental Protection Agency.

USEPA (1980d). Ambient water quality criteria for lead, Springfield, VA, National Technical Information Service, No. PB 81-117681, U.S. Environmental Protection Agency.

USEPA (1980e). Ambient water quality criteria for nickel, Springfield, VA, National Technical Information Service, No. PB 81-117715, U.S. Environmental Protection Agency.

USEPA (1980f). Ambient water quality criteria for silver, Springfield, VA, National Technical Information Service, PB 81-117822, U.S. Environmental Protection Agency.

Van Ordstrand, H. S., Hughes, R., and Carmody, M. G. (1943). Chemical pneumonia in workers extracting beryllium oxide. *Cleveland Clin. Q.* **10**:10-18.

Vorwald, A. J. (1959). Experimental pulmonary cancer in monkeys. *Progress Report, U.S. Public Health Service Grant C-2507 (C4) SEOH, 1959.*

Vorwald, A. J., Reeves, A. L., and Urban, E. C. J. (1966). Experimental beryllium toxicology. In *Beryllium: Its Industrial Hygiene Aspects.* Edited by H. E. Stokinger. New York, Academic Press, pp. 201-229.

Waters, M. D., Gardner, D. E., Aranyi, C., and Coffin, D. L. (1975). Metal toxicity for rabbit and alveolar macrophages *in vitro. Environ. Res.* **9**:32-47.

Weibel, E. R. (1984). *The Pathway for Oxygen, Structure and Function in the Mammalian Respiratory System.* Cambridge, MA, Harvard University Press.

Willeke, K. (1980). Generation of aerosols and facilities for exposure experiments. Ann Arbor, MI, Ann Arbor Science Publishers, Inc.

5

Diagnostic Imaging in Inhalation Lung Injury

CAROLINE CHILES, LAURENCE W. HEDLUND, and CHARLES E. PUTMAN

Duke University Medical Center
Durham, North Carolina

Lung injury may occur following acute inhalation of a toxic gas or fume, or following chronic exposure to pulmonary irritants (Fitzgerald et al., 1973). Many chemical agents are responsible for acute inhalation injury (Seaton and Morgan, 1984; Summer and Haponik, 1981; Yockey et al., 1980) and the number of people with occupational exposure to these toxic gases continues to increase. However, because of the difficulty in performing controlled clinical studies, much of our present knowledge of inhalation injury has been gathered from burn units throughout the world. Pulmonary insufficiency is a major cause of death in burn victims, and has been shown to result from inhalation of toxic products of combustion including the oxides of sulfur and nitrogen, and aldehyde gases, rather than from thermal injury (Trunkey, 1978; Zikria et al., 1972). Since the lung has a fairly uniform response to chemical injury, the radiographic approach to burn victims and industrial accident victims is similar.

The choice of imaging studies and the information sought in the patient with a history of inhalation of a toxic gas varies according to the time elapsed since the acute event. During the first 24 hr, the goal of the radiologist is to document the extent of injury and to determine whether the toxic gas has been inhaled deeply, or whether laryngospasm has confined the injury to the upper airway (Berkman, 1980). A normal chest radiograph at the time of hospital admission may be valuable as a baseline for subsequent radiographs. A normal chest radiograph does not rule out the presence of parenchymal or airway injury, which may only be radiographically evident 24-48 hr after the acute event. In the subacute stage, imaging studies are directed toward monitoring complications in the hospitalized patient. In the patient who has survived the acute epidose and is receiving long-term follow-up care, or in the patient who has chronic exposure to a low concentration of a noxious gas, imaging studies may be oriented toward the diagnosis of bronchiolitis obliterans and pulmonary fibrosis.

In burn victims, the incidence of pulmonary complications ranges from 15 to 42%. Because the presence of pulmonary complications is associated with a significant increase in mortality, ranging from 50 to 89%, early diagnosis of pulmonary injury is important for both therapeutic prognostic considerations (Teixidor et al., 1983a).

Imaging studies that can be performed on patients following acute inhalation include chest radiographs, radionuclide studies, pulmonary angiography, computed tomography (CT), and magnetic resonance imaging (MR). However, because of the often unstable condition of these patients, chest radiographs, obtained at the patient's bedside with a portable unit, remain the most frequently used imaging modality.

I. Acute Phase

During the first 24 hr following inhalation of smoke and/or toxic gases, the chest radiograph may or may not demonstrate pulmonary parenchymal manifestations of direct inhalational injury. In contrast to the patient whose injury is limited to the upper airway with resulting chemical tracheobronchitis and in whom the chest radiograph is normal, the patient who has inhaled a noxious fume deeply often develops radiographic abnormalities within the first 24 hr (McArdle and Finlay, 1975; Pruitt, 1975). However, a normal chest radiograph does not exclude parenchymal injury (Moylan et al., 1972; Teixidor et al., 1983b). The chest radiograph may remain normal despite clinical evidence of parenchymal injury, including arterial hypoxemia and elevated carboxyhemoglobin levels (Putman et al., 1977).

Focal opacities or diffuse patchy opacities may be seen. If the acute phase is not complicated by adult respiratory distress syndrome, these opacities typically clear within 3 days (Kangarloo et al., 1977) (Fig. 1). The temporal relationship between the inhalation episode and the development and clearing of these opacities suggests that they are most likely due to atelectasis (Fig. 2). Possible

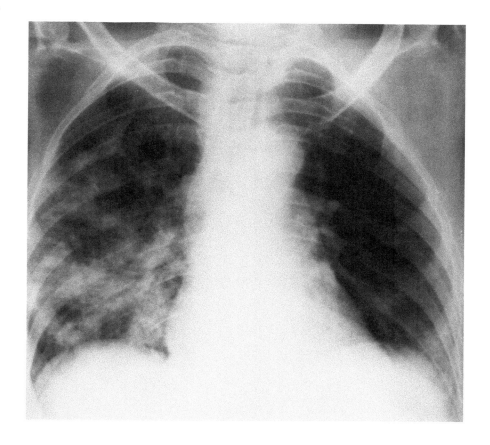

Figure 1 Asymmetrical pattern of airspace disease, greater in the right lung, with-in 24 hr of smoke inhalation.

causes of atelectasis include decreased mucociliary clearance with inspissation of secretions within bronchi and bronchioles, reflex bronchoconstriction, and sur-factant inactivation (Trunkey, 1978). Animal models of smoke inhalation have been used to observe atelectasis in vivo, and to measure surface tension in lung samples as an indicator of surfactant activity (Nieman et al., 1980). Gross atel-ectasis was seen within seconds of the onset of smoke exposure, and was invari-ably present at the end of a 5 min period of smoke inhalation. Cinephotomi-

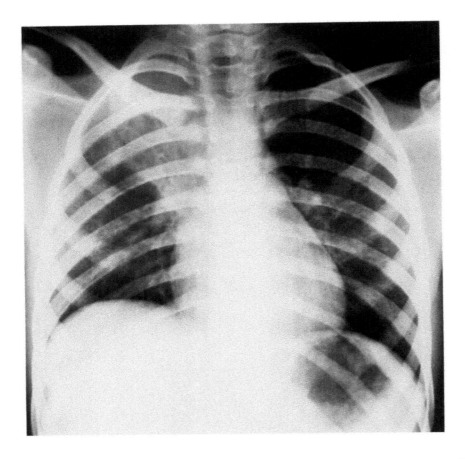

Figure 2 Right upper lobe atelectasis in a 10-year-old boy developed within 4 hr of smoke inhalation. Chest radiograph was normal 24 hr later.

croscopy suggested that the alveolar walls became unstable, and minimum surface tension measurements increased from 6.8 to 22 dynes/cm. This suggests either a decrease in available surfactant or inactivation of the surfactant present.

Bilateral diffuse alveolar opacities more likely represent noncardiogenic pulmonary edema, which develops as a result of damage to both the alveolar epithelium and the capillary endothelium (Fig. 3a). This damage results in increased permeability of the alveolar-capillary membrane, with resultant transudation of fluid

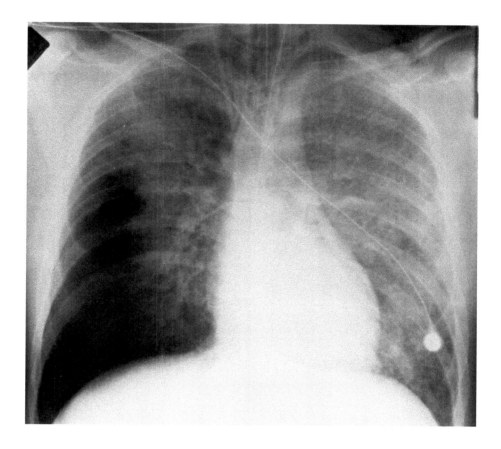

Figure 3a Bilateral airspace disease resembling pulmonary edema with relative sparing of right lower lobe occurred within 6 hr of sulfuric acid inhalation in a 20-year-old man. Intubation and positive pressure ventilation resulted in pneumomediastinum and subcutaneous emphysema.

into the alveolar spaces. In some patients, the radiographic appearance of interstitial edema, manifested by indistinct pulmonary vessels and peribronchial cuffing, may be the first sign of parenchymal injury (Teixidor et al., 1983b). The involvement is often asymmetrical. In the acute phase, pleural effusions, cardiomegaly, and septal lines are typically absent.

During the first 24 hr following the acute event, complications related to

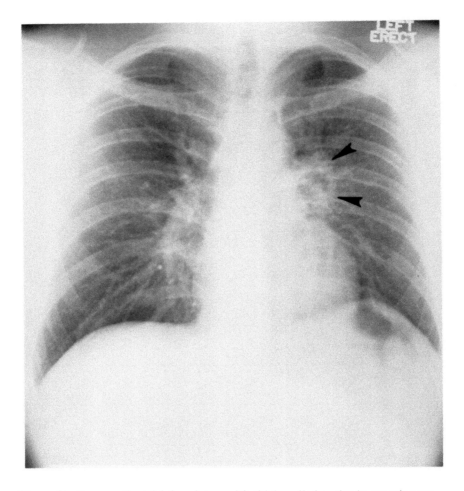

Figure 3b Same patient 16 days later, with thick-walled cavity in superior segment of left lower lobe representing lung abscess resulting from aspiration.

therapeutic intervention may also be apparent on chest radiographs. The placement and optimal positioning of central venous lines and endotracheal and nasogastric tubes can be monitored on chest radiographs. The rapid appearance of pleural or mediastinal fluid after venous line placement should raise the possibility of arterial injury or aberrant line placement with subsequent infusion of fluid (Fig. 4). Positioning of the endotracheal tube in a mainstem bronchus can result in collapse of the opposite lung, a potentially life-threatening complication in a

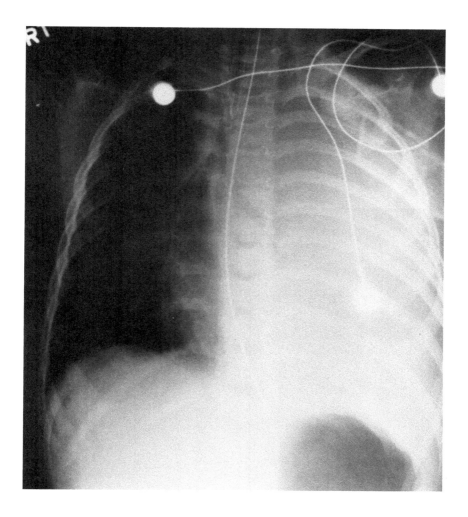

Figure 4 Opacification of left hemithorax with shift of the mediastinum to the right occurred in a 4-year-old burn patient following inadvertent puncture of the pleura during subclavian line placement, with subsequent infusion of fluid.

patient with pre-existing lung injury. In addition, barotrauma related to mechanical ventilation may first be detected by chest radiographs (Fig. 3a). Chest radiographs in critically ill patients are often obtained using a portable unit with the patient supine. Attention should be directed to the highest portions of the tho-

rax, the anterior costophrenic sulci in the supine patient, when pneumothorax is
suspected.

II. Subacute Phase

Imaging studies may be of greatest value in the subacute phase of inhalation injury, defined here as the patient's hospitalization following the first 24 hr after
the acute event. During this period, the goal of the radiologist is to detect second-

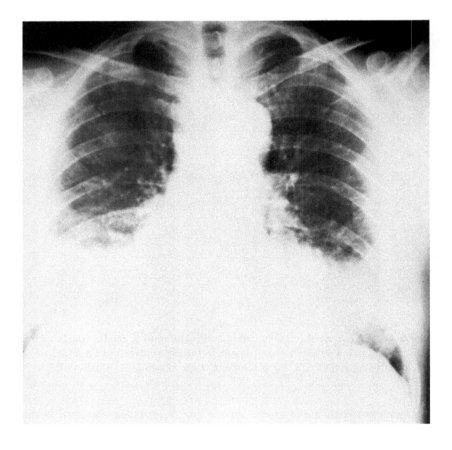

Figure 5a Bibasilar airspace opacities were present within 8 hr of phosgene gas
inhalation.

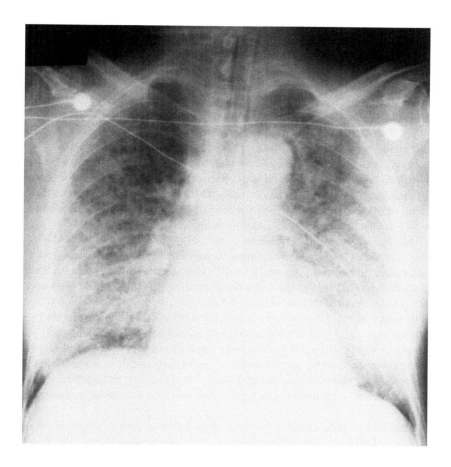

Figure 5b Same patient 8 hr later with diffuse bilateral pattern of noncardiogenic pulmonary edema.

ary pulmonary complications, including infection, barotrauma, and fluid overload. The abnormal chest radiograph in the subacute phase of inhalation injury can be considered an example of adult respiratory distress syndrome (ARDS), ARDS is the final pathway of acute lung injury caused by a variety of agents, including inhaled toxins, aspiration, and infection (Greene et al., 1983). In many cases of ARDS the chest radiograph may be normal during the initial 24 hr despite the presence of clinical signs of respiratory distress. After 24 hr, diffuse bilateral lung opacification is noted. Focal areas of spared lung may be present initially, yielding to widespread involvement (Fig. 5). In this setting, radiographic detection of superimposed intravenous fluid overload, infection, or pulmonary hemorrhage may be difficult.

Septic complications are the principal cause of death in 54% of burn patients (Curreri et al., 1980). The radiographic appearance of cavitation, increased focal opacity, or bulging interlobar fissures suggests infection. After an initial increase in extravascular lung water (EVLW) following the inhalation injury, the development of sepsis causes a further increase in pulmonary capillary membrane permeability (Peitzman et al., 1981; Tranbaugh et al., 1980). This results in increased diffuse alveolar edema 24-48 hr after the clinical onset of sepsis.

In patients who have sustained thermal injury over a large percentage of the body surface area, large volumes of intravenous fluid are often required to compensate for fluid loss from the skin surface. This may result in inadvertent fluid overload. Radiographic distinction of pulmonary edema due to fluid overload from that due to increased capillary permeability is difficult.

Overhydration pulmonary edema commonly produces a central perihilar pattern of airspace opacity, accompanied by prominent pulmonary vessels, and cardiomegaly. In addition, the width of the vascular pedicle (measured on the posteroanterior chest radiograph from the point at which the superior vena cava crosses the right mainstem bronchus to the midline, and from the midline to the point of origin of the left subclavian artery from the aorta) is increased above the normal range of 43-53 mm on an erect posteroanterior chest radiograph (Milne et al., 1985). Capillary permeability edema has a more peripheral distribution of airspace opacity, accompanied by pulmonary vessels of normal caliber, normal heart size, and vascular pedicle width. However, since mixed patterns are common, additional studies may be required to document parenchymal injury.

Clearance of radionuclides from the lungs has been used to diagnose inhalation injury (Lull et al., 1980; Moylan et al., 1972; Moylan and Chan, 1978; Schall et al., 1978). Intravenous injection of 10 mCi ^{133}Xe dissolved in saline is followed by serial gamma camera imaging of the lungs at 30 sec intervals (Fig. 6). In a normal person, there is complete clearing of the xenon from the lungs at 90-150 sec after injection. Delayed clearance of xenon identifies inhalation injury, although false-positive studies occur in patients with underlying pulmonary diseases (emphysema, asthma, chronic bronchitis, bronchiectasis) or as a result of other acute pulmonary disease, including pneumonia. Delayed clearance of xenon corresponding to inhalation injury may be detected before the chest radiograph demonstrates abnormality. A perfusion scan, obtained using a 4 mCi dose of ^{99m}Tc] macroaggregated albumin (MAA), can be obtained to detect perfusion abnormalities related to pulmonary emboli.

More recently, ^{99m}Tc] diethylenetriamine pentaacetate (Tc-99m-DTPA) has been used to differentiate cardiogenic from noncardiogenic pulmonary edema

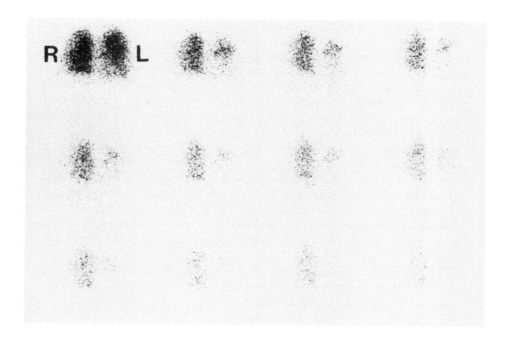

Figure 6 Xenon 133 ventilation scan performed after intravenous injection of 4 mCi [133] Xenon dissolved in saline. The washout images show retention of xenon in the entire right lung and the left midlung. The patient is a 21-year-old female burn victim. Her lungs were clear on the chest radiograph, and perfusion scan revealed normal perfusion to both lungs. The focal retention of xenon in the left lung is consistent with inhalation injury, but the diffuse retention in the right lung raises concern about underlying pulmonary disease, foreign body aspiration, or mucous plugging of central bronchi. (Case provided by Paul Christian, M.D., University of Utah Medical Center, Salt Lake City, Utah.)

(Mason et al., 1985). The radionuclide is dissolved in saline and delivered as an aerosol, which is then inhaled by the patient. Serial images of the lungs are obtained with a scintillation camera at 30 sec intervals. The rate of clearance of [99mTc] DTPA over electronically defined regions of interest is calculated over a 7 min washout interval and expressed as percent decline per minute. In the normal population, the radionuclide is cleared at an average rate of 1.3%/min. In patients with noncardiogenic edema, the clearance is accelerated to 5.1%/min (in a study of nine patients). Although the clearance is also increased in patients with cardiogenic edema, the average rate is only 2.9%/min (in a study of six patients).

Exposure to smoke or noxious gases can result in asphyxia, and the resulting loss of consciousness predisposes the patient to aspiration of gastric contents. Aspiration may be superimposed on the lung injury primarily related to inhalation, or it can mimic inhalation injury. Focal disease in the presence of a resolving pattern of edema may be due to pneumonia or aspiration. [111]Indium-labeled white cell scanning may help to document the presence of pulmonary infection. Pulmonary infection can progress to lung abscess, often in the dependent areas of the lungs (Fig. 3b).

In the presence of **ARDS**, the decreased compliance of the lungs in association with mechanical ventilation may result in the rupture of an alveolus, with subsequent dissection of air along bronchovascular sheaths into the mediastinum. Radiographic evidence of pneumomediastinum may be followed by the appearance of subcutaneous emphysema, pneumothorax, and, rarely, pneumopericardium.

Pulmonary embolus also occurs in this setting. Because of coexisting pulmonary disease, ventilation-perfusion scans may be indeterminate, requiring pulmonary angiography for diagnosis.

III. Chronic Injury

In the months to years following the acute inhalational event, patients may continue to exhibit upper airway and pulmonary dysfunction. The chronic sequelae of inhalation injury include bronchiolitis obliterans, bronchiectasis, and tracheal stenosis. Tracheal stenosis can occur as a result of chemical irritation of the tracheobronchial mucosa, and also as a result of tracheostomies performed during the patient's hospitalization (Perez-Guerra et al., 1971; Pruitt et al., 1975). This lesion is best evaluated by bronchoscopy or linear tomography, but may sometimes be visualized on chest radiographs (Fig. 7). CT may also demonstrate tracheal stenosis, but often overestimates the severity of the stenosis (Gamsu and Webb, 1982).

The pathologic diagnosis of bronchiolitis obliterans is made when plugs of granulation tissue or organized purulent secretions are found obliterating the lumina of the bronchioles and alveolar ducts. This may be accompanied by emphysema and pulmonary fibrosis that further engulfs vessels and terminal airways. Organizing pneumonia, manifested by variable degrees of interstitial infiltration by mononuclear cells, may also be present (Epler et al., 1985). Although broncholitis obliterans is frequently idiopathic in origin, it is also associated with identified causes, including exposure to toxic fumes (Seggey et al., 1983).

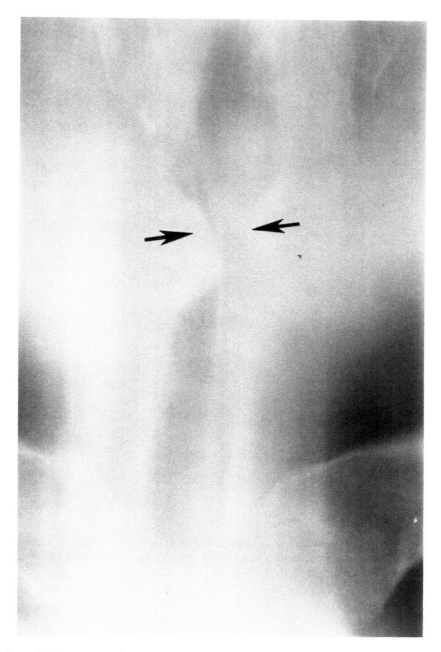

Figure 7 Narrowing of the trachea secondary to prior tracheostomy can be visualized with conventional linear tomography.

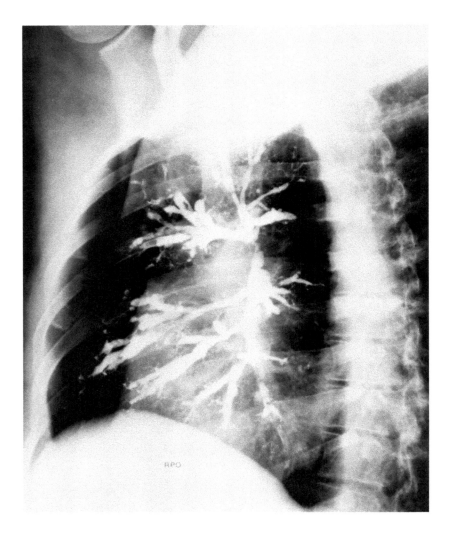

Figure 8 Bronchogram reveals cylindrical and saccular bronchiectasis in a 28-year-old fireman, 9 months after acute smoke inhalation. (Reproduced with permission from Putman et al., 1977.)

The chest radiograph in bronchiolitis obliterans is variable, but most frequently demonstrates bilateral patchy "ground-glass" or alveolar opacities, often lobar or segmental in distribution (Gosink et al., 1973). Hyperinflation, unilateral disease, cavitation, and pleural effusions are infrequent.

Bronchiectasis involving the segmental bronchi has also been described (Perez-Guerra et al., 1971). Bronchography using oily Dionosil (propyliodine) as a contrast medium, may reveal cylindrical and saccular bronchiectasis, with plugs of granulation tissue preventing filling of the more peripheral airways (Fig. 8).

Cylindrical bronchiectasis is manifested by mild tubular dilatation of the bronchi. Saccular, or cystic, bronchiectasis, representing advanced disease, includes markedly dilated bronchi with ballooned terminations. Fewer bronchi are visualized since small branches are destroyed and obliterated by fibrosis.

IV. Experimental Methods

Experimental studies in animals have helped to define more clearly some of the very early radiographic changes that occur following lung injury. CT has been particularly useful because of its sensitivity in detecting small increases in lung density associated with pulmonary edema, which often follows acute lung injury (Hedlund and Putman, 1985; Hedlund et al., 1983).

Regional analysis of density change in the axial, or cross-sectional, CT image has shown distinct patterns occurring with different forms of pulmonary edema. For instance, following 2 hr of elevated left atrial pressure (>28 mmHg) in dogs, increased CT density is seen primarily in central and dependent areas of the axial lung image (Hedlund et al., 1984). On the other hand, the embolic-hemorrhagic injury from vascular infusion of oleic acid results in a patchy, primarily peripheral, pattern of increased lung density in dogs (Hedlund et al., 1982, 1985) and in sheep. Significant increases in lung density can be detected with CT within 15-30 min after a single infusion of oleic acid (dogs, 0.05 ml/kg; sheep, 0.03 ml/kg). Lung injury can be detected earlier with CT than with conventional chest films. A similar pattern and time course of oleic acid injury has been observed in dogs with magnetic resonance spin echo images (Hedlund et al., 1986). By comparison to oleic acid, alloxan infusion in dogs produces a more uniform increase in lung CT density both peripherally and centrally (Putman et al., 1984). The differences between these three forms of pulmonary edema (hydrostatic, embolic-hemorrhagic, capillary leak) reflect in part differences in dispersal of toxic agents in the pulmonary vasculature (Chiles et al., 1986; Tarver et al., 1986) and the response of the lungs to elevated vascular pressures (Hedlund et al., 1984).

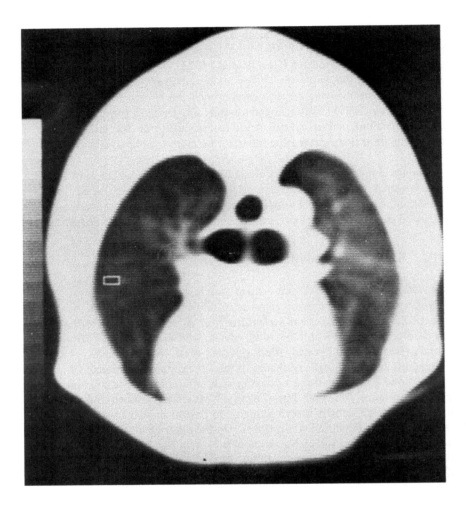

(a)

Figure 9 CT scans of the thorax of a prone dog before (a, left) and 48 hours after a 4 hr exposure to 1 ppm of phosgene gas (b, right). Both scans were obtained with the lungs at functional residual capacity. Overall density of the lung parenchyma, determined by an automated method (Hedlund et al., 1983) increased 35% (77 HU) from −780 HU (220 density units) during baseline (a) to −703 HU (297 density units) after phosgene exposure (b).

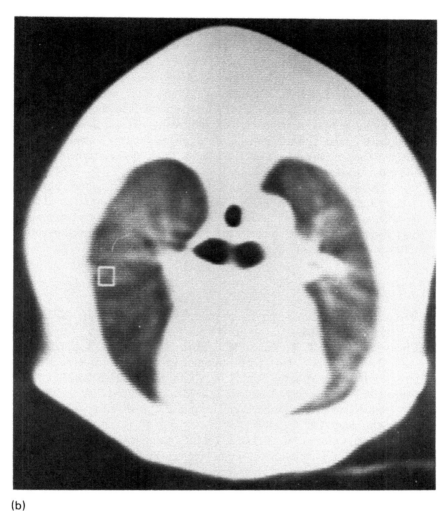

(b)

Figure 9 (continued)

Preliminary animal studies with CT and MR have shown that these modalities are also useful for revealing regional changes in the lungs following inhalational injury. Following exposure to phosgene gas (concentration X time ranging from 240 to 350 ppm X min), CT scans of the canine thorax showed diffusely increased lung density, with both central and perivascular/peribronchial predominance (Fig. 9) (Hedlund and Putman, 1985). Spin echo MR images of baboons exposed to 98% oxygen for 4 days showed diffusely increased signal intensity in the lung parenchyma. Signal intensity was also elevated in peribronchial, perivascular, and subpleural areas suggesting the development of interstitial edema. These observations correlated well with physical assessments of edema and observations at autopsy.

These results suggest that carefully controlled animal studies using transaxial modalities such as CT and MR may help to evaluate parenchymal injury in patients following acute inhalation of a toxic gas. These experimental studies may also help us to develop better methods for early lesion detection and for following the course of injury and treatment.

References

Berkman, Y. M. (1980). Aspiration and inhalation pneumonias. *Semin. Roentgenol.* **15**:73-84.

Chiles, C., Hedlung, L. W., Kubek, R. T., Harris, C., Sullivan, D. C., Tsai, J. C., and Putman, W. E. (1986). Distribution of 15- and 37-μ diameter microspheres in the dog lung in the axial plane. *Invest. Radiol.* **21**:618-621.

Curreri, P. W., Luterman, A., Braun, D. W. Jr., and Shires, G. T. (1980). Burn injury: analysis of survival and hospitalization time for 937 patients. *Ann. Surg.* **192**:472-478.

Epler, G. R., Colby, T. V., McLoud, T. C., Carrington, C. B., and Gaensler, E. A. (1985). Bronchiolitis obliterans organizing pneumonia. *N. Engl. J. Med.* **312**:152-158.

Fitzgerald, M. X., Carrington, C. B., and Gaensler, E. A. (1973). Environmental lung disease. *Med. Clin. North Am.* **57**:593-622.

Gamsu, G., and Webb, W. R. (1982). Computed tomography of the trachea: normal and abnormal. *Am. J. Roentgenol.* **139**:321-326.

Gosink, B. B., Friedman, P. J., and Liebow, A. A. (1973). Bronchiolitis obliterans: roentgenologic-pathologic correlation. *Am. J. Roentgenol.* **117**: 816-832.

Greene, R., Jantsch, H., Boggis, C., Strauss, H. W., and Lowenstein, E. (1983). Respiratory distress syndrome with new considerations. *Radiol. Clin. North Am.* **21**:699-703.

Hedlund, L. W., and Putman, C. E. (1985). Methods for detecting pulmonary edema. *Toxicol. Indust. Health* **1**:59-68.

Hedlund, L. W., Effman, E. L., Bates, W., Beck, J., Goulding, P., and Putman, C. (1982). Pulmonary edema: a CT study of regional changes in lung density following oleic acid injury. *J. Comput. Assist. Tomogr.* **6**:939-946.

Hedlund, L. W., Vock, P., and Effmann, E. (1983). Computed tomography of the lung: densitometric studies. *Radiol. Clin. North Am.* **21**:775-788.

Hedlund, L. W., Vock, P., Effmann, E. L., Lischko, M. M., and Putman, C. E. (1984). Hydrostatic pulmonary edema: an analysis of lung density changes by computed tomography. *Invest. Radiol.* **19**:254-262.

Hedlund, L. W., Vock, P., Effmann, E. L., and Putman, C. E. (1985). Morphology of oleic acid-induced lung injury: observations from computed tomography, specimen radiography, and histology. *Invest. Radiol.* **20**: 2-8.

Hedlund, L. W., Deitz, J., Herfkens, R., Nassar, R., Effmann, E., and Putman, C. (1986). Magnetic resonance imaging of pulmonary edema following oleic acid injury. *Am. Rev. Respir. Dis.* **133**:A403.

Kangarloo, H., Beachley, M. C., and Ghahreman, G. G. (1977). The radiographic spectrum of pulmonary complications in burn victims. *Am. J. Roentgenol.* **128**:441-445.

Lull, R. J., Anderson, J. H., Telepak, R. J., Brown, J. M., and Utz, J. A. (1980). Radionuclide imaging in the assessment of lung injury. *Semin. Nucl. Med.* **10**:302-310.

Mason, G. R., Effros, R. M., Uszler, J. M., and Mena, I. (1985). Small solute clearance from the lungs of patients with cardiogenic and noncardiogenic pulmonary edema. *Chest* **88**:327-334.

McArdle, C. S., and Finlay, W. E. I. (1975). Pulmonary complications following smoke inhalation. *Br. J. Anaesth.* **47**:618-622.

Milne, E. N. C., Pistolesi, M., Minati, M., and Guintini, C. (1985). The radiologic distinction of cardiogenic and non-cardiogenic edema. *Am. J. Roentgenol.* **144**:879-894.

Moylan, J. A., and Chan, C-K (1978). Inhalation injury—an increasing problem. *Ann. Surg.* **188**:34-37.

Moylan, J. A., Wilmore, D. W., Mouton, D. E., and Pruitt, B. A. (1972). Early diagnosis of inhalation injury using Xenon-133 lung scan. *Ann. Surg.* **176**:477-484.

Nieman, G. F., Clark, W. R. Jr., Wax, S. D., and Webb, W. R. (1980). The effect of smoke inhalation on pulmonary surfactant. *Ann. Surg.* **191**: 171-181.

Peitzman, A. B., Shires, G. T. III., Corbett, W. A., Curreri, P. W., and Shires

G. T. (1981). Measurement of lung water in inhalation injury. *Surgery* **90**: 305-312.

Perez-Guerra, F., Walsh, R. E., and Sagel, S. S. (1971). Bronchiolitis obliterations and tracheal stenosis: late complications of inhalation burn. *JAMA* **218**:1568-1570.

Pruitt, B. A., Erickson, D. R., and Morris, A. (1975). Progressive pulmonary insufficiency and other pulmonary complications of thermal injury. *J. Trauma* **15**:369-379.

Putman, C. E., Loke, J., Matthay, R. A., and Ravin, C. E. (1977). Radiographic manifestations of acute smoke inhalation. *Am. J. Roentgenol.* **129**:865-870.

Putman, C. E., Hedlund, L. W., Tsai, J., and Effmann, E. L. (1984). Pulmonary edema: a comparison of regional differences in the lung in three animal models. *Chest* **86**:338 (abstr).

Schall, G. L., McDonald, H. D., Carr, L. B., and Capozzi, A. (1978). Xenon ventilation-perfusion lung scans: the early diagnosis of inhalation injury. *JAMA* **240**:2441-2445.

Seaton, A., and Morgan, W. K. C. (1984). Toxic gases and fumes. In *Occupational Lung Diseases,* 2nd ed. Philadelphia, W. B. Saunders, pp. 609-642.

Seggev, J. S., Mason, U. G. III, Worthen, S., Stanford, R. E., and Fernandez, E. (1983). Bronchiolitis obliterans: report of three cases with detailed physiologic studies. *Chest* **83**:169-174.

Summer, W., and Haponik, E. (1981). Inhalation of irritant gases. *Clin. Chest Med.* **2**:273-287.

Tarver, R., Tsai, J., Hedlund, L. W., Sullivan, D., Lischko, M., Harris, C. C., Effmann, E., and Putman, C. (1986). Regional pulmonary distribution of iodine-125-labeled oleic acid: its relationship to the pattern of oleic acid edema and pulmonary blood flow. *Invest. Radiol.* **21**:102-107.

Teixidor, H. S., Novick, G., and Rubin, E. (1983a). Pulmonary complications in burn patients. *J. Can. Assoc. Radiol.* **34**:264-270.

Teixidor, H. S., Rubin, E., Novick, G. S., and Alonso, D. R. (1983b). Smoke inhalation: radiologic manifestations. *Radiology* **149**:383-387.

Tranbaugh, R. F., Lewis, F. R., Christensen, J. M., and Elings, V. B. (1980). Lung water changes after thermal injury: the effects of crystalloid resuscitation and sepsis. *Ann. Surg.* **192**:479-487.

Trunkey, D. D. (1978). Inhalation injury. *Surg. Clin. North Am.* **58**:1133-1140.

Yockey, C. C., Eden, B. M., and Byrd, R. C. (1980). The McConnell missile accident: clinical spectrum of nitrogen dioxide exposure. *JAMA* **244**:1221-1223.

Zikria, B. A., Ferrer, J. M., Floch, H. F. (1972). The chemical factors contributing to pulmonary damage in "smoke poisoning." *Surgery* **71**:704-709.

6

Bronchoalveolar Lavage in Inhalation Lung Toxicity

K. RANDALL YOUNG, JR.

National Institute of Allergy
   and Infectious Diseases
National Institutes of Health
Bethesda, Maryland

HERBERT Y. REYNOLDS

Yale University School of Medicine
New Haven, Connecticut

Over the past decade, as fiberoptic bronchoscopy has become an increasingly useful tool in the evaluation of airway and parenchymal lung disease, bronchoalveolar lavage (BAL) has emerged as a valuable technique for sampling cellular and soluble components of the lower respiratory tract for clinical and research purposes (Hunninghake et al., 1979; Young and Reynolds, 1984). In a clinical setting, BAL has proven useful in the diagnosis of infectious lung disease, the diagnosis of some forms of interstitial lung disease, and in the "staging" of sarcoidosis and idiopathic pulmonary fibrosis. As a research tool, BAL has provided a relatively noninvasive means of sampling secretions of the lower respiratory tract; the soluble and cellular constituents of these secretions can then be subjected to a wide variety of analyses in the laboratory. The general categories of tests that can be performed on BAL fluid are summarized in Table 1.

This chapter will review BAL as a clinical and research tool applicable to the study of inhalational lung disease. We will discuss practical aspects of BAL technique, review in detail the basic properties of the more important cellular and protein constituents of BAL, and finally discuss studies dealing with the clinical and research utility of BAL as applied to patients and animal models with inhalational lung disease.

Table 1 Research Applications of BAL

Cellular components
  Total and differential counts
  Determination of cell viability
  Determination of lymphocyte subpopulations with monoclonal antibodies
  Ultrastructural studies of cells
  Functional studies of cells
    Macrophages
      Receptor functions
      Phagocytosis
      Mediator release (e.g., interleukin 1, leukotrienes)
      Antigen processing and presentation
    Lymphocytes
      Immunoglobulin production
      Proliferative responses to antigens and antigens
      Mediator release (e.g., interleukin 2, gamma-interferon)
  Molecular studies of gene expression
Soluble components
  Total protein quantitation
  Immunoglobulins
    Total and subclass (IgG and IgA) determination
    Opsonic activity
  Assessment of integrity of alveolar-capillary membrane by analyzing protein
  size, partition coefficient
  Lipid components: phospholipid profile

Our discussion of the applicability of **BAL** to clinical and research issues in inhalational toxicology will focus on three critical questions:

1. How might **BAL** help assess the burden of inhaled material in the lung and thus quantitate intensity of exposure?

2. What role may **BAL** play in determining the presence or absence of injury and in estimating its severity?

3. How can **BAL** contribute to therapy, either directly as a therapeutic

modality itself or by providing information that might influence decisions regarding treatment and assist in evaluating the response?

These questions will have relevance in both clinical inhalational toxicology and animal models that attempt to reproduce certain aspects of the clinical situation.

I. History

While fiberoptic bronchoscopy has been in increasingly widespread use in Japan, the United States, and Europe since the 1960s, direct cannulation of the lower respiratory tract dates to the mid-19th century, when Green's report of bronchial catheterization was met with scorn and derision (Gee and Fick 1980; Patterson, 1926). Chevalier Jackson of Philadelphia pioneered the practical use of rigid bronchoscopy in the 1920s for airway examination and removal of foreign bodies. In 1922, bronchial lavage was used to treat a patient with phosgene gas poisoning (Gee and Fick, 1980), and beginning approximately 50 years ago the practice of washing out a portion of the lung to remove accumulated secretions or to treat intractable asthma was first practiced (Crystal et al., 1986). Whole lung lavage remains a viable treatment modality for patients with pulmonary alveolar proteinosis. These lavages were usually accomplished using a large-bore double-lumen Carlens tube. Also practical were pulmonary washings obtained through smaller flexible catheters, such as a 19 Fr Metras catheter (Finley et al., 1967). Using this technique, Finley and co-workers successfully obtained alveolar lining fluid and cells from the lungs of seven young healthy volunteers and four patients with obstructive lung disease. In addition, they diagnosed histoplasmosis in a patient with resolving nodular lung infiltrations whose lavage fluid cell block contained yeast-like organisms and whose histoplasmin skin test became positive and complement-fixation test for antibodies to *H. capsulatum* increased in titer. Harris and colleagues, using similar methods, performed bronchoalveolar lavage on smokers and nonsmokers and studied the phagocytic capabilities, glucose utilization, and ultrastructure of alveolar macrophages obtained from these individuals. They demonstrated ultrastructural differences and a significant increase in the rate of baseline glucose use in smokers' cells compared to those from nonsmokers (Harris, 1970).

The advent of fiberoptic bronchoscopy as a common pulmonary diagnostic technique in the 1970s greatly facilitated bronchoalveolar lavage, and the technique is now performed routinely in the clinical evaluation of inflammatory and infectious lung disease. Numerous investigations have helped to clarify the interrelationships among the various soluble and cellular components of the alveolar lining fluid (as will be discussed below), to elucidate some of the pathogenetic processes leading to lung injury, and to suggest a potential clinical role for BAL in staging and following interstitial lung disease (Reynolds, 1974; Reynolds et al., 1977; Weinberger et al., 1978; Calvanico, 1980; Crystal et al., 1981; Hunninghake et al., 1980, 1981; Hunninghake and Crystal, 1981; Hunninghake, 1980; Merrill and Reynolds, 1982, 1983).

While the precise place of BAL in the clinical armamentarium of the pulmonary physician is still being debated (Fulmer, 1982), the technique appears to be safe and well-tolerated by most patients (Strumpff et al., 1981; Goldenheim, 1984; Rankin et al., 1984). Occasional patients will experience fever, and some will exhibit reversible impairment of measured pulmonary function, but with careful patient selection and appropriate technique performed by experienced operators, the mortality is zero and the morbidity is very low.

II. Technique

BAL technique varies from one institution to another, especially in such details as the size of aliquots of lavage fluid used and total volume infused; however, the basic method is fairly standard and some general guidelines to the procedure will be presented here.

As noted above, patient selection is an important factor in limiting the morbidity and mortality of the BAL procedure. Although the lavage may be performed through an endotracheal tube with the patient under general anesthesia (e.g., before performing an open lung biopsy), the procedure is most commonly done in the awake patient under local anesthesia; thus, the patient should be able to cooperate with the procedure and understand simple instructions (such as breath holding) during the test.

No firm guidelines exist on abnormalities in pulmonary function that may preclude the safe performance of BAL. However, extreme caution should be exercised in performing BAL in patients with advanced restrictive or obstructive defects evident on pulmonary function testing. Similarly, significant hypoxemia that cannot be corrected with supplemental oxygen may preclude BAL or mandate that the procedure be performed through an endotracheal tube with good airway control and the capacity to administer high flow oxygen and positive pressure ventilation. A guideline we have used is that BAL should be performed in an intensive care unit through an endotracheal tube in any patient in whom the arterial pO_2 cannot be raised above 70 mmHg by the administration of supplemental nasal oxygen.

BAL is usually performed with the subject in the supine position, although the sitting position is also acceptable. Supplemental oxygen is administered via a nasal cannula or face mask, and electrocardiographic monitoring is performed throughout the procedure. Of course, all necessary emergency and resuscitative equipment should be immediately available.

In our usual procedure, the subject is premedicated with intramuscular atropine (0.6-0.8 mg) and codeine (60 mg) 30-60 min before the bronchoscopy. Additional sedation, if necessary, may be achieved by the administration of intravenous diazepam in 5-10 mg increments. The nares and pharynx are anesthetized with a spray or topical application of 1 or 2% lidocaine. Following adequate anesthesia of the pharynx, the fiberoptic bronchoscope is passed transnasally or transorally to a point just above the epiglottis and larynx. Additional 1% lidocaine may then be administered through the suction channel directly onto the vocal cords and into the trachea. Since lidocaine is readily absorbed from the respiratory mucous membranes, an important concern is the total dose of lidocaine administered during the procedure. A reasonable guideline appears to be a maximum total of approximately 300 mg lidocaine (30 ml of a 1% solution) (Credle et al., 1974).

Once adequate anesthesia of the trachea is obtained, the bronchoscope is advanced into the major bronchi. Following careful inspection of the entire tracheobronchial tree, the bronchoscope is wedged gently but firmly into a third- or fourth-generation bronchial segment. The choice of lavage location may be dictated by several concerns, chiefly the anatomical distribution of the lung disease as judged radiographically. If possible, segments of the middle lobe or lingula should be chosen, because their anterior location favors fluid recovery in the supine subject. However, adequate return of infused solution should be possible from virtually any region of the lung. Additional lidocaine may be infused into the segment chosen for lavage to minimize coughing in response to instillation of the lavage fluid.

In a typical lavage procedure, sterile isotonic saline is infused through the bronchoscope in 30-50 ml aliquots; following instillation of each aliquot, the fluid is gently aspirated back through the bronchoscope using a syringe or gravity drainage. This alternating procedure is continued until a predetermined total of instilled volume is reached (see below). Fluid recovery is initially poor as the lung segment is filled with saline but improves quickly; typically 55-75% of the infused volume is recovered from the lung. The remainder is rapidly absorbed into the circulation and is no longer detectable (at least radiographically) within 24 hr of the procedure.

Volumes as great as 300 ml may be infused into each of two lung segments in normal volunteers without noticeable symptoms or postbronchoscopy complications. However, in patients with lung disease, we commonly limit the infused volume to no more than 150-200 ml. In hypoxemic patients, only one segment is lavaged. Lavage volumes smaller than 150 ml may be employed, but use of excessively small amounts tends to sample predominantly the larger airways and not sample adequately the alveoli and smaller airways (Lee et al., 1981; McGuire et al. 1982). Merrill et al. (1982) have shown that use of lavage volumes of 100 ml or more yields results on protein analysis that are reproducible and comparable to those obtained by other laboratories.

With respect to sampling of cellular populations, a number of investigators have found that the first of serial lavage aliquots tends to have a larger percentage of neutrophils and airway epithelial cells than do subsequent aliquots, presumably due to preferential sampling of larger airways (Babal, 1984; Voisin, 1984; Yasuoka, 1984).

III. Processing of BAL Fluid

The method by which BAL fluid is processed will be determined largely by the questions being asked in each individual clinical or research setting. Virtually all protocols, however, will involve separation of the recovered instillate into fluid and cellular components. Our protocol will be discussed here, with comments on important modifications added when necessary.

The recovered fluid is filtered through sterile gauze to remove any large particulate matter and then centrifuged at 500 X g to pellet the cellular fraction. The fluid is then decanted and prepared for subsequent analysis of relevant substances (see below). Some or all of the fluid may be concentrated by positive pressure ultrafiltration through a membrane of approximately 10,000 dalton molecular weight cut-off and frozen for later measurement of proteins and other macromolecular constituents. Small molecules should be measured on the unconcentrated fluid.

The cell pellet obtained from the initial centrifugation step is washed, and a count of total cells is performed using a hemacytometer. Cell viability is assessed using exclusion of trypan blue or other nonvital dye, and the percentage of red blood cells is given as an estimate of the degree of contamination of lavage fluid by blood during the lavage procedure. Cytocentrifuge preparations made from the lavage cell pellet are stained with a Wright-Giemsa or analogous stain (such as Diff-Quick) to determine counts of various cell types present.

The optimal method for enumerating different cell populations in BAL has been the topic of some debate (Crystal et al., 1986). Differential counting of Wright-Giemsa-stained cytocentrifuge preparations has been the standard in most laboratories. However, Saltini and co-workers (1984) noted that the proportion of small cells in the original BAL cell suspension was greater than the percentage of lymphocytes identified on cytocentrifuge preparations, and they developed a method for quantitating cell populations collected on Millipore filters and stained with hematoxylin-eosin. Using both filter and cytocentrifuge methods, they examined BAL fluid from 10 normal volunteers and 39 patients with interstitial lung disease. They found that the percentage of lymphocytes identified on cytocentrifuge preparations was lower than that on filter preparations in 88% of the 49 individuals studied. On average, the proportion of lymphocytes determined from cytocentrifuge preparations was 73% of that quantitated on filter preparations. The filter technique was validated on cell mixtures of alveolar macrophages and highly purified lymphocytes and in that setting yielded values that closely approximated the predicted value. The cytocentrifuge method, in contrast, underestimated the percentage of lymphocytes by an average of 36%, with apparent losses of lymphocytes of up to 50% in some cases. These authors also noted that repeated "washing" and centrifugation of cells led to an average loss of 22% of cells present in the original lavage suspension.

Mordelet-Dambrine and colleagues (1984) also investigated the effect of BAL processing on cell counts and found that the percentage of macrophages determined by staining with neutral red was slightly lower than that found when May Grunwald Giemsa staining was used. Additionally, these investigators noted that cell counts decreased by 34% after two washings and that speed of cytocentrifugation altered the percentage of lymphocytes found, with more lymphocytes found after centrifugation at 90 g than at 23 g.

These findings highlight the importance of considering the role of laboratory processing when interpreting lavage findings and comparing results between and among different laboratories.

A persistent problem in the interpretation of lavage findings lies in the fact that the amount of alveolar epithelial lining fluid sampled in a given BAL procedure is unknown and there is thus no reliable denominator against which amounts of proteins and numbers of cells may be standardized. For this reason, protein concentrations are frequently expressed in relation to the amount or concentration of albumin retrieved and cell counts are expressed in absolute numbers or in number of cells per volume of lavage fluid recovered.

In an effort to circumvent this difficulty and to estimate the relative dilution of the epithelial lining fluid (ELF) by BAL fluid, Rennard and co-workers (1986) used urea as a marker of dilution. By measuring urea concentrations in plasma and BAL fluid and assuming that the concentration of urea in the ELF equals that of plasma and that the diffusion of urea into BAL fluid is negligible during the short duration of the procedure, these investigators estimated that the volume of ELF recovered is approximately 1.0 ml/100 ml lavage fluid recovered. Using this value they calculated that the density of inflammatory and immune effector cells on the alveolar epithelial surface was approximately 21,000 cells/μl.

The utility of the urea method for calculating ELF volume has been questioned by other investigators. Marcy et al. (1987) found that while there was a successive decrease in total protein and IgG concentrations in serial BAL aliquots, the concentration of urea increased, suggesting that the diffusion of urea into BAL fluid is not negligible and may introduce significant artifacts into the

Table 2 Factors Influencing BAL Recovery of Soluble and
Cellular Components

Temperature, pH, divalent cation content of instilled fluid

Aliquot size and number; total instilled volume

Presence of obstructive lung disease

Processing of lavage material

  Number of centrifugations in washing

  Cytocentrifuge versus filter preparations for differential counting

  Method of concentration of fluid phase of BAL

Trauma to airways

Adequacy of wedge of bronchoscope in airway

estimation of ELF volume. These attempts, however, represent useful approaches to advancing our understanding of the manner in which ELF is sampled by BAL and should lead to methods by which more accurate quantitation and standardization of BAL protein and cellular components may be achieved.

Recovery of instilled BAL fluid and protein and cellular components can be influenced by the specific details of the BAL protocol used (Crystal et al., 1986). Some of the important factors affecting concentrations are listed in Table 2.

IV. Soluble Components of BAL Fluid

The list of noncellular components identified in BAL fluid is long and ever-increasing. Most of these substances are proteins or lipids. They represent both materials that transude from the serum and substances that may be synthesized locally in the lung. Many of the proteins identified in BAL are important constituents of the inflammatory and immunologic processes or are important in protecting the lung from assault by digesting enzymes (e.g., alpha-1-antiprotease). The major substances identified in BAL are listed in Table 3, together with the estimated percentage of total protein in the BAL sample that they constitute.

Proteins in respiratory secretions come from two major sources: transudation across the barrier between capillaries and the alveolar epithelial surface (the blood-air barrier), and local synthesis by cells lining the bronchial and alveolar epithelial surfaces. These latter cells include the epithelial cells of the lung, such as type II pneumocytes and columnar cells, and immune effector cells, such as B lymphocytes, plasma cells, and alveolar macrophages.

Table 3 Immunologic Substances in Normal Lower Airway and Alveolar Lining Fluids as Sampled by **BAL**

Component	Estimated percentage of total protein in **BAL** sample
Serum-derived	
Albumin	30
Transferrin	0.1
Immunologic proteins	
IgA	5
11S Dimeric (with bound secretory component and J-chain constitutes about 90% of IgA) Monomeric IgA (<10%)	
IgG	14
IgE	0.00001
IgM	<0.1
IgD	?
Complement components C_4, C_3, C_6	
Properdin factor **B**,	—
Lactoferrin	
Carcinoembryonic antigen	
Epithelial cell products	
Free secretory component	1.0
Enzyme inhibitors	
α_1-Antitrypsin	0.7
α_2-Macroglobulin	0
Low-molecular-weight trypsin inactivator	—
Enzymes (metalloprotease, serine proteases, collagenase, angiotensin convertase, lysozyme)	—
Vasoactive mediators	
Surfactant	
Structural proteins	
Fibronectin	—
	~52% of total protein identified

From Young and Reynolds (1984) with permission.

The amount of protein that transudes from blood into the epithelial lining fluid of the lung depends on the size of the particular protein in question, its electric charge and molecular configuration, and the integrity of the alveolar-capillary barrier. The integrity of this barrier may be affected by such diverse factors as hydrostatic pressure in the pulmonary capillaries and damage from inflammatory processes occurring on either the endothelial surface of the capillary or the epithelial surface of the lung. Substances of low molecular weight (e.g., electrolytes, sugars, urea) and smaller proteins such as albumin (molecular weight approximately 69,000) pass relatively unhindered across the normal alveolar-capillary barrier. There appears to be little impairment of diffusion for proteins up to molecular weights of approximately 200,000, while above this size there is significant restriction of transudation.

A variety of insults to either side of the blood-air barrier can result in its increased permeability to serum proteins and cellular components. For example, inhalation of toxic fumes or aspiration of gastric contents may damage the epithelial layer of the bronchoalveolar surface, or initiation of the inflammatory process and activation of complement components or polymorphonuclear neutrophils in the bloodstream may injure the endothelial surface of the pulmonary capillary. Mechanisms by which host defense mechanisms may contribute to acute and chronic lung injury have recently been reviewed (Ward, 1986). While a number of investigators have used various techniques (including measurement of radiolabeled albumin, influx of erythrocytes, and clearance of dextran molecules of known size into the airways) to measure alveolar capillary permeability in experimental models and human ARDS (Sibbald et al., 1981), there is not yet available a practical and reproducible method for doing this in routine clinical practice.

As shown in Table 3, the principal protein identified in BAL fluid is albumin, which accounts for approximately 30% of the total protein identified. Since albumin is synthesized solely by the liver and enters the epithelial lining fluid of the lung only by transudation, it provides a useful marker of serum protein entry into the lung and is frequently used as the denominator against which concentrations of other proteins are normalized.

Transferrin, another serum-derived protein, is frequently identifiable in BAL samples. Lactoferrin, an iron-binding protein synthesized and secreted by neutrophils, is also present in BAL and may have important bacteriostatic properties (Weinberg, 1978), rising in concentration in conjunction with the influx of neutrophils into the lung in response to an inflammatory or infectious insult.

Immunoglobulins and complement components make up a large group of immunologically important molecules routinely found in significant concentrations in the epithelial lining fluid of the lung (Reynolds and Newball, 1974). Immunoglobulin G (IgG) is the immunoglobulin present in the largest amount in the epithelial lining fluid and accounts for approximately 14% of the total protein in BAL fluid. IgG in respiratory secretions appears to be derived from both active secretion in the lung and passive transudation across the blood-air barrier. The IgG/albumin ratio in BAL closely approximates that in serum (0.33 versus 0.31) in normal nonsmokers (Merrill et al., 1980a; Reynolds and Merrill, 1981), suggesting the roughly equal transudation of these two molecules, both of which are smaller than the above-noted 200,000 dalton threshold below which diffusion occurs relatively unhindered.

There is preliminary evidence, however, that IgG and other immunoglobulin species may be secreted locally in the lung, especially during inflammatory activity. Lawrence and co-workers (1978, 1980) and Rankin et al. (1983) have studied immunoglobulin production by airway lymphocytes in normal subjects and patients with interstitial lung disease. While there was no correlation between IgG concentrations and numbers of IgG-secreting cells in BAL in normal individuals, in patients with sarcoidosis there was a highly significant correlation between these two parameters (Rankin et al., 1983), which substantiates the hypothesis that during active inflammation a major portion of airway IgG is secreted locally. Hunninghake and Crystal (1982) have suggested that activation of T lymphocytes in the lung and concomitant polyclonal B-cell activation may contribute to high serum levels of IgG as well.

IgG is actually a family of four proteins, termed IgG subclasses (Schur, 1972). Merrill and co-workers (1985a) have quantitated IgG subclasses in the serum and lavage fluid of normal subjects and found that BAL levels of IgG_1 and IgG_2 approximated those in serum, while concentrations of IgG_4 were increased in comparison to serum levels. BAL levels of IgG_3 were variable, with some subjects having increased levels compared to serum and others having concentrations similar to serum values. The significance of the relative concentrations of IgG subclasses in normal persons and in those with disease (Merrill et al., 1985b) is not yet clearly understood; however, these molecules have differing properties with respect to complement fixation, cell surface receptor attachment, opsonic activity, and sensitization of cells for mediator release and thus may each modulate airway inflammatory processes in a unique fashion.

Immunoglobulin A, the major immunoglobulin in human external secretions, is detectable in all BAL specimens and constitutes approximately 5% of all BAL protein (Reynolds and Newball, 1974; Reynolds and Merrill, 1981). More than 90% of this IgA is typical secretory IgA (dimeric with attached secretory component) in contrast to human serum IgA, which is nearly all monomeric. The size of dimeric IgA (approximately 380,000 daltons), the presence of secretory piece (which is produced by airway epithelial cells), and the fact that the BAL IgA/albumin ratio exceeds that in serum all suggest that a considerable proportion of airway IgA is produced locally in the lung (Merrill et al., 1980a).

Immunoglobulin E is detectable in very minute amounts in the BAL of some normal individuals (Merrill et al., 1980b), and sensitive assays can quantitate small amounts of IgM in some samples of normal BAL. Reynolds and colleagues (1977) noted that elevated values of BAL IgM could be measured in individuals with hypersensitivity pneumonitis.

Delacroix and colleagues (1985) have recently studied carefully the concentrations of various proteins in the BAL fluid of normals and patients with interstitial lung disease using sensitive immunonephelometric and immunoradiometric assays. They then calculated relative coefficients of excretion for alpha-2-macroglobulin and monomeric and polymeric IgA and IgM. These investigators found evidence of either local secretion of polymeric IgA and small amounts of IgM in the bronchial lamina propria or the active transepithelial transport of these molecules. In patients with active interstitial lung disease, they noted that seepage from serum probably accounted for most of the rise in the concentration of polymeric IgA, while there was evidence for active secretion of monomeric IgA, IgG, alpha-2-macroglobulin, and IgM.

A number of complement components may be identified in BAL fluid (Robertson et al., 1976). These may enter by diffusion or be synthesized locally by alveolar macrophages (Pennington et al., 1981; Scherzer et al., 1980). The presence of these proteins is likely of importance in the generation of complement component fragments with chemotactic and proinflammatory activity (e.g., C3a and C5a). There remains some controversy surrounding the question of whether the lung is an active site of immunoglobulin synthesis under normal and/or diseased conditions. The data cited above support a role for airway lymphocytes in the local secretion of immunoglobulin, but Hance and colleagues (1984), using a technique that detected direct immunoglobulin synthesis from radiolabeled precursors, found only small amounts of immunoglobulin secretion in patients with interstitial lung disease and virtually none in normal individuals. A definitive answer to this crucial question must await further investigations.

Merrill and colleagues have studied proteins produced by bronchial epithelial cells and have investigated the roles of these substances as correlates of histopathologic airway changes in smokers and patients with lung carcinoma. They demonstrated a significant decrease in the amount of free secretory component recovered in the lung lavage of 20% of cigarette smokers and postulated that low levels of this glycoprotein may indicate biochemical dysfunction of epithelial cells after inhalant exposure to cigarette smoke (Merrill et al., 1980a). In a more recent investigation (Merrill et al., 1984) they analyzed levels of secretory component and keratins in BAL. They found a decrease in free secretory component in BAL from symptomatic smokers compared to nonsmokers and asymptomatic smokers and noted detectable levels of keratin proteins only in symptomatic smokers. Furthermore, they noted an inverse relationship between tissue free secretory component and keratins in immunohistochemical studies of lung sections from patients with pulmonary carcinoma. This relationship was borne out in analysis of the concentrations of these proteins in lavage fluid from cancer patients. These investigators postulated that smokers with altered levels of free secretory component and keratins in BAL fluid may be at increased risk of smoking-associated lung disease.

As can be seen in Table 3, a variety of additional molecules can be identified in normal BAL fluid. These include important antiproteases, crucial to the defense of the lung against digestion by the ubiquitous proteolytic enzymes of inflammatory cells and invading microorganisms, and the lipid lining material of the alveolus (surfactant), which probably has important antiinfectious and immunomodulatory properties in addition to its well-described effects on surface tension in the alveolus (Juers et al., 1976; LaForce, 1976; Ansfield and Benson, 1980).

V. Cellular Components in BAL Fluid

In the typical BAL of a normal nonsmoker, 10-20 million respiratory cells are recovered; this number may be increased four- or fivefold in BAL from individuals who smoke. There is a rough correlation between cell recovery and the intensity of smoking history. Table 4 lists cell retrieval and average differential counts of respiratory cells from nonsmokers and people with a history of smoking.

As discussed above, differential counts of respiratory cells obtained by bronchoalveolar lavage may be performed on stained cytocentrifuge preparations or by using stained filters on which cells have been collected. Analysis of the differential counts of BAL cells has been found to provide useful clinical information in a variety of pulmonary disorders, especially the granulomatous and nongranulomatous interstitial lung disorders. The literature on this topic is extensive and has been carefully reviewed (Hunninghake and Mosely, 1984; Merrill and Reynolds, 1983; Hunninghake et al., 1979; Crystal et al., 1981; Reynolds, 1984; Turner-Warwick and Haslam, 1986). Our discussion of respiratory cells in this chapter will be confined to important aspects of individual cell types found in the normal and damaged lung and the relation of these cells to inhalational lung injury.

A. Alveolar Macrophages

Approximately 90% of the cells recovered in normal lavage fluid are alveolar macrophages (see Table 4). These large vacuolated cells are the pulmonary component of the reticuloendothelial system, similar to the mononuclear phago-

Table 4 Respiratory Cells in Lung Washings from Smokers and Nonsmokers

Group	Age (yr) sex	Smoking HX pack-yr	Cell count (10^6)	AMs	Differential, % PMNs	Lymphs	Eo/baso[b]
Nonsmokers ($n = 44$)	27.2 ± 1.2[a] 27M 17F	0	19.5 ± 2.3 (3-59)[c]	87.4 ± 1.3 (77-99)	1.5 ± 0.2 (0-5)	9.3 ± 0.8 (0-23)	—
Marijuana smokers ($n = 7$)	20.3 ± 0.7 6M 1F	?	63.4 ± 10.0 (27-99)	88.5 ± 2.6 (76-100)	3.7 ± 0.9 (0-10)	7.7 ± 2.2 (0-20)	—
Light smokers (<10 pack-years) ($n = 18$)	23.4 ± 0.7 11M 7F	6.4 ± 0.6	58.2 ± 5.8 (27-110)	$93 \;\pm 0.9$ (79-99)	3.3 ± 0.9 (0-17)	4.0 ± 0.5 (0-10	—
Moderate smokers (10-20 pack-years) ($n = 14$)	25.8 ± 0.9 7M 7F	15.8 ± 0.9	91.1 ± 16.3 (27-234)	95.7 ± 0.7 (85-99)	2.4 ± 0.4 (1-9)	2.5 ± 0.4 (0-6)	—
Heavy smokers (>20 pack-years) ($n = 20$)	38.2 ± 2.3 12M 8F	41.1 ± 5.9	102.0 ± 12.1 (15-200)	$92 \;\pm 0.5$ (75-99)	3.5 ± 0.6 (1-18)	3.7 ± 0.5 (1-10)	—

[a]Mean ± SEM.
[b]Less than 1 percent in all differential counts.
[c]Range observed.
From Reynolds and Merrill (1981) with permission.

cytes found in other tissues throughout the body (such as the Kupffer's cells in the liver, dendritic cells in the spleen, and Langerhans' cells in the skin). The alveolar macrophage is derived from promonocytes in the bone marrow (Thomas et al., 1976) and appears to have a very long life span in the lung.

The principal activity classically associated with the macrophage is phagocytosis of microorganisms and other foreign particles in the alveolus. This constitutes the first line of phagocytic defense against infection and airway assault by inhalation or aspiration. The surface of the macrophage has been found to possess a wide array of membrane receptors for the Fc portion of IgG, IgG subclasses and complement components (Reynolds et al., 1975; Naegel et al., 1984). Through these membrane receptors, the alveolar macrophage binds and internalizes opsonized organisms and particulate matter.

It has been recognized increasingly over the past decade that, in addition to its well-developed phagocytic capabilities, the macrophage plays an important effector role in the modulation of immune and inflammatory responses in the lower respiratory tract (Nathan et al., 1980). Macrophages express class II (or Ia) antigens of the major histocompatibility complex on their membranes and process and present antigens to lymphocytes for the initiation and development of cell- and antibody-mediated immune responses (Unanue, 1980). In addition, they secrete a vast array of products that modulate various aspects of lung inflammatory and immune responses (Table 5) (Fels and Cohn, 1986). Among these substances are certain toxic elements such as reactive oxygen species and proteases that likely play an important role in mediating lung damage in response to an inhalational injury (Ward, 1986) and chemotactic factors for neutrophils, which influence the migration of these secondary inflammatory cells into the lung under certain infectious or toxic conditions (Hunninghake et al., 1978, 1980; Merrill et al., 1980c).

B. Lymphocytes

Lymphocytes make up 8-10% of cells recovered from the lung by BAL. As noted above, the differential count of lymphocytes may be significantly underestimated by cytocentrifuge counting of cells compared to filtration methods (Saltini et al., 1984), especially when the percentage of lymphocytes in a given BAL sample is increased. Lymphocyte percentage tends to fall in BAL from smokers' lungs, but the absolute number of lymphocytes is usually increased due to the significant rise in total cell recovery. As in blood, airway lymphocytes may be classified as T (or thymus-derived) cells, B (or "bursal" or bone marrow-derived) cells, or null cells on the basis of functional characteristics and surface properties.

Numerous investigators have used monoclonal antibodies directed against lymphocyte surface antigens to analyze the phenotypic characteristics of airway

Table 5 Secretory Products of Mononuclear Phagocytes that Modulate the Inflammatory and Immune Response

Complement components	Other enzymes (continued)
C1	Deoxyribonucleases
C4	Phosphatases
C2	Glycosidases
C3	Sulfatases
C5	Arginase
Factor B	Lipoprotein lipase
Factor D	Enzyme inhibitors
Properdin	Plasmin inhibitors
C3b inactivator	α_2-Macroblobulin
β1H	Binding proteins
Coagulation factors	Transferrin
X	Transcobalamin II
IX	Fibronectin
VII	Apolipoprotein E[a]
V	Oligopeptides
Thromboplastin	Glutathione
Prothrombin	Bioactive lipids
Prothrombinase	Arachidonate metabolites
Other enzymes	Prostaglandin E_2
Lysozyme[a]	Prostaglandin $F_{2\alpha}$
Neutral proteases	6-Ketoprostaglandin $F_{1\alpha}$ (from prostacyclin)
Plasminogen activator	Thromboxane A_2
Collagenase	Leukotrienes B, C, D, E
Elastase	Monohydroxyeicosatetraenoic acids (5-, 12-, 15-)
Angiotensin converting enzyme	Dihydroxyeicosatetraenoic acids
Acid hydrolases	Platelet-activating factors
Proteases	
Lipases	

Table 5 (continued)

Nucleosides and metabolites	Growth-promoting factors
Thymidine	Lymphocytes (T- and B-cells)
Uracil	Myeloid precursors (colony-stimu-
Uric acid	lating factors, factor inducing
	monocytopoiesis)
Reactive metabolites of O_2	Erythroid precursors
Superoxide anion	Fibroblasts
Hydrogen peroxide	Capillaries (angiogenesis factor)
Hydroxyl radical	
Singlet oxygen (?)	Factors inhibiting growth of:
	Lymphocytes
Chemotactic factors	Myeloid precursors
For neutrophils	Tumor cells
For fibroblasts	Viruses (α- and β-interferons)
Factors regulating synthesis of	Other hormone-like factors
proteins by other cells	Endogenous pyrogens (two mol wt
Hepatocytes	species)
Serum amyloid A	Insulin-like activity
Haptoglobin	Thymosin B_4
Synovial-lining cells	
Collagenase	
Prostaglandins	
Plasminogen activator	
Adipocytes	
Lipoprotein lipase	

[a]Major bulk products.
From Fels and Cohn (1986), with permission.

T lymphocytes obtained by BAL of normal individuals and patients with a variety of respiratory disorders (Hunninghake and Crystal, 1981; Leatherman et al., 1984; Young et al., 1985). While functional status may not always be inferred reliably from such surface marker data, there may be characteristic changes in lymphocyte subpopulations in certain disease states. For example, there is an increase in cells reacting with the OKT_4 antibody (usually denoting helper-inducer cells) in the

BAL of patients with active sarcoidosis, and increases in cells with the suppressor-cytotoxic phenotype (OKT_8+) in hypersensitivity pneumonitis, another granulomatous lung disorder. Functional studies performed on T cells from the airways of patients with interstitial lung disease have helped to elucidate the pathogenic mechanisms underlying the alveolitis and lung injury in these disorders (Pinkston et al., 1983; Robinson et al., 1985).

Airway B lymphocytes mature into immunoglobulin-secreting cells under the influence of factors secreted by T cells. Numbers of immunoglobulin secreting cells for different immunoglobulin isotypes may be determined by use of a reverse hemolytic plaque assay and are increased in patients with interstitial lung disease (Lawrence et al., 1978, 1980; Rankin et al., 1983) and in other conditions, such as acquired immunodeficiency syndrome (Young et al., 1985).

C. Neutrophils

The polymorphonuclear neutrophil is not usually found in the BAL of normal lungs in large numbers (see Table 4). As discussed above, the neutrophil may migrate into the lung under the influence of several chemotactic factors, including the activated complement component C5a and substances secreted by alveolar macrophages (Merrill et al., 1980c; Hunninghake et al., 1980). Once present in the airways, the neutrophil may help to augment the phagocytic capabilities of the alveolar macrophage but it may also participate in the process of injuring the lung through its ability to secrete toxic oxygen species and proteolytic enzymes (Ward, 1986). Idiopathic pulmonary fibrosis (IPF) and asbestosis are characterized by the presence of a "neutrophil alveolitis" (Reynolds et al., 1977), in contrast to the "lymphocyte alveolitis" of sarcoidosis and hypersensitivity pneumonitis. In addition to its role in mediating chronic lung injury in disorders such as IPF, the neutrophil likely participates in damaging the alveolar capillary membrane in acute lung injury states (such as ARDS) as well (reviewed in Glauser and Fairman, 1985).

D. Other Respiratory Tract Cells

In addition to macrophages, lymphocytes, and neutrophils, other respiratory tract cells may be found in small numbers in BAL fluid. Eosinophils and basophils are rare in normal persons and generally make up less than 1% of the lavage cell population. However, eosinophils may be found in increased numbers in patients with disorders such as IPF and the various eosinophilic pneumonias or after allergen challenge in asthmatic subjects (De Monchy et al., 1985). Ciliated respiratory epithelial cells and erythrocytes may also be seen in normal BAL fluid. The number and percentage of erythrocytes will increase dramatically in patients with airway trauma or in association with pulmonary hemorrhage.

E. BAL as a Reflection of Lung Histology

An important assumption underlying the use of BAL to reflect the status of the airways and alveoli is that the cellular components in BAL fluid accurately represent those cells found on the epithelial surface of the lower respiratory tract and in the lung parenchyma. A number of investigators have attempted to ascertain how well BAL cell data reflect lung histology.

Davis and colleagues (1978) found that, as expected, lavage lymphocyte counts correlated better with airway lymphocytosis than with cells in the interstitial spaces. Hunninghake and co-workers (1981) isolated immune and inflammatory cells from lung tissue obtained from patients with IPF and sarcoidosis and patients undergoing resection of solitary pulmonary nodules and compared those values to cell populations found in bronchoalveolar lavage fluid from the respective groups. They found that cell populations obtained from tissue specimens, when grouped by disease and analyzed, were very similar to those seen in the respective bronchoalveolar lavage. They did not, however, compare values on an individual patient by patient basis.

Turner-Warwick and Haslam (1986) point out that important differences between tissue histology and BAL cell counts should be remembered. For example, while neutrophils and eosinophils predominate in BAL from IPF (or cryptogenic fibrosing alveolitis) patients, the predominant inflammatory cells in the interstitial tissue in this disorder are lymphocytes and plasma cells.

While the above-mentioned studies have attempted to validate BAL as a sampling technique in chronic lung disease, its utility in acute lung injury remains relatively undefined. Using a dog model of acute lung injury caused by intravenous injection of phorbol myristate acetate (a potent neutrophil activator), Weiland and colleagues (1985) found a strong correlation between lavage neutrophil count and the number of neutrophils measured in lung sections. Furthermore, there was a good correlation between BAL neutrophilia and two physiological parameters of lung injury: alveolar-arterial oxygen gradient and alveolar-capillary permeability as estimated by BAL protein content.

Thus, while BAL provides a valuable and fairly noninvasive tool for sampling inflammatory and immune effector cells from the lower respiratory tract, attempts should be made to correlate BAL findings with actual histologic findings whenever possible.

VI. BAL as a Method of Assessing Toxin Exposure

While BAL can theoretically sample the lower respiratory tract and retrieve respired particles deposited during previous exposures, the utility of this application is limited by the solubility of some respiratory toxins and their transient residence in the epithelial lining fluid. BAL has been applied to the investigation of exposure to asbestos, an insoluble fibrous mineral, in which particles might be expected to remain intact for a considerable length of time. De Vuyst et al. (1982) performed BAL on 82 patients with suspected asbestos-related diseases, 2 patients with known asbestos exposure but without related disease, and 40 control subjects with a variety of non-asbestos-related lung disorders. Asbestos bodies were detected in BAL from most of the individuals with known or suspected exposure, in 5 of 8 patients without known exposure but with suspicious asbestos-related disease, and among 5 of 40 controls. Quantitative results showed higher asbestos body counts in patients with interstitial disease than in those with benign or malignant pleural disease.

Thus, while BAL may help detect exposure to certain respirable toxins, its utility is limited and it cannot reliably be used to assess the type or extent of previous toxic inhalational exposures.

VII. BAL in the Detection of Inhalational Lung Injury

General aspects of the application of BAL to the quantitation of airway and parenchymal damage have been carefully reviewed by Brain and Beck (1985) and Henderson (1984) and Henderson et al. (1985). As these investigators have demonstrated, the utility of BAL as a means of assessing respiratory tract injury from toxic inhalation relies on the accumulation of inflammatory cells and the release of cellular and serum constituents into the epithelial fluid following an inhalational injury.

Henderson (1984) has systematically reviewed the various constituents of BAL fluid that may be used to assess airway damage. Total protein may rise in response to damage to the alveolar-capillary membrane with subsequent transudation of serum proteins into the epithelial lining fluid of the lung. Lactate dehydrogenase (LDH) is a cytoplasmic enzyme involved in catalysis of glycolytic reactions. When there is significant damage to cell membranes, leakage of LDH into the extracellular milieu may lead to accumulation of detectable levels of the enzyme in BAL fluid. Other cytoplasmic enzymes such as glucose-6-phosphate dehydrogenase, glutathione peroxidase, and glutathione reductase may be measured as indicators of similar cellular damage. Release of hydrolases such as beta-glucuronidase and arylsulfatase implies damage to phagocytic cells (neutrophils or macrophages) or type II pneumocytes. Henderson et al. (1979b) and De Nicola et al. (1981) have suggested that elevations of alkaline phosphatase levels in BAL may indicate type II pneumocyte injury or proliferation; isoenzyme patterns should be determined to distinguish lung-derived from serum-derived alkaline phosphatase. Changes in cellular populations in BAL may also be used as indicators of lung injury, with increases in neutrophils and/or macrophages being seen in both acute and chronic inflammatory reactions.

An early study by Henderson and co-workers (1978) established the utility of measuring LDH in BAL fluid as an index of lung injury. They determined LDH activity in the lavage of the lungs of Syrian hamsters exposed to increasing concentrations of the detergent Triton X-100. The results of their investigation showed that LDH activity increased with increasing Triton exposure (correlation coefficient of 0.98), and the isoenzyme pattern of LDH in BAL fluid resembled that of lung tissue, thus supporting the hypothesis that the LDH was derived from damaged lung rather than from lysis of red blood cells. This study validated the use of LDH as a marker of pulmonary epithelial injury.

In a subsequent investigation, Henderson et al. (1979b) examined the response of hamster lungs to inhalation of two different metal salts: $CdCl_2$, a known toxin, and $CrCl_3$, an innocuous salt. While $CrCl_3$ exposure caused minimal biochemical or cytologic change, inhalation of $CdCl_2$ was accompanied by a dose-dependent release of LDH and hydrolases into BAL fluid, tissue morphologic and biochemical changes that lagged behind airway changes, and an acute accumulation of neutrophils in lavage fluid.

Padmanabhan et al. (1982), in a rat model of cadmium inhalation, detected elevations in BAL elastase and lysyloxidase activities and neutrophil numbers.

Using methodology similar to that in their previous studies, Henderson and co-workers (1979a) extended their observations on cadmium and chromium salts to include additional salts. On the basis of BAL measurements of enzymatic activities, sialic acid, protein content, and differential cell counts, they determined the relative toxicity of the compounds to be $CdCl_2 > SeO_2$, NH_4VO_3, $NiCl_2 > CrCl_3$.

Exposure to oxygen in pharmacologic concentrations is well-known to be toxic to the lung (Deneke and Fanburg, 1980; Frank and Massaro, 1980; Jackson, 1985). A number of investigators have used BAL methodology to study the pathogenesis of pulmonary oxygen toxicity.

Fox and colleagues (1981) investigated the mechanism leading to accumulation of neutrophils in the lung of rats exposed to 100% oxygen. They found that chemoattractant activity in the lavages of rats exposed to hyperoxia was increased approximately 10-fold compared to control animals and that this chemoattractant activity correlated closely with neutrophil counts in BAL from exposed animals. Pretreatment of the animals with cobra venom factor to deplete them of complement did not alter the results, which suggests that products of complement activation were likely not the only chemoattractant substances present in their model.

Another investigation of the role of complement in mediating pulmonary oxygen toxicity was performed by Parrish et al. (1984), who compared BAL analysis, lung histologic findings, and survival following hyperoxic exposure of mice that were genetically deficient or sufficient in the fifth component of complement. They noted that neutrophils migrated into the lungs of both groups of animals, suggesting that chemoattractant substances other than complement components play a role in mediating hyperoxic lung injury. However, the time course of the lung injury was considerably delayed in the C5-deficient mice, and this group exhibited a significant reduction in mortality compared to the C5-sufficient group. These studies suggest an important, but not exclusive, role for complement-derived chemotactic substances in mediating the neutrophil influx and subsequent lung damage in animals exposed to high inspired oxygen tensions.

Davis et al. (1983) used BAL to examine changes in the permeability of the alveolar-capillary membrane and factors secreted by bronchoalveolar cells after exposure of normal human subjects to 95% oxygen for 17 hr. They noted increased amounts of albumin and transferrin in BAL fluid, suggesting an increase in permeability of the blood-air barrier in response to hyperoxic exposure. Furthermore, they noted that alveolar macrophages from these individuals secreted more fibroblast growth factor and more fibronectin than control macrophages, suggesting that an increased macrophage-dependent stimulus to formation of fibrous tissue may be important in mediating the pathogenesis of oxygen-induced lung fibrosis. There were no consistent changes in total number or differential count of cells obtained by BAL.

Kelley and Hartman (1985) examined the release of macrophage-derived growth factors into the alveolar lining fluid in rats exposed to 100% oxygen for variable periods of time. They noted a biphasic pattern with continued O_2 exposure, with growth factor activity in lavage falling to approximately 20% of control values after 2.5 days of exposure but rebounding to three to four times baseline after 10 days of hyperoxia.

In contrast to the well-recognized adverse clinical effects of very high inspired oxygen tensions, conventional clinical wisdom has deemed lower concentrations (21-50% FiO_2) to be safe. Griffith and colleagues (1986) performed baseline and follow-up BAL and [^{99m}Tc] DTPA clearance studies on normal individuals before and after exposure to normal "therapeutic" oxygen concentrations. They observed that permeability of the blood-air barrier, as judged by BAL albumin concentration, was increased after breathing concentrations of oxygen of 30% or higher for a mean duration of 45 hr. Lung clearance of the isotope was significantly increased in the group who breathed 50% oxygen, and in these individuals there was a trend toward an increased percentage of BAL neutrophils. In none of the individuals was there bronchoscopic evidence of lung inflammation or biochemical evidence of lung tissue injury as judged by BAL concentrations of LDH, alkaline phosphatase, potassium, or several eicosanoids. These findings suggest that even concentrations of oxygen widely considered to be "safe" have the potential for causing subtle but potentially important alterations in lung structure.

A number of investigators have noted that hyperoxia may augment other forms of lung injury. Rinaldo and co-workers (1984) examined the combined effect of endotoxemia and hyperoxia on rats, and found that previous exposure to 100% oxygen potentiated the development of neutrophil chemotactic activity in BAL fluid and accelerated and intensified the neutrophil alveolitis seen in these animals. The mechanism whereby hyperoxia worsened the endotoxin injury was not clear from their investigation.

Another oxygen species, ozone, is known to cause airway inflammation and hyperresponsiveness. Holtzman and colleagues (1983) had previously demonstrated a correlation between inflammation in large conducting airways in ozone-exposed dogs and airway hyperresponsiveness to acetylcholine. In a more recent study, this same group (Fabbri et al., 1984) extended their findings to more distal airways and found that airway hyperresponsiveness is accompanied by an influx of neutrophils into smaller airways and the desquamation of airway epithelial cells. Although their BAL findings do not prove conclusively a cause and effect relationship between airway inflammation and hyperreactivity, they suggest that they may be pathogenetically related and argue that BAL may play an important role in studying the mechanisms of airway responses to ozone exposure.

Acute smoke inhalation is a source of significant morbidity and mortality from airway obstruction, bronchitis, pneumonitis, and respiratory failure. Loke and colleagues (1984) examined pathologic changes in the airways of smoke-exposed and control rabbits and analyzed BAL from these animals. They noted severe loss of tracheal epithelium, denudation of airway epithelium, ciliary flattening, and alteration in the shape of alveolar macrophages in smoke-exposed animals. Distal alveolar epithelium was well preserved. There were no significant alterations in total BAL cell counts, differential cell counts, or macrophage viability between control and smoke-exposed animals. In another study (Fick et al., 1984), these same investigators demonstrated a functional impairment of bactericidal and phagocytic capability of alveolar macrophages obtained from smoke-exposed rabbits, suggesting that smoke-induced alterations in macrophage function may leave the lung increasingly susceptible to infection after this type of injury.

Bowen and colleagues (1985) characterized a urokinase-type plasminogen activator molecule in the alveolar macrophages and BAL fluid of humans and hamsters. They found that, despite the widely recognized effect of cigarette smoking on macrophage activation, there was no difference in plasminogen activator activity between smoke-exposed and control humans and hamsters.

Diller et al. (1985) used BAL to examine changes in the blood-air barrier occurring in response to exposure of rats to low concentrations of phosgene, an important chemical intermediate used for the synthesis of plastics, dyes, pharmaceuticals, and agricultural chemicals. They found BAL protein concentration to be a sensitive marker of alveolar injury as judged histologically, and they noted that the BAL changes correlated with the degree of morphologic alteration.

In summary, BAL is an extremely useful tool for the relatively noninvasive evaluation of inhalational injury of the lung by a wide variety of substances in both humans and in animal preparations. By choosing appropriate indices of altered tissue integrity, blood-air barrier permeability, and inflammatory cell activation, the investigator can gather important insights into pathologic processes affecting the lower respiratory tract.

VIII. BAL in Therapy and Therapeutic Decision Making

One of the first uses of bronchoalveolar lavage was in the treatment of phosgene poisoning at Yale in 1922 (Gee and Fick, 1980). Since that time, the therapeutic utility of BAL (or, more appropriately, whole lung lavage through a double-lumen endotracheal tube) has been extended under certain circumstances in pulmonary alveolar proteinosis, cystic fibrosis, and asthma. Whole-lung lavage remains virtually the only therapeutic intervention available for alveolar proteinosis.

There is at present no apparent role for BAL in the treatment of acute or chronic inhalational lung disease. Perhaps more importantly, however, there may be on the horizon a role for BAL in staging clinical inhalational injury and in guiding decisions about therapy, similarly to the manner in which BAL is used by many clinicians today in treating interstitial lung diseases. The full realization of this possibility, however, must await our better understanding of the contribution of the various components of the respiratory immune and inflammatory systems to inhalational lung injury and delineation of factors with important prognostic implications.

IX. Conclusion

Bronchoalveolar lavage provides a sensitive, reproducible, and relatively noninvasive means of sampling the cellular and humoral milieu of the lower respiratory tract. This technique is finding an increasingly important place in the armamentarium of the inhalational toxicologist in studying lung injury induced by inhaled substances in both human subjects and experimental animals. As our understanding of the interplay among inhaled toxins and the complicated immune and inflammatory systems of the lower respiratory tract advances, BAL will likely provide valuable insights into the ways in which this mode of injury can be modified or prevented.

References

Ansfield, M. J., and Benson, B. J. (1980). Identification of the immunosuppressive components of canine pulmonary surface active material. *J. Immunol.* **125**:1093-1098.

Babal, P., Soler, P., Georges, R., Saumon, G., and Basset, F. (1984). Additional data on cell differentials in bronchoalveolar lavages. Presented at International Conference on Bronchoalveolar Lavage, Columbia, MD, May 1984.

Bowen, R. M., Hoidal, J. R., and Estensen, R. D. (1985). Urokinase-type plasminogen activator in alveolar macrophages and bronchoalveolar lavage fluid from normal and smoke-exposed hamsters and humans. *J. Lab. Clin. Med.* **106**:667-673.

Brain, J. D., and Beck, B. D. (1985). Bronchoalveolar lavage. In *Toxicology of Inhaled Materials.* Edited by H. Witschi and J. D. Brain. New York, Springer-Verlag, pp. 203-226.

Calvanico, N. J., Ambegaonkar, S. P., Schleuter, D. P. et al. (1980). Immunoglobulin levels in bronchoalveolar lavage fluid from pigeon breeders. *J. Lab. Clin. Med.* **96**:129-140.

Credle, W. F., Smiddy, J. F., and Elliott, R. C. (1974). Complications of fiberoptic bronchoscopy. *Am. Rev. Respir. Dis.* **109**:67-72.

Crystal, R. G., Gadek, J. E., Ferrans, V. J., Fulmer, J. D., Line, B. R., and Hunninghake, G. W. (1981). Interstitial lung disease: Current concepts of pathogenesis, staging and therapy. *Am. J. Med.* **70**:542-567.

Crystal, R. G., Reynolds, H. Y., and Kalica, A. R. (1986). Bronchoalveolar lavage—the report of an international conference. *Chest* **90**:122-131.

Davis, G. S., Brody, A. R., and Craighead, J. E. (1978). Analysis of airspace and interstitial mononuclear cell populations in human diffuse interstitial lung disease. *Am. Rev. Respir. Dis.* **118**:7-15.

Davis, W. B., Rennard, S. E., Bitterman, P. B., and Crystal, R. G. (1983). Pulmonary oxygen toxicity. Early reversible changes in human alveolar structures induced by hyperoxia. *N. Engl. J. Med.* **309**:878-883.

De Monchy, J. G. R., Kauffman, H. F., Venge, P., et al. (1985). Bronchoalveolar eosinophilia during allergen-induced late asthmatic reactions. *Am. Rev. Respir. Dis.* **131**:373-376.

De Vuyst, P., Jedwab, J., Dumortier, P., Vandermoten, G., Vande Weyer, R., and Yernault, J. C. (1982). Asbestos bodies in bronchoalveolar lavage. *Am. Rev. Respir. Dis.* **126**:972-976.

Delacroix, D. L., Marchandise, F. X., Francis, C., and Sibille, Y. (1985). Alpha-2-macroglobulin, monomeric and polymeric immunoglobulin A, and immunoglobulin M in bronchoalveolar lavage. *Am. Rev. Respir. Dis.* **132**:829-835.

Deneke, S. M., and Fanburg, B. L. (1980). Normobaric oxygen toxicity of the lung. *N. Engl. J. Med.* **303**:76-86.

DeNicola, D. B., Rebar, A. H., and Henderson, R. F. (1981). Early damage indicators in the lung. V. Biochemical and cytological response to NO_2 inhalation. *Toxicol. Appl. Pharmacol.* **60**:301-312.

Diller, W. F., Bruch, J., and Dehnen, W. (1985). Pulmonary changes in the rat following low phosgene exposure. *Arch. Toxicol.* **57**:184-190.

Fabbri, L. M., Aizawa, H., Alpert, S. E., et al. (1984). Airway hyperresponsiveness and changes in cell counts in bronchoalveolar lavage after ozone exposure in dogs. *Am. Rev. Respir. Dis.* **129**:288-291.

Fels, A. O. S., and Cohn, Z. A. (1986). The alveolar macrophage. *J. Appl. Physiol.* **60**:353-369.

Fick, R. B., Paul, E. S., Merrill, W. W., et al. (1984). Alterations in the antibacterial properties of rabbit pulmonary macrophages exposed to wood smoke. *Am. Rev. Respir. Dis.* **129**:76-81.

Finley, T. N., Swenson, E. W., Curran, W. S., et al. (1967). Bronchopulmonary lavage in normal subjects and patients with obstructive lung disease. *Ann. Intern. Med.* **66**:651-658.

Fox, R. B., Hoidal, J. R., Brown, D. M., and Repine, J. E. (1981). Pulmonary inflammation due to oxygen toxicity: involvement of chemotactic factors and polymorphonuclear leukocytes. *Am. Rev. Respir. Dis.* **123**:521-523.

Frank, L., and Massaro, D. (1980). Oxygen toxicity. *Am. J. Med.* **69**:117-126.

Fulmer, J. D. (1982). Bronchoalveolar lavage. *Am. Rev. Respir. Dis.* **126**:961-963.

Gee, J. B. L., and Fick, R. B. (1980). Bronchoalveolar lavage. *Thorax* **35**:1-8.

Glauser, F. L., and Fairman, R. P. (1985). The uncertain role of the neutrophil in increased permeability pulmonary edema. *Chest* **88**:601-607.

Goldenheim, P. D., Tilles, D. S., Ginns, L. C., Hales, C. A., and Kazemi, H. (1984). Bronchoalveolar lavage (BAL) causes deterioration in lung function. Presented at International Conference on Bronchoalveolar Lavage, Columbia, MD, May 1984.

Griffith, D. E., Holden, W. E., Morris, J. F., Min, L. K., and Krishnamurthy, G. T. (1986). Effects of common therapeutic concentrations of oxygen on lung clearance of ^{99m}Tc DTPA and bronchoalveolar lavage albumin concentration. *Am. Rev. Respir. Dis.* **134**:233-237.

Hance, A. J., Zimmerman, R., and Crystal, R. G. (1984). Is the human lung a site of immunoglobulin synthesis? *Am. Rev. Respir. Dis.* **129**:A6.

Harris, J. O., Swenson, E. W., and Johnson, J. E. (1970). Human alveolar macrophages: comparison of phagocytic ability, glucose utilization, and ultrastructure in smokers and nonsmokers. *J. Clin. Invest.* **49**:2086-2096.

Henderson, R. F. (1984). Use of bronchoalveolar lavage to detect lung damage. *Environ. Health. Perspect.* **56**:115-129.

Henderson, R. F., Damon, E. G., and Henderson, T. R. (1978). Early damage indicators in the lung I. Lactate dehydrogenase activity in the airways. *Toxicol. Appl. Pharmacol.* **44**:291-297.

Henderson, R. F., Rebar, A. H., and DeNicola, D. B. (1979a). Early damage indicators in the lungs. IV. Biochemical and cytologic response of the lung to lavage with metal salts. *Toxicol. Appl. Pharmacol.* **51**:129-135.

Henderson, R. F., Rebar, A. H., Pickrell, J. A., and Newton, G. J. (1979b). Early damage indicators in the lung. III. Biochemical and cytological response of the lung to inhaled metal salts. *Toxicol. Appl. Pharmacol.* **50**: 123-136.

Henderson, R. F., Benson, J. M., Hahn, F. F., et al. (1985). New approaches for the evaluation of pulmonary toxicity: bronchoalveolar lavage fluid analysis. *Fund. Appl. Toxicol.* **5**:451-458.

Holtzman, M. J., Fabbri, L. M., O'Byrne, P. M., et al. (1983). Importance of airway inflammation for hyperresponsiveness induced by ozone. *Am. Rev. Respir. Dis.* **127**:686-690.

Hunninghake, G. W., and Crystal, R. G. (1981). Pulmonary sarcoidosis: a disorder mediated by excess helper T-lymphocyte activity at sites of disease activity. *N. Engl. J. Med.* **305**:429-434.

Hunninghake, G. W., and Crystal, R. G. (1982). Mechanisms of hypergammaglobulinemia in pulmonary sarcoidosis: site of increased antibody production and role of T-lymphocytes. *J. Clin. Invest.* **67**:86-92.

Hunninghake, G. W., and Moseley, P. L. (1984). Immunological abnormalities of chronic noninfectious pulmonary diseases. In *Immunology of the Lung and Upper Respiratory Tract.* Edited by J. Bienenstock. New York, McGraw-Hill, pp. 345-364.

Hunninghake, G. W., Gallin, J. I., and Fauci, A. S. (1978). Immunologic reactivity of the lung: the *in vivo* and *in vitro* generation of a neutrophil chemotactic factor by alveolar macrophages. *Am. Rev. Respir. Dis.* **117**:15-23.

Hunninghake, G. W., Gadek, J. E., Kawanami, O., Ferrans, V. J., and Crystal, R. G. (1979). Inflammatory and immune processes in the human lung in health and disease: evaluation by bronchoalveolar lavage. *Am. J. Pathol.* **97**:149-206.

Hunninghake, G. W., Gadek, J. E., Fales, H. M., et al. (1980). Human alveolar macrophage-derived chemotactic factor for neutrophils: stimuli and partial characterization. *J. Clin. Invest.* **66**:473-483.

Hunninghake, G. W., Kawanami, O., Ferrans, V. J., Young, R. C., Roberts, W. C., and Crystal, R. G. (1981). Characterization of the inflammatory and immune effector cells in the lung parenchyma of patients with interstitial lung disease. *Am. Rev. Respir. Dis.* **123**:407-412.

Jackson, R. M. (1985). Pulmonary oxygen toxicity. *Chest* **88**:900-905.

Juers, J. A., Rogers, R. M., McCurdy, J. B., et al. (1976). Enhancement of bactericidal capacity of alveolar macrophages by human alveolar lining material. *J. Clin. Invest.* **58**:271-275.

Kelley, J., and Hartman, A. (1985). Growth factor release during hyperoxic pulmonary injury in young rats. *Fed. Proc.* **44**:921.

LaForce, F. M. (1976). Effect of alveolar lining material on the phagocytic and bactericidal activity of lung macrophages against *Staphylococcus aureus.* *J. Lab. Clin. Med.* **88**:691-699.

Lawrence, E. C., Blaese, R. M., Martin, R. R., et al. (1978). Immunoglobulin secreting cells in normal human bronchial lavage fluids. *J. Clin. Invest.* **62**: 832-835.

Lawrence, E. C., Martin, R. R., Blaese, R. M., et al. (1980). Increased bronchoalveolar IgG-secreting cells in interstitial lung diseases. *N. Engl. J. Med.* **302**:186-1189.

Leatherman, J. W., Michael, A. F., Schwartz, B. A., and Hoidal, J. R. (1984). Lung T cells in hypersensitivity pneumonitis. *Ann. Intern. Med.* **100**:390-392.

Lee, C. T., Fein, A. M., Lippmann, M., et al. (1981). Elastolytic activity in pulmonary lavage fluid from patients with adult respiratory distress syndrome. *N. Engl. J. Med.* **304**:192-196.

Loke, J., Paul, E., Virgulto, J. A., and Smith, G. J. W. (1984). Rabbit lung after acute smoke inhalation. *Arch. Surg.* **119**:956-959.

Marcy, T. W., Merrill, W. W., Rankin, J. A., and Reynolds, H. Y. (1987). Limitations of using urea to quantify epithelial lining fluid recovered by bronchoalveolar lavage. *Am. Rev. Respir. Dis.* **135**:1276-1280.

McGuire, W. W., Spragg, R. G., Cohen, A. B., et al. (1982). Studies on the pathogenesis of the adult respiratory distress syndrome. *J. Clin. Invest.* **69**:543-553.

Merrill, W., O'Hearn, E., Rankin, J., et al. (1982). Kinetic analysis of respiratory tract proteins recovered during a sequential lavage protocol. *Am. Rev. Respir. Dis.* **126**:617-620.

Merrill, W. W., and Reynolds, H. Y. (1982). Applied immunology of the lung. *Curr. Pulmonol.* **4**:167-188.

Merrill, W. W., and Reynolds, H. Y. (1983). Bronchial lavage in inflammatory lung disease. *Clin. Chest. Med.* **4**:71-84.

Merrill, W. W., Goodenberger, D., Strober, W., et al. (1980a). Free secretory component and other proteins in human lung lavage. *Am. Rev. Respir. Dis.* **122**:156-161.

Merrill, W. W., Naegel, G. P., and Reynolds, H. Y. (1980b). Reaginic antibody in the lung lining fluid—analysis of normal human bronchoalveolar lavage fluid IgE and comparison to immunoglobulins G and A. *J. Lab. Clin. Med.* **96**:494-500.

Merrill, W. W., Naegel, G. P., Matthay, R. A., et al. (1980c). Alveolar macrophage-derived chemotactic factor: kinetics of *in vitro* production and partial characterization. *J. Clin. Invest.* **65**:268-276.

Merrill, W. W., Barwick, K. W., Madri, J., et al. (1984). Bronchial lavage proteins as correlates of histopathologic airway changes in healthy smokers and patients with pulmonary carcinoma. *Am. Rev. Respir. Dis.* **130**:905-909.

Merrill, W. W., Naegel, G. P., Olchowski, J. J., and Reynolds, H. Y. (1985a). Immunoglobulin G subclass proteins in serum and lavage fluid of normal subjects. *Am. Rev. Respir. Dis.* **131**:584-587.

Merrill, W. W., Rankin, J. A., Naegel, G. P., Young, K. R., and Reynolds, H. Y. (1985b). Immunoglobulin G subclasses in broncholaveolar lavage and serum of normals and patients with inflammatory lung diseases. *Clin. Res.* **33**:508A.

Mordelet-Dambrine, M., Arnoux, A., Stanislas-Leguern, G., Sandron, D., Chretien, J., and Huchon, G. (1984). Processing of lung lavage fluid causes variability in bronchoalveolar cell count. *Am. Rev. Respir. Dis.* **130**:305-306.

Naegel, G. P., Young, K. R., and Reynolds, H. Y. (1984). Receptors for human IgG subclasses on human alveolar macrophages. *Am. Rev. Respir. Dis.* **129**:413-418.

Nathan, C. F., Murray, H. W., and Cohn, Z. A. (1980). The macrophage as an effector cell. *N. Engl. J. Med.,* **303**:622-626.

Padmanabhan, R. V., Gudapaty, S. R., Liener, I. E., and Hoidal, J. R. (1982). Elastolytic acitivty in the lungs of rats exposed to cadmium aerosolization. *Environ. Res.* **29**:90-96.

Parrish, D. A., Mitchell, B. C., Henson, P. M., and Larsen, G. L. (1984). Pulmonary response of fifth component of complement-sufficient and -deficient mice to hyperoxia. *J. Clin. Invest.* **74**:956-965.

Patterson, E. J. (1926). History of bronchoscopy and esophagoscopy for foreign body. *Laryngoscope* **36**:157-175.

Pennington, J. E., Matthews, W. J., Rossing, T. H., et al. (1981). Local regulation of complement biosynthesis by human alveolar macrophages. *Clin. Res.* **29**:450A.

Pinkston, P., Bitterman, P. B., and Crystal, R. G. (1983). Spontaneous release of interleukin-2 by lung T lymphocytes in active pulmonary sarcoidosis. *N. Engl. J. Med.* **308**:793-800.

Rankin, J. A., Naegel, G. P., Schrader, C. E., Matthay, R. A., and Reynolds, H. Y. (1983). Air-space immunoglobulin production and levels in bronchoalveolar lavage fluid or normal subjects and patients with sarcoidosis. *Am. Rev.*

Respir. Dis. **127**:442-448.

Rankin, J. A., Snyder, P. E., Schachter, E. N., and Matthay, R. A. (1984). Bronchoalveolar lavage—its safety in subjects with mild asthma. *Chest* **85**: 723-728.

Rennard, S. I., Basset, G., Lecossier, D., et al. (1986). Estimation of volume of epithelial lining fluid recovered by lavage using urea as marker of dilution. *J. Appl. Physiol.* **60**:532-538.

Reynolds, H. Y. (1984). Classification, definition and correlation between clinical and histologic staging of interstitial lung diseases. *Sem. Respir. Dis.* **6**: 1-19.

Reynolds, H. Y., and Newball, H. H. (1974). Analysis of proteins and respiratory cells obtained from human lungs by bronchial lavage. *J. Lab. Clin. Med.* **84**:559-573.

Reynolds, H. Y., Atkinson, J. P., Newball, H. H., and Frank, M. M. (1975). Receptors for immunoglobulin and complement on human alveolar macrophages. *J. Immunol.* **114**:1813-1819.

Reynolds, H. Y., Fulmer, J. D., Kazmierowski, J. A., et al. (1977). Analysis of cellular and protein content of bronchoalveolar lavage fluid from patients with idiopathic pulmonary fibrosis and chronic hypersensitivity pneumonitis. *J. Clin. Invest.* **59**:165-175.

Reynolds, H. Y., and Merrill, W. W. (1981). Pulmonary immunology: humoral and cellular immune responsiveness of the respiratory tract. *Curr. Pulmonol.* **3**:381-422.

Rinaldo, J. E., Dauber, J. H., Christman, J., and Rogers, R. M. (1984). Neutrophil alveolitis following endotoxemia—enhancement by previous exposure to hyperoxia. *Am. Rev. Respir. Dis.* **130**:1065-1071.

Robertson, J., Caldwell, J. R., Castle, J. R., et al. (1976). Evidence for the presence of components of alternative (properdin) pathway of complement activation in respiratory secretions. *J. Immunol.* **117**:900-903.

Robinson, B. W. S., McLemore, T. L., and Crystal, R. G. (1985). Gamma interferon is spontaneously released by alveolar macrophages and lung T-lymphocytes in patients with pulmonary sarcoidosis. *J. Clin. Invest.* **75**:1488-1495.

Saltini, C., Hance, A. J., Ferrans, V. J., Basset, F., Bitterman, P. B., and Crystal, R. G. (1984). Accurate quantification of cells recovered by bronchoalveolar lavage. *Am. Rev. Respir. Dis.* **130**:650-658.

Scherzer, H. H., Kreutzer, D. L., Varani, J., et al. (1980). Demonstration of the synthesis of the third and fifth components of complement by human alveolar macrophages. *Am. Rev. Respir. Dis.* **121**:92A.

Schur, P. H. (1972). Human gamma-G subclasses. *Prog. Clin. Immunol.* **1**:71-104.

Sibbald, W. J., Anderson, R. R., Reid, B., et al. (1981). Alveolar capillary permeability in human septic ARDS—effect of high dose corticosteroid therapy.

Chest **79**:133-142.

Strumpf, J. J., Feld, M. K., Cornelius, M., et al. (1981). Safety of fiberoptic broncholaveolar lavage in evaluation of interstitial lung disease. *Chest* **80**: 268-271.

Thomas, E. D., Ramberg, R. E., Sale, G. E., et al. (1976). Direct evidence for a bone marrow origin of the alveolar macrophage in man. *Science* **192**:1016-1017.

Turner-Warwick, M. E., and Haslam, P. L. (1986). Clinical applications of bronchoalveolar lavage: an interim view. *Br. J. Dis. Chest* **80**:105-121.

Unanue, E. R. (1980). Cooperation between mononuclear phagocytes and lymphocytes in immunity. *N. Engl. J. Med.* **303**:977-985.

Voisin, C., Wallaert, B., Fournier, E., et al. (1984). Cell population analysis of the first broncho-alveolar lavage (BAL) sample in interstitial lung diseases. Presented at International Conference on Bronchoalveolar Lavage, Columbia, MD, May 1984.

Ward, P. A. (1986). Host-defense mechanisms responsible for lung injury. *J. Allergy Clin. Immunol.* **78**:373-378.

Weiland, J. E., Dorinsky, P. M., Davis, W. B., Mohammed, J. R., Lucas, J., and Gadek, J. E. (1985). Validity of bronchoalveolar lavage (BAL) in the assessment of acute lung injury. *Am. Rev. Respir. Dis.* **131**:A29.

Weinberg, E. D. (1978). Iron-infection. *Microbiol. Rev.* **42**:45-66.

Weinberger, S. E., Kelman, J. A., Elson, N. A., et al. (1978). Bronchoalveolar lavage in interstitial lung disease. *Ann. Intern. Med.* **89**:459-466.

Yauoka, S., and Tsubura, E. (1984). Comparative analysis of cellular and biochemical components of bronchoalveolar lavage fluid (BALF) and bronchial lavage fluid (BLF). Presented at International Conference on Bronchoalveolar Lavage, Columbia, MD, May 1984.

Young, K. R., and Reynolds, H. Y. (1984). Bronchoalveolar washings: proteins and cells from normal lungs. In *Immunology of the Lung and Upper Respiratory Tract*. Edited by J. Bienenstock. New York, McGraw-Hill, pp. 157-173.

Young, K. R., Rankin, J. A., Naegel, G. P., Paul, E. S., and Reynolds, H. Y. (1985). Bronchoalveolar lavage cells and proteins in patients with the acquired immunodeficiency syndrome. An immunologic analysis. *Ann. Intern. Med.* **103**:522-533.

7

Diagnosis and Treatment of Inhalation Injury in Burn Patients

KHAN Z. SHIRANI

U.S. Army Institute of Surgical Research
Fort Sam Houston, San Antonio, Texas

BASIL A. PRUITT, JR.

U.S. Army Institute of Surgical Research
Fort Sam Houston, San Antonio, Texas

JOSEPH A. MOYLAN, JR.

Duke University Medical Center
Durham, North Carolina

I. Introduction

Man has known the toxic potential of smoke for ages. The Romans, millennia ago, executed their war criminals by exposing them to smoke prepared from the burning of green wood (Dressler et al., 1976). The recent interest in smoke as a prime contributor to burn mortality stems from clinical observations made on the victims of catastrophic events such as the Cleveland Clinic fire in 1929, the Cocoanut Grove fire in 1942, the Hartford Circus fire in 1944, and the S. S. Noronic fire in 1949. The high mortality in victims of these disasters was closely associated with the presence of pulmonary injury (Terrill et al., 1978). These and other similar events provided an impetus to the systematic studies of the toxicology of smoke. A detailed investigation of those fires along with experimental animal work in the 1940s soon indicated that the inhalation of the

The opinions or assertions contained herein are the private views of the authors and are not to be construed as official or as reflecting the views of the Department of the Army or the Department of Defense.

products of incomplete combustion, not the temperature of the inspired smoke, was responsible for the pulmonary damage sustained in fires (Moritz et al., 1945).

Recent advances in the treatment of burn injury (Demling, 1985), particularly in the area of postburn fluid therapy (Cope and Moore, 1947; Harkens, 1942; Evans et al., 1952; Moyer et al., 1965; Pruitt and Mason, 1971) and burn wound management (Lindberg et al., 1965; Pruitt, 1984), have resulted in improved patient survival (Monafo et al., 1978; Demling, 1983). As the incidence of hypovolemic burn shock, prerenal azotemia, and acute renal failure has declined and the frequency of burn wound invasion and sepsis has receded, the pulmonary complications of thermal injury have emerged as the prime determinants of postburn mortality (Phillips and Cope, 1962a,b; Foley et al., 1968).

Of the victims of fires, approximately one-third sustain inhalation injury and one-third among those with inhalation injury develop pneumonia. A recent review of over 1,000 burn patients treated at this Institute during the past 5 years indicated that inhalation injury increased mortality by about 20% beyond that expected for any given age and burn size (unpublished data). Since inhalation injury adumbrates the development of subsequent pulmonary complications and portends a high mortality, its diagnosis in the patient with cutaneous burns assumes considerable import. As means of support in patients with pulmonary insufficiency have become routinely available, most of the arcane complications of mechanical ventilation in the patient with burns (Foley et al., 1968; Morris, 1973; Teplitz et al., 1964; Epstein et al., 1963), similar to those described for the unburned patient (Stauffer et al., 1981; Lewis et al., 1977), have been frequently recognized.

II. Diagnosis of Inhalation Injury

A. Anatomical Distribution of Inhalation Injury

The anatomical site of injury to the respiratory tract influences symptoms, clinical course, and the treatment of a burn patient. The respiratory tract can be divided into three functionally distinct anatomical compartments: the upper respiratory tract (nose to epiglottis), the lower respiratory tract (vocal folds to terminal bronchioles), and the pulmonary parenchyma. The pulmonary parenchyma, or the functional gas exchange unit, encompasses the respiratory bronchioles, alveolar ducts, atria, alveoli, and alveolar sacs. These arbitrary anatomical compartments are helpful in describing the topographic distribution of the respiratory tract damage sustained with inhalation injury.

B. Mechanisms of Injury

Essential to the diagnosis of inhalation injury and imperative to prognosis in the patient with pulmonary insult is an understanding of the basic mechanisms of smoke-induced pulmonary damage. Combustion, as a rule, is an incomplete process. The products of incomplete combustion, commonly known as smoke, consist of irritant gases and airborne particles that may be liquids or solids. The nature and concentrations of the products of combustion in a fire depend on the type of material ignited and on the location as well as the timing of sampling of an environment. Combustion in unvented structures commonly results in oxygen depletion and carbon monoxide production besides smoke, a combination thought to be particularly lethal. The ignition of wood framing and mattresses yields high concentrations of carbon dioxide and particulate matter; the burning of chemically treated materials and plastics, such as interior wall coverings, kitchen cabinets, and wood floors, produces high concentrations of hydrogen chloride, hydrogen cyanide, acetaldehyde, acrolein, and benzene. The latter contaminant is also an important constituent of fires that result from ignition of petroleum products (Grand et al., 1981). Both hydrogen cyanide and hydrogen chloride are potent toxins and have been incriminated in fire-related deaths (Dyer and Esch, 1976). In 70% of 256 fire fatalities in Maryland between 1975 and 1977, the blood cyanide levels exceeded the normal range (0.00-0.25 μg/ml), indicating prevalence of this fatal gas in fire environments (Caplan, 1977). The combustion of wool, silk, and nylon fabrics yields ammonia, an intense mucous membrane irritant, and generates, to a lesser extent, nitrogen dioxide and other oxides of nitrogen.

Exposure to these irritant gases produces pulmonary edema due to both alveolar epithelial cell damage (Dowell et al., 1971) and endothelial cell damage that results in an increased capillary permeability (Sherwin and Richters, 1971). The exposure to nitrogen dioxide, in addition, impairs alveolar macrophage function, which has obvious clinical implications as related to the later development of pneumonia (Sherwin and Richters, 1971). The burning of sulfur-containing products yields sulfur dioxide, a strong mucous membrane irritant. The pyrolysis of cellulosics, wood, paper, and cotton produces acrolein, a potent mucosal irritant, inhalation of which by human volunteers in concentrations as low as 0.8 parts per million (ppm) produced intense lacrimation and irritation of all exposed mucous membranes (Sim and Pattle, 1957). Exposure of dogs to wood smoke, a rich source of acrolein, lead to pulmonary congestion and edema and death (Zikria et al., 1972b). Burning of polyvinyl chloride, a material used commonly to insulate wires and in upholstery and bedding, produces hydrogen cyanide, hydrogen chloride, chlorine, phosgene, benzene, toluene, xylene, and naphthalene (Bowes, 1974; Terrill et al., 1978). These products are strong pulmonary toxicants in low concentrations and lethal when inhaled in sufficient doses. The symptoms of pulmonary involvement, such as dyspnea, cyanosis, and acute respiratory failure, may be delayed in onset for up to 6 hr after exposure to polyvinyl chloride fumes (Dyer and Esch, 1976).

Table 1 Short-Term Lethal Concentrations for Products of
Incomplete Combustion in Fires

Contaminant gas	Short-term lethal concentration (ppm)[a]
Acrolein	30-100
Toluene diisocyanate (TDI)	~100
Nitrogen dioxide (NO$_2$)	>200
Hydrogen cyanide (HCN)	350
Hydrogen chloride (HCl)	>500
Hydrogen bromide (HBr)	>500
Sulfur dioxide (SO$_2$)	>500
Ammonia (NH$_3$)	>1,000

[a]Parts per million for a 10 min exposure.

Distribution of contaminants within the fire environment is nonhomogeneous and varies according to the location and the phase of the fire. In general, despite considerable overlap, the concentrations of particulate matter and hydrogen chloride are higher during the initial phases of the fire while levels of carbon monoxide and carbon dioxide are elevated during the knockdown or suppression phase (Grand et al., 1981). Urban fires, which commonly involve poorly ventilated structures such as skyscrapers and cellars, compared with rapidly evolving fires of highly vented structures in suburban settings (Grand et al., 1981), contain higher concentrations of contaminants such as acrolein, hydrogen chloride, and particulate materials (Burgess et al., 1979). A few among the host of toxic chemicals emitted in fires are hydrogen chloride, acetaldehyde, acrolein, benzene, hydrogen cyanide, ammonia, nitrogen dioxide, and sulfur dioxide. Table 1 lists the lethal concentrations of some of the more common contaminants. These gases, even in sublethal doses, are potent mucosal irritants and their inhalation results in extensive chemical airway damage.

The most abundant gas generated in fires, carbon monoxide, on the other hand, has no direct cytotoxic properties but causes injury through the production of systemic hypoxemia. Carbon monoxide causes a leftward shift in the oxygen dissociation curve, which accentuates tissue hypoxia and leads to cell injury. Both hypoxia and hypothermia cause a suppression of membrane-based adenosine triphosphate synthesis rate that is unmatched by a reciprocal reduction in the intracellular metabolic processes. Such imbalance in the supply and demand of energy results in uncoupling of the metabolic and membrane cell functions, increased membrane permeability, and irreversible cell damage (Hochachka, 1986).

Prevalent in a combustion atmosphere are smoke at exceedingly high temperatures and a gallimaufry of irritant gases, the toxic effects of which have been previously discussed. Another very important cause of smoke-induced pulmonary damage besides direct heat and irritant gases, of course, is the aerosolized liquid and solid particles of heterogeneous size that are well saturated with the toxic combustion products that prevail in a burning environment. These airborne, superheated, chemically contaminated particles serve not only as a vehicle of heat transfer but also as a medium of transport of combustion products to the far reaches of the respiratory apparatus. The size, solubility, and degree of contamination of those particles as well as the duration of exposure and the minute ventilation of an individual at the time of exposure determine the extent and anatomical site of injury to the respiratory tract. As the size of the aerosolized particles decreases, their ability to travel within the respiratory tract increases. Particles smaller than 0.06 μm bypass the upper airway and are deposited exclusively in the lower respiratory tract and pulmonary parenchyma, where they produce thermochemical damage. For a patient inhaling predominantly smaller particles, it is possible to sustain trivial or no airway injury, but extensive pulmonary damage. Particles 2 μm in diameter, on the other hand, are deposited with equal frequency in the upper airway, the lower respiratory tract, and the pulmonary parenchyma. The larger the particle's size, the greater its tendency to be trapped in the upper airway (Brain and Valberg, 1974). With progression in size, the deposition of these particles in the upper airway increases to the extent that particles 10 μm in size or greater are predominantly deposited in the nasopharynx (Hatch and Gross, 1964). Implicit from these findings is the fact that a patient with extensive carbonaceous deposits in the nasopharynx and upper airway does not always have significant pulmonary damage.

It is interesting that the normal breathing frequency of 15-20 breaths/min confers a remarkable degree of immunity against inhalation injury. With a normal breathing pattern, the overall deposition of particles in the respiratory tract is minimal. In contrast, both higher and lower rates of breathing potentiate overall particle deposition in the respiratory tract. Both hyperventilation in a fire victim due to pain, panic, or pyrexia and hypoventilation because of impaired mentation from the use of drugs or as a result of oxygen depletion and carbon monoxide excess in the burning environment will increase the intensity of particle deposition in the respiratory tract and promote diffuse inhalation injury (Task Group on Lung Dynamics, 1966; American Conference of Governmental Industrial Hygienists, 1983).

The toxicity of the products of incomplete combustion, inhalation of which results in local and systemic toxicity including chemical injury to the respiratory tract, can be assessed in terms of established safety standards that are applicable to toxic industrial products (American Conference of Governmental Industrial Hygienists, 1983; Terrill et al., 1978).

Taken together, fires produce respiratory tract damage through three basic mechanisms: direct heat, irritant gases, and contaminated particles. Tissue damage, depending on concentrations of offending agents and mechanism of injury, manifests itself predominantly in the form of injury to the upper respiratory or the lower respiratory tract, which may produce upper airway obstruction or tracheobronchitis, respectively (Achauer et al., 1972; Stone and Martin, 1969; Petroff and Pruitt, 1979). When, however, the brunt of the injury is borne by the pulmonary parenchyma, progressive pulmonary insufficiency ensues (Aub et al., 1943; Pruitt et al., 1975).

C. Pathophysiology

Understanding of the pulmonary response to noxious stimuli is central to rational therapy of inhalation injury. The typical responses of the lung to a host of pernicious stimuli are manifested by disruption of the alveolar capillary membranes with resultant leakage of a protein-rich exudate of plasma and cellular elements of the blood into the pulmonary interstitium and alveoli.

The most prevalent among the toxic gases produced in a fire is carbon monoxide, generally causally linked to fire-related deaths. The affinity of hemoglobin to combine with carbon monoxide to form carboxyhemoglobin is over 200 times greater than its affinity to combine with oxygen. Both duration of exposure and prevailing carbon monoxide concentrations at the time of exposure regulate the rate of carboxyhemoglobin formation.

In an autopsy study of New York City fire victims during 1966 and 1967, of all victims who died during the first 12 hr postburn, 70% had sustained inhalation injury and 59% among those tested had significant to lethal levels of carbon monoxide in their blood (Zikria et al., 1972a). In one study of 14 patients with carboxyhemoglobin levels above 19%, the mean alveolar-arterial oxygen difference was abnormally increased to 55 torr, suggesting that carbon monoxide interferes with pulmonary gas exchange (Whorton, 1976). Several clinical reports have suggested that patients with acute carbon monoxide poisoning and inhalation injury develop abnormal findings, both on physical examination of the chest (Smith and Brandon, 1970; Meigs and Hughes, 1952) and on chest x-rays (Sones et al., 1974), due to the development of interstitial and interalveolar pulmonary edema (Drinker, 1938). At postmortem pathologic examination, pulmonary edema and hemorrhages are characteristic findings in patients dying of carbon monoxide intoxication (Finck, 1966). Experimental animals exposed to carbon monoxide concentrations that raise carboxyhemoglobin levels above 60% exhibit a reduction in dynamic lung compliance, increased airway resistance, progressive hypoxemia, and a significant increase in alveolar-epithelial membrane permeability (Fein et al., 1981). Fisher et al. (1969) selectively exposed one lung of the dog to carbon monoxide and found no changes in the diffusing capacity of the lungs, pressure-volume (PV) curves, or lung morphology in dogs with blood carboxyhemoglobin concentrations in the range of 8-18%. However, dogs with 60% carboxyhemoglobin saturation developed intense congestion, pulmonary edema, and hemorrhages of the lungs, findings similar to that reported for humans as mentioned above. Pulmonary changes in the dog were thought to be the systemic manifestations of hypoxemia produced by the leftward shift of the oxygen dissociation curve caused by the carboxyhemoglobin.

Inhalation injury in experimental animals causes a prolonged rise in airway pressures (Clark and Lambertson, 1971), reduced lung compliance, hypoxemia, increased shunt, loss of surfactant activity, and atelectasis (Nieman et al., 1980). Atelectasis develops early after smoke inhalation and has been explained on the basis of nonobstructive causes, which include reduced surfactant activity and intense bronchospasm. Histologic sections of the atelectatic lung fail to demonstrate any plugging of the bronchioles with mucosal debris (Nieman et al., 1980).

Hyperinflation of the excised lung as well as the in vivo lung reduces pulmonary surfactant activity, which can be restored by the application of positive end-expiratory pressure (PEEP) (Fariday et al., 1966; McClenahan and Urtnowski, 1967). Hyperinflation of the lung in the adult cat releases surfactants, but they are rapidly inactivated. The application of 2.5 cm H_2O PEEP in those animals, however, preserves surfactant activity and prevents atelectasis (Wyszogrodski et al., 1975). Within 5 min after induction of smoke inhalation injury in the dog, surfactant activity declines and animals develop a diffuse nonobstructive atelectasis that persists despite the application of 5 cm H_2O PEEP and responds only partially to 10 cm H_2O. It appears that, in burn patients, both the inhalation injury (Zikria et al., 1968) and hypoventilation as well as their treatment with mechanical ventilation result in surfactant loss and promote atelectasis, which is preventable with low-level PEEP.

During the initial 24 hr postburn in humans with modest inhalation injury, studies have shown that ventilation increased predominantly to a high ventilation-perfusion compartment, indicating either a reduced blood flow due to pulmonary vasospasm, or increased dead space ventilation, or both. This abnormal pattern resolved gradually over 72 hr and when, by the third postburn day, perfusion to a low ventilation-perfusion compartment increased, the arterial oxygen pressure/inspired flow of oxygen (PaO_2/FIO_2) ratios declined to the hypoxic range (200-300), suggesting bronchiolar constriction due to bronchospasm or peribronchial edema. The true intrapulmonary shunt, however, remained unchanged during the entire 72-hr study period (Robinson et al., 1981). Since blood flow to edematous or injured, and thus hypoventilated and hypoxic, lung segments is reduced (Goldzimer et al., 1974), this latter finding is consistent with the notion that reduction in blood flow to the injured lung is a compensatory mechanism that serves to improve ventilation-perfusion matching and guards against systemic hypoxia. Failure of the lung to divert blood flow from the injured regions, on the other hand, can lead to profound and irreversible hypoxemia and culminate in death.

Pulmonary injury, with its increased pulmonary capillary permeability, may be assessed by estimating extravascular leakage of radiolabeled macromolecules (Gorin et al., 1978, 1980) or by identifying an increase in pulmonary lymph flow and protein content (Staub et al., 1975; Erdmann et al., 1975; Brigham et al., 1976). However, these techniques cannot separate changes due to increased permeability from those due to reduction in the surface area of pulmonary microvasculature that partakes in gas exchange. In this regard, the measurement of lung permeability-surface are using ^{14}C-labelled urea appear to be useful. In humans with acute respiratory failure, changes in the permeability-surface area but not lung water correlated with the severity of abnormalities in pulmonary gas exchange and patient outcome. In patients who died of respiratory failure, the permeability-surface area remained persistently elevated and the initially low permeability–surface area in survivors gradually returned to normal with improvement in pulmonary function (Brigham et al., 1983). Both severity and the extent of pulmonary damage influence pulmonary function after inhalation injury.

D. Pulmonary Damage Due to Cutaneous Burns

Another important factor that compounds the adverse effects of inhalation injury on the pulmonary system is the presence of cutaneous burns. Thermal trauma to skin, even in the absence of inhalation injury, can cause pulmonary damage. Activation of complement has been observed within 1 hr of 30% scald burns in the rat. As C5a-related chemotactic activity in the serum increased, the animals became profoundly neutropenic and concomitantly developed an increase in lung permeability. In these animals, an appreciable protection against lung damage was achieved when they were depleted either of neutrophils or complement prior to injury. Pretreatment of the animals with catalase or superoxide dismutase also offered a partial protection, indicating the involvement of oxygen radicals in burn-induced pulmonary damage (Till et al., 1983). It appears that a burn activates complement (Fjellstrom and Arturson, 1963; Bjornson et al., 1977; Heideman, 1979; Till et al., 1983). As a consequence, neutrophils are activated (O'Flaherty et al., 1977b; Till et al., 1982) and sequestered in the pulmonary circulation (Craddock et al., 1977, 1979; O'Flaherty et al., 1977b, 1978; Haslam et al., 1980; Nusbacher et al., 1978). The complement-activated neutrophils produce capillary endothelial cell damage through the release of oxygen metabolites (Sacks et al., 1978; Till et al., 1982).

In vivo microscopic examination of the pulmonary circulation in the rat after remote cutaneous burns has revealed pulmonary vasoconstriction acting as a "catch trap" for masses of aggregated red blood cells (Knisely and Knisely,

1954). Direct cinematographic observations of the pulmonary microcirculation has revealed, within 10-60 min following a cutaneous burn, an intense vasoconstriction involving most of the pulmonary arterioles and venules. This leads to intravascular aggregation of red cells, causing total occlusion of some and partial obstruction of other capillaries. Despite this, pulmonary blood flow remained rapid and continuous because of the opening of a large number of shunts between the arterioles and venules (Hayashi et al., 1979).

Another mechanism by which burns, without inhalation injury, cause pulmonary dysfunction has been explained on the basis of alterations in the pulmonary microvascular integrity (Demling et al., 1978; Morgan et al., 1978). In sheep, for at least 72 hr postburn, both lymph flux and lymph to plasma protein ratios are elevated in the burned skin. The nonburned skin manifests similar changes, but only for 12 hr. These changes reflect an increased permeability of the skin for proteins. On the other hand, in the absence of changes of pulmonary artery or pulmonary capillary wedge pressures, an increased lung lymph flow was observed that lasted for 24-36 hr, indicating that the increased lymph flow was due to the increased hydrostatic pressure. The vasoconstriction of the pulmonary venules in response to vasoactive peptides released after burns has been postulated to cause the increased hydrostatic pressure (Harms et al., 1982).

The pulmonary insufficiency of burns is of multifactorial origin. Direct cytotoxic damage due to a multitude of products of incomplete combustion, hypoxic cellular degeneration caused by exposure to oxygen-deficient fire atmospheres or carbon monoxide poisoning, smoke-induced pulmonary epithelial injury, pulmonary surfactant inactivation, oxygen radical-dependent pulmonary damage, and microvascular changes due either to aggregation of cellular elements of blood or release of vasoactive substances are but some of the mechanisms responsible for pulmonary insufficiency of burns. The magnitude of pulmonary response depends on the intensity of the insult. With a limited initial insult and in the absence of secondary complications, an experimental pulmonary injury resolves in a 2 to 3 week period (Walker et al., 1981).

E. Incidence of Inhalation Injury

Of the various methods of diagnosis of inhalation injury, none is impeccable and all have limitations. A diagnosis of inhalation injury ideally is based on historical events and clinical presentation and includes the results of routine laboratory investigations such as arterial blood gases, chest roentgenogram, bronchoscopy, xenon 133 lung scan, and pulmonary function studies. Such a diagnosis is comprehensive, precise, and reliably estimates the true incidence of airway damage sustained in fires. The reported incidence of inhalation injury, however, will vary depending on the thoroughness of investigation and the sensitivity and specificity of the tests used in establishing its diagnosis. A diagnosis that was based on clinical criteria alone yielded a 2.9% incidence of clinically significant respiratory tract injury in patients treated in a burn center (DiVincenti et al., 1971), while more comprehensive workup of patients, to include bronchoscopy, xenon 133 lung scan, and pulmonary function tests, improved the diagnostic accuracy to 96% and raised the incidence of inhalation injury to 43% in a similar population (Agee et al., 1976).

F. Clinical Presentation

A reduction in the oxygen-carrying capacity of the blood, proportional to its carboxyhemoglobin content, produces tissue hypoxia and leads to the symptoms of carbon monoxide poisoning that range from a slight headache to coma and death.

The susceptibility of a person to carbon monoxide toxicity is greatly ininfluenced by individual variations and by physical status at the time of exposure. Patients with carbon monoxide intoxication often present with lightheadedness, increased light perception, tingling of the lips and extremities, and cherry red discoloration of the skin. The diagnosis of carbon monoxide poisoning can be made by determining the carboxyhemoglobin saturation of the blood. Carboxyhemoglobin concentrations below 10% in normal individuals are generally well tolerated, but, based on individual patient variations, carboxyhemoglobin concentrations below 5% in otherwise healthy individuals are known to have been poorly tolerated (Drinkwater et al., 1974; Aronow et al., 1974). On the other hand, patients with preexisting cardiovascular disease are extremely susceptible to carbon monoxide toxicity and may become symptomatic even at concentrations as low as 3% (Ayres et al., 1970; Aronow and Cassidy, 1975). Carboxyhemoglobin concentrations of the blood above 15% are generally considered toxic and those above 50% are usually lethal (Table 2).

In victims of fire, injury to the respiratory tract results both from the application of direct heat and the inhalation of smoke. Extensive burns about the head and neck region extending beyond the level of skin with a direct laryngeal or tracheal involvement are infrequent in clinical practice since most patients with such an extensive injury die at the scene of the fire. Inhalation of superheated smoke may inflict a direct thermal injury to the respiratory tract. However, this form of injury is rare because of the reflex laryngospasm precipitated by the inhalation of the particulate material (Widdicombe et al., 1962), extreme efficiency of the cooling mechanisms of the labyrinthine respiratory apparatus, and the relatively low heat-carrying capacity of the dry air of a burning environment (Moritz et al., 1945). A direct injury to the respiratory tract due to dry heat is mainly confined to the upper airway structures and the lower respiratory tract escapes this kind of damage. The inhalation of superheated steam, on the other hand, because of its 4,000 times greater heat-carrying capacity than dry

Table 2 Clinical Symptoms of Carbon Monoxide Toxicity

Carboxyhemoglobin concentrations (%)	Clinical symptoms
5-10	Impaired visual acuity, progressive impairment of mental function
11-20	Generalized vasodilation, flushing of the skin, and progressively severe headache
21-30	Nausea, throbbing headache, and impaired manual dexterity
31-40	Vomiting, dizziness, syncope
41-50	Tachypnea and tachycardia (response to systemic hypoxia)
>50	Coma, convulsions, and death

air (Moritz et al., 1945), is capable of producing extensive thermal damage that may involve the lower respiratory tract.

A clinical presentation that may often alert the physician to the possibility of inhalation injury includes a history of injury in a closed environment, impaired alertness at the time of the accident, prolonged exposure to smoke, facial burns, hoarseness, carbonaceous sputum, and physical signs such as rales and wheezing on chest auscultation. These symptoms may be present on admission but, in a majority of patients, are first evident on the second postburn day and may be delayed for several days (Pruitt, 1979). While about 95% of patients with inhalation injury present with facial burns and most have been injured in closed space fires, the converse does not hold true. Not all patients with facial burns sustain inhalation injury and not all inhalation injuries occur in patients burned in closed environments. Outdoor fires, particularly those due to petroleum products and natural gas explosions, account for 10-15% of the cases of inhalation injury (Hunt et al., 1975).

G. Diagnostic Modalities

In patients with inhalation injury, the admission blood gases on room air often reveal a mild hypoxemia with PaO_2 in the 60-70 torr range (Petroff et al., 1976). The initial chest x-ray is usually normal in these individuals and thus is of little diagnostic value since it does not rule out the presence of inhalation injury (DiVincenti et al., 1971). Earlier reports in patients with acute carbon monoxide poisoning and inhalation injury have suggested that physical examination

of the chest and chest x-rays in these individuals may reveal abnormal findings
(Smith and Brandon, 1970; Meigs and Hughes, 1952; Sones et al., 1974) due to
the development of interstitial and interalveolar pulmonary edema (Drinker,
1938), but the appearance of these findings (usually focal or diffuse pulmonic
infiltrates) is usually delayed for 24-36 hr and they are also nonspecific (Putman
et al., 1977). Besides the history, clinical findings, and the results of arterial
blood gas determinations, which are essential to the work-up of any injured patient, the accurate diagnosis of inhalation injury often requires use of specialized tests.

Bronchoscopy

Foremost among these diagnostic procedures is bronchoscopy, a procedure that
allows a detailed inspection of the tracheobronchial tree to assess mucosal damage. This is a relatively innocuous bedside procedure that can be performed in
the awake patient under topical anesthesia or with minimal sedation (Hunt et al.,
1975). Once the nasal and pharyngeal mucosa and supraglottic larynx have been
adequately anesthetized, a flexible, 5-7 mm external diameter fiberoptic bronco-
scope is gently inserted through one of the nostrils and guided through the nasopharynx. The instrument is maneuvered and advanced under direct vision to the
level of the epiglottis where the vocal cords are visualized and their mobility observed. In patients with stridor and impending obstruction, a nasotracheal tube
of appropriate size should be passed over the bronchoscope and then both advanced as a single unit. In the patient exhibiting boggy and edematous, sluggish,
or immobile vocal cords, the nasotracheal tube is further advanced into the trachea to secure the airway. Tracheal intubation is easy to perform during inspiration when the vocal cords are maximally abducted. To prevent hypoxia during
bronchoscopy, the examination period should be limited to about 10 min.
Should the signs and symptoms suggestive of hypoxia, such as unexplained agitation or irregularity of the cardiac rate and rhythm develop, the procedure
should be terminated and the patient ventilated with 100% oxygen. To safe-
guard further against hypoxia, all patients undergoing bronchoscopy should
be allowed to breathe 100% oxygen for 3-5 min before the procedure is begun.
    Depending on the prevailing concentrations of the airborne chemicals
and on the duration of exposure of an individual, a spectrum of mucosal damage
ranging from erythema, edema, blister formation, and focal submucosal hemorrhages to frank ulceration and pseudomembrane formation may be evident on
bronchoscopy. Specks of carbonaceous material are often seen deposited on or
in the mucosa of the nasopharynx and tracheobronchial tree in approximately
half of the patients with inhalation injury.
    In extreme cases, there may be sloughing of the mucosal lining of the en-
tire tracheobronchial tree that results in the formation of endobronchial casts

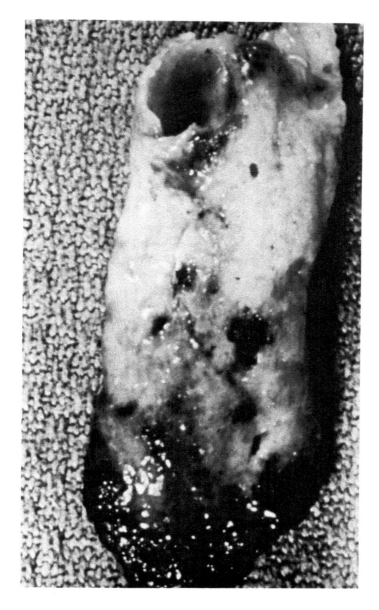

Figure 1 This bronchial cast, composed of necrotic mucosa and inflammatory exudate, exceeded 2 cm in greatest diameter and caused acute airway obstruction. The cast was extracted using the rigid bronchoscope. Note embedded carbon particles causing focal areas of dark discoloration.

(Fig. 1) which, when dislodged, may cause an acute airway obstruction, a condition that is life-threatening if diagnosis and intervention are delayed.

The principal advantages of bronchoscopy are the technical ease with which the procedure can be accomplished and utility of the procedure that allows direct visualization of the major airways to assess the extent of mucosal damage, to remove mucosal debris, endobronchial casts, and inspissated mucous in patients with atelectasis or respiratory distress due to bronchial obstruction, and to monitor the progress of repair. The chief limitation of the procedure is the disproportion between the size of currently available instruments and the lumina of the bronchial tree. Even with the smallest scope, the external diameter of which is 3.7 mm, visualization of the first-order bronchus, that is 4 mm in internal diameter, is possible but inspection of the secondary and tertiary bronchi, which are 2 mm or less in diameter, is not possible. Particles 1 μm in diameter or less are preferentially deposited in the distal airway; their trapping, which is 5-10 times greater in the pulmonary compartment than the lower respiratory tract, implies that small size particles predominantly injure lung parenchyma inaccessible to bronchoscopy. This explains falsely negative results of bronchoscopy in some patients with an abnormal xenon 133 lung scan. Since bronchoscopic diagnosis of inhalation injury relies solely on the demonstration of mucosal abnormalities, the intense vasoconstriction in hypovolemic patients will mask mucosal changes and also give rise to false-negative results. Bronchoscopy, despite these limitations, is an excellent diagnostic tool with an accuracy rate of 86% and an acceptably low 13% false-negative rate (Agee et al., 1976).

Xenon 133 Lung Scan

As opposed to bronchoscopy that allows visual assessment of airway damage, the other two diagnostic techniques, xenon 133 lung scan and pulmonary function tests, are based on identification of the pathophysiological changes in the airways and pulmonary circulation following injury. The xenon 133 lung scan is a useful diagnostic modality used frequently in conjunction with bronchoscopy in the diagnosis of inhalation injury (Moylan et al., 1972). Inhalation injury causes heterogeneity of ventilation-perfusion ratios of the lung. The detection of ventilation-perfusion mismatch with the xenon 133 lung scan forms the basis of this diagnostic test. After intravenous injection of 6-10 μCi xenon 133, its washout from the lungs is monitored sequentially with timed scintiphotographs. A negative study consists of the absence of localized trapping of the isotope and a complete washout of radioactivity from the lungs in 90 sec, while a positive study is indicated by a regional or generalized delay in isotope washout beyond 90 sec.

Coexistent unrelated pulmonary pathology that perturbs the normal ventilation-perfusion arrangement of the lung will give rise to false-positive results.

A preexisting chronic obstructive pulmonary disease and asthma or the presence of atelectasis or pneumonia in a burn patient will give false-positive results. Postburn hyperventilation accelerates clearance of the radiolabeled gas and produces false-negative results. This limits the applicability of the procedure to the first, 72 hr postburn, beyond which time minute ventilation is markedly increased. False-negative results are also obtained in patients with upper airway damage in the absence of pulmonary parenchymal injury. The diagnostic accuracy of the procedure is 87%, with 8% false-positive and 5% false-negative rates (Agee et al., 1976).

Pulmonary Function Tests

With current techniques, an accurate determination of the extent and severity of lung damage in terms of volume or surface area of the injury is not possible; however, impairment in pulmonary function is amenable to assessment. Patients with inhalation injury exhibit marked changes in the maximum expiratory flow volume curve and in pulmonary resistance. These changes correlate well with xenon 133 lung scan findings in patients with inhalation injury (Petroff et al., 1976). Characteristically, patients with inhalation injury exhibit a decreased peak flow, a reduced flow at 25, 50, and 75% of vital capacity, and an enhanced pulmonary resistance (Table 3). The unique features of these studies are the reliability with which one can assess physiological reserve and pulmonary function impairment in patients with inhalation injury. The accuracy of pulmonary function studies in making a diagnosis of inhalation injury approximates 91%.

When all three tests, bronchoscopy, xenon 133 lung scan, and pulmonary function studies, are included in the workup of a patient suspected of having inhalation injury, the overall diagnostic accuracy rate is increased to 96%. Moreover, this battery of tests eliminates virtually all of the false-negative results.

H. Differential Diagnosis

A few potentially avoidable and frequently manageable conditions capable of precipitating acute respiratory failure in the burn patient, irrespective of the status of inhalation injury, that respond best to more specific therapies than the support of ventilation need be kept in mind.

Inhalation injury with cutaneous burns reportedly increases fluid requirements during resuscitation and thus increases the risk of pulmonary edema during the first postburn week (Morgan et al., 1978). Beyond the second postburn day, an acute airway obstruction due to laryngeal edema is infrequent. However, acute respiratory insufficiency in patients with pre-existing cardiopulmonary disease, particularly the elderly, can result from the mobilization of edema fluid about the fourth to fifth postburn day (Pruitt et al., 1976). The tendency for

Table 3 Pulmonary Function Tests (Mean Values) with Inhalation Injury

	Inhalation injury	
	Present (n=7)	Absent (n=8)
Arterial PaO$_2$ (torr)	69.4	85.5
Ventilation-perfusion gradient (torr)	37.4	27.2
Resistance (cm H$_2$O/liter/sec)	4.85	3.05
Peak flow (percent of predicted value)	61.9	99.1
Flow at 75% vital capacity (percent of predicted value)	47.7	120.1

fluid retention in these individuals will be indicated by inappropriate weight change and will be evident in the 24-hr fluid balance. Hemodynamic monitoring under these conditions using a flow-directed pulmonary artery catheter is helpful in assessing cardiac function and in estimating the volume status. An elevated pulmonary capillary wedge pressure and normal to elevated cardiac output points to a noncardiogenic cause, while an elevated pulmonary capillary wedge pressure and a reduced cardiac output suggest cardiac failure as an underlying cause of pulmonary edema. The estimation of the protein content of edema fluid is helpful in differentiating the cardiogenic from noncardiogenic variety of pulmonary edema. A ratio of edema fluid protein to plasma protein of less than 5 suggests transudation based on increased osmotic pressure gradient, while a ratio above 5 indicates exudation due to an inflammatory process (Mathru et al., 1983b). Cardiogenic pulmonary edema and associated systemic hypotension in these volume-overexpanded individuals are best managed by inotropic support with dopamine or dobutamine used individually or in combination (Colucci et al., 1986).

Other causes of respiratory insufficiency in the postburn period include aspiration pneumonia (Teabeaut, 1952), tension pneumothorax, massive atelectasis, pleural effusion, pulmonary embolism, and pneumonia. The diagnosis and therapy of these ailments are no different in the burn patient than in any other acutely ill patient.

III. Treatment

A. Carbon Monoxide Poisoning

Carbon monoxide poisoning may play a central role in the hypoxemia of inhalation injury. The initial carboxyhemoglobin levels, in addition, reflect the exposure of an individual to a spectrum of noxious gases and therefore serve as a useful guide in assessing the severity of inhalation injury. Patients with carbon monoxide poisoning benefit from oxygen therapy. An increased alveolar oxygen tension facilitates carbon monoxide elimination from the blood through the mass effect. Patients with abnormally elevated carboxyhemoglobin saturation, or those who are symptomatic at carboxyhemoglobin concentrations under 10%, should receive supplemental oxygen. In the spontaneously breathing patient, 100% oxygen may be given through a well-fitting, nonrebreathing face mask, while patients with pulmonary insufficiency or those who are unconscious are best treated with 100% oxygen delivered through an endotracheal tube by a mechanical ventilator until carboxyhemoglobin levels drop below 20%. Carboxyhemoglobin levels should be monitored during oxygen treatment to assess the response to therapy. The uptake of carbon monoxide depends on individual variations and its disposal on intra-alveolar oxygen concentrations (Stadie and Martin, 1925). In individuals inspiring room air at sea level, carboxyhemoglobin concentrations fall to half of their initial values in 250 min (Forbes et al., 1945), while comparable results can be achieved in less than 1 hr with the inhalation of pure oxygen (Mellins and Park, 1975).

Hyperbaric oxygen at 2 atmospheres absolute (ATA) has been shown to increase survival of carbon monoxide-poisoned rodents. Improved survival of the mice in that study was attributed to an increase in the dissolved oxygen content of the plasma that occurred with hyperbaria and provided a mechanism to circumvent the oxygen transport deficit produced by carbon monoxide poisoning (Haldane, 1895). In normal individuals breathing room air, the whole body arterial to venous oxygen content difference is 5-6 vol % with dissolved oxygen content of plasma of only 0.3 vol %. The inhalation of 100% oxygen at normal atmospheric pressures can raise the dissolved oxygen content of the plasma to 2.09 vol %, approximating one-third of the tissue oxygen demands. When one is breathing oxygen at 2.5 ATA, the dissolved oxygen content of plasma can rise to 5.62 vol %, an amount that is sufficient to meet the oxygen needs of the entire body (Winter and Miller, 1976). Additionally, hyperbaric oxygen increases the rate of elimination of carbon monoxide from the blood, which makes more hemoglobin available for oxygen transport. Administration of 100% oxygen to a canine subject with carbon monoxide poisoning reduced the half-time for carbon monoxide elimination from 35 min at 1 ATA to 17 min at 2 ATA. Moreover, the hyperbaric oxygen at 2 ATA also abrogated the rebound rise in carboxyhemoglobin levels that results from the release of tissue-bound carboxyhemoglobin into the circulation (Peirce et al., 1972).

To accelerate carbon monoxide elimination and to reverse tissue hypoxia, hyperbaric oxygen has been used with success in patients with carbon monoxide poisoning (Smith and Brandon, 1970). In six unconscious carbon monoxide-intoxicated patients who were indifferent to previous treatment with normobaric 100% oxygen, the use of pure oxygen at 2.8-3 ATA was considered to have improved their neurologic recovery. Hyperbaric oxygen therapy in those individuals was given over a 46-161 min period. In all but one of those patients, hyperbaric oxygen therapy was repeated once in the ensuing 6-8 hr. All patients survived and five made apparently full neurologic recovery (Myers et al., 1981).

Conversely, Ogawa et al. (1972) found that 17 of 72 patients (24%) with severe carbon monoxide poisoning (unconscious on admission) expired within 1 week (7) or showed little or no change in level of consciousness (10) following a 1-hr treatment with oxygen at 2 ATA once a day for 3 days. Marked acidosis on admission was prognostic of a fatal outcome in those patients. In normal adults, it appears that up to 4 hr of exposure to oxygen at 2.5 ATA is well tolerated except for the occasional development of seizures due to the central nervous system toxicity of oxygen. High concentrations of oxygen in premature infants, on the other hand, are extremely toxic and should be avoided (Winter and Smith, 1972). From these reports, it appears that hyperbaric oxygen at 2.5-3 ATA may be used for short periods as an adjunctive therapy in severe carbon monoxide poisoning. In the absence of rigorously controlled clinical studies, the effectiveness of hyperbaric oxygen therapy remains uncertain.

The long-term side effects of carbon monoxide poisoning are those due to nervous system damage as a result of cerebral hypoxia. The level of cerebral hypoxia parallels carboxyhemoglobin concentrations. Furthermore, inspiration of carbon monoxide augments both cerebral perfusion and cerebral capillary permeability which leads to cerebral edema, increased intracranial pressure, and brain hypoxia (Root, 1965; Grunnet, 1976). The residual neurologic sequelae may be in the form of encephalopathy, chorioathetosis, hemiparesis, and peripheral neuropathy (Zikria et al., 1975).

B. Upper Respiratory Tract Injury

The mainstay of the therapy of inhalation injury is the support of ventilation, although not all patients require this prescription. A vast majority of patients sustain minimal to moderate airway damage and can be managed by general supportive measures that reduce laryngeal edema formation and by vigilant observation to detect early signs of pulmonary insufficiency that require prompt intervention. Prophylactic intubation of patients with inhalation injury of the upper airway has been advocated (Venus et al., 1981) to avoid possible complications of upper airway obstruction, but we believe that an otherwise unimpaired patient, even with hoarseness of voice due to nonobstructing laryngeal edema, may be safely observed. In these individuals, nebulization of 0.5% racemic epinephrine or neosynephrine every 4 hr appears to be beneficial in reducing vocal cord edema and preventing the development of complete airway obstruction. Another frequently used effective measure that optimizes lymphatic drainage of the head and neck region is the nursing of a hemodynamically stable patient in a head propped-up position.

Humidified, oxygen-rich air prevents dessication of the acutely inflamed tracheobronchial mucosa and should be administered, preferably through a face mask, in patients with inhalation injury (Pruitt, 1979). Most patients with limited upper airway damage respond to the above outlined conservative measures. Patients with progressive airway occlusions and imminent obstruction should be promptly intubated until such time as the upper airway edema recedes sufficiently to permit extubation. A thorough physical examination of these patients needs to be performed on a daily basis and supplemented when indicated by arterial blood gases and chest x-ray to assess their ventilation and oxygenation status and to detect the development of atelectasis or pneumonia.

Soft tissue swelling of the airway passages may parallel the generalized body edema that accompanies fluid resuscitation. This reaches an apogee at approximately 24 hr postburn, and previously asymptomatic patients with mild to moderate inhalation injury may develop respiratory distress at this time. Fluid intake in these individuals will require careful regulation, often in the form of fluid restriction. In patients manifesting signs of acute volume expansion with resultant respiratory and cardiovascular embarrassment, the use of a loop diuretic is indicated. The progress of upper airway edema should be monitored on a scheduled basis by a direct laryngoscopic examination, both to assess the need for a translaryngeal artificial airway in patients with impending laryngeal obstruction due to progressive laryngeal edema and also to determine the timing of safe extubation when airway edema has sufficiently resolved. Deep breathing, coughing, and early mobilization help prevent atelectasis and should be encouraged. Most patients with limited upper airway damage recuperate in a week to 10 days with no residual sequelae.

C. Artificial Airway

In the physiologically sound, young individual, a modest airway injury without respiratory compromise may be safely observed. On the other hand, patients with large burns and massive airway damage, the elderly, and those with associated skeletal or visceral injuries or pre-existing cardiopulmonary disease are extremely vulnerable to the ravages of hypoxia. The development of pulmonary insufficiency in these individuals with limited physiological reserve often calls for early and, at times, urgent support of ventilation.

The indications for translaryngeal intubation in a burn patient are similar to any other patient with trauma and fall under two broad categories: mechanical obstruction of the airway and pulmonary insufficiency. The usual signs suggestive of upper airway obstruction include cyanosis, dyspnea, stridor, the use of the accessory muscles of breathing, and paradoxical movements of the diaphragm.

Arterial blood gases that indicate the need for intubation and mechanical ventilation will reveal hypoxemia (PaO_2 less than 50 torr on room air), hypercarbia (arterial carbon dioxide pressure [$PaCO_2$] greater than 49 torr), and acidosis with a hydrogen ion concentration (pH) less than 7.35. A transnasally placed artificial airway is preferred over the transoral intubation because a nasotracheal tube interferes less with oral hygiene, is less prone to distortion while coursing through the nasopharynx, is less susceptible to indentation and occlusion by the patient's teeth, stimulates the gag reflex less frequently, and, even in the awake patient, is generally well tolerated. However, certain risks peculiar to the transnasal route are pressure necrosis of the nasal septum and alae and impaired drainage of the maxillary sinus which can lead to sinusitis. Tubes with cuffs that have high volume and low pressure cause less tracheal damage and are recommended (Grillot et al., 1971).

Translaryngeal intubation initially is the preferred mode of securing airway patency. The endotracheal tubes can be safely left in place for at least 3 weeks (Lund et al., 1985) and possibly even longer (Via-Reque and Rattenborg, 1981). However, when the need for an artificial airway to provide mechanical ventilation to patients with protracted pulmonary insufficiency continues beyond the arbitrary 3-week limit, a tracheostomy is generally considered a reasonable alternative to long-term translaryngeal intubation. Tracheostomy cannulae appear to be as likely to inflict tracheal trauma as translaryngeal tubes and, in both instances, the duration of intubation as well as the intratracheal tube cuff pressures seem to determine the extent of airway damage. Tracheostomy cannulae are generally of a larger caliber than translaryngeal tubes and, hence, on a comparative basis, are a more effective route for tracheobronchial toilet, especially in patients with pulmonary infection and with viscous and copious endotracheal secretions. The adequate removal of secretions in individuals with pneumonia forms an integral part of therapy. In addition, tracheostomy in patients with severe inhalation injury and massive necrosis of the tracheobronchial mucosa with resultant mucosal sloughing and endobronchial cast formation is particularly valuable since it provides a ready access to the trachea for frequent suctioning, pulmonary toilet, and extraction of endobronchial casts under direct vision using a rigid bronchoscope.

D. Lower Respiratory Tract Injury

Patients with severe airway damage and extensive necrosis of the tracheobronchial mucosa usually require intubation early in their postburn course. In these individuals, an abrupt dislodgement of necrotic mucosal fragments or of endobronchial casts can occur during the first 2 weeks postinjury. This may precipitate an acute airway obstruction that requires relief by the expeditious removal of such endotracheal debris using a flexible catheter or a rigid bronchoscope. Depending upon the extent of mucosal damage and the ability of the patient to clear endobronchial debris, once or even twice daily bronchoscopic toilet of the tracheobronchial tree to extract intraluminal debris may be necessary. To facilitate removal of viscid or copious bronchial secretions, to extract devitalized mucosa and endobronchial casts, and particularly in anticipation of the need for prolonged ventilatory support, a tracheostomy is indicated. The endotracheal secretions at the time of endoscopy for pulmonary toilet may be sampled for surveillance cultures to identify the colonizing bacteria of the respiratory tract.

E. Pulmonary Insufficiency

The extent of pulmonary damage determines the severity of respiratory failure and the acuteness of need for support of ventilation (Table 4). Pulmonary insufficiency will usually be manifested by reduction in vital capacity below 4 ml/kg (normal: 12-15 ml/kg), tachypnea (a respiratory rate greater than 40/min), and alveolar hypoventilation ($PaCO_2$ greater than 49 torr). A convenient method of monitoring pulmonary function is frequent analysis of arterial oxygen tension (PaO_2). It is generally accepted that patients with a PaO_2 of less than 50-60 torr while breathing room air should be provided with ventilatory support. In patients receiving mechanical ventilation, every effort should be made to maintain PaO_2 greater than 70 torr while keeping inspired oxygen concentrations (FIO_2) under 0.5. Ordinarily, the ventilation-perfusion inequality of the lung determines PaO_2 values. Under conditions where oxygen delivery lags behind oxygen consumption, such as in patients with hypovolemia, severe anemia, and congestive heart failure, a drastic reduction in the central venous oxygen tension may occur. Under these circumstances, the degree of pulmonary venous unsaturation, not a ventilation-perfusion mismatch, appears to be the prime determinant of PaO_2 (Philibin et al., 1970). This implies that hypoxemia in patients with inadequate perfusion responds best to volume expansion or support of a failing myocardium, depending on the underlying pathologic process.

Determinations of the physiological shunt fraction, Qsp/Qt, can be useful in assessing the adequacy of ventilation and circulation and can be used to guide adjustments of oxygen and fluid therapy in patients on mechanical ventilation (Kirby et al., 1975; Suter et al., 1975). In clinical practice, a ventilation-perfusion ratio of 20 is commonly used as an upper limit. Patients with Qsp/Qt above 20 require support of ventilation; PEEP and FIO_2 are accordingly adjusted to achieve Qsp/Qt values below 20. Although changes in Qsp/Qt adequately reflect impairment in pulmonary function, its measurement requires mixed venous sampling through a pulmonary artery catheter, its calculations are tedious, and extrapulmonary variables, such as both low-flow and hyperdynamic states, influence the results (Dantzker, 1982; Martyn et al., 1979). A simple extrapolation of ar-

Table 4 Indications for Mechanical Ventilatory Support

	Normal range	Criteria for intubation	Criteria for extubation
Mechanics			
Respiratory rate (per minute)	12–20	>40	<30
Vital capacity (ml/kg/body wt)	12–15	<10	>10
FEV_1 (ml/kg/body wt)	50–60	<10	>10
Inspiratory force (cm H_2O)	75–100	<25	>25
Oxygenation			
PaO_2 (mmHg on room air)	75–100	50–60	>70 (on FIO_2 <0.3)
P (A-aDO_2) (mmHg)	25–65	>450	<350
PaO_2/FIO_2 (mmHg)	300–500	<200	>250
Ventilation			
$PaCO_2$ (mmHg)	35–45	>49	<49
Dead space to tidal volume ratio (Vd/Vt)	0.2–0.4	>0.6	<0.6

terial blood gas data that correlates well (r = 0.9) with Qsp/Qt greater than 20 is the PaO_2/FIO_2 ratio of less than 200. A PaO_2/FIO_2 ratio of less than 200 rather than a Qsp/Qt of more than 20 can be used as an indication for instituting mechanical ventilatory support and in guiding respirator adjustments (Covelli et al., 1983). Since its introduction (Horowitz et al., 1974), the PaO_2/FIO_2 ratio has been successfully used in the management of patients with pulmonary insufficiency (Kirby et al., 1975; Venus et al., 1979, 1981; Pollack et al., 1980).

F. Pulmonary Parenchymal Injury

The maintenance of airway patency as well as initiation of ventilation take precedence over the support of other systems. Pulmonary insufficiency in the burn patient, with or without inhalation injury, requires mechanical support of ventilation with PEEP or continuous positive airway pressure (CPAP) added as needed. In normal individuals, the inspiratory and expiratory static pressure-volume (PV) curves are concave below the functional residual capacity (FRC) and exponential above that point. The concavity of the PV curve indicates airway closure (Mead, 1961). The inflection point where a transition in the shape of the PV curve occurs corresponds with the closing volume (Hughes et al., 1970; Burger and Macklem, 1968; Demedts et al., 1975): that lung volume at which closure of terminal bronchioles and small airways of 0.4 to greater than 0.9 mm i.d. begins. In the presence of pulmonary edema, the concave portion of the PV curve extends above the FRC, that is, the closing volume exceeds the FRC, indicating persistence of significant airway closure throughout inspiration (Pontoppidan et al., 1972; Lemaire et al., 1979). This results in ventilation-perfusion inequalities, impaired gas exchange, and hypoxemia.

The use of PEEP in patients with adult respiratory distress syndrome (ARDS) increases FRC, prevents airway closure, and improves oxygenation (Kumar et al., 1970; McIntyre et al., 1969). The "best PEEP," although subject to individual variations, is one that permits the highest values for oxygen transport, mixed venous oxygen pressure, and static compliance (Suter et al., 1975). To determine the optimal PEEP for any given patient in clinical practice, the level of PEEP is raised on a scheduled basis, for example, every 2 hr, in increments of 3-5 cmH_2O to obtain maximum oxygenation. A further increase in the PEEP beyond the optimal level for that particular individual will either minimally improve arterial blood gases or cause actual deterioration.

The use of controlled mechanical ventilation (CMV) combined with PEEP may adversely influence cardiac performance, particularly in patients with intravascular volume contraction (Uzawa and Ashbaugh, 1969; Colgan et al., 1971). The adverse effects of PEEP depend on elevations of the intrathoracic pressures produced by this procedure, which in turn impede venous return and lead to a depressed cardiac output (Sykes et al., 1970; Qvist et al., 1975). A reduction in left ventricular distensibility occurs with PEEP and has been explained on the basis of ventricular interdependence, that is, the volume distention of the right ventricle leading to reduced distensibility of the left ventricle through a shift in interventricular septum (Cassidy et al., 1979). Recently, however, it has been suggested that the ventricular dysfunction following use of PEEP may result from stiff ventricles. Application of 20 cmH$_2$O PEEP in the normovolemic or volume-expanded dog reduces both right and left ventricular diastolic distensibility, indicating the requirement of higher transmural end-diastolic pressures for any given end-diastolic volume in order to distend the ventricles. Such biventricular reduction in compliance has been attributed to impaired ventricular filling due to both increased lung volume and lung stiffness as a result of application of PEEP (Santamore et al., 1984). PEEP, despite undesirable cardiovascular effects, obviously holds a prominent place in the management of patients with respiratory failure.

Intermittent mandatory ventilation (IMV), first introduced as a weaning technique (Downs et al., 1973), is much preferred over the CMV mode for providing ventilatory support in the spontaneously breathing patient exhibiting respiratory insufficiency. Since IMV produces lower inflation pressures and permits a lesser number of CMV breaths per unit time, it interferes less with the normally negative intrapleural pressures and thus impedes venous return and cardiac output to a lesser degree (Downs et al., 1977; Kirby et al., 1975). In spontaneous breathing, ventilation and perfusion are closely matched and the dependent regions of the lung are preferentially perfused (West, 1974). Thus IMV, which allows spontaneous respiration, permits an optimal ventilation-perfusion matching, reduces intrapulmonary shunt, and improves oxygenation.

The use of CPAP technique, originally developed to treat the respiratory distress syndrome in infants (Gregory et al., 1971), has, in recent years, been successfully used in treating patients with ARDS (Civetta et al., 1972; Grag and Gill, 1975; Glasser et al., 1975). In spontaneously breathing normal athletes, the application of PEEP increased the total mechanical lung work in a linear fashion, producing a stepwise increase with each increment in PEEP level. However, with the use of CPAP in those individuals, the total work per minute remained unchanged even up to the CPAP level of 20 cmH$_2$O (Gherini et al., 1979). For CPAP to be effective, airway pressures must remain constant throughout inspiration and expiration; otherwise, the work of breathing increases. In one clinical study, mean airway pressures in patients with ARDS requiring ventilatory assistance remained lower in those receiving CPAP compared to those treated with PEEP (Shah et al., 1977). In patients with pulmonary insufficiency, the use of optimal CPAP that ranged from 10 to 25 cmH$_2$O was shown to increase forced vital capacity and reduce both the intrapulmonary shunt and respiratory rate without adversely altering the cardiac output or the arterial-mixed venous oxygen content difference (Venus et al., 1979). It has also been reported that CPAP as compared to PEEP has been well tolerated in treating pulmonary insufficiency in a patient with blast injury (Uretzky and Cotev, 1980).

Any form of mechanical ventilation may cause overdistention of respiratory bronchioles and alveoli with rupture due to so-called barotrauma (Kumar et al., 1973). Extra alveolar air can then travel along the perivascular spaces into the mediastinum and can dissect along the pleural reflections of the large intrathoracic vessels into the fascial planes of the head and neck region, pericardium, and retroperitoneal space (Macklin, 1939; Macklin and Macklin, 1944). The use of IMV in infants (Moylan and Alexander, 1978) and IMV with CPAP in adults (Mathru et al., 1983) reportedly protects patients with respiratory insufficiency against the development of barotrauma. From these studies, it appears that IMV combined with CPAP is a suitable way of supporting respiratory failure in the critically ill individual, including the patient with inhalation injury.

Ventilator settings should be adjusted in terms of FIO_2, tidal volume, respiratory rate, and CPAP/PEEP to maintain Qsp/Qt below 20, FIO_2/PaO_2 above 200, PaO_2 above 60-70 torr, pH above 7.35, and $PaCO_2$ below 45 torr. FIO_2 should be kept under 0.5 to reduce oxygen toxicity. Hyperoxia of even less than 24 hr duration in normal volunteers has been shown to injure the alveolar-capillary membrane (Davis et al., 1983) and the exposure of humans to high concentrations of oxygen for 2-3 days results in permanent pulmonary parenchymal injury and fibrosis of the alveolar wall (Nash et al., 1967; Katzenstein et al., 1976). In addition, a high FIO_2 promotes alveolar collapse, particularly in low Qsp/Qt regions (0.1-0.001) of the lung, that produces atelectasis (Wagner et al., 1974). Alveolar hypoventilation, when evident by rising $PaCO_2$, should be treated by increasing minute ventilation as can be achieved by the addition of a minimum number of mechanical breaths or by increasing the tidal volume. Patients with a translaryngeal airway should receive at least minimal PEEP of 2.5 cmH_2O, which has been shown to protect against surfactant loss and prevent the development of atelectasis which accompanies lung distention (Wyzsogrodski et al., 1975).

Since ventilator settings in these critically ill individuals are guided by the results of arterial blood gases, a vascular access to facilitate sampling as well as monitoring may be gained through an arterial line. The use of an arterial line eliminates the trauma of repeated arterial puncture, a particular consideration in the elderly in whom intimal injury and perivascular extravasation of blood may aggravate a pre-existing compromised flow through an arteriosclerotic vessel and cause limb ischemia. Additionally, perivascular hematomas have the potential for becoming infected. In critically ill patients, the results of arterial blood gases correlate well with those obtained by noninvasive devices that detect transcutaneous oxygen and carbon dioxide tensions. With certain limitations, such as slow response time and inaccuracy of results at low flow states (Tremper et al., 1980a), these electronic sensors are a viable alternative to direct blood gas measurements in monitoring pulmonary function (Hansen and

Tooley, 1979; Tremper et al., 1979, 1980b; Rowe and Weinburg, 1979; Salmenperä and Heinonen, 1984).

The ultimate goal of ventilatory support in the seriously ill patient is a successful extubation with return of adequate pulmonary function. A spontaneously breathing conscious patient with no acute roentgenographic pulmonary changes and with no evidence of cardiovascular instability may be considered for extubation. A vital capacity in excess of 10 ml/kg (Bendixen et al., 1965), a respiratory rate less than 30/min, arterial blood pH above 7.35, a $PaCO_2$ less than 45 torr, an arterial PaO_2 over 60 torr with an FIO_2 of 0.4 or less and a PEEP/CPAP of 5 cmH_2O or less (Gallagher et al., 1978), a maximal voluntary ventilation to minute ventilation ratio of 2, a peak negative pressure of 20-30 cmH_2O (Sahn and Lakshminarayan, 1973), an alveolar-arterial PaO_2 gradient of 350 torr on 100% oxygen, a dead space to tidal volume ratio of 0.6 or less (Pontoppidan et al., 1970), and a PaO_2/FIO_2 of more than 300 (Kirby et al., 1975) generally indicate a patient who can maintain adequate spontaneous ventilation. One should keep in mind that the administration of an excessive glucose load in the hypermetabolic and septic patient can result in increased carbon dioxide production (Askanazi et al., 1980), which may interfere with the weaning process.

In preparation for extubation, weaning begins by gradual reduction of FIO_2, reduction in the IMV rate, and reduction of the level of PEEP or CPAP over a period of several hours. Following such ventilator changes, blood gases should be monitored and, if the patient meets the criteria indicating adequate pulmonary function, he or she should be extubated. After extubation, patients should receive humidified oxygen supplements at flow rates of 8 liters/min with a FIO_2 of approximately 0.3-0.4. Close observation of these individuals to detect signs of respiratory insufficiency is essential. Using conventional criteria of extubation, it has been found that 15-20% of patients with ARDS require reintubation because of deterioration in their pulmonary function (Hilberman et al., 1976; Sahn and Lakshminarayan, 1973; Tahvanainen et al., 1983). In this regard, measurements of blood oxygen half-saturation pressure of hemoglobin (P-50) (Abermann et al., 1975) values in patients who were on IMV with added CPAP (range, 0-5) and FIO_2 (range, 0.21-0.4) were found to be helpful in discriminating between those who tolerated or did not tolerate extubation. All patients in that study exhibiting P-50 of 25 or less required reintubation, while extubation in those with P-50 values of 27 and above was well tolerated (Tahvanainen and Nikki, 1983). All the above mentioned criteria of pulmonary sufficiency serve at best as guides to the timing of extubation of a patient. They are not meant to substitute for astute clinical judgment and careful assessment of individual patient variations.

G. Complications

The magnitude of the pulmonary responses to inhalation injury depends on the intensity of insult. Time heals. With limited initial damage and in the absence of secondary complications, the inhalation injury is repaired in 2-3 weeks. Inhalation injury in experimental animals that survive heals in 3 weeks (Walker et al., 1981); similarly, the airway damage in humans with inhalation injury who subsequently came to autopsy was found to have completely resolved in 2 weeks (Hunt et al., 1975). In a clinical study of convalescent burn patients from this Institute, Morris and Spitzer (1973) determined that inhalation injury in burn patients seldom caused long-term impairment of pulmonary function.

Mechanical airway trauma and pulmonary infection constitute major complications in a patient with inhalation injury (Pruitt, 1970). In nonburn patients, the late complications of an artificial airway are more frequent and severe in patients with prolonged intubation and those requiring high cuff pressures to maintain an effective seal around the tube (Stauffer et al., 1981). Tracheal stenosis may occur at the site of the tracheostomy stoma and, in one series, occurred in 85% of the patients studied (Stoeckel, 1970). In a prospective evaluation of 41 burn patients with respiratory insufficiency at this Institute, 35 of whom had a severe inhalation injury, tracheal stenosis developed in 4 patients and tracheal scar granuloma formation in another 5. The intratracheal tube cuff pressures were above 25 cmH$_2$O in three patients, two of whom subsequently developed tracheal stenosis and one a granuloma at the tracheostomy site. The tracheostomy patients, on an average, remained intubated longer than those with transnasal or transoral tubes (49 days versus 10 days), and the complication rate beyond 21 days of intubation rose sharply. Twelve patients came to autopsy; all had evidence of mild to severe tracheobronchitis (Lund et al., 1985). The airway sequelae in these patients reflected the severity of initial pulmonary pathology that had prompted institution of ventilatory support and were related to the duration rather than the route of intubation. Burn patients with extensive pulmonary damage are likely to require prolonged intubation and artificial ventilation and the decreased pulmonary compliance in certain of these individuals will necessitate high cuff pressures to obtain an effective seal and thus increase the risk of mechanical injury of the tracheal wall.

Respiratory tract infection is the most common complication of inhalation injury (Pruitt et al., 1975). The global immunosuppression of burn patients (Miller and Baker, 1979; Constantian, 1978; Stratta et al., 1986) compounded by the local anatomical and functional defects (Loke et al., 1984; Demarset et al., 1979) in the respiratory tract of patients with inhalation injury increases their risk of developing pulmonary infection. Surgical procedures (Slade et al., 1975; Lanser et al., 1986; Tønnesen et al., 1984; Ryhänen et al., 1984) and use of inhalational anesthetics (Hole, 1984a,b,c), frequently required in the care of these patients, are also immunosuppressive and may further enhance susceptibility to infection in such patients.

In an attempt to reduce the intensity of tracheobronchial inflammation subsequent to inhalation injury, the use of steroids has been recommended because of their well-known anti-inflammatory properties (Phillips and Cope, 1962; Dressler et al., 1976). In a prospective randomized study of 30 burn patients treated at this Institute in whom inhalation injury was diagnosed on bronchoscopy, 15 patients were given dexamethasone (20 mg, intravenously) daily for 3 days and 15 were given placebo. Pulmonary functions were tested before and 48 hr after the steroid or saline treatment. Patients in both treatment groups had a similar incidence of pulmonary complications, pulmonary function deterioration, and overall mortality (Levine et al., 1978). Likewise, in a retrospective analysis of pulmonary complications in victims of hotel fires in Las Vegas, steroid therapy was found to exert no beneficial effect on patients with inhalation injury (Robinson et al., 1982). The use of steroids, even in humans with other forms of acute lung injury, has been shown to be either ineffective (Calderwood et al., 1975; Glauser et al., 1979; Wynne et al., 1981) or actually harmful (Wynne et al., 1979; Smith and Brody, 1981; Moylan et al., 1972).

The use of prophylactic antibiotics has also been advocated in an effort to reduce the rate of septic pulmonary complications in patients with inhalation injury. In another trial at this Institute, 12 of 30 patients with inhalation injury received a 10-day course of aerosolized gentamycin (80 mg dissolved in 2 ml saline) every 8 hr and the other 18 received aerosolized saline on a similar schedule. The rate of pulmonary complications, as indexed by the development of pneumonia or the need for and the duration of ventilatory support, and the average postburn day of death as well as the overall mortality among the patients of these two treatment groups were not significantly different (Levine et al., 1978). The recovery of *Pseudomonas* organisms from the tracheobronchial tree (considered an index of gram-negative flora) was not even altered by such therapy. On the basis of those studies, neither prophylactic aerosolized antibiotics nor prophylactic systemic steroids are recommended in the management of patients with inhalation injury.

In our recent review of 1,058 burn patients treated at this Institute during the past 5 years, inhalation injury was diagnosed in 35% of the patients, and of those, 38% developed pneumonia, while the incidence of pneumonia in patients without inhalation injury was only 9%. Upon further analysis, the contributions of pneumonia and inhalation injury to the age and burn size-specific patient mortality were found to be independent as well as additive. The age and burn size-specific patient mortality increased by up to 20% with the presence of inhalation injury, by up to 40% with pneumonia, and by up to 60% when both inhalation injury and pneumonia were present in a given patient. It is imperative, therefore, that the burn patient with inhalation injury be protected from infections, specifically pneumonia. Sterility of gloves, catheters, saline, etc., should be ensured during the performance of pulmonary toilet to minimize the risk of contaminating the chemically injured tracheobronchial tree of a patient with inhalation injury.

Bronchoscopy and suctioning should be accomplished with the utmost care and gentleness, without inflicting tracheal trauma. Tracheal aspiration and routine cannula care should proceed under aseptic conditions to reduce contamination of the respiratory tract.

The maintenance of proper oral hygiene is also crucial in reducing the risk of airway contamination. Since significant changes occur across time in both the burn wound flora and in the bacterial species endemic to a given environment (Pruitt, 1984), most burn centers resort to surveillance cultures of burn patients to identify trends in bacterial ecology and to monitor antibiotic sensitivity patterns of colonizing bacterial. The organisms that cause pulmonary infection in the burn patient are generally those that colonize the burn wound. Respiratory tract flora of intubated patients should be monitored by Leuken's tube cultures of the endotracheal secretions obtained on a regular basis, that is, every second or third day depending on pulmonary symptoms and severity of tracheobronchial injury. Such surveillance cultures should be used to guide initial antibiotic treatment in a patient who develops clinical and roentgenographic signs of pneumonia. Antibiotic therapy of pneumonia in these patients should be modified as necessary once culture and sensitivity results become available.

IV. Summary

Fires are inexorable enemies of life. Most fire-related fatalities occur in dwellings and often involve physically or mentally impaired individuals. Of burn patients treated at burn centers, approximately one-third suffer from inhalation injury. Three fire-related factors—direct heat, poisonous gases, and particulate material— alone or in combination, inflict damage to the upper airway, tracheobronchial tree, or pulmonary parenchyma and, respectively, produce upper airway obstruction, tracheobronchitis, and pulmonary dysfunction. Inhalation injury may be suspected on the basis of historical events and diagnosed by bronchoscopy, xenon 133 lung scan, and pulmonary function studies. Treatment consists of securing the airway and providing ventilatory support. Complications of an artificial airway are related to the duration of intubation and intratracheal cuff pressures. About one-third of those with inhalation injury subsequently develop pneumonia, which should be treated with antibiotics effective against the predominant organisms recovered from endobronchial secretions. Prophylactic antibiotics and steroids are ineffective in preventing pulmonary sepsis. Both inhalation injury and pneumonia sharply increase burn mortality and warrant further research to improve survival.

Acknowledgment

The authors are grateful to Ms. Christine C. Davis for her editorial assistance and review.

References

Abermann, A., Cavanilles, J. M., Weil, M. H., and Shubin, H. (1975). P_{50} calculated from a single measurement of pH, PO_2, and SO_2. *J. Appl. Physiol.* **38**:171-176.

Achauer, B. M., Allyn, P. A., Furnas, D. W., and Bartlett, R. H. (1972). Pulmonary complications of burns: the major threat to the burn patient. *Ann. Surg.* **177**:311-319.

Agee, R. N., Long, J. M. III, Hunt, J. L., Petroff, P. A., Lull, R. J., Mason, A. D. Jr., and Pruitt, B. A. Jr. (1976). Use of [133]Xenon in early diagnosis of inhalation injury. *J. Trauma* **16**:218-224.

American Conference of Governmental Industrial Hygienists. (1983). *Annals of the American Conference of Governmental Industrial Hygienists*, Cincinnati.

Aronow, W. S., and Cassidy, J. (1975). Effect of carbon monoxide on maximal treadmill exercise. A study in normal persons. *Ann. Intern. Med.* **83**: 496-499.

Aronow, W. S., Stemmer, E. A., and Isbell, M. W. (1974). Effect of carbon monoxide exposure on intermittent claudication. *Circulation* **49**:415-417.

Askanazi, J., Carpentier, Y. A., Elwyn, D. H., Nordenstrom, J., Jeevanandam, M., Rosenbaum, S. H., Gump, F. E., and Kinney, J. M. (1980). Influence of total parenteral nutrition on fuel utilization in injury and sepsis. *Ann. Surg.* **191**:40-46.

Aub, J. C., Pittman, H., and Brues, A. M. (1943). The management of the Cocoanut Grove burns at the Massachusetts General Hospital. The pulmonary complications: a clinical description. *Ann. Surg.* **117**:118-834.

Ayres, S. M., Gianelli, S. Jr., and Mueller, H. S. (1970). Myocardial and systemic responses to carboxyhemoglobin. *Ann. N. Y. Acad. Sci.* **174**:268-293.

Bendixen, H. H., Egbert, L. D., Hedley-Whyte, J., Laver, M. B., and Pontoppidan, H. (1965). Management of patients undergoing prolonged artificial ventilation. In *Respiratory Care*. St. Louis, C. V. Mosby, p. 149.

Bjornson, A. B., Altemeier, W. A., and Bjornson, H. S. (1977). Changes in humoral components of host defense following burn trauma. *Ann. Surg.* **186**:88-96.

Bowes, P. C. (1974). Smoke and toxicity hazards of plastics in fire. *Ann. Occup. Hyg.* **17**:143-157.

Brain, J. D., and Valberg, P. A. (1974). Models of lung retention based on ICRP Task Group Report. *Arch. Environ. Health* **28**:1-11.

Brigham, K. L., Bowers, R. E., and Owen, P. J. (1976). Effects of antihistamines on the lung vascular response to histamine in unanesthetized sheep. Diphenhydramine prevention of pulmonary edema and increased permeability. *J. Clin. Invest.* **58**:391-398.

Brigham, K. L., Kariman, K., Harris, T. R., Snapper, J. R., Bernard, G. R., and Young, S. L. (1983). Correlation of oxygenation with vascular permeability-surface area but not with lung water in humans with acute respiratory failure and pulmonary edema. *J. Clin. Invest.* **72**:339-349.

Burger, E. J. Jr., and Macklem, P. (1968). Airway closure: demonstration by breathing 100% O_2 at low lung volumes and by N_2 washout. *J. Appl. Physiol.* **25**:139-148.

Burgess, W. A., Treitman, R. D., and Gold, A. (1979). *Air Contaminants in Structural Firefighting.* Boston, Harvard School of Public Health.

Calderwood, H. W., Modell, J. H., and Ruiz, B. C. (1975). The ineffectiveness of steroid therapy for treatment of fresh water near-drowning. *Anesthesiology* **43**:642-650.

Caplan, Y. H. (1977). *Fire Problems Program. Relationship of Cyanide to Deaths Caused by Fire.* Laurel, MD, The John Hopkins University.

Cassidy, S. S., Eschenbacher, W. L., Robertson, C. H. Jr., Nixon, J. V., Blombquist, G., and Johnson, R. L. Jr. (1979). Cardiovascular effects of positive-pressure ventilation in normal subjects. *J. Appl. Physiol.* **47**:453-461.

Civetta, J. M., Brons, R., and Gabel, J. D. (1972). A simple and effective method of employing spontaneous positive pressure ventilation. *J. Thorac. Cardiovasc. Surg.* **63**:312-317.

Clark, J. M., and Lambertson, C. J. (1971). Pulmonary oxygen toxicity: a review. *Pharmacol. Rev.* **23**:37-133.

Colgan, F. J., Barrow, R. E., and Fanning, G. L. (1971). Constant positive-pressure breathing and cardiorespiratory function. *Anesthesiology* **34**:145-151.

Colucci, W. S., Wright, R. F., and Braunwald, E. (1986). New positive inotropic agents in the treatment of congestive heart failure. Mechanisms of action and recent clinical developments. *N. Engl. J. Med.* **314**:290-299.

Constantian, M. B. (1978). Association of sepsis with an immunosuppressive polypeptide in the serum of burn patients. *Ann. Surg.* **188**:209-215.

Cope, O., and Moore, F. D. (1947). The redistribution of body water and fluid therapy of the burned patient. *Ann. Surg.* **126**:1010-1045.

Covelli, H. D., Nessan, V. J., and Tuttle, W. K. III (1983). Oxygen derived variables in acute respiratory failure. *Crit. Care Med.* **1**:646-649.

Craddock, P. R., Fehr, J., Dalmasso, A. P., Brigham, K. L., and Jacob, H. S. (1977). Hemodialysis leukopenia: pulmonary vascular leukostasis resulting from complement activation by dialyzer cellophane membranes. *J. Clin. Invest.* **59**:879-888.

Craddock, P. R., Hammerschmidt, D. E., Moldow, C. F., Yamada, O., and Jacob, H. S. (1979). Granulocyte aggregation as a manifestation of membrane interactions with complement: possible role in leukocyte margination, microvascular occlusion, and endothelial damage. *Semin. Hematol.* **16**: 140-147.

Dantzker, D. R. (1982). Gas exchange in the adult respiratory distress syndrome. *Clin. Chest Med.* **3**:57-67.

Davis, W. B., Rennard, S. I., Bitterman, P. B., and Crystal, R. G. (1983). Pulmonary oxygen toxicity. Early reversible changes in human alveolar structures induced by hyperoxia. *N. Engl. J. Med.* **309**:878-883.

Demarset, G. B., Hudson, L. D., and Altman, L. C. (1979). Impaired alveolar macrophage chemotaxis in patients with acute smoke inhalation. *Am. Rev. Respir. Dis.* **119**:279-286.

Demedts, M., Clement, J., Sanescu, D. C., and Van de Woestijne, K. P. (1975). Inflexion point on transpulmonary pressure-volume curves and closing volume. *J. Appl. Physiol.* **38**:228-235.

Demling, R. H. (1983). Improved survival after massive burns. *J. Trauma* **23**: 179-184.

Demling, R. H. (1985). Burns. *N. Engl. J. Med.* **313**:1389-1398.

Demling, R. H., Will, J. A., and Belzer, F. O. (1978). Effect of major thermal injury on the pulmonary microcirculation. *Surgery* **83**:746-751.

DiVincenti, F. C., Pruitt, B. A. Jr., and Reckler, J. M. (1971). Inhalation injuries. *J. Trauma* **11**:109-117.

Dowell, A. R., Kilburn, K. H., and Pratt, P. C. (1971). Short-term exposure to nitrogen dioxide. *Arch. Intern. Med.* **128**:74-80.

Downs, J. B., Klein, E. F., Desautels, D., Modell, J. H., and Kirby, R. R. (1973). Intermittent mandatory ventilation: a new approach to weaning patients from mechanical ventilators. *Chest* **64**:331-335.

Downs, J. B., Doublas, M. E., Sanfelippo, P. M., Stanford, W., and Hodges, M. R. (1977). Ventilatory pattern, intrapleural pressure, and cardiac output. *Anesth. Analg.* **56**:88-96.

Dressler, D. P., Skornik, W. A., and Kupersmith, S. (1976). Corticosteroid treatment of experimental smoke inhalation. *Ann. Surg.* **183**:46-52.

Drinker, C. K. (1938). *Carbon Monoxide Asphyxia.* New York, Oxford University Press, pp. 88, 90-97, and 126.

Drinkwater, B. L., Raven, P. B., Harvath, S. M., Gliner, J. A., Ruhling, R. O. Bolduan, N. W., and Taguchi, S. (1974). Air pollution, exercise, and heat stress. *Arch. Environ. Health* **28**:177-181.

Dyer, R. F., and Esch, V. H. (1976). Polyvinyl chloride toxicity in fires. Hydrogen chloride toxicity in fire fighters. *J.A.M.A.* **235**:393-397.

Epstein, B. S., Rose, L. R., Teplitz, C., and Moncrief, J. A. (1963). Experiences with low tracheostomy in the burn patient. *J.A.M.A.* **183**:966-968.

Erdmann, J., Vaughan, T., Brigham, K. L., Woolverton, W., and Staub, N. (1975). Effect of increased vascular pressure on lung fluid balance in unanesthetized sheep. *Circ. Res.* **37**:271-284.

Evans, E. I., Pernell, O. J., Robinette, P. W., Batchelor, A., and Martin, M. (1952). Fluid and electrolyte requirements in severe burns. *Ann. Surg.* **135**:804-817.

Fariday, E. E., Permutt, S., and Riley, R. L. (1966). Effect of ventilation on surface forces in excised dogs' lungs. *J. Appl. Physiol.* **21**:1453-1462.

Fein, A., Grossman, R. F., Jones, J. G., and Hoeffel, J. (1981). Effect of major burns on alveolar-epithelial permeability in rabbits. *Crit. Care Med.* **9**:669-671.

Finck, P. A. (1966). Exposure to carbon monoxide: a review of the literature and 567 autopsies. *Milit. Med.* **131**:1513-1539.

Fisher, A. B., Hyde, R. W., Baue, A. E., Reif, J. S., and Kelly, D. F. (1969). Effect of carbon monoxide on function and structure of the lung. *J. Appl. Physiol.* **26**:4-12.

Fjellstrom, K. E., and Arturson, G. (1963). Changes in the human complement system following burn trauma. *Acta Pathol. Microbiol. Scand.* **59**:257-270.

Foley, F. D., Moncrief, J. A., and Mason, A. D. Jr. (1968). Pathology of the lung in fatally burned patients. *Ann. Surg.* **167**:251-264.

Forbes, W. H., Sargent, F., and Roughton, F. J. W. (1945). The rate of carbon monoxide uptake by normal men. *Am. J. Physiol.* **143**:594-608.

Gallagher, T. J., Civetta, J. M., and Kirby, R. R. (1978). Terminology update: optimal PEEP. *Crit. Care Med.* **6**:323-326.

Gherini, S., Peters, R. M., and Virgilio, R. W. (1979). Mechanical work on the lungs and work of breathing with positive end-expiratory pressure and continuous positive airway pressure. *Chest* **76**:251-256.

Glasser, K. L., Civetta, J. M., and Flor, R. J. (1975). The use of spontaneous ventilation with constant-positive airway pressure in the treatment of salt water near drowning. *Chest* **67**:355-357.

Glauser, F. L., Millen, J. E., and Falls, R. (1979). Increased alveolar epithelial permeability with acid aspiration: the effects of high-dose steroids. *Am. Rev. Respir. Dis.* **120**:1119-1123.

Goldzimer, E., Donopta, R., and Moser, K. (1974). Reversal of the perfusion defect in experimental canine lobar pneumococcal pneumonia. *J. Appl. Physiol.* **37**:85-91.

Gorin, A., Weidner, W., Demling, R., and Staub, N. (1978). Noninvasive measurements of pulmonary transvascular protein flux in sheep. *J. Appl. Physiol.* **45**:225-233.

Gorin, A. B., Kohler, J., and DeNardo, G. (1980). Noninvasive measurement of pulmonary transvascular protein flux in normal man. *J. Clin. Invest.* **66**:869-877.

Grag, G. P., and Gill, G. E. (1975). The use of spontaneous continuous positive airway pressure (CPAP) for reduction of intrapulmonary shunting in adults with acute respiratory failure. *Can. Anaesth. Soc. J.* **22**:284-290.

Grand, A. F., Kaplan, H. L., and Lee, G. H. II (1981). *Investigation of Combustion Atmospheres in Real Building Fires.* San Antonio, Southwest Research Institute.

Gregory, G. A., Kitterman, J. A., Phibbs, R. H., et al. (1971). Treatment of the idiopathic respiratory distress syndrome with continuous positive airway pressure. *N. Engl. J. Med.* **284**:1333-1340.

Grillot, C., Cooper, J. D., Gefin, B., and Pontoppidan, H. (1971). A low-pressure cuff for tracheostomy tubes to minimize tracheal injury. A comparative clinical trial. *J. Thorac. Cardiovasc. Surg.* **62**:898-907.

Grunnet, M. L. (1976). Long-term nervous system effects resulting from carbon monoxide exposure. In *Proceedings of Symposium on Physiological and Toxicological Aspects of Combustion Products, University of Utah, Salt Lake City, Utah, March 1974.* Washington, DC, National Academy of Sciences, pp. 119-129.

Haldane, J. (1895). The relation of the action of carbonic oxide to oxygen tension. *J. Physiol.* **18**:201-217.

Hansen, T. N., and Tooley, W. H. (1979). Skin surface carbon dioxide in sick infants. *Pediatrics* **64**:942-945.

Harkens, H. H. (1942). *The Treatment of Burns.* Springfield, Chas. C Thomas.

Harms, B. A., Bodai, B. I., Kramer, G. C., and Demling, R. H. (1982). Microvascular fluid and protein flux in pulmonary and systemic circulations after thermal injury. *Microvasc. Res.* **23**:77-86.

Haslam, P. L., Townsend, P. J., and Branthwaite, M. A. (1980). Complement activation during cardiopulmonary bypass. *Anaesthesia* **25**:22-26.

Hatch, T. F., and Gross, P. (1964). *Pulmonary Deposition and Retention of Inhaled Aerosols.* New York, Academic Press, pp. 29-142.

Hayashi, M., Bond, T. P., Guest, M. M., Linares, H., Wells, C. H., and Larson, D. L. (1979). Pulmonary microcirculation following full-thickness burns. *Burns* **5**:227-235.

Heideman, M. (1979). The effect of thermal injury on hemodynamic, respiratory, and hematologic variables in relation to complement activation. *J. Trauma* **19**:239-243.

Hilberman, M., Kamm, B., Lamy, M., Dietrick, H. P., Martz, K., Osborn, J. J. (1976). An analysis of potential physiological predictors of respiratory adequacy following cardiac surgery. *J. Thorac. Cardiovasc. Surg.* **71**:711-720.

Hochachka, P. W. (1986). Defense strategies against hypoxia and hypothermia. *Science* **231**:234-241.

Hole, A. (1984a). Pre- and postoperative monocyte and lymphocyte functions: effects of sera from patients operated under general or epidural anaesthesia. *Acta Anaesthesiol. Scand.* **28**:287-291.

Hole, A. (1984b). Pre- and postoperative monocyte and lymphocyte functions: effects of combined general and epidural anaesthesia. *Acta Anaesthesiol. Scand.* **28**:367-371.

Hole, A. (1984c). Depression of monocytes and lymphocytes by stress-related humoral factors and anaesthetic-related drugs. *Acta Anaesthesiol. Scand.* **28**:280-286.

Horowitz, H. H., Carrico, C. J., and Shires, G. T. (1974). Pulmonary response to major injury. *Arch. Surg.* **108**:349-355.

Hughes, J. M. B., Rosenzweig, D. Y., and Kivitz, P. B. (1970). Site of airway closure in excised dog lungs: histologic demonstration. *J. Appl. Physiol.* **29**:340-344.

Hunt, J. L., Agee, R. N., and Pruitt, B. A. Jr. (1975). Fiberoptic bronchoscopy in acute inhalation injury. *J. Trauma* **15**:641-649.

Katzenstein, A-L. A., Bloor, C. M., and Leibow, A. A. (1976). Diffuse alveolar damage—the role of oxygen, shock, and related factors. *Am. J. Pathol.* **85**:210-228.

Kirby, R. R., Perry, J. C., Calderwood, H. W., Ruiz, B. C., and Lederman, D. S. (1975). Cardiorespiratory effects of high positive end-expiratory pressure. *Anesthesiology* **43**:533-539.

Kirby, R. R., Downs, J. B., Civetta, J. M., Modell, J. H., Dannemiller, F. J., Klein, E. F., and Hodges, M. (1975). High level positive end expiratory pressure (PEEP) in acute respiratory insufficiency. *Chest* **67**:156-163.

Knisely, W. H., and Knisely, M. H. (1954). Preliminary observations of the catch-trap architecture of pulmonary artery tips and their responses following distant somatic burns. *Anat. Rec.* (Abstr.) **118**:320.

Kumar, A., Falke, K. J., Geffin, B., et al. (1970). Continuous positive-pressure ventilation in acute respiratory failure: effects on hemodynamics and lung function. *N. Engl. J. Med.* **283**:1430-1436.

Kumar, A., Pontoppidan, H., Falke, K., Wilson, R. S., and Laver, M. B. (1973). Pulmonary barotrauma during mechanical ventilation. *Crit. Care Med.* **1**:181-186.

Lanser, M. E., Brown, G. E., Mora, R., Coleman, W., and Siegel, J. H. (1986).

Trauma serum suppresses superoxide production by normal neutrophils. *Arch. Surg.* **121**:157-162.

Lemaire, F., Simoneau, G., Harf, A., Rivara, D., Teisseire, B., Atlan, G., and Rapin, M. (1979). Static pulmonary pressure-volume curve, positive end expiratory pressure, and gas exchange in acute respiratory failure. *Am. Rev. Respir. Dis.* (Abstr.) **119**:328.

Levine, B. A., Petroff, P. A., Slade, L. C., and Pruitt, B. A. Jr. (1978). Prospective trials of dexamethasone and aerosolized gentamycin in the treatment of inhalation injury in the burned patient. *J. Trauma* **18**:188-193.

Lewis, F. R., Schiobohm, R. M., and Thomas, A. N. (1977). Prevention of complications from prolonged tracheal intubation. *Am. J. Surg.* **135**:452-457.

Lindberg, R. R., Moncrief, J. A., Switzer, W. E., Order, S. E., and Mills, W. Jr. (1965). The successful control of burn wound sepsis. *J. Trauma* **5**:601-616.

Loke, J., Paul, E., Virgulto, J. A., and Smith, G. J. W. (1984). Rabbit lung after acute smoke inhalation: cellular responses and scanning electron microscopy. *Arch. Surg.* **119**:956-959.

Lund, T., Goodwin, C. W., McMannus, W. F., Shirani, K. Z., Stallings, R. J., Mason, A. D. Jr., and Pruitt, B. A. Jr. (1985). Upper airway sequelae in burn patients requireing endotracheal intubation or tracheostomy. *Ann. Surg.* **201**:374-382.

Macklin, C. (1939). Transport of air along sheaths of pulmonic blood vessels from alveoli to mediastinum. *Arch. Intern. Med.* **64**:913-926.

Macklin, M. T., and Macklin, C. (1944). Malignant interstitial emphysema of the lungs and mediastinum as an important occult complication in many respiratory diseases and other conditions: an interpretation of the clinical literature in the light of laboratory equipment. *Medicine* **23**:281-358.

Martyn, J. A. J., Aikawa, N., Wilson, R. S., Szyfelbein, S. K., and Burke, J. F. (1979). Extrapulmonary factors influencing the ratio of arterial oxygen tension to inspired oxygen concentration in burn patients. *Crit. Care Med.* **7**:492-496.

Mathru, M., Rao, T. L. K., and Venus, B. (1983a). Ventilator-induced barotrauma in controlled mechanical ventilation versus intermittent mandatory ventilation. *Crit. Care Med.* **11**:359-361.

Mathru, M., Venus, B., Rao, T. L. K., and Matsuda, T. (1983b). Noncardiac pulmonary edema precipitated by tracheal intubation in patients with inhalation injury. *Crit. Care Med.* **11**:804-806.

McClenahan, J. B., and Urtnowski, A. (1967). Effect of ventilation on surfactant and its turnover rate. *J. Appl. Physiol.* **23**:215-220.

McIntyre, R. W., Laws, A. K., and Ramchandran, P. R. (1969). Positive expiratory pressure plateau: improved gas exchange during mechanical ventilation. *Can. Anaesth. Soc. J.* **16**:477-486.

Mead, J. W. (1961). Mechanical properties of lungs. *Physiol. Rev.* **41**:281-330.

Meigs, J. W., and Hughes, J. P. W. (1952). Acute carbon monoxide poisoning: analysis of 105 cases. *Arch. Industr. Hyg.* **6**:344-356.

Mellins, R. B., and Park, S. (1975). Respiratory complications of smoke inhalation in victims of fires. *J. Pediatr.* **87**:1-7.

Miller, C. L., and Baker, C. C. (1979). Changes in lymphocyte activity after thermal injury: the role of suppressor cells. *J. Clin. Invest.* **63**:202-210.

Monafo, W. W., Robinson, H. N., Yoshioka, T., and Ayvazian, V. H. (1978). "Lethal" burns: a progress report. *Arch. Surg.* **113**:397-401.

Morgan, A., Knight, D., and O'Connor, N. (1978). Lung water changes after thermal burns: an observational study. *Ann. Surg.* **187**:288-293.

Moritz, A. R., Henriques, F. C. Jr., and McLean, R. (1945). The effects of inhaled heat on the air passages and lungs: an experimental investigation. *Am. J. Pathol.* **21**:311-331.

Morris, A. H. (1973). Nebulizer contamination in a burn unit. *Am. Rev. Respir. Dis.* **107**:802-808.

Morris, A. H., and Spitzer, K. W. (1973). Lung function in convalescent burn patients. *Am. Rev. Respir. Dis.* **108**:989-993.

Moyer, C. A., Margraft, H. W., and Monafo, W. W. Jr. (1965). Burn shock and extravascular sodium deficiency—treatment with Ringer's solution with lactate. *Arch. Surg.* **90**:799-811.

Moylan, J. A., and Alexander, L. G. Jr. (1978). Diagnosis and treatment of inhalation injury. *World J. Surg.* **2**:185-191.

Moylan, J. A. Jr., Wilmore, D. W., Mouton, D. E., and Pruitt, B. A. Jr. (1972). Early diagnosis of inhalation injury using [133]xenon lung scan. *Ann. Surg.* **176**:477-484.

Myers, R. A. M., Snyder, S. K., Linberg, S., and Cowley, R. A. (1981). Value of hyperbaric oxygen in suspected carbon monoxide poisoning. *J.A.M.A.* **246**:2478-2480.

Nash, G., Blennerhassett, J. B., and Pontoppidan, H. (1967). Pulmonary lesions associated with oxygen therapy and artificial ventilation. *N. Engl. J. Med.* **276**:368-374.

Nieman, G. F., Clark, W. R., Wax, S. D., and Webb, W. R. (1980). The effect of smoke inhalation on pulmonary surfactant. *Ann. Surg.* **191**:171-181.

Nusbacher, J., Rosenfeld, S. I., Macpheerson, J. L., Thiem, P. A., and Leddy, J. P. (1978). Nylon fiber leukapheresis: associated complement component changes and granulocytopenia. *Blood* **51**:359-365.

O'Flaherty, J. T., Kreutzer, D. L., and Ward, P. A. (1977a). Neutrophil aggregation and swelling induced by chemotactic agents. *J. Immunol.* **119**: 232-239.

O'Flaherty, J. T., Showell, H., and Ward, P. A. (1977b). Neutropenia induced by systemic infusion of chemotactic factors. *J. Immunol.* **118**:1586-1589.

O'Flaherty, J. T., Craddock, P. R., and Jacob, H. S. (1978). Effect of intravascular complement activation on granulocyte adhesiveness and distribution. *Blood* **51**:731-739.

Ogawa, M., Tamura, H., Katsurada, K., and Sugimoto, T. (1972). Respiratory changes in carbon monoxide poisoning with reference to hyperbaric oxygenation. *Med. J. Osaka Univ.* **22**:251-258.

Peirce, E. C. II, Zacharias, A., Alday, J. M. Jr., Hoffman, B. A., and Jacobson, J. H. II (1972). Carbon monoxide poisoning: experimental hypothermic and hyperbaric studies. *Surgery* **72**:229-237.

Petroff, P. A., Hander, E. W., Clayton, W. H., and Pruitt, B. A. Jr. (1976). Pulmonary function studies after smoke inhalation. *Am. J. Surg.* **132**:346-351.

Petroff, P. A., and Pruitt, B. A. Jr. (1979). Pulmonary disease in the burn patient. In *Burns. A Team Approach.* Philadelphia, Saunders, pp. 95-106.

Philibin, D. M., Sullivan, S. F., Bowman, F. O. Jr., Malm, J. R., and Papper, E. M. (1970). Postoperative hypoxemia: contribution of the cardiac output. *Anesthesiology* **32**:136-142.

Phillips, A. W., and Cope, O. (1962a). Burn therapy. I. Concealed process due to a shifting battlefront. *Ann. Surg.* **152**:767-776.

Phillips, A. W., and Cope, O. (1962b). Burn therapy. II. The revelation of respiratory tract damage as a principal killer of the burned patient. *Ann. Surg.* **155**:1-19.

Pollack, M. M., Fields, A. I., Holbrook, P. R. (1980). Cardiopulmonary parameters during high PEEP in children. *Crit. Care Med.* **8**:372-376.

Pontoppidan, H., Laver, M. B., and Geffin, N. (1970). Acute respiratory failure in surgical patients. In *Advances in Surgery,* Volume 4. Edited by C. E. Welch. Chicago, Year Book Med. Pub., p. 163.

Pontoppidan, H., Geffin, B., and Lowenstein, E. (1972). Acute respiratory failure in the adult. *N. Engl. J. Med.* **287**:690-806.

Pruitt, B. A. Jr. (1979). The burn patient: I. Initial care. *Curr. Probl. Surg.* **16**:4-62.

Pruitt, B. A. Jr. (1984). The diagnosis and treatment of infection in the burn patient. *Burns* **11**:79-91.

Pruitt, B. A. Jr., Flamma, R. J., DiVincenti, F. C., Foley, F. D., and Mason, A. D. Jr. (1970). Pulmonary complications in burn patients. *J. Thorac. Cardiovasc. Surg.* **59**:7-20.

Pruitt, B. A. Jr., and Mason, A. D. Jr. (1971). Hemodynamic studies of burn patients during resuscitation. In *Research in Burns.* Edited by P. Matter, T. L. Barclay, and Z. Konickova. Bern, Hans Huber.

Pruitt, B. A. Jr., Erickson, D. R., and Morris, A. (1975). Progressive pulmonary insufficiency and other pulmonary complications of thermal injury. *J. Trauma* 15:369-379.

Pruitt, B. A. Jr., Mason, A. D. Jr., and Hunt, J. L. (1976). Burn injury in the aged or high risk patient. In *The Aged and High Risk Surgical Patient.* Edited by J. H. Siegel and P. D. Chadoff. New York, Grune & Stratton, pp. 523-546.

Putman, C. E., Loke, J., Matthay, R. A., and Ravin, C. E. (1977). Radiographic manifestations of acute smoke inhalation. *Am. J. Roentgenol.* 129:865-870

Qvist, J., Pontoppidan, H., Wilson, R. S., Lowenstein, E., and Laver, M. B. (1975). Hemodynamic responses to mechanical ventilation with PEEP: the effect of hypervolemia. *Anesthesiology* 42:45-55.

Robinson, N. B., Hudson, L. D., Robertson, H. T., Thorning, D. R., Carrico, C. J., and Heimbach, D. M. (1981). Ventilation and perfusion alterations after smoke inhalation injury. *Surgery* 90:352-363.

Robinson, N. B., Hudson, L. D., Riem, M., Miller, E., Willoughby, J., Ravenholt, O., Carrico, C. J., and Heimbach, D. M. (1982). Steroid therapy following isolated smoke inhalation injury. *J. Trauma* 22:876-879.

Root, W. S. (1965). Carbon monoxide. In *Handbook of Physiology,* Volume II. Edited by W. O. Fenn and H. Rahn. Washington, DC, American Physiological Society, p. 1987.

Rowe, M. I., and Weinburg, G. (1979). Transcutaneous oxygen monitoring in shock and resuscitation. *J. Pediatr. Surg.* 14:773-778.

Ryhänen, P., Huttunen, K., and Ilonen, J. (1984). Natural killer cell activity after open-heart surgery. *Acta Anaesthesiol. Scand.* 28:490-492.

Sacks, T., Moldow, C. F., Craddock, P. R., Bowers, T. K., and Jacob, H. S. (1978). Oxygen radical mediated endothelial cell damage by complement-stimulated granulocytes: an *in vitro* model of immune vascular damage. *J. Clin. Invest.* 61:1161-1167.

Sahn, S. A., and Lakshminarayan, M. B. (1973). Bedside criteria for discontinuation of mechanical ventilation. *Chest* 63:1002-1005.

Salmenperä, M., and Heinonen, J. (1984). Transcutaneous oxygen measurement during one-lung anaesthesia. *Acta Anaesthesiol. Scand.* 28:241-244.

Santamore, W. P., Bove, A. A., and Heckman, J. L. (1984). Right and left ventricular pressure-volume response to positive end-expiratory pressure. *Am. J. Physiol.* 246:H114-H119.

Shah, D. M., Newell, J. C., Dutton, R. E., and Powers, S. R. (1977). Continuous positive airway pressure versus positive end-expiratory pressure in respiratory distress syndrome. *J. Thorac. Cardiovasc. Surg.* 74:557-562.

Sherwin, R. P., and Richters, V. (1971). Lung capillary permeability. *Arch. Intern. Med.* **128**:61-68.

Sim, V. M., and Pattle, R. E. (1957). Effect of possible smog irritants on human subjects. *J.A.M.A.* **165**:1908-1913.

Slade, M. S., Simmons, R. L., Yunis, E., and Greenberg, L. J. (1975). Immuno-depression after major surgery in normal patients. *Surgery* **78**:363-372.

Smith, J. S., and Brandon, D. (1970). Acute carbon monoxide poisoning: three years experience in a defined population. *Postgrad. Med. J.* **46**:65-70.

Smith, L. J., and Brody, J. S. (1981). Influence of methylprednisolone on mouse alveolar type 2 cell response to acute lung injury. *Am. Rev. Respir. Dis.* **123**:459-464.

Sones, F. M., Higashihara, T., Kotake, T., Morimoto, S., Miura, T., Ogawa, M., and Sugimoto, T. (1974). Pulmonary manifestations of carbon monoxide poisoning. *Am. J. Roentgenol.* **120**:865-871.

Stadie, W. C., and Martin, K. A. (1925). The elimination of carbon monoxide from the blood. A theoretical and experimental study. *J. Clin. Invest.* **2**: 77-91.

Staub, N., Bland, R., Brigham, K. L., Demling, R., Erdmann, J., and Woolverton, W. (1975). Preparation of chronic lung lymph fistulas in sheep. *J. Surg. Res.* **19**:315-320.

Stauffer, J. L., Olson, D. E., and Petty, T. L. (1981). Complications and conse-quences of endotracheal intubation and tracheotomy. A prospective study of 150 critically ill adult patients. *Am. J. Med.* **70**:65-76.

Stoeckel, H. (1970). Late complications after tracheostomy. In *Progress in Anaesthesiology: Proceedings of the Fourth World Congress of Anaes-thesiologists.* Edited by T. B. Boulton et al. Amsterdam, Excerpta Medica, pp. 825-830.

Stone, H. H., and Martin, J. D. (1969). Pulmonary injury associated with ther-mal burns. *Surg. Gynecol. Obstet.* **129**:1242-1246.

Stratta, R. J., Warden, G. D., Ninnemann, J. L., and Saffle, J. R. (1986). Im-munologic parameters in burned patients: effect of therapeutic interven-tions. *J. Trauma* **26**:7-17.

Suter, P. M., Fairley, H. B., and Isenberg, M. D. (1975). Optimum end-expira-tory airway pressure in patients with acute pulmonary failure. *N. Engl. J. Med.* **292**:284-289.

Sykes, M. K., Adams, A. P., Finlay, W. E. I., McCormick, P. W., and Economides, A. (1970). The effects of variations in end-expiratory inflation pressure on cardiopulmonary function in normal hypo- and hypervolemic dogs. *Br. J. Anaesth.* **42**:669-677.

Tahvanainen, J., and Nikki, P. (1983). The significance of hypoxemia with low inspired O_2 fraction extubation. *Crit. Care Med.* **11**:708-711.

Tahvanainen, J., Salmenperä, M., and Nikki, P. (1983). Extubation criteria after weaning from intermittent mandatory ventilation and continuous positive airway pressure. *Crit. Care Med.* 11:702-707.

Task Group on Lung Dynamics (1966). Deposition and retention models for internal dosimetry of the human respiratory tract. *Health Phys.* 12:173-207.

Teabeaut, J. R. II. (1952). Aspiration of gastric contents. An experimental study. *Am. J. Pathol.* 28:51-67.

Teplitz, C., Epstein, B. S., Rose, L. R., and Moncrief, J. A. (1964). Necrotizing tracheitis induced by tracheostomy tube. *Arch. Pathol.* 77:6-19.

Terrill, J. B., Montgomery, R. R., and Reinhardt, C. F. (1978). Toxic gases from fires. *Science* 200:1343-1347.

Till, G. O., Johnson, K. J., Kunkel, R., and Ward, P. A. (1982). Intravascular activation of complement and acute lung injury: dependency on neutrophils and toxic oxygen metabolites. *J. Clin. Invest.* 69:1126-1135.

Till, G. O., Beauchamp, C., Menapace, D., Tourtellottee, W. Jr., Kunkel, R., Johnson, K. J., and Ward, P. A. (1983). Oxygen radical dependent lung damage following thermal injury of rat skin. *J. Trauma* 23:269-277.

Tønnesen, E., Huttel, M. S., Christensen, N. J., and Schmitz, O. (1984). Natural killer cell activity in patients undergoing upper abdominal surgery: relationship to the endocrine stress response. *Acta Anaesthesiol. Scand.* 28:654-660.

Tremper, K. K., Waxman, K., and Shoemaker, W. C. (1979). Effects of hypoxia and shock on transcutaneous PO_2 values in dogs. *Crit. Care Med.* 7:526-531.

Tremper, K. K., Waxman, K., Bowman, R., and Shoemaker, W. C. (1980a). Continuous transcutaneous oxygen monitoring during respiratory failure, cardiac decompensation, cardiac arrest, and CPR. *Crit. Care Med.* 8:377-381.

Tremper, K. K., Mentelos, R. A., and Shoemaker, W. C. (1980b). Effect of hypercarbia and shock on transcutaneous carbon dioxide at different electrode temperatures. *Crit. Care Med.* 8:608-612.

Uretzky, G., and Cotev, S. (1980). The use of continuous positive airway pressure in blast injury of the chest. *Crit. Care Med.* 8:486-489.

Uzawa, T., and Ashbaugh, D. G. (1969). Continuous positive-pressure breathing in acute hemorrhagic pulmonary edema. *J. Appl. Physiol.* 26:427-432.

Venus, B., Jacobs, H. K., and Lim, L. (1979). Treatment of the adult respiratory distress syndrome with continuous positive airway pressure. *Chest* 76:257-261.

Venus, B., Matsuda, T., Copiozo, J. B., and Mathru, M. (1981). Prophylactic intubation and continuous positive airway pressure in the management of inhalation injury in burn victims. *Crit. Care Med.* **9**:519-523.

Via-Reque, E., and Rattenborg, C. C. (1981). Prolonged oro- or nasotracheal intubation. *Crit. Care Med.* **9**:637-639.

Wagner, P. D., Saltzman, H. A., and West, J. B. (1974). Measurement of continuous distribution of ventilation-perfusion ratios: theory. *J. Appl. Physiol.* **36**:588-599.

Walker, H. L., McLeod, C. G., and McManus, W. F. (1981). Experimental inhalation injury in the goat. *J. Trauma* **21**:962-964.

West. J. B. (1974). Blood flow to the lung and gas exchange. *Anesthesiology* **41**:124-138.

Whorton, M. D. (1976). Carbon monoxide intoxication: a review of fourteen patients. *J.A.C.E.P.* **5**:505-509.

Widdicombe, J. G., Kent, D. C., and Nadel, J. A. (1962). Mechanism of bronchoconstriction during inhalation of dust. *J. Appl. Physiol.* **17**:613-616.

Winter, P. M., and Miller, J. N. (1976). Carbon monoxide poisoning. *J.A.M.A.* **236**:1502-1504.

Winter, P. M., and Smith, G. (1972). The toxicity of oxygen. *Anesthesiology* **37**:210-241.

Wynne, J. W., Reynolds, J. C., Hood, C. I., Auerback, D., and Ondrasick, J. (1979). Steroid therapy for pneumonitis induced in rabbits by aspiration of foodstuff. *Anesthesiology* **51**:11-19.

Wynne, J. W., DeMarco, F. J., and Hood, C. I. (1981). Physiological effects of corticosteroids in foodstuff aspiration. *Arch. Surg.* **116**:46-49.

Wyszogrodski, I., Kyei-Aboagye, K., Taeusch, H. W. Jr., and Avery, M. E. (1975). Surfactant inactivation by hyperventilation: conservation by end-expiratory pressure. *J. Appl. Physiol.* **38**:461-466.

Zikria, B. A., Sturner, W. Q., Astarjian, N. K., Fox, C. L. Jr., Ferrer, J. M. Jr. (1968). Respiratory tract damage in burns: pathophysiology and therapy. *Ann. N. Y. Acad. Sci.* **150**:618-626.

Zikria, B. A., Weston, G. C., Chodoff, M., and Ferrer, J. M. (1972a). Smoke and carbon monoxide poisoning in fire victims. *J. Trauma* **12**:641-645.

Zikria, B. A., Ferrer, J. M., and Floch, H. F. (1972b). The chemical factors contributing to pulmonary damage in "smoke poisoning." *Surgery* **71**:704-709.

Zikria, B. A., Budd, D. C., Floch, F., and Ferrer, J. M. (1975). What is clinical smoke poisoning? *Ann. Surg.* **181**:151-156.

8

Battlefield Chemical Inhalation Injury

JOHN S. URBANETTI

Yale University School of Medicine
New Haven, Connecticut

Warfare has never been "humane," but rather extrahuman in nature, and certainly destructive. Often called the "failure of statesmen," war has been the last refuge of failed communications. As recorded by Thucydides, Sparta was one of the earliest users of chemical warfare (423 B.C.). While they were attacking Athenian cities, a combination of pitch, sulfur, and naptha was burned to produce a cloud of toxic SO_2. Since that time the adversarial use of chemicals has surfaced in sporadic conflicts.

The French, who were already familiar with the use of tear gas in various civilian demonstrations, were possibly the first World War I combatants to use chemicals. In 1914, the French began use of tear gas grenades against the Germans. Shortly thereafter the Germans retaliated with tear gas artillery shells. On 22 April, 1915, in Ypres, Belgium, the Germans, using chlorine, launched what was to be the single most destructive gas attack of the war. The difficulties of chemical warfare were graphically described by an American physician, Dr. G. W. Norris, who detailed his first-hand observations at a Philadelphia medical meeting:

> A field hospital full of freshly and badly gassed men is, in the estimation of all who have had an opportunity of seeing it, the most horible and ghastly sight of the war. Even the man who has received multiple and severe wounds,

when he has been splinted, put to bed, and given his morphine, is relatively comfortable; but to see a hundred or more men, hale and hearty a few hours before, slowly strangling to death from pulmonary edema with gradually increasing dyspnea, cyanosis and pallor, making futile efforts to expectorate and to assist their breathing by voluntary effort and muscular contortions, until exhausted, they pass from semidelirium into stupor, collapse, and death, is a never-to-be-forgotten sight, a sight which makes one clench one's teeth and curst the Hun who started this dastardly infamy. This is phosgene! But can nothing be done? Yes! The cyanotic cases are promptly bled, one pint, sometimes two. The ward looks like a shambles because in hurrying from bed to bed, twenty to thirty in a row, the spurting blood has left its trace upon bed and floor and linen. Meanwhile oxygen is being administered to greedy mouths while hands are loath to loose the bag when their five minutes of respite are over. For never are there enough bags for all, and the precious gas we must not waste, for it has been no small task to bring these great iron tanks up to the front. Opium we dare not use, for it checks an often life-saving cough. But the gray cases, what of them? Lying about with a clammy skin, too weak to move or even care. Some venturous spirits say that one should bleed and then transfuse, but most that we should not meddle (Norris, 1919).

Chemical warfare continued to be of both theoretical and practical interest in the years after World War I. By 1923 a joint German-Soviet company was formed for the development and manufacture of chemical agents. In 1929 the Japanese began chemical warfare research and development activities and subsequently produced substantial quantities of a variety of poison gases, mustard gases among them. Because of the secrecy surrounding such manufacture, gas-production employees were often not well informed or protected in their work environment. The neoplastic hazard of long-term/multiple exposures to mustard was thereby identified. Mustard gases were apparently used by the Japanese in their military encounters with the Chinese in the late 1930s and by the Italians in Ethopia in 1936. Mustards and a variety of other agents were prepared and stockpiled in strategic locations by the allies during World War II. The Germans, meanwhile, had developed and stockpiled a new group of toxic gases, the organophosphates. Because of the neurologic toxicity of the organophosphates, they came to be known as "nerve agents." Neither the Allies or the Germans, for reasons that remain unclear, used chemical agents in any military campaign during World War II.

Most nations have a chemical defense group that is actively investigating the subject of chemical toxicity. In the United States, the United States Army Medical Research Institute of Chemical Defense at Aberdeen Proving Ground, Maryland, has been at the forefront of such chemical defense investigation since its establishment as an Army Medical Department Laboratory by Congressional act in 1915. One of the primary missions of this facility is the education and training of medical personnel in chemical defense. Much of the data here are the result of such careful medical research interest.

Agents with a particular respiratory toxicity or a primary inhalational route of entry have been selected from a wider range of potential biologic poisons. Both chemical and "natural" toxins are included. All data reported in this chapter derive from literature in the public domain. The selection of agents and specific therapies represent the views of the author and does not reflect official policy or position of the Department of the Army, Department of Defense, or the U.S. government.

I. General Principles and Treatment

A. Military Use

A wide variety of chemical exposures both intentional (belligerent) and unintentional (accidental), may occur in battlefield conditions. Military preparedness training focuses on prevention of exposures by appropriate warning, use of masking techniques, and use of prophylactic medications where available.

Military technology is sufficiently well developed to permit the delivery of virtually any chemical into nearly any setting or environment by means of artillery shells, rockets, grenades, or vehicle- or aircraft-mounted sprays. Exposure may result from contact with droplets or vapors in the immediate area of exploding munitions or from dermal contact or inhalational exposure to more persistent agents that may continue to contaminate the environment. Because chemical exposures occur primarily by either respiratory or dermal routes (or a combination of the two), adequate protection requires the development of sophisticated masks and protective clothing. Suspicion of exposure may result from observing suspicious smokes, fumes, vapors, odors, or liquids; aircraft spray attack; otherwise unexplained clinical signs in associates. Practical protection includes continuous use of protective clothing if there is even a suspicion of impending chemical attack.

B. Agents

Agents are grouped here by their general categories, with recognition that their use has a primary military aim.

Riot Control Agents

These chemicals of short effect, designed to be used at a specific site to disrupt purposeful behavior, have mild to moderate self-limited respiratory effects, unless there is a severe exposure. Chloroacetophenone, chlorobenzylidene, dibenzoxazepine, and diphenylaminochlorarsine are described below as examples of these agents.

Choking Agents

These chemicals of primary respiratory toxicity with more severe and damaging effects are designed to incapacitate severely or kill. Onset of symptoms may vary from immediate contact to days, depending on agent and degree of exposure. Examples include phosgene, diphosgene, chlorine, and chlorpicrin.

Blood Agents

These chemicals are transported by the blood, blocking oxygen transport and ultimately blocking cellular respiration. Cyanide and cyanogen chloride are discussed.

Nerve Agents

Chemicals thought to affect acetyl cholinesterase and thereby ultimately much of the nervous system interfere with bodily control mechanisms. Death generally occurs as a result of respiratory failure. Examples include sarin, soman, tabun, and VX.

Incapacitants

These chemicals affect the CNS in a fashion that interferes with higher centers and causes thought processes/emotions to become disordered (BZ).

Blister Agents

Blister agents are chemicals primarily developed for their dermal toxicity, with resulting vesicant damage to the skin. Most are also found to have severe respiratory toxicity in vapor form. These include sulfur mustard, nitrogen mustard, lewisite, and phosgene oxime.

Organic Toxins

This additional group of chemicals with significant respiratory toxicity or risk of inhalation includes botulinus toxin, staphylococcal enterotoxin B, and ricin.

C. Treatment

Removal/Escape

Escape from exposure is generally not practical in a military environment. A variety of protective environments have been developed. These range from individual protective suits to specially sealed vehicles, free-standing tent-like enclosures that are fully sealed with a filtered air supply, tentlike devices that can be set up within buildings, and specific rooms isolated from the external environment.

Medical Triage

Immediate decisions regarding the likelihood of medical salvage of exposed individuals must be made. Generally this triage is performed by the most senior medical officer present. Such decisions require (1) understanding of the medical/ surgical importance of both chemical and "conventional" injuries (2) and understanding of the capabilities of the support facilities to care for a given injury (e.g., a single severe phosgene-induced respiratory failure may occupy personnel and resources otherwise able to care for multiple nerve agent casualties).

Emergency Support

Airway

In the event of continued environmental exposure, a gas mask will be required by the injured person. If upper airway occlusion occurs that is not relieved by head extension, laryngospasm is then presumed. Because a gas mask precludes normal endotracheal tube placement, tracheostomy/cricothyroidotomy should be considered. Such a procedure is undertaken if resolution of the laryngospasm does not occur within a few minutes. Devices have been developed to accomplish this easily and simultaneously provide a connection to a small, portable (possibly jet/high-frequency) ventilator. If there is no continued environmental exposure, in practiced hands an endotracheal tube can generally be placed even in the event of laryngospasm.

Breathing

Respiratory failure with nerve agents is generally fully reversible and artificial respiration should be employed. Respiratory failure with all other exposures is of such serious consequence that the casualty may be considered beyond practical assistance unless an intensive care unit is readily available.

Circulation

Circulatory failure in a situation of chemical or mixed (chemical and "conventional") exposure is generally of such serious consequence that the casualty may be considered beyond practical assistance unless an intensive care unit is readily available.

Decontamination

Careful decontamination by well-established procedures and using standard powder/solutions is an extremely important next step. Failure at this point propagates the casualties' illness and endangers the health of all subsequent health care personnel. Lack of attention to this detail has been the cause of many unfortunate exposures to mustards during World War I and more recently, during the Iran/Iraq conflict, where aircraft personnel evacuating mustard casualties themselves became casualties.

Specific Therapy (see Agents)

In certain circumstances, specific therapy may be begun, coincident with the exposure (see section on nerve agents).

II. Riot Control Agents

Lacrimatory agents are generally potent irritators of all mucous membranes, causing severe pain and copious secretions. At higher doses, distal portions of the respiratory tract may be affected as well. Aside from general "crowd" riot control, some of these agents have been advocated for use in specific antipersonnel situations.

A. Chloroacetophenone

Synonyms for chloroacetophenone (CN) include alpha-chloroacetophenone, "tear gas," phenylacyl chloride, phenyl chloromethyl ketone, chloromethyl phenyl ketone, Mace, Cap, 1-chloroacetophenone, O-chloroacetophenone. Its formula is $C_6H_5COCH_2Cl$; vapor density 5.2 (air = 1); specific gravity 1.32 (water = 1); melting point: 59°C. CN is colorless to grey solid with a sharp irritating odor that is often described as "orange-blossom like." Since the odor threshold is substantially below lethal levels, the substance is considered to have adequate warning properties. Dissemination is generally accomplished by "burning munitions," such as lacrimatory candles or grenades that produce a blue/white cloud.

Toxicity: Thresholds and Limits

Concentration (ppm)	Effect	References
0.02	Odor threshold	NIOSH, 1981
0.05	Permissible exposure limit (OSHA 8 hr average)	NIOSH, 1981
0.05-0.07	Lacrimation threshold	NIOSH, 1981
140	Lethal (10 min)	Stein and Kirwan, 1964

Chemical Effects

This substance is thought to act chemically as an alkylating agent for sulfhydryl-containing enzymes, and to denature tissue proteins as well (Cucinell et al., 1971; Louvre and Cucinell, 1970). A rapid and noncompetitive inhibition of cholinesterase (ChE) has also been described. This observation possibly explains the rapid onset of lacrimation (Castro, 1968).

Respiratory Effects

Clinical

An incident of exposure reported by Thorburn (1982) typifies the respiratory effects of this agent. In a reported prison riot, 44 prison cells, each with a separate inhabitant, were sprayed with CN aerosol, some more than once. The inmates showered while clothed and there was no subsequent change of clothing. Acute respiratory effects included a burning sensation in the eyes, nose, and throat, salivation, rhinorrhea, dyspnea, sore throat, pharyngeal edema, and cough. Although symptoms persisted for 1-2 days, there were no reported deaths or long-term injuries.

Lacrimatory symptoms generally abate within 10-20 min of withdrawal from exposure. Conjunctivitis may persist for up to 24 hr. Higher doses of CN that have produced pharyngeal edema may precipitate a persistent hoarseness that can last for up to a week. Dyspnea may be more prominent in this setting. At particularly high doses death can occur within 10-12 hr primarily due to pulmonary edema. This pulmonary edema is most likely to occur as a result of exposure in a confined space if escape is not possible. Five deaths are reported in this setting (Chapman and White, 1978; McNamara et al., 1969; Stein and Kirwan, 1964).

After a single exposure, cough may persist for several days. A follow-up of a volunteer exposure group at Edgewood Arsenal (Maryland) showed no evidence of long-term respiratory effects (National Research Council, 1984).

Pathology

Animals exposed to large doses (a monkey study using 280 ppm for 5.5 min) showed pulmonary edema and parenchymal hemorrhage at 24-72 hr. Animals that survived this exposure demonstrated no pathologic abnormalities to light microscopy at 30 days (Striker et al., 1967a). Oral ingestion of this substance (in rat and rabbit) produces histologically evident pulmonary congestion which, if the animal survives, remits entirely by 3 weeks (Ballantyne and Swanston, 1978).

In humans with acute exposures, oropharyngeal erythema and pharyngeal edema are seen without stridor (Thorburn, 1982). If, after severe exposure, the patient survives the pulmonary edema and intraalveolar hemorrhage, there is necrosis of respiratory mucosa and formation of grey pseudomembranous exudates. Bronchopneumonia may appear on the 3rd-4th day (Stein and Kirwan, 1964; Chapman and White, 1978; McNamara et al., 1969).

Therapy

There is no specific prophylactic or chemical therapy available for exposure to this agent. Respiratory tract symptoms are treated symptomatically, generally simply by removal from exposure. Because this substance is used in a powder/ dust formulation, it may persist as a skin or clothing contaminant after the subject is removed from an area of exposure. Further personal decontamination can be accomplished by flushing the skin with copious quantities of water or preferably by washing with a 5 or 10% sodium bicarbonate (water) solution (U.S. Dept. of the Army, 1968).

B. Chlorobenzylidene

Synonyms for chlorobenzylidene (CS) include OCBM, ortho-chlorobenzylidene, 2-chlorobenzylidene malonitrile, and o-chlorobenzalmalononitrile. Its formula is $C_{10}H_5ClN_2$; specific gravity greater than 1; vapor density 6.5; melting point: 93-95°C. CS is white crystalline solid with a faint peppery odor.

Toxicity: Thresholds and Limits

Concentration (ppm)	Effect	References
0.005	Minimal detectible irritant level	Himsworth, 1971a,b
0.05	Permissible exposure limit (OSHA 8 hour average)	NIOSH, 1981
0.2	Headache (90 min exposure) and lacrimation	National Research Council, 1984
0.5-0.8	Tolerance limit (only if gradually attained, 30 min)	NIOSH, 1981
1.3	Field concentration for troop dispersal	Himsworth, 1971
300-1800	Lethal (10 min) by animal extrapolation	WHO Consultants, 1970; McNamara et al., 1969

Chemical Effects

CS has been shown to cause alkylation of sulfydryl-containing enzymes. There is a specific inhibition of lactic dehydrogenase and documented reaction with a variety of nucleophilic compounds such as glutathione and lipoic acid (Louvre and Cucinell, 1970). CS-induced inhibition of lactic dehydrogenase can be reversed with sodium thiosulfate in dogs. Rats poisoned with lethal doses of CS can be saved by injections of sodium thiosulfate (Cucinell et al., 1971). This observation has not been reported in humans.

Respiratory Effects

Clinical

Acute exposure with CS produces lacrimation with a peppery sensation in the eyes, as well as copious rhinorrhea and salivation. With increasing doses there is chest tightness, dyspnea, coughing, and sneezing (Owens and Punte, 1963). These symptoms remit spontaneously within 30 min after cessation of exposure (Ballantyne, 1977b), although a photophobia may persist up to 1 hr. At still higher concentrations, cyanosis may be present with severe respiratory distress followed by pulmonary edema. A case of an infant with a confined space exposure of 2-3 hr (unknown concentration) is reported. Initial examination showed only first-degree cheek burns; however, cyanosis was noted on day 2, resolving by day 3, only to be followed by pneumonia, which delayed hospital discharge to day 28 (Park and Giammona, 1972). Another child unable to escape a confined exposure in a bedroom (Londonderry riots) was found to be crying and gasping for breath. There was pallor and lacrimation but rapid recovery after removal from exposure (Himsworth, 1971a).

Acute exposures have been shown to produce no changes in chest x-ray findings, peak flow rate, tidal volume, vital capacity, or airway resistance (Punte et al., 1963; Beswick et al., 1972). Further physiological studies with experimental exposure showed no significant effect on gas transfer or alveolar volume. However, a small reduction in exercise ventilation volume could be shown (Cotes et al., 1972a,b). Tolerance to this substance may develop with repeat low-dose exposures (Himsworth, 1971a). This tolerance is decreased with exercise, hyperventilation, and increasing temperature and humidity (Punte et al., 1963). Individuals with asthma and chronic bronchitis may suffer acute exacerbations of their underlying illness as a result of exposure (Ballantyne, 1977b; Himsworth, 1971a,b).

Long-Term Effects

Individuals with preexisting chronic bronchitis are thought to be at some increased risk of superimposed acute bronchitis or bronchial pneumonia after exposure. Although a causal relationship between CS exposure and asthma attacks has not been clearly established, CS smoke is thought to represent an adjunctive irritant to otherwise susceptible individuals. There was no significant long-term effect noted in two follow-up assessments of otherwise healthy exposed populations (National Research Council, 1984; Himsworth, 1971a). Also, there is no report of human death attributable to CS exposure.

CS has been shown to be a potent skin sensitizer, causing allergic contact dermatitis in a high percentage of subjects.

Pathology

There are no human pathologic reports available. Monkey data show severe edema, emphysematous change, and bronchiolitis at 600-1,000 ppm exposure over 10 min (Striker, 1967). Animal studies attempting to evaluate carcinogenicity of this substance show that subchronic animal exposure (rats: 65 exposures of 6 hr each at 0.2 ppm or higher) show epithelial hyperplasia and squamous metaplasia of the trachea and larynx. No tumors were identified (McNamara et al., 1969). In long-term exposure studies rats develop bronchial pneumonia at 2-3 weeks (with exposures of 80 min/day, 9 days at 15 ppm) (Ballantyne and Calloway, 1972).

Therapy

See discussion of chloroacetophenone.

C. Dibenzoxazepine

Synonyms for dibenzoxazepine (CR) include dibenz[b,f]-[1,4]oxazepine and dibenzoxazepine. Its melting point is 72°C. CR is a pale yellow solid with a sharp irritating odor. Since the odor threshold is substantially below lethal levels, the substance is considered to have adequate warning properties.

Toxicity: Thresholds and Limits

Concentration (ppm)	Effect	References
0.003	Eye irritation	Ballantyne and Swanston, 1974
4	Tolerance limit	Ballantyne and Swanston, 1974
>75000	Lethal (10 min) (animal extrapolation)	National Research Council, 1984

Chemical Effects

CR is thought to act on specific sensory units of the amyelinate nerve fibers (Foster and Ramage, 1975). An observed postexposure pressor effect is thought to be due to release of norepinephrine from adrenergic nerve endings. This effect is short-term and is considered to be limited by rapid metabolism of CR (Lundy and McKay, 1975). When CR is administered by the aerosol route, rats have been shown to absorb ^{3}H-labeled CR rapidly. Blood levels are detectable within 15 sec of onset of exposure and a plasma half-life is calculated at approximately 5 min. The authors believe that such rapid absorption implies that systemic effects contribute to the symptoms demonstrated with CR (Leadbeater and Maidment, 1973; Bandman and Savateyer, 1977).

Clinical Respiratory Effects

The location of the acute effects of riot control agents is thought to be somewhat dependent on particle size. The larger- (greater than 60 μm) diameter particles produce predominantly ocular effects and smaller particles produce primarily respiratory irritative effects (Punte, 1962). The respiratory effects of CR include rhinorrhea, salivation, nasal irritation and stuffiness, choking, dyspnea, and tachypnea. Eye irritation and upper airway irritation generally resolved 15-20 min after removal from exposure.

One long-term study (at Edgewood Arsenal, Maryland) reported that dyspnea and tachypnea appeared commonly with aerosol exposure. These symptoms abated spontaneously. There was no evidence of long-term effects or skin sensitization (National Research Council, 1982).

The few available human physiological studies focus on the observation that there is a brief pressor effect, seen most commonly after bodily drenching with a solution of CR. It was concluded that a CR drench presented no more of a hazard for blood pressure increase than did exercise alone (Ballantyne, 1977a,b).

Therapy

See section on chloroacetophenone.

D. Diphenylaminochlorarsine

Synonyms for diphenylaminochlorasine (DM) include Adamsite, 10 chloro 5,10, dihydrophenarsazine, diphenyl amino chlorarsine, "Blue Cross," "mask breaker," and "sneeze agent." The formula is $C_6H_5ClA_s$, and melting point, 195°C. Adamsite (DM) appears as a canary yellow crystalline solid that can be disseminated as a spray or aerosol from solution or as a dust. When volatilized by grenade or bomb it produces a canary yellow smoke with the odor of burning fireworks. Since the

odor threshold is substantially below toxic levels, this material is considered to
have good warning properties.

Toxicity: Thresholds and Limits

Concentration (mg/m^3)	Effects	References
0.38	Threshold, throat irritation	Owens et al., 1967
0.5-0.75	Threshold, lower respiratory tract (cough)	Owens et al., 1967
22-92	1 min toleration	McNamara et al., 1969
1000-2000	30 min lethal	McNamara et al., 1969

Chemical Effects

Specific chemical interactions with biological systems have been reported in limited fashion. Adamsite has been found to be an active inhibitor of chlorinesterase.
This observation has led to speculation that the clinically observed lacrimation
and rhinorrhea are due to this effect (Castro, 1968).

Respiratory Effects

Clinical

At low doses, the effects of an aerosol exposure include severe irritation of both
the upper respiratory tract and the eyes, and a milder skin irritation. At high
doses the respiratory effects are even more prominent with nasal tickling, sneezing
acute nasal and sinus pain, violent cough, choking, and thick viscous mucous production. Recovery generally occurs within 1-2 hr of cessation of exposure.
Hoarseness and aphonia may appear and persist for 3-5 days. Laryngitis and
tracheitis are prominent. The patient may expectorate foamy mucopurulent
material. A frontal headache may be almost unbearable and chest pain may be
oppressive with substantial dyspnea (WHO Consultants, 1970; Ballantyne, 1977b).
Typically the onset of symptoms is delayed several minutes after the exposure,
hence a greater quantity of agent may be absorbed before one is aware of the exposure, resulting in more severe symptoms and more delayed recovery.

Later (2-4 hr) effects of a severe exposure may include severe tiredness
and toxic pulmonary edema. One accidental death has been reported to have occurred with an exposure of uncertain time (5-30 min) at an ambient concentration estimated to be 1130-2260 mg/m^3 (McNamara et al., 1969). Generally,
however, recovery is complete 1-2 hr after removal from exposure. A subsequent

feeling of depression is thought to be primarily psychological (Gates et al., 1946). Human studies at Edgewood Arsenal, Maryland, reported the above clinical findings, but some effects lasted for several hours.

Pathology

Only animal data are available. A range of monkey exposures have been reported, with low doses shown to produce a superficial tracheitis and edema of the tracheal and bronchial mucosa. At moderate doses pulmonary edema and focal parenchymal hemorrhage are seen. This increases with time, peaks at 24 hr, and gradually clears thereafter. High-dose exposures may produce death within 24 hr and typically show early bronchopneumonia, pulmonary edema, emphysematous change, and ulcerated tracheobronchial mucosa within 24-48 hr if death does not occur (Striker et al., 1967a,b).

Therapy

See discussion of CN.

III. Choking Agents

Agents that severely irritate the tracheobronchial tree and also commonly produce pulmonary edema are generally classed as choking agents. This section will include phosgene (Moore and Gates, 1946a) (also diphosgene) and chlorine as typical examples of choking agents found in battlefield exposure.

Although choking agents are generally very effectively screened by a properly worn and maintained gas mask, substantial toxicity may be encountered before the individual becomes consciously aware of an exposure and dons a mask. The earliest evidence of a toxic exposure may only be tachypnea or dyspnea, a presentation that may confuse the triage officer and be (unfortunately) regarded as hysterical or malingering. This is a particularly serious problem since the physical findings of abnormal lung sounds, radiologic evidence of infiltrate, or blood gas abnormalities may appear as late as 2-6 hr after a lethal exposure. It is therefore imperative that complaints of dyspnea be seriously considered as evidence of possible toxic inhalational exposure until at least 4-6 hr of otherwise sign-free time have passed and there is no further evidence of impending pulmonary edema as evidenced by both chest x-ray and arterial blood gas measurements.

A. Phosgene

Synonyms for phosgene (CG) include carbonyl chloride, carbonoxychloride, chloroforml chloride, Green Cross. Its formula is $COCL_2$; vapor density 3.4 (gas); specific gravity 1.4 (liquid); boiling point 8.2°C. Phosgene in low concentration has

an odor of new-mown or musty hay or green corn. An odor threshold of 1.5
ppm has been reported. Even with training, this threshold is not consistently observed. There is also a rapid olfactory adaptation, which further limits odor as
a useful warning. Consequently, odor threshold does not provide adequate warning of toxic exposure. Phosgene appears as a gas, hydrolyzing sufficiently in the
air to produce a white cloud that typically hugs the ground (trenches in World
War I) (Bunting, 1945a).

Toxicity: Thresholds and Limits

Concentration (ppm)	Effects	References
0.5	Permissible exposure limit (OSHA 8 hour average)	NIOSH, 1981
1.5	Odor threshold	Wells et al., 1938
2-4	Eye irritation	NIOSH, 1981
5	Cough	Bunting, 1945a
50-100	Lethal (30 minutes)	WHO Consultants, 1970)

Chemical Effects

Phosgene was originally thought to be toxic to the lung through the mechanism
of hydrolysis and production of topically toxic (hydrochloride) HCl. Subsequent
studies suggest that this is not the case since free inhaled HCl is approximately
1/800 times as toxic as phosgene (Buscher, 1931) and ketene, a substance with a
similarly available carbonyl group (but that does not hydrolyze to HCl), is almost
equally as toxic as phosgene.

Phosgene's carbonyl group ($C = 0$) reacts promptly with a variety of primary
amines and hydroxyl groups, subsequently affecting cell wall stability with particular effect on capillary membrane permeability (Bunting, 1945a). The effect is a
local/topical one and is evidenced by the protective effects of bronchial plugging
and the lack of transfer of disease by cross-circulation experiments (Tobias et al.,
1949).

Possible additional effects include interference with cellular energy supply
(glycolysis is disrupted) and with polypeptide formation (Bunting, 1945a). A
demonstration that thromboplastin is destabilized may also contribute to increased
cellular/capillary permeability (Gerard, 1948; Simon and Potts, 1945). More recent studies suggest that phosgene triggers a sympathetic reflex, producing a neurogenic (hypoactive sympathetic) pulmonary edema (Frosolono, 1974; Ivanhoe and

Meyers, 1964; Gregory, 1970). Some conflicting reports suggest that vagotomy protects (Buscher, 1931) and does not protect (Bunting, 1945a) a phosgene-exposed lung from the development of pulmonary edema.

Phosgene is primarily toxic in the more peripheral airways. This is presumably due in part to the relatively low rate of hydrolysis, which limits its absorption in the upper airways. It may also be in part due to the physiological effect of an eightfold volume dilution of gas entering the alveolar ducts from the terminal bronchioles. Such dilution delays local clearance of inhaled gases/fumes and promotes local toxicity (Gross et al., 1967).

Respiratory Effects

Clinical (Everett and Overholt, 1968; Manufacturing Chemists Assoc., 1970)

Acute Effects. At low concentrations a mild cough may be seen initially. At moderate concentrations lacrimation may first be noted and an observation that tobacco has an unpleasant or objectionable taste is made (Underhill, 1920). At very high concentration a severe cough with laryngospasm may lead to sudden death (Buscher, 1931). This may possibly be due to the local effect of larger quantities of HCl liberated by hydrolysis.

Subacute Effects. At 30 min to 12 hr after exposure (depending on dose) there may appear substernal tightness, cough, and progressive dyspnea leading to overt pulmonary edema. Pneumonia may appear on the 3rd-4th day.

Long-Term Effects. After a severe acute exposure, exercise hypoxia may be seen from months to years later (Pearce, 1920). A detailed study was made of six workers, each of whom survived a single phosgene exposure severe enough to produce pulmonary edema. The author considered that changes typical of pulmonary emphysema were typical sequelae of phosgene exposure. However, in that study pulmonary histories (particularly smoking) were not taken and all individuals had normal chest x-rays (without hyperinflation). Only three of the six individuals had abnormal gas mixing. Of these three, two had normal exercise pO_2 (and one was not studied) (Galdston et al., 1947a). There are no other studies showing classic emphysema to be a sequela of acute phosgene exposure (Cucinell, 1974).

Chronic Effects. The only available report studying individuals with multiple small dose phosgene exposure describes five workers with repeated small exposures over an 18-42 month period. Findings (interpreted by the author as consistent with emphysema) were reported to include decreased vital capacity, impaired gas mixing, and hyperinflated chest radiograph. However, arterial blood gases on exercise were abnormal only in two of the five workers, and in those two there was a history consistent with hyperreactivity of the airways (Galdston et al., 1974b). There are no other studies showing classic emphysema as a result of chronic phosgene exposure.

A variety of epidemiologic studies of long-term, low-dose phosgene exposures show no evidence of chronic pulmonary toxicity. However, pulmonary function testing are not available in those studies (Levina et al., 1966; Levina and Kurando, 1967).

Physiology

Shortly after exposure, radiologic increases in lung volume can be identified, suggesting air trapping with early bronchiolitis (Ardran, 1964; Glass et al., 1971). Clinical evidence for such early air trapping was also provided by Buscher (1931).

A group of six patients studied 3-14 months after exposure showed no exercise hypoxia despite complaints of shortness of breath and precordial chest pain after exertion. There were no other consistent changes in lung volumes, dead space, maximal breathing capacity, arterial blood gases, rest or exercise oxygen uptake, or carbon dioxide production. The authors commented on a pattern of rapid shallow breathing that was thought to be typical of phosgene exposure (Galdston et al., 1947a). Long and Hatch (1961) demonstrated in an animal study that decreased diffusing capacity is a reliable early test of lung irritant effect (rats show diffusing capacity change at phosgene exposures of 0.5-5 ppm for 30 min). Diffusing capacity diminishes progressively for 6-8 hr subsequent to phosgene exposure followed by gradual recovery. Diffusing capacity abnormalities are seen at 0.5 ppm exposures, even though the lung appears normal at postmortem.

Animal studies show prolongation of circulation time that is improved with atropine injections. A widened $(A-a)O_2$ gradient is noted, and may be due in part to altered ventilation/perfusion relationships with increases in bronchomotor tone. Some studies show that a histamine-like substance is released in guinea pigs after exposure; however, there is no evidence that phosgene pulmonary effects are mediated by bloodborne substances. Other data suggest that increased bronchomotor tone is only seen in animals with sufficiently high exposure to have encountered topical effects of HCl.

Hypoxia occurs due to effects of the pulmonary edema, further compromising myocardial function.

Pathology (Bruner and Coman, 1945; Buscher, 1931; Clay and Rossing, 1964; Coman et al., 1947; Delepine, 1923; Gross et al., 1965; Winternitz, 1919)

Description of the pathologic effects of phosgene is best undertaken chronologically and is drawn primarily from animal studies. There is an immediate effect (30 min or less) and in a severe exposure there is bronchiolar constriction, swelling, necrosis, and perivascular edema. During the early effects (0.5-6 hr) with moderate exposure, bronchiolar constriction, and pulmonary arteriolar constriction with dilatation/engorgement of capillaries and veins are noted. In addition, polymorphonuclear leukocytes move into interstitial spaces and emphysematous change is seen particularly at lung margins and in areas showing prior bronchial constriction. In severe exposure, interstitial edema is seen as early as 30-45 min and noted after perivascular edema. Also bronchiolar epithelial sloughing with plugging by necrotic cells or mucus is noted. Eight to 24 hr after mild exposure there is perivascular and interstitial edema; with moderate and severe exposures bronchiolar dilatation and bronchiolar epithelial sloughing is seen. During the first 3 days, edema peaks and begins to resolve, and right heart failure is seen. During the repair period (days 4 and later), bronchopneumonia may appear. There is resolution of edema and bronchiolar inflammation and repair of mucosal sloughing.

General Therapy

The possible prophylaxis of phosgene exposures has long been studied. Early attempts to bind phosgene chemically led to the discovery that certain amine derivatives were effective in animal studies (e.g., taurine, hexamethylenetetramine [HMT]). HMT was used in World War I gas masks in an attempt to absorb phosgene (Buscher, 1931) and there was some prophylactic effect if administered before exposure. This substance had subsequently been studied in a variety of animal settings (Schultz, 1945; Diller, 1978). Available human data, however, are anecdotal with poor controls (Shohl and Deming, 1920; Braker et al., 1977; Stavrakis, 1971).

The clinical effects of phosgene toxicity are those of "noncardiac pulmonary edema." Early attempts at therapy with venesection (Bramwell, 1915) have given way to more "modern" approaches. There are no unique therapies for phosgene exposure that are not already routinely applied in other situations of "noncardiac pulmonary edema."

Two therapeutic subjects bear brief statement:

1. Although steroids have been used in a number of phosgene exposures, and specific inhalational steroid therapy is regarded as doctrine by some military services, there are insufficient human data to support such therapy (Brand, 1971).

2. Early application of positive airway pressure has been shown to delay, ameliorate, and possibly prevent some of the phosgene-induced pulmonary edema. Dr. R. V. Christie first suggested the specific use of positive pressure for phosgene intoxication in 1937. The first use of positive pressure respiration was reported by Longcope (Longcope et al., 1943) and studied shortly thereafter by others (Chasis et al., 1944).

In considering therapy of a phosgene exposure, particular attention should be paid to the apparent delay in onset of clinical symptoms after exposure. A period of 2-6 hr after exposure may occur before symptoms of pulmonary edema appear. Such a delayed onset of symptoms does not imply a mild exposure. The earliest clinical index of pulmonary edema is the patient's own sense of dyspnea. Subsequently, changes in $(A-a)O_2$ gradient, pulmonary auscultation, and chest radiograph are seen in that order. Resolution of phosgene-induced illness generally follows the reverse order.

Specific Therapy

Remove subject from contamination, institute immediate control of airway, and evaluate the cardiopulmonary system. In less severe exposures (alert, oriented without dyspnea), assess the chest by auscultation: bibasilar crackles and obstructive airway sounds may be early indices of impending pulmonary edema. If abnormal arterial blood gases are also obtained, institution of positive pressure ventilation is indicated using a positive end-expiratory pressure (PEEP) mask for alert individuals and endotracheal intubation with PEEP or positive pressure ventilation for others. Individuals who appear otherwise normal by physical examination or evaluation of arterial blood gases should be carefully observed for 4-6 hr after exposure. At the end of this observation period, a repeat physical examination, arterial blood gas measurement, and chest x-ray should be performed. With abnormality of any one of these parameters, the possibility of rapidly progressive and lethal pulmonary edema must still be considered, and further careful observation for a minimum of 24 hr should be undertaken. An individual who is under observation should be followed to resolution of symptoms of dyspnea, clearance of physical examination, and normalization of both arterial blood gas and radiologic abnormalities before being discharged.

Abnormal arterial blood gases and significant dyspnea occurring within an hour of exposure suggest that intubation is likely to be required. PEEP appears effective as an adjunct to routine positive pressure ventilation. The possible benefits of negative extrathoracic ventilation have not been explored in toxic inhalational exposure of phosgene.

There is no indication for routine prophylactic antibiotics or steroids in this setting. In the absence of infectious complications, resolution of a severe phosgene exposure generally occurs over 2-4 days. Generally, with resolution of the acute symptoms and in the absence of complications of superinfection, long-term follow-up studies need not extend past 1 year, if arterial blood gas and lung function test including diffusing capacity are normal at that time. Complaints of dyspnea on exertion may necessitate exercise testing.

B. Diphosgene

Synonyms for diphosgene (DP) include perstoff, superpalite, trichloromethyl chloroformate, and perchlormethyl formate. Its formula is CCl_3OCOl; specific gravity 1.65; vapor density 6.9; boiling point 128°C. Diphosgene is generally spread as a vapor. It is less volatile than phosgene (droplet evaporation may take up to 3 hr) (Buscher, 1931) and hence is toxic over a longer period.

Chemical Effects

One mole of diphosgene in aqueous solution produces 2 mol phosgene with a chemical action fully equivalent to the released phosgene. If fact, most chemical research with phosgene in both aqueous solution and living cell suspension is done using aqueous solutions of diphosgene for convenience. The chemical effects of diphosgene are identical to those of phosgene.

Clinical Respiratory Effects

The respiratory effects of diphosgene are basically identical to those of phosgene. However, with initial exposure, diphosgene produces a more impressive lacrimation/burning.

Therapy

Treatment is identical to that for phosgene (see Phosgene).

C. Chlorine

The formula for chlorine (Cl) is Cl_2; density 2.5; specific gravity 1.41; boiling point -34.1°C. Chlorine appears as a greenish yellow gas with an acrid, pungent, characteristic odor. Since the odor threshold is substantially below the toxic limit, this substance is considered to have good warning properties. With chronic and repeated exposure, however, some threshold adaptation occurs (Beck, 1959). A progressive olfactory inhibition has been described. This progressive loss of sensitivity is thought to be the reason that chlorine workers suffer more frequent and more severe exposures in the later months and years of their work history, ostensibly because of the "warning" threshold of their olfactory sensitivity (Laciak and Sipa, 1958).

Chemical Action

Chlorine exists in elemental form at a pH of less than 2. In the less acid environment of human tissue it becomes hypochlorous acid (HOCl), a molecular form

Toxicity: Thresholds and Limits

Concentration (ppm)	Effects	References
0.01-0.2	Odor threshold range	May, 1966
0.5	Nasal irritation	NIOSH, 1981
1	Permissible exposure limit (OSHA 15 min average)	NIOSH, 1981
1-3	Eye irritation	International Labor Office, 1971
3-6	Sneezing, coughing, bloody, nose intolerable after a few minutes	Zielhuis, 1970
35+	Lethal 60-90 minutes	Freitag, 1940

that easily penetrates cell walls, reacting with cytoplasmic proteins to form N-chloro derivatives that are toxic to the cell structure (National Research Council, 1976). Cell wall damage occurs early (edema formation). Interaction with sulfhydryl groups and consequent interference with sulfhydryl-dependent enzymes has been suggested (Knox et al., 1948). RNA inactivation may be important as well (Griffin, 1976; Oliver et al., 1973).

Chlorine added to the water that contains nitrogenous materials forms chloramines, with some systemic toxicity related to this compound as well.

Respiratory Effects

Clinical

With low-dose exposures, immediate ocular irritation is followed shortly by spasmodic coughing and a choking sensation. Mild shortness of breath with substernal tightness is apparent. Minimal to mild cyanosis may be evident with exertion and exertional dyspnea may be prominent. Persistent cough on deep inspiration is also common.

Moderate dose exposure results in immediate cough and a choking sensation with a prominent complaint of suffocation. Hoarseness or an inability to speak may be present. There is severe substernal pain. Symptoms and signs of pulmonary edema may appear at 2-6 hr (earlier with higher doses). The radiologic changes of pulmonary edema are commonly seen somewhat later than the clinical symptoms. Retching and vomiting of gastric material with an odor of chlorine may occur.

With more severe exposures, pulmonary edema may appear earlier. Copious tracheobronchial secretions are seen beginning at a rate of 50-10 ml/hr, and then increasing further, with one fatal case reported to have produced 2 liters of tracheal secretions within 75 min. Dyspnea is extreme. A hyperinflated chest with subcutaneous emphysema may be noted. Coma may appear early. Shock is more typically seen in the older patient exposed to high doses. Of the deaths that occur, 81% occur within 24 hr and 92% occur within 48 hr of the initial exposure (Bunting, 1945b). A massive exposure may produce sudden death without obvious pulmonary lesions at postmortem. This is thought to be due to laryngospasm (Gilchrist and Matz, 1933).

Bronchospasm may appear in a variable degree within 10-12 hr. It occurs earlier with higher doses and in individuals with predisposing airway diseases, such as asthma, bronchitis. It is uncertain whether airway edema or neurogenic reflex is the precipitating factor. Resolution of the respiratory distress and substernal pain generally occurs with 36-72 hr. This resolution is typically delayed in individuals with underlying respiratory disorders. Cough may be particularly prominent on deep inspiration and may resolve at 10-14 days. Individuals with a more severe exposure may continue to demonstrate cyanosis with exertion for 1-2 weeks. Acute bronchitis may supervene at 3-5 days. Pneumonia may then appear in 4-7 days.

Ciliary activity has been studied in animals subsequent to chlorine exposure. Temporary ciliostasis has been observed after exposure to 20 ppm for 2.5 min and permanent cessation of ciliary activity has been observed at exposures of 20 ppm for 10 min or 30 ppm for 5 min (Cralley, 1942).

Animal studies show changes in respiratory rhythm (transient respiratory arrest) (Shultz, 1918b) and cardiac arrest (Shultz, 1918a); both effects are prevented by sectioning of the vagus prior to study.

Shortly after a single exposure there may be an increase in closing volume (Callaway et al., 1974). Bronchoconstriction is occasionally seen as a result of aggravation of underlying asthma subsequent to even low concentration exposures to chlorine. Ingestion of chlorinated water has been shown to create bronchospasm in some instances (Watson and Kibler, 1933). Bronchospasm may be precipitated by chlorine-containing air in the vicinity of a swimming pool or sauna (Sheldon and Lovell, 1949).

Multiple or prolonged low dose or repeated exposures to chlorine result in inflammation of the nasal mucous membrane and possibly result in increased susceptibility to respiratory infections (NIOSH, 1981). One study of chlorine workers showed somewhat poorer respiratory function compared to a cohort of sulfur dioxide workers. However, both groups showed a lower prevalence of respiratory disease than in a matching local male population group (Ferris et al., 1967). Another review showed a decrease in the maximal midexpiratory flow rates of an exposed group. Smoking appeared to be a major contributing factor as well

(Chester et al., 1969). A group of 332 chlorine cell workers (with generally less than 1 ppm chronic exposure) showed no significant long-term effects (Patil et al., 1970).

Pathology

With mild exposure there is a reddened oropharynx with some endothelial inflammation extending peripherally to the level of the smaller airways. As exposure increases, the oropharynx becomes more intensely injected. There is edema of the epiglottis and larynx as well as the base of the tongue. A sharp line of demarcation may be seen separating the pharyngeal injection from the pale uninvolved esophagus. Pleural effusions may be seen in association with developing pulmonary edema. With even more severe exposures there are distended pulmonary lymphatics with a dense, heavy edematous consolidation of lung. Subcutaneous emphysema is common. A fibrinous exudate may be seen lining the bronchi at 1-2 days. There may be epithelial necrosis. With moderate exposures a purulent bronchitis may be seen with small areas of pneumonic consolidation that became larger with increasing severity of exposure. Infarction and gangrene have been reported by the French but is not a common finding in other pathologic reviews (Bunting, 1945c).

Bronchiectatic changes in a setting of chronic bronchitis have been described subsequent to World War I exposures. More recent studies do not show a significant incidence of chronic airways disease subsequent to a single chlorine exposure (Chasis et al., 1947; Hoveid, 1956; Kowitz et al., 1967; Weill et al., 1969).

Therapy

There is no specific prophylactic therapy for the effects of chlorine exposure. Acute postexposure therapy is nonspecific and identical to that undertaken for phosgene (Hardy and Barach, 1946). There is no evidence that acute chlorine-induced laryngotracheitis or bronchitis responds to corticosteroid therapy. Bronchodilators and corticosteroids are useful in individuals with underlying bronchospastic airway disease.

Pulmonary edema is treated in the same manner as other causes of noncardiac pulmonary edema. There is no evidence that "prophylactic" antibiotic therapy is of specific value unless an underlying bacterial bronchitis or pneumonitis can be specifically identified.

Long-term postexposure therapy is nonspecific and identical to that for phosgene. There is no evidence that corticosteroid therapy or prophylactic antibiotic therapy modifies the long-term effects of an exposure to chlorine, unless the individual has a preexisting respiratory disorder.

D. Chloropicrin

Synonyms for chloropicrin (PS) include klop, "vomiting gas," Green Cross (when combined with diphosgene in artillery shell), nitrochloroform, trichloro-nitromethane, nitrotrichloromethane, and chloropicrin. Its formula is $CCl_2 NO_2$; vapor density 5.7; specific gravity 1.64; boiling point 112°C. Chloropicrin is a colorless, oily liquid with a penetrating pungent odor that immediately causes tears. The odor threshold is considered sufficiently low to serve as an adequate warning with respect to toxicity. This substance is used as an insecticide and sterilizing agent, especially for cereals in ship holds. It is also used as a warning agent in other fumigants because of its strong odor. Thermal decomposition of this product can produce additional toxic substances in the form of various oxides of nitrogen, as well as phosgene, Cl_2, and CO.

Toxicity: Thresholds and Limits

Concentration (ppm)	Effects	References
0.1	Permissible exposure limit (OSHA 8 hr average)	NIOSH, 1981
0.3	Eye irritation	NIOSH, 1981
1.1	Odor threshold	NIOSH, 1981
15	Tolerated 1 minute	NIOSH, 1981
119	Lethal in 30 minutes	NIOSH, 1981, Vettorrazi, 1977

Chemical Effects

Data regarding specific chemical effects of this substance are not available. This substance has been thought to induce a susceptibility that leads to asthma in the event of reexposure to smaller doses (Bunting, 1945b).

Respiratory Effects

Clinical

At low doses, effects include cough, lacrimation, rhinorrhea, nausea, and vomiting. With higher doses dyspnea, cyanosis, and signs of pulmonary edema appear, with death occurring in a few hours. Survivors of acute exposures show persistent dyspnea and exertional cyanosis. Death might occur at 3-5 days, generally as a result of superinfection (Winternitz, 1920). Methemoglobinemia has also been reported in association with exposure, but the clinical significance of this observation is uncertain (Vettorazi, 1977).

In a study of farm-fumigant exposure of several hundred workers, headache and fatigue persisting for several hours after the exposure were noted. Coughing and lacrimation persisted for 1-3 days. There was a positive correlation between age and symptoms, with older individuals demonstrating more severe symptoms (Okada et al., 1970).

Long-term effects have not been reported. Follow-up studies of volunteer exposures show no evidence of long-term effects (National Research Council, 1984).

Pathology

Animal data show that massive exposures produce early pathologic changes of pulmonary edema. Edema fluid with a characteristically high fibrin content is reported. With less severe exposures a mild tracheal injury with an inflammatory bronchitis is seen. There may be focal bronchial occlusions with inflammatory cells. Bronchitis and bronchopneumonia may ensue at 3-5 days. As the traumatized epithelium regenerates and there is organization of necrotic bronchial changes, scar formation may occur (Underhill, 1920).

Other Effects

Chloropicrin liquid has a corrosive action on the skin. Dermabrasions exposed to chloropicrin gas often become septic, with local abscess formation. Small amounts of the agent may be systemically absorbed through the skin but there is no evidence that this has significant respiratory effects (National Research Council, 1984).

Therapy

There is no specific chemical prophylaxis or therapy developed for this substance. Symptomatic therapy is similar to that given for chlorine and phosgene.

IV. Blood Agents

Several chemicals may act primarily on the oxygen transport system of the body, thereby inhibiting basic respiratory processes and ultimately damaging vital organ systems. Cyanide and cyanogen chloride are the two examples cited.

The French were perhaps the first to use cyanide during World War I. Animal studies (dogs) performed by the French showed cyanide to be exceptionally toxic while animal studies (goats) done by the British showed much less toxicity. Professor Joseph Barcroft conducted a study showing that the human was less sensitive than the dog to cyanide. He entered an exposure chamber, unmasked, with a dog. A subsequent exposure to cyanide killed the dog but left Barcroft only with brief periods of residual dizziness that occurred whenever he turned his head suddenly (Cookson and Nottingham, 1969).

A. Cyanide

Synonyms for cyanide (AC) include hydrocyanic acid, hydrogen cyanide, and prussic acid. Its formula is HCN; vapor density 0.93; specific gravity 0.69; boiling point 25.7°C. Cyanide is a colorless gas (or liquid) with a peach-kernel or bitter-almond odor. Although it can be detected by trained observers at slightly less than toxic levels, because of the rapidity of onset of toxic symptoms this substance is regarded as having poor warning properties (Braker et al., 1977).

Toxicity: Thresholds and Limits

Concentration (ppm)	Effects	References
50	Tolerated 1 hr	Friedberg, 1968
110	Fatal 1 hr	Braker et al., 1977
180	Fatal 10 min	Braker et al., 1977
270	Fatal immediately	Braker et al., 1977

Chemical Effects

Cyanide forms exceptionally stable complexes with the metals in a variety of metal-containing enzymes. Cyanide may combine with metalloporphyrins in concentrations as low as 33 μM. As early as 1929, cytochrome oxidase was identified as the most significantly inhibited metalloporphyrin due to its primary position in electron transfer to molecular oxygen. Because of the widespread distribution of cytochrome oxidase in the body, inhibited function as a result of cyanide binding interrupts cellular respiration in nearly all aerobic cells. Historically, therapy has been directed towards attempted binding of cyanide to other noncritical molecules such as methemoglobin. However, recent clinical studies showing that amyl nitrite reverses both the respiratory and cardiac effects of cyanide before significant methemoglobin is formed suggest that the classic theory regarding cytochrome oxidase inhibition may not be the primary lethal effect of cyanide (Vick and Froehlich, 1985). Because of the observed vasodilatory effect of amyl nitrite, further study of other vasoactive substances in cyanide poisoning has been undertaken.

While cyanide is percutaneously absorbed, it is only toxic in massive doses. A somewhat slow absorption rate makes this a route of relatively minor risk (Friedberg, 1968; Bastian and Mercker, 1959).

Respiratory Effects

Clinical

Most exposures and therefore most effects are acute. At low doses, hyperpnea, headache, vertigo, nausea, trismus, and weakness may be observed. Recovery is generally complete within 15-20 min of cessation of exposure. With more intense exposures severe nausea, vomiting, dyspnea, coma, and convulsions may occur. If there is recovery at this point, occasional evidence of prolonged neurologic damage is seen. Individuals may demonstrate irrationality and unsteady gait, and animal studies document a variety of focal neurologic lesions. With more severe exposure, respiratory failure and death supervene. The venous blood is typically bright red because of peripheral cell failure to utilize the transported oxygen.

Clinical effects of chronic toxicity are of some concern, particularly when there may be multiple environmental exposures added to small systemic accumulations of cyanide available from dietary cyanogens (Seigler, 1977) smoking (smoke may contain 1600 ppm) (Towill et al., 1978), and some gastrointestinal bacterial release (Adams et al., 1966). A "cyanide syndrome" has been described with toxic effects of chronic cyanide exposure primarily involving the central nervous system, gastrointestinal tract, and thyroid (Poulton, 1983). Pulmonary edema has been reported in humans, probably due to left ventricular failure as a result of direct toxic effect of cyanide on the myocardium (Way et al., 1984).

Animal studies show that minute ventilation is stimulated by cyanide (both increased frequency and tidal volume). This may be due to a combination of both central and extracranial mechanisms other than those related to the carotid or aortic chemoreceptors (Solomonson, 1981; Brodie, 1959; Levine, 1975). Respiration is immediately stimulated 7-10 times baseline values. This stimulus lasts for 15-20 sec, making breath-hold exceptionally difficult for even a trained individual while he or she is attempting to don a gas mask or escape a contaminated area (Loevenhart et al., 1918).

Pathology

With large exposure, the sudden death that results leaves no obvious histopathologic changes. With smaller, multiple, or prolonged exposure and/or recovery from a near lethal dose, animals may show hemorrhage of the thymus gland. Other typically posthypoxic lesions may be seen in the cerebrum and cerebellum. Intense exposure occasionally produces pulmonary edema prior to death, although this is more commonly seen with cyanogen chloride (Moore and Gates, 1946b).

Therapy

Artificial respiration was first suggested as a specific therapy in 1839 (Blake, 1840a,b). Subsequent attention to chemical therapy resulted from K. K. Chen's report of the antidotal combination of amyl nitrite, sodium nitrite, and sodium thiosulfate (Chen et al., 1933). This combination was thought to be effective because of selective cyanide sequestration. Adjunctive use of oxygen, however, is clearly synergistic, with the combination of oxygen and nitrite-thiosulfate producing physiological (reversal of EEG effects) (Burrows et al., 1973) and biochemical (reversal of cytochrome oxidase inhibition (Ison et al., 1982) improvement.

The observation that amyl nitrite reversed both respiratory and cardiac effects in dogs before significant methemoglobin was formed suggested at least that methemoglobin formation was not the most significant therapeutic effect of amyl nitrile and that perhaps the classic cytochrome oxidase-inhibition may not be the primary lethal effect (Vick and Froehlich, 1985). The observed vasodilating effect of amyl nitrite prompted further investigation of other vasoactive substances.

Alpha-Blocking Agents

Phenoxybenzamine (and chlorpromazine) are not individually effective in CN toxicity but show substantial synergism with sodium-thiosulfate (Burrows and Wag, 1970; Burrows et al., 1977).

Sulfane Pool Expansion

Mammalian tissues contain the enzymes and substrates to convert CN to SCN, a very much less toxic substance that is excreted in the urine. Studies are currently directed toward analyzing and manipulating these substances as a therapeutic intervention in cyanide toxicity (Westley, 1984).

Aminothiols

A variety of aminothiols are under intense study. These substances are thought to act in combination as CN scavengers, either through addition to the bodily sulfane pool or through an alpha-blocking effect (Davidson et al., 1984).

CN Scavengers

Cobalt compounds (especially cobalt-EDTA) have been shown to form a stable cyanide complex (Paulet, 1957, 1958). Although hydroxycobalamin and cobalt-EDTA have been used in cyanide poisoning, questions of a possible toxic effect of cobalt on the myocardium remain (Naughton, 1974). Other metalloporphyrins and gold-containing compounds may be effective and are undergoing further study (Hambright et al., 1984).

Other Methemoglobin Formers

Dimethylaminophenol (DMAP) has been studied (and is deployed in Germany) as a more rapid methemoglobin former than the nitrites (Kiese and Weger, 1969). This substance may have a minor advantage in that it is available as an intramuscular as well as intravenous preparation. Clear superiority to nitrite therapy has not been shown.

Development of prophylactic therapy has been of increasing military concern, largely because of the rapid effect of this agent. Consequently, studies are underway to increase the body's natural store of cyanide scavengers (e.g., by increasing the sulfane pool and producing significantly protective levels of methemoglobin, etc.) and to study thiol compounds that have alpha-adrenergic blocking activity and would perhaps mimic the vasodilatory effects of amyl nitrite.

Postexposure therapy consists of the following. Remove the subject from the contaminated environment immediately. Amyl nitrite (pearls, ampules), one or two crushed and held near nose/mouth for inspiration repeated every 5 min (to a maximum of eight ampules until recovery). Apneic individuals should immediately receive artificial respiration (possibly with a device to administer amyl nitrite via one-way valve). Oxygen therapy should be added immediately if available. Moderate hypotension may occur with this therapy but is rarely of clinical significance. Sodium nitrite/thiosulfate is then administered: parenteral injection of 10 ml 3% sodium nitrite solution over 1 min followed with 50 mil 25% sodium sulfate solution over 5 min. As part of the post-acute therapy, individuals should be observed for evidence of hypoxic damage (Norris et al., 1984) to critical organs. There is no evidence that antioxidants or antiinflammatory agents are of specific value. Individuals who survive (without coma or convulsions) an exposure for the time necessary to begin parenteral therapy are very likely to have survived without such therapy. This therapy is primarily indicated for other than inhalational exposures where absorption may continue over a prolonged period (e.g., swallowed CN salts, severe dermal/ocular exposure).

B. Cyanogen Chloride

The formula for cyanogen chloride (CK) is ClCN. Its vapor density is 2.0; specific gravity 1.19; boiling point 12.6°C. Cyanogen chloride is a strongly irritating gas that is easily detected at 20 mg/m^3 by its irritant effects on the eyes and nose (Moore and Gates, 1946b). Some observers are able to detect eye irritation at concentrations as low as 2 mg/m^3. The substance is fully metabolized to cyanide very quickly after inhalation and all subsequent systemic effects are primarily attributable to the hydrogen cyanide thereby produced.

Toxicity: Thresholds and Limits

Concentration (ppm)	Effects	References
48	Fatal at 30 min.	Moore and Gates, 1946b
159	Fatal at 10 min.	Moore and Gates, 1946b

Respiratory Effects

Clinical

The clinical effects of this substance are due to a combination of systemic clinical effects of cyanide and the topical irritant effects of cyanogen chloride. At low dose there is immediate irritation of the eyes and nose with a sense of substernal tightness and cough. At moderate dose cough and increasing dyspnea may appear in association with dizziness. At higher dose unconsciousness with convulsions and ultimate respiratory failure will occur. If there is immediate survival of the cyanide effects of this higher dose, persistent cough with frothy sputum, rales, and persistent cyanosis is seen. These effects are the result of a toxic pulmonary edema caused by the topical irritant effects of cyanogen chloride.

Pathologic

There are no reported human studies available. Histologic studies in animals show a mild bronchiolitis with typical changes of pulmonary edema noted after more intense exposures. The damage to the central nervous system may be relatively greater as a result of the added hypoxia of the pulmonary edema.

Therapy

See discussion of cyanide.

V. Organophosphorus Compounds (Nerve Agents)

A. Chemical Effects

The toxicity of organic phosphorus (OP) compounds is thought to be primarily due to inhibition of cholinesterase (Holmstedt, 1959). OP compounds are classed as esters. When absorbed, their immediate interaction is with esterases, which in the human are classified into three groups: A, B, C. Of these, the A and B esterases interact with OP compounds; C esterases do not. A-esterases (e.g., phosphoryl phosphatase) rapidly interact with OP compounds and detoxify them by hydrolysis. Such hydrolysis is generally complete within 1-2 hr, releasing free A-esterases for further reaction. B-esterases (e.g., cholinesterase) react equally well with OP compounds. Hydrolysis is less rapid, however, and, depending on the particular compound, it may take from 1 to greater than 1000 hr. Additionally, certainly OP compounds become progressively irreversibly bound ("aged"), resulting in permanent inhibition of the cholinesterase.

Although a variety of esterases are known to interact with OP compounds, cholinesterase is the only esterase whose function is understood, and whose inhibition is known to be clinically significant.

Cholinesterase functions in the exceptionally rapid metabolism of acetylcholine, reacting completely with that substance within a few microseconds (Wilson, 1951). Such rapid metabolism of acetylcholine maintains the very delicate balance necessary for the cholinergic aspects of the nervous system.

Acetylcholine functions as the chemical mediator for motor nerves to striated (skeletal) muscle, postganglionic sympathetic and parasympathetic fibers (to their respective end organs, including sweat glands and visceral musculature), preganglionic to postganglionic nerve transmission in both sympathetic and parasympathetic systems, and some nerve functions within the central nervous system (of uncertain anatomy and function). More complete discussions of cholinergic mechanisms can be found in the texts of Waser (1975) and Goldberg and Hanin (1976).

OP compounds inhibit cholinesterase by the binding of the organic phosphorus atom to the cholinesterase enzyme site, which is normally occupied by acetylcholine. While the normal cholinesterase-acetylcholine reaction is complete within a few microseconds (Wilson, 1951), the toxic cholinesterase-OP reaction and bond-breaking may take much longer (Austin and James, 1970). Depending on the specific OP compound, the breaking of the cholinesterase-OP bond may take from 1 to more than 1000 hr. This spontaneous regeneration of free cholinesterase can be chemically accelerated in some instances. Certain OP agents (soman) form a bond with cholinesterase that becomes progressively resistant to regeneration over a period of time ("aging"). The agents that show "aging" are less easily treated with standard oxime therapy, even if it is instituted very early.

After absorption of an OP compound, esteratic degradation proceeds at a rate primarily dependent on the type of OP compound. Ultimately, the A-esterases will detoxify the OP compound. However, until that detoxification, cholinesterase (a B-esterase) is also inhibited. As a result, acetylcholine accumulates in excess quantities at its sites of production. As acetylcholine accumulates, there is an initial stimulation of neural function followed shortly thereafter by an inhibitory effect. Such progression from stimulation to inhibition is most clearly seen in skeletal muscle, with progression from twitching and fasciculation to weakness and ultimate paralysis. The initial stimulatory effect of acetylcholine on smooth muscle and glands generally persists even after skeletal muscle has progressed to acetylcholine inhibition.

Toxicity: Thresholds and Limits

Concentration (mg min/m³)					
Tabun	Sarin	Soman	VX	Effects	References
0.3	-	-	-	Chest constriction (1 min) (vapor)	Gates and Renshaw, 1946
3.2	2.4	-	-	Pupillary (constriction 2 min) (vapor)	Gates and Renshaw, 1946
14-21	-	-	-	Severe headache, visual effects 2-15 days (vapor)	Gates and Renshaw, 1946; U.S. Dept. of Army, 1968
40-100	35-55	20-25	5	Severe dyspnea (vapor)	U.S. Dept. of Army, 1968; Dick, 1981
200-400	70-100	70	36	Lethal (1-5 min)$_{50}$ (vapor)	U.S. Dept. of Army, 1968; Dick, 1981
1-1.5g	1.7g	0.35g	0.01-0.7g	Lethal$_{50}$ (vapor)	WHO Consultants, 1970; Sidell and Groff, 1974; Dutreau et al., 1950

B. Respiratory Effects

Clinical

Respiratory effects of the organophosphate (OP) compounds depend to some degree on route of exposure as well as the amount of exposure.

Signs and symptoms of exposure generally are limited to the effects of cholinesterase inhibition. Generally within minutes of a topical exposure and within 30 sec or less of an inhalational exposure symptoms of nervousness, headache, blurred vision, weakness, nausea, intestinal cramping, diarrhea, chest tightness, and incoordination may be seen. The signs of excessive oropharyngeal secretions, tearing, sweating, increased respiratory secretions, vomiting, muscle twitching, cyanosis, muscle weakness, convulsions, loss of sphincter competence, areflexia, heart block, and cardiac arrest are seen. There may be rapid progression through these signs and symptoms to death within 5-15 min. Alternatively, with lower dose exposure and, depending on degree and competence of medical support, life may be sustained for days to weeks with ultimate full recovery unless a major organ system (liver, kidney, heart, CNS) has suffered hypoxic damage.

It is difficult to separate the effects of atropine from the effects of OP compound on the quantity of saliva. Furthermore, the contribution of such thick saliva to the observed respiratory obstruction has not been well evaluated. Bronchospasm secondary to OP exposures has been shown to increase pulmonary resistance and decrease dead space. A report of severe dyspnea without measurable increase in airways resistance was thought to be due to changes in chest wall mechanics. Respiratory center inhibition may be of relatively short duration.

Paralysis of respiratory muscles is likely the most mechanically significant effect of OP agents. Paralysis of the diaphragm, rectus, and intercostals persists until restoration of acetylcholinesterase activity. The additional clinical sequelae of muscle twitching, seizures, and vomiting may further complicate the respiratory abnormalities. The specific contributions of each of these factors to respiratory failure depends to a large extent on both intensity and route of exposure (Hayes, 1982; Grob, 1956; Elam et al., 1956). There are insufficient data to allow assessment of the effects of OP agents on the biochemical function of the lung or lung defense mechanisms (Leith et al., 1983; Hayes, 1982; Elam et al., 1956).

Human laboratory studies that detail the physiological effects of "nerve gases" are limited to low-dose exposure (Freeman et al., 1952) and reports of the occasional accidental exposure (Ward, 1962). Respiratory physiological studies of humans exposed to the "nerve agents" have rarely been reported. Clements studied human exposure to sarin vapor. Descriptions of dyspnea were not accompanied by significant changes in airway resistance (Clements et al., 1952). Studies by Grob (Grob et al., 1950) report symptoms of dyspnea that were attributed to bronchial constriction, but airway function measurements were not available. However, an extensive animal literature has been accumulated. Significant difficulties with the use of animal models include variable response to nerve agents in different species (deCandole et al., 1952; Johnson et al., 1958); and variable results in animal experimentation with and without anesthesia (particularly since anesthesia prevents OP-induced seizures, which themselves contribute significantly to the mortality) (Fredriksson et al., 1960).

Pathologic

With acute exposure, excessive respiratory secretions and mucous inspissation may be seen. Pulmonary edema has been reported (Hayes, 1982). However, death typically occurs without significant light microscopic changes. A myopathy has been reported in exposures to some OP compounds, with electron microscopic changes in the end-plate region of striated muscle (xwelling, eosinophilia, loss of striations). Such changes are seen in rats as early as 30 min after OP exposure (Laskowski et al., 1976). Similar lesions have been reported in the diaphragm of a human supported on a respirator for 9 days after a severe OP compound exposure (DeReuck and Willems, 1975).

Some postmortem studies of primates show air trapping and bullae at the edges of the lobes (Berdine et al., 1983).

C. Therapy

Chemical Therapy: General Considerations

A variety of chemical techniques have been considered and developed to prevent cholinesterase-OP binding, accelerate its regeneration, and minimize the effects of accumulated acetylcholine while awaiting regeneration (deJong, 1985; Dept. of the Army et al., 1974; Durham and Hayes, 1962).

Binding Prevention

Various chemical compounds may be used to occupy temporarily the active site of cholinesterase, thus preventing its phosphorylation by OP agents until the A-esterases (e.g., phosphoryl phosphatase) detoxify the absorbed OP. Among various substances under consideration, the carbamates (especially physostigmine) have been primarily considered (Wannarka, 1984).

Anti-OP Antibodies

The possibility of developing a specific antiorganophosphate antibody has been considered.

Regeneration of Cholinesterase

Reactivation of the inhibited enzyme with serine- (cholinesterase active site) directed nucleophiles has been accomplished using quaternary oximes. A wide variety of oximes has been studied. Of these, 2-PAM-Cl (pralidoxime chloride), P2S (pralidoxime methanesulfonate). Toxogonin, and TMB-4 have been most intensively studied (National Research Council, 1984). These substances speed the separation of the phosphorus atom from the active cholinesterase site, freeing the cholinesterase for acetylcholine binding. This process is more difficult if "aging" has occurred, hence the oximes are less effective with OP compounds that age rapidly (e.g., sarin, soman). In the absence of reactivation of the inhibited enzyme, normal metabolic regeneration of fresh cholinesterase must occur. Blood cholinesterase is regenerated at the rate of new red blood cell entry into the peripheral circulation since resynthesis does not occur in circulating red blood cells. Tissue cholinesterase is regenerated more quickly (Austin and James, 1970; Funckes, 1960; Grob and Johns, 1958; Namba and Hiraki, 1958).

Treatment of Accumulated Acetylcholine

The primary respiratory effects of accumulated acetylcholine include excessive secretions and bronchospasm. Both of these effects are responsive to atropine in doses that may have to be as high as 2 g/24 hr. Adequacy of atropinization should be judged by secretion rate and bronchospasm control. Excessive heart rate may be moderated by the adjunctive use of propranolol. Cardiac arrhythmias have been occasionally observed with the use of atropine during severe hypoxia. This has prompted the suggestion that atropine should not be given to a severely cyanotic patient (Wood, 1950). However, the absence of reports of sudden death following atropine suggests that this agent should not be withheld. A suggestion that theophylline is contraindicated (Johns et al., 1951) comes from the observation that convulsions occur with organophosphate compounds and the consideration that other agents that may affect seizure threshold should not be administered concurrently. However, with adequate oxygenation and immediate availability of respiratory support and Valium, theophylline should not be withheld if otherwise indicated. For the previously normal (nonasthmatic) patient, atropine alone should be sufficient for the induced bronchospasm. A concern that individuals with asthma are more sensitive to OP agents has not been supported by epidemiologic studies of other non-"nerve gas" OP agents that are found to not potentiate asthma (Hayes, 1982). Combination atropine and oxime therapy is suggested.

Specific Chemical Therapy for OP Poisoning

The lethality and rapidity of onset of effects of the "nerve gases" make any postexposure chemical therapy unlikely to be effective, unless trained individuals are available. Principles of therapy include immediate isolation from source of exposure. This can be accomplished either by removal from source or donning of protective equipment, including gas masks, and fully protective skin covering (in the presence of liquid toxins). Immediately upon suspicion of exposure, the prompt administration of 2 mg atropine intramuscularly with subsequent doses by the intravenous route should be given. If there is no exposure, a mild degree of atropinization will persist for 1-6 hr. In mild exposure with miosis, rhinorrhea, and bronchospasm, an additional 2 mg atropine may be required. Intramuscular atropine has peak effects at 15-25 min; hence the intravenous route (peak 10-15 min) may be preferred. Atropine (2 mg) may be given every 15 min to maintain moderate atropinization for at least 24 hr in moderate to severe exposure and in certain instances intravenous atropine (2 mg) may be given every 1-5 min. Higher dose OP exposures shorten the duration of effect of atropine. Up to 2 g atropine/24 hr has been given and therapy should continue for at least 24 hr subsequent to return of spontaneous respiration. Because of the direct effects of OP agents on the eye, pupillary dilation cannot be used as an index of adequate atropinization. One g 2 PAM Cl is also given intravenously (1 g in 150 ml normal saline or 5% dextrose in water over 10-20 min). In the absence of nerve agent exposure, the administration of 2 PAM Cl will occasionally produce headache, dizziness, blurred vision, or diarrhea. Occasional hypertension may require use of phentolamine (5 mg). For mild exposure a single injection of 2 PAM Cl will suffice while for moderate to severe exposure a second dose of 2 PAM Cl at 1 hr should be followed by hourly 1 g doses until spontaneous respiration returns. Immediate ventilatory assistance should be applied with cessation of spontaneous respiration and the administration of oxygen. Laryngospasm may occur but resolve quickly with the giving of atropine; the latter is also useful for the excess secretions. Severe muscle twitching, fasciculations, and convulsions are best controlled with parenteral (preferably intravenous) Valium in doses of 5-10 mg as needed to maintain seizure control (Jones et al., 1984).

A variety of other therapeutic interventions including various vitamins, particularly vitamin C, potassium chloride, and ganglionic blocking agents may be of value (Lapushkov, 1973; Luzhnikov, 1966). Additional reports suggest that corticosteroids (Lopez, 1970), purified human cholinesterase (Klose and Gutensohn, 1976), and hemoperfusion against charcoal (Luzhnikov et al., 1977) or soy bean oil (Jax et al., 1977) would be useful. These therapies have been suggested for the longer-acting insecticides, which typically have somewhat more delayed onset of action. There is one recommendation that oximes be administered sublingually for first aid (Luzhnikov and Pankov, 1969).

Because the literature suggests that central apnea is an early finding and perhaps a major factor in organophosphate-induced respiratory failure, mechanical ventilation may be required. If the casualty is wearing a gas mask, the Holger-Neilsen back pressure arm lift method may suffice for brief periods and may be particularly useful in allowing excess secretions to drain from the oropharynx. Devices to permit assisted ventilation through a gas mask have generally not been found effective. Consideration has been given to the development of a cricothyroidotomy cannula. This device allows the site of laryngospasm to be bypassed, thus allowing maintenance of the patients' masked status and allows connection to a mechanical respirator. Several types of mechanical respirators have been or are under development for field use, with recent interest directed toward high-frequency jet ventilation and high-frequency oscillatory ventilation. These techniques permit more compact ventilators to be used in a field setting.

Although analeptics have been suggested for central stimulation, such agents would be considered effective only in patients with early respiratory insufficiency.

D. Tabun

Synonyms for tabun (GA) include gelan, dimethylaminocyanophosphoric acid ethyl ester, ethyl dimethylamidocyanophosphate (MCE), dimethylamidoethoxy phosphoryl cyanide, ethyl phosphorodimethylamide cyanidate, ethyl-M-dimethyl-phosphoroamido cyanate, ethyl-M, N-dimethylphosphoramidocyanidate, Trilon

83, Substance 83, Le 100, and Taboon A. Its formula is $C_5H_{11}N_2O_2P$; vapor density 5.6; specific gravity 1.08; boiling point 230-245°C (depending on purity). Pure Tabun is both colorless and odorless as a gas. Slight impurities in production may lend a faintly fruity aroma and brown color to the liquid. This odor does not constitute an adequate warning for the presence of toxic levels of the gas. The combustion and hydrolysis of Tabun causes the production of hydrogen cyanide. Calcium hypochlorite should not be used as a decontaminant because it leads to the production of cyanogen chloride.

Clinical Respiratory Effects

The route of exposure to this agent has little effect on the order in which signs and symptoms of intoxication appear. Aside from local muscle fibrillation with topical exposures, various routes of exposure only vary the time of onset of symptoms. Inhalational exposures may become symptomatic and lethal within 1-10 min. Ocular exposures may act nearly as rapidly. Unless the dose is very large, percutaneous exposures are somewhat slower in onset of action, with lethal effects seen as late as 2 hr after exposure.

Therapy

Tabun is more responsive to oxime therapy than the other OP agents reported.

E. Sarin

Synonyms for Sarin (GB) include T46, Trilon 46, methylfluorophosphoric acid isopropyl ester, isopropyl methanefluorophosphonate (MFI), isopropyl methylphosphonofluoridate, and isopropoxy-methylphosphoryl fluoride. Its formula is $C_4H_{10}FO_2P$; vapor density 4.8; specific gravity 1.09; boiling point 158°C. Sarin is a colorless and odorless substance that may be disseminated by spray or explosion (in liquid form). Although it has a soil persistence of up to 14 days, it is generally regarded as a relatively nonpersistent agent when it contaminates hard surfaces.

Clinical Respiratory Effects

With acute exposures, the effects of this agent (Grob and Harvey, 1958) are similar to Tabun although effective at lower doses. Generally full respiratory recovery is obtained with appropriate support unless there has been hypoxic damage to the central nervous system. With vapor inhalations, wheezing will appear rapidly and, if not lethal, may persist for 1-2 days. Systemic absorption (oral, dermal), if not lethal, may result in residual wheezing for several days. Individuals with mild, low-level, or chronic exposures show increased sensitivity to recurrent exposures.

Therapy

See discussion of general therapy above.

F. Soman

Synonyms for Soman (GD) include fluoromethypinacolyloxy phosphine oxide, methylfluorophosphoric acid pinacol ester, pinacoloxy-methylphosphoryl fluoride, and pinacolyl methylphosphonofluoridate. Its formula is $C_7H_{16}FO_2P$; vapor density 6.3; specific gravity 1.02; and boiling point 167-198°C (depending on the degree of purity). Soman is a colorless liquid with an occasionally slightly fruity odor. The threshold for this odor does not constitute an adequate warning for this substance. This agent may be disseminated as a liquid in vapor or aerosol format.

Since combustion of Soman produces other toxic substances such as HF and various oxides of phosphorus, decontamination methods other than heat are usually applied.

Clinical Respiratory Effects

The respiratory control center (guinea pig studies) shows spontaneous return of function approximately 1 hr after poisoning. Loss of function at this center does not disappear with repeat dosing with Soman, suggesting that this depressant effect is not AChE-mediated. Soman is particularly rapidly toxic when exposure is by the percutaneous route, with the rate of onset of toxicity approaching that of the inhalational route. Ocular exposures are rapidly toxic as well (Adams et al., (1972).

Therapy

Since Soman is somewhat resistant to the reactivating effects of oximes, and is in addition, more toxic than Sarin, more prolonged respiratory support may be needed.

G. VX

Synonyms for VX include tammelin ester and S-(2-diisopropylaminoethyl)o-ethyl methylphosphonothiolate. Its formula is $C_{11}H_{26}NO_2PS$; vapor density 9.2; specific gravity 1.008; boiling point 298°C. VX is an odorless liquid with a relatively low volatility. Consequently, liquid droplets may persist on the skin, thereby facilitating absorption. Since combustion produces both H_3PO_4 and H_2SO_4, other methods of decontamination are undertaken.

Chemical Effects on Biological Systems

Studies of VX in relationship to AChE show that this substance ages less rapidly than GB and that there is spontaneous reactivation of the enzyme at the rate of approximately 1%/hr (Sidell and Groff, 1974).

Respiratory Effects

The respiratory effects of this substance are essentially identical to GB but occur at substantially lower doses. Onset of effect depends on dosage and may be as rapid as GB but death can be delayed up to 20 hr.

Therapy

Combination atropine and oxime therapy is effective for VX (Jules and Popa, 1966; Aquilonius et al., 1964; WHO Consultants, 1970; Sidell and Groff, 1974).

VI. Incapacitating Agents: BZ

Attempts to develop "humane" weapons have led to the investigation of a variety of substances termed "incapacitating agents." Optimally, the effective dose of such agent will produce a significant but nonfatal and temporary incapacitation, limiting the combatant ability of the enemy soldier.

A wide variety of agents have been studied as incapacitants. Generally these are categorized as physical incapacitants—substances that create muscle tremors and paralysis, hyperthermia, hypotension, and severe diarrhea—and psychochemical incapacitants, which include a wide variety of psychotomimetics of which BZ is an example.

BZ is also called QNB, 3-Quinuclidinyl benzilate, and EA 2277. BZ is a white crystalline solid whose thermal stability permits aerosols to be produced using pyrotechnic methods. Dissemination may also be by dust or spray. Toxic doses can be absorbed through the skin as well as by inhalation, although the dermal absorption rate is slow.

A. Chemical Effects

BZ acts similarly to atropine, competing with atropine for specific central nervous system binding sites and binding more strongly and with longer duration in peripheral muscarinic receptors (Yamamura et al., 1974; Sidell, undated).

Focal central nervous system binding is shown by autoradiographic studies to occur prominently in the occipital cortex, cortex of the cingulate gyrus, and the striate body. The motor and sensory cortices were prominently labeled as well (in rats and cats, Snyder et al., 1975). Different techniques of determining central

Toxicity: Thresholds and Limits

Concentration (mg.min/m^3)	Effects	References
66-124	Mild incapacitation (some slowing of thought)	National Research Council, 1982
102-152	Moderate incapacitation (hallucinations, incoherent)	National Research Council, 1982
110-165	Severe incapacitation (stupor, coma)	National Research Council, 1982
5.7-6.7 mg/kg	Lethal dose (LD$_{50}$)	National Research Council, 1982

nervous system distribution of this agent give somewhat differing results, but most studies show the caudate nucleus to be a site of very prominent localization (Yamamura et al., 1974). Homogenate studies of caudate and other tissues that strongly bind BZ show the greatest activity in the mitochondrial fractions. Oxygen consumption of these organelles is reduced. The sites of prominent localization correspond to areas of normally intense choline uptake and choline acetyltransferase activity. Postsynaptic muscarinic sites bind BZ with a very high degree of affinity (K_d = 10-11 M) (National Research Council, 1982).

B. Respiratory Effects

Clinical

At low doses, beginning 15-30 min after exposure there is increased heart rate, dry mouth, restlessness, decreased gastric mobility, inhibition of sweating, flushed skin, pupillary dilatation, and loss of accommodation, as well as mild sedation and mental slowness. At higher doses, there is rapid onset of discoordination and confusion, which progresses to hallucinations, incoherent speech, stupor, and coma, all of which may last for several hours. Unpredictable behavior can be seen up to 96 hr with gradual return to normal over the ensuing 2-4 days. The duration of effect is generally related to dose. No long-term effects have been reported in follow-up studies several years after a series of volunteer experiments at Edgewood Arsenal (National Research Council, 1982).

Because of inhibition of sweating, exposure to this agent is thought to carry a greater risk in hot climate. BZ produces the changes of belladonna alkaloid poisoning. Children are particularly susceptible to the toxic delerium and psychosis of atropine and might be expected to show similar increased sensitivity to BZ (Rumack, 1973).

Pathologic

There are no reported BZ-death-related pathologic studies available.

C. Therapy

Specific therapy with physostigmine salicylate should be given promptly in the presence of hallucinatory and delirious behavior with signs of atropinism (flushed dry skin, dry mouth, tachycardia, hyperthermia). Three milligrams is given intramuscularly (or 1 mg intravenously) and repeated if necessary in 40 min. Subsequent oral maintenance is recommended with 2-5 mg physostigmine salicylate every 1-2 hr. Heart rate is thought to be the best indicator of adequate therapy; and pulse rate should be maintained between 70 and 80 beats/min, and the medication is reduced for heart rate below 70 per min.

VII. Vesicants

A. Mustards

For a variety of military reasons, mustard became the principal battle gas during the last year of World War I. However, because of a relatively low volatility, vapor concentrations were generally low in the battlefield. Consequently, the death rate was very low among those gassed (less than 1%). More military disability resulted from direct contact that caused skin and or ocular toxicity.

Mustard Gas: Sulfur Mustards

Synonyms for sulfur mustards (H, HD, HQ, HT, dichlorodiethylsulfide, bis (B-chloroethyl) sulfide, S-Yperite, sulfur mustard, "Yellow Cross," and Schwefellost. Its empirical formula is $C_4H_8Cl_2S$ and it is used as an oily liquid with a boiling point of 214-215°C (with low vapor pressure). A garlic-like odor is just detectable at concentrations of 0.0006 mg/liter although a faint residual sulfide odor can still be detected even after evaporation of the active H. Since this level of olfactory detection does not adequately warn against the respiratory effects of this agent, mustard is considered to have poor warning properties.

Chemical Effects

Mustard acts by alkylation and consequent degradation of DNA (Fox and Scott, 1980; Davis and Ross, 1947). Mouse studies show that sulfur mustard is systemically absorbed to reach germinal tissue and induce lethal mutations (Rozmiarek et al., 1973). Specific extrapolation of this data to humans is difficult. However, extensive review of available literature has led to World Health Organization to conclude that there are adequate data associating mustards with cancer induction (Bartsch et al., 1982; International Agency for Research on Cancer, 1975).

Toxicity: Thresholds and Limits

Concentration (mg/m^3)	Effects	References
0.6	Odor threshold	Gates et al., 1946
100-200	Lethal 10 min (vapor)	Gates et al., 1946
100	Serious visual impairment 24-48 hr (1 min exposure)	Gates et al., 1946
200	Temporary blindness 1 week or more (1 min exposure)	Gates et al., 1946

Clinical Respiratory Effects

Clinical effects of mustard are very dependent on dose and ambient conditions. The unprotected individual will suffer eye, skin, and respiratory effects almost simultaneously (Gates et al., 1946). The specific chemical and cytologic toxic effects occur within minutes of exposure, but clinical presentation of symptoms typically occurs only after a latent period of a few hours up to 24 hr.

Very low dose inhalational exposures (such as those experienced by chemical workers in the general vicinity of mustard) may create a sense of chest oppression 2-4 hr after exposure. With more intense exposures, symptoms may appear within 30 min-3 hr and include sneezing, lacrimation, rhinorrhea, nasal bleeding, sore throat, hoarseness, hacking cough, or a toneless voice. At 4-16 hr sinus tenderness may appear and cough may be persistent for 16-48 hr. There may be aphonia, tachypnea, and signs of early pulmonary edema. At 36-48 hr, hemorrhagic pulmonary edema is prominent and after 48 hr bronchopneumonia may supervene.

Twelve percent of mustard-exposed British soldiers were awarded disability for respiratory disorders thought due to gas exposures during combat (total of approximately 19,000) (Gilchrist, 1928). Among these soldiers, bronchitis was the predominant complaint. Emphysema and asthma were also reported to a minor degree (Gilchrist and Matz, 1933). However, the quality of the epidemiologic studies of the relationship between gas exposure and subsequent respiratory disability was severely limited for several reasons:

1. Individuals had often experienced multiple combined exposures to mustards and other chemical agents.

2. Influenza and other respiratory ailments were often misdiagnosed as mustard gas injury.

3. There was lack of epidemiologic control for smoking and postexposure environmental and occupational histories (Beebe, 1960).

Some studies have supported the suggestion of an increase in respiratory tract cancer in individuals whose only exposure to mustard was in the military service. An increase in cancer of approximately 40% over control has been observed. In another study, however, even this increase was not considered statistically significant (Beebe, 1960; Norman, 1975). The chronic exposure of mustard workers in chemical factories shows a more clear-cut disease relationship. Of one group of workers 82% were said to develop chronic cough within a year of commencing work (Kurozumi et al., 1977). Individuals with prior mustard exposure show a mortality with pneumonia approximately twice that of controls (Beebe, 1960). Laryngeal and bronchial carcinoma is substantially increased in this population as well (Manning et al., 1981; Nakamura, 1956; Wada et al., 1968). Others have demonstrated the close association between chronic repetitive exposures and carcinomas of the respiratory tract (Case and Lea, 1955; Cowles, 1983).

Depending on ambient concentrations, chronic low dose mustard exposure may present with loss of taste and smell, nose bleed, sore throat, chest pain, wheezing, and dyspnea. Both Morgenstern et al. (1947) and Buscher (1931) emphasize that chronic low-dose exposure leads to a lingering bronchitis, bronchial asthma, hoarseness, aphonia, and hypersensitivity to smoke, dust, and fumes. Even after discontinuing work in such an environment, men typically showed persistent disability with increased susceptibility to respiratory tract infections and persistent evidence of bronchitis and bronchiectasis.

Pathologic Respiratory Effects

Acute toxic effects of mustard include edematous changes in the pharynx and tracheobronchial tree. With higher concentrations, pseudomembranous changes occur in the airways and, with severe exposure, necrotic changes occur throughout the airways. At postmortem, alveolar and pleural hemorrhage are seen. In persons who survive the acute effects of exposure, secondary bacterial infection of the lung is seen at 48-72 hr. Pulmonary abscess or gangrene may appear.

Mustard is highly vesicant in topical (skin) exposures, producing blisters and necrotic sloughs with exceptionally delayed healing. Extensive skin absorption may be lethas as a result of bone marrow suppression.

Therapy

There is no specific prophylactic or therapeutic intervention reported for inhalational mustard exposures. The tracheobronchitis may respond to nonspecific demulcents. Codeine seems particularly effective for the barking cough. Dexamethasone inhalation combined with parenteral corticosteroids have been recently recommended; again, adequately controlled data are not available (Weger, 1975).

Nitrogen Mustards: *Nitrogen mustard, N-Yperite*

Among the various nitrogen mustards, the ethyl-bis (HN_1), the methyl-bis (HN_2), and tris (HN_3) forms have been most extensively studied. Of these the HN_1 and HN_3 forms showed sufficient stability and toxicity to be considered as alternatives to the sulfur mustards for special uses.

HN_1 has a faintly fishy or soapy odor and HN_3 has a faint geranium odor. The odor threshold of these substances approximates 15 μg/liter. This level is substantially higher than that of the sulfur mustards (0.6 μg/liter), resulting in a much more serious hazard of incapacitating exposure prior to olfactory awareness.

Aside from differences in physical properties of the agents and their relative toxicities, the effects of these agents are considered similar to the sulfur mustards with typically delayed inflammatory and necrotic effects.

B. Lewisite I, II, III

Physical Characteristics

	Lewisite I	Lewisite II	Lewisite III
Formula	$ClCH{=}CHAsCl_2$	$(ClCH{=}CH)_2 AsCL$	$(ClCH{=}CH)_3 As$
Molecular weight	203	232	258
Specific gravity	1.89	1.7	-
Vapor density	7.1	-	-
Boiling point (°C)	77-78	130-133	151-155

Appearance

Manufacture of lewisite results in the production of one or a combination of three very similar arsenicals, depending on the specific chemical process used. These similar products have been identified, labeled, and studied as lewisite I, II, and III.

Lewisite I appears as a colorless oil that becomes gradually more yellow eith increasing time and increasing impurity content. Lewisite II in pure form appears as an oil as clear as water but also quickly takes on a yellow-brown color with increasing concentration of impurities. Lewisite III is an oily liquid with a somewhat yellowish tint. Aside from mild differences in their physical properties, the three lewisites act almost identically. Lewisite can be spread as an aerosol, but this requires low-altitude (100 feet) application because of the rapid evaporation rate of the droplets. A thickened format was developed using methyl methacrylate (and/or similar substances) to stabilize and provide the thickening (improving adherence to surfaces). As a result, droplet evaporation is slowed. The thickened droplet form appears to have a decreased toxicity, however, possibly due to surface development of the relatively nontoxic lewisite oxide. Lewisite has a very penetrating odor of geraniums that may persist for hours to days after exposure. Personnel working with this substance often remain aromatic long after leaving the workplace. Nasal irritation and odor detection occur at a level substantially below toxic levels, thus this substance would be described as having adequate vapor warning properties. Respiratory complications of exposure would be relatively minor compared to its topical vesicant effects unless exposure were to occur in a closed environment without possible escape. Lewisite III has little effect on either the skin or the respiratory system.

Toxicity: Thresholds and Limits

Concentration			
Vapor (mg.min/m^3)	Liquid (mg)	Effects	References
6-8		Nasal irritation	Gates et al., 1946
14-23		Odor detection	Gates et al., 1946
1200-1500	0.014	Skin vesication	Gates et al., 1946
1200-1500		Death by inhalation	Gates et al., 1946
100,000	2800	Death in 30 min (body exposure)	Vedder, 1925

Respiratory Effects

Clinical

Human inhalational effects have been reported in groups of workers who, after handling this material in closed environments, developed bronchitis characterized by a thick viscus mucus with a sweetish taste. Respiratory exposures typically produce a prominent nasal burning sensation with diffuse rhinorrhea and sneezing. These effects are of such an immediate and intense nature that masking or escape is generally accomplished before serious respiratory exposure occurs. Data regarding more substantial exposures is reported for animals only.

Animal studies (dogs) initially show sneezing, coughing, lacrimation, copious salivation, vomiting, and retching. At higher concentrations pseudomembrane formation and signs of pulmonary edema are seen. Cough and secretions may be so copious as to produce casts of the trachea and bronchi. Hemoconcentration has been reported as a prominent finding, presumably due to the quantities of alveolar fluid produced (Harrison, 1944).

This substance is primarily injurious as a topical vesicant with toxic effects similar to the sulfur mustards but with onset of a severe burning sensation almost immediately after application. A single layer of clothing has a substantial protective effect against lewisite vapor, hence this substance would be a hazard primarily as a liquid in this setting. Despite some evidence for systemic absorption in the case of liquid or vapor applications to the skin, significant respiratory effects of lewisite are only seen in the case of inhalational (nonmasked) exposures.

Pathologic

There are no human data available. Dog exposures are reported to produce pseudomembranes: thick, fibrinous membranes with necrotic mucosa in the nares, larynx, trachea, and large bronchi. The membrane may detach from the wall of the trachea leading to a ball-valve type obstruction with resulting obstruction, emphysema, or obstructive atelectasis. Pulmonary edema and occasional pleural effusions are also seen (Vedder, 1925). Hemoconcentration with shock is seen (dogs) with high-concentration exposure. Death typically occurs at 10-24 hr (Harrison, 1944). Although fatty liver and degenerative change of the lymphatic system have been observed and are thought to demonstrate systemic absorption of lewisite, these changes do not contribute materially to the animal's death (Harrison, 1944). Animals (dogs) surviving inhalational exposure show only areas of squamous metaplasia or patchy atelectasis.

Therapy

The rapidity of onset of topical (burning) symptoms (within minutes of exposure) allows identification of this substance.

For topical exposures the administration of chloride of lime or other alkylating agents is useful for skin exposures, effectively decomposing the agent if applied shortly (minutes) after exposure. Earlier topical therapy is more beneficial; however, some benefit may still be obtained prior to blister formation (blisters may appear as early as 5 minutes). Retention of the blister as a "protective bandage" may speed healing (Buscher, 1931). The discovery in 1941 of 2,3-dimercaptopropanol-1 (British antilewisite; BAL, DTH) resulted in the production of an effective agent to minimize the damage of lewisite. Application of the topical ointment to the eyes within 10 min or to the skin within 1 hr after exposure minimized the topical effects of lewisite.

Inhalational and systemic exposures could be treated by parenteral use of BAL as well (10% in oil). Suggested dose (by deep intramuscular injection) is 0.02 ml/lb up to 4 ml maximum given every 4 hr for a total of four doses. In dog studies, earlier injections are more beneficial, with virtual absence of effect 90 min after exposure (Harrison, 1944).

C. Phosgene Oxime

Synonyms for phosgene oxide (CX) include nettle gas, Red Cross, and dichloroform oxime. Its formula is CCl_2NOH; melting point 39-40°C; and boiling point 129°C. This substance appears as colorless crystals (or colorless liquid) with a pungent penetrating odor.

Animal inhalational exposure is reported (Tschanatschev, 1957), with a lethal dose reported at 1.5-2 mg/liter for 30 min.

Toxicity: Thresholds and Limits

Concentration	Effects	References
1.5-2 g/m³	Inhalational lethal (dogs)	Tschanatschev, 1957
.01 g/kg	Parenteral lethal (dogs)	Tschanatschev, 1957
25 mg/kg	Percutaneous lethal (guinea pig)	Cookson and Nottingham, 1969

Respiratory Effects

Clinical

This substance is primarily active as a topical agent with local application producing skin necrosis at the site of contact. There is early blanching followed by erythematous changes surrounding the area of blanching. Within 30 min a wheal appears and within 24 hr the original area of blanching acquires brown pigmentary changes. Subsequently an eschar forms that will slough off in 3-4 weeks. Itching is typically persistent throughout this period. Healing may be delayed to more than 2 months (U.S. Dept. of the Army, 1968). Topical absorption of this material in one reported human case led to dyspnea, which was thought to be an early sign of toxic pulmonary edema (Tschanatschev, 1958).

Pathologic

Available animal data (parenteral exposures only) show hemorrhagic inflammatory change of the large intestine with bloody diarrhea, pulmonary edema with emphysematous change, hemorrhagic gastritis, and hemorrhagic pulmonary edema (Tschanatschev, 1957).

Therapy

Specific prophylactic or therapeutic intervention is not available. This substance is rapidly degraded in an alkaline solution; however, its rapid reaction with tissue reduces the effectiveness of decontamination. The pulmonary edema should be treated as "noncardiac" pulmonary edema (Tschanatschev and Dronsin, 1964).

VIII. Organic Toxins

Biologically manufactured molecules (biotoxins), are among the most potent toxic substances known. These substances are manufactured by biological systems rather than chemical systems, which constitutes the chief distinction between chemical and biologic warfare.

Because of the relative ease with which biotoxins can be produced, such agents are likely to represent a new range of warfare agents. Concern has already been expressed regarding the possible active use of one example of such a biotoxin: T_2 mycotoxin (known more popularly as "yellow rain") (Seeley et al., 1985).

A. Staphylococcal Enterotoxin B

Staphylococcal enterotoxin B (SEB) has a molecular weight of 35,300 daltons and is composed of a single chain of 19 amino acids (Spero et al., 1965). SEB may be sprayed or dusted as a powder. The toxin is relatively heat-resistant and is not destroyed by 30 min of boiling, freezing, or by the normal concentrations of chlorine in public water treatment (United Nations Report, 1970).

Toxicity: Thresholds and Limits

Concentration (mg/kg)	Effects	References
0.1	Intravenous: minimal to diarrhea (monkeys)	Lamanna and Carr, 1967
0.9	Oral: minimal to diarrhea (monkeys)	Lamanna and Carr, 1967
0.03	Inhalational: minimal to nausea (monkeys)	Lamanna and Carr, 1967

Chemical Effects

Staphylococcal cultures may produce a number of biologically active compounds that include one or more enterotoxins. Four distinct antigenic groups of enterotoxins are described (A, B, C, D). These enterotoxins are simple proteins, of which the type B toxin has been most extensively studied (Wagman et al., 1965; Lamanna and Carr, 1967).

After oral ingestion, symptoms typically begin after 1/2-6 hr, appearing as sudden and violent emesis. There is evidence for a direct irritant action on the gastrointestinal tract, with high doses leading to sufficient diarrhea to produce shock and death. Nausea and vomiting appear to result from stimulation of the medullary emetic center via abdominal vagi and sympathetic nerves. Section of these nerves or ablation of the emetic center prevents nausea and vomiting (Sugiyama and Hayama, 1965).

Studies with ^{131}I-labeled enterotoxin injected intravenously (monkeys) show some leukocyte binding. These cells subsequently sequester in the lung (Crawley et al., 1966). The relationship of this observation to pulmonary edema is unclear. Pulmonary edema is seen in Rhesus monkeys exposed to aerosols. The edema is assumed to result from vagal stimulus to vagal nuclei, which in turn neurogenically alter the permeability of the pulmonary vessels.

Respiratory Effects

Clinical

Inhalation of SEB is likely to produce systemic effects more quickly than ingestion (WHO Consultants, 1970). Inhalation has been shown to produce systemic effects in monkeys (Lamanna, 1961).

Systemic effects of this substance appear at 1/2-6 hr after exposure, with increased salivation as a cardinal sign. Nausea, vomiting, crampy abdominal pain, and watery diarrhea ensue. Temperature elevation and hypotension may follow, depending on the degree of diarrhea. Recovery is typically spontaneous and occurs within 24 hr.

Pathologic

Inhalational exposures have not been reported for humans. Monkey studies show pulmonary edema to be a common mode of death (Soto and Roessler, 1965).

Therapy

Spontaneous recovery typically occurs within 24 hr. The mortality rate is higher in infants and debilitated persons. An antitoxin has been developed that may be useful in patients at higher risk of mortality (Casman and Bennett, 1964). A toxoid that is effective in providing immunoprophylaxis for Rhesus monkeys has been developed (Bergdoll, 1966). The relative infrequency of SEB infection in the general population would make such immunoprophylaxis impractical. However, its immunoprophylaxis in the military population could be considered.

B. Botulinus Toxin

This has a molecular weight of 894,589 daltons and is a single polypeptide chain with 7,754 amino acids (Buehler et al., 1947). Of six antigenically distinctive toxins, only type A has been crystallized. The crystalline solid is white, tasteless, and odorless. Both crystalline and noncrystalline toxins are stable for weeks in cold water and for months in food. Destruction of this toxin requires boiling for 5-10 min, formaldehyde precipitation, or specific antitoxin precipitation.

A dosage of 2×10^7 mg is estimated to be lethal (Lamanna and Carr, 1967).

Chemical Effects

Six antigenically distinguishable botulinal toxins have been identified (A, B, C, D, E, F). A given strain of *Clostridium botulinum* produces only one of the toxin types. Of these types A, B, C, D, F are fully active as produced. Type E has been shown to be produced in a precursor form, which is toxic itself. However, further activation of the precursor form occurs prior to intestinal absorption, possibly as a result of exposure to trypsin and increasing its toxicity up to 200-fold (Bulatova, 1964). The toxin is absorbed from the gut via the intestinal lymphatics (May and Whaler, 1958). Growth of *Clostridia* in the intestine is not essential to toxicity and mucosal membrane can absorb the toxin. Although normal skin represents a barrier, shaving or plucking hair opens the skin to increased toxin absorption (Geiger and Fellow, 1924).

Respiratory (inhalational) exposures are more toxic than oral exposures by at least 1 order of magnitude (May and Whaler, 1958), presumably because of some gastric degradation of ingested toxin (Lamanna and Carr, 1967).

Botulinal toxin acts by irreversible binding at all cholinergic portions of the peripheral nervous system, including pre- and postganglionic autonomic fibers and postganglionic muscle junctions. The toxin appears to act by inhibiting acetylcholine release at presynaptic sites since both nerve conduction and post-synaptic muscle fiber excitability have been shown to be normal (Tyler, 1963a,b). Intact muscle fiber excitability can be shown by direct application of electrical current causing muscle contraction, which differentiates botulin from curariform poisoning (Guyton and MacDonald, 1947). While there is some suggestion of a central (midbrain) toxic effect of this substance that might contribute to respiratory failure (Abrosimov, 1956), the predominant lethal effect results primarily from toxic paralysis of the respiratory musculature.

Clinical Respiratory Effects

Symptoms of exposure may appear as early as 6 or as late as 72 or more hr after exposure. Symptoms may be more rapid in onset with respiratory exposure, and include dizziness, fatigue, weakness, severe headache, blurred vision, diplopia, and dysphagia (Holzer, 1962). Examination will show loss of accommodation, weakness of extraocular and facial muscles, and later weakness of peripheral and respiratory musculature. Progressive weakening of the respiratory musculature results, with most deaths due to respiratory failure. Even with respiratory assistance there may be lethal cardiac arrhythmias.

Paralysis of the respiratory center is thought by some authors to be at least a contributory factor. After toxin exposure, efferent inspiratory fibers of the brainstem are not responsive to normal stimuli (Ado and Abrosimov, 1964). One study using parenteral toxin shows depression of cortical electrical activity in monkeys with otherwise stable vital signs just before respiratory failure and may suggest a direct central nervous system toxicity of botulinal toxins (Polley et al., 1965).

Therapy

Specific therapy has been well described (Dolman, 1963; Hill and Chesney, 1966). A pentavalent toxoid (against A, B, C, D, E) has been successfully developed (Flock et al., 1963). After diagnosis some modification of severity of the disease may result from use of guanidine hydrochloride (animal reports) or a polyvalent antisera that is available at state health departments. With appropriate therapy, recovery is often complete at 1-2 weeks. Occasional cases requiring months of ventilation are reported (Stares, 1983; Kao et al., 1976; WHO Consultants, 1970; Lamanna and Carr, 1967; Hill and Chesney, 1966; Tyler, 1963a,b; Flock et al., 1963; Velikanov, 1934).

C. Ricin (Castor Bean Poison)

This is a complex protein with a molecular weight of approximately 85,000 daltons. When purified, an odorless crystalline material can be produced that can subsequently be milled into 6-8 μm particles, spray-dried 3-6 μm particles, or atomized (solution to 1.4-3 μm particles).

Toxicity: Thresholds and Limits

Concentration	Effects	References
0.3 mg/kg	Lethal ingestion (human; equivalent to two castor beans)	Cope et al., 1946
100 mg/min/m^3	$L(CT)_{50}$: monkey inhalation	Cope et al., 1946
0.3 mg/kg	Lethal inhalation (human) estimated	Cope et al., 1946

Chemical Effects

Ricin has been shown to produce severe hypoglycemia (convulsive levels) just before death. However, provision of glucose does not prevent death. An observation that ricin hydrolyzes adenosine triphosphate (ATP), thereby interfering in metabolic energy transfer, has not been confirmed in subsequent frog or rat experiments. Inhalational toxicity is greater with smaller particles (range of comparison 1.4-10 μm).

Respiratory Effects

Clinical

Inhalational exposures appear to produce a biphasic response, with both immediate and delayed toxic effects. Immediate effects occur within minutes after exposure with protracted sneezing, subsequent violent cough and retching, progressing occasionally to severe asthma. These symptoms resolve in 1 hr. Individuals who have the immediate response have no detectable antiricin in their serum and show a dramatic hypersensitivity to toxoid injected intradermally. Other individuals may not demonstrate an immediate response. The more severe type of reaction shows a delayed reaction (4-8 hr) with fever, tracheitis, cough, diffuse joint pains, nausea, severe dyspnea, coma, convulsions, and death.

Many fatal cases of poisoning have been reported in humans as a result of ingestion of this substance, with more severe ingestions showing nausea, vomiting, epigastric pain, tachypnea, hyperthermia, and followed by coma and convulsions. Symptoms could appear as early as 1 hr, but could be delayed from 2 to 14 days. Parenteral exposure produces a similar clinical picture of a delayed febrile illness with convulsions, coma, or sudden death.

Individuals who survive the initial febrile response and other acute symptoms show a resolution of the illness with profuse sweating and followed by rapid relief of the other symptoms, although tracheitis and cough may persist for several weeks.

Pathologic

Inhalational pathologic changes as reported in various animals is confined almost entirely to the thorax. Lungs are congested and densely edematous. Occasionally, the liver shows mild fatty degeneration and necrosis. Parenteral administration may produce a prominent pulmonary edema.

Therapy

Ricin toxoids have been prepared by formaldehyde precipitation. Antiricin sera have produced in horses and other animals. Subsequent globulin fractionation results in a hyperimmune serum that might be of clinical utility in case of accidental exposure. No report of use of such serum in humans is available.

Antiserum is most effective if administered immediately after exposure. It is not completely effective in preventing pulmonary complications, even with immediate use, but it reduces death rates if given within 6 hr. Specific toxoid immunization has not been developed because of the system toxicity of the toxoid and local necrotizing effects of its injection.

References

Abrosimov, V. N. (1956). Mechanism of action of botulinal toxin on respiration. *Arkh, Pat. Moskva* **18**:86-91.

Adams, G. K., Yamamura, H. I., and O'Leary, J. F. (1972). Spontaneous recovery of central respiratory function after an irreversible AChE inhibitor. *Eur. J. Pharmacol.* **20**:377-380.

Adams, J. H., Blackwood, W., and Wilson, J. (1966). Further clinical and pathological observations on Leber's optic atrophy. *Brain* **89**:15-26.

Ado, A. D., and Abrosimov, V. N. (1964). The specific effect of bacterial toxins on the nervous regulation of respiration. *J. Hugiene Epidemiol.* **8**:433-441.

Aquilonius, S. M., Fredriksson, T., and Sundwall, A. (1964). Studies on phosphorylated thiocholine and choline derivatives. *Toxicol. Appl. Pharmacol.* **6**:269-279.

Ardran, G. M. (1964). Phosgene poisoning. *Br. Med. J.* **1**:375.

Austin, L., and James, K. A. C. (1970). Rates of regeneration of acetylcholinesterase in rat brain subcellular fractions following DFP inhibition. *J. Neurochem.* **17**:705-707.

Ballantyne, B. (1977a). The acute mammalian toxicology of dibenz(B.f)-1:4-oxazepine. *Toxicology* **8**:347-379.

Ballantyne, B. (1977b). Riot control agents. In *The Medical Annual.* Edited by R. B. Scott and J. Fraser. Bristol, John Wright, pp. 7-14.

Ballantyne, B., and Calloway, S. (1972). Inhalation toxicology and pathology of animals exposed to O-chlorobenzylidene malonitrile (CS). *Med. Sci. Law* **12**:43-65.

Ballantyne, B., and Swanston, D. W. (1974). The irritant effects of dilute solutions of dibenzoxazepine (CR) on the eye and tongue. *Acta Pharmacol. Toxicol.* **35**:412-423.

Ballantyne, B., and Swanston, D. W. (1978). The comparative acute mammalian toxicity of 1-chloroacetophenone (CN) and 2-chlorobenzylidene malonitrile (CS). *Arch. Toxicol.* **40**:75-79.

Bandman, A. L., and Savateyev, N. V. (1977). Toxicology of CR. *Voen. Med. Zh.* **3**:84-86.

Bartsch, H., Tomatis, L., and Malaveille, C. (1982). Qualitative and quantitative comparisons between mutagenic and carcinogenic activities of chemicals. In *Mutagenicity: New Horizons in Genetic Toxicology.* Edited by J. A. Heddle. New York, Academic Press, pp. 35-72.

Bastian, G., and Mercker, H. (1959). On the question of the usefulness of amylnitrite in the treatment of cyanide poisoning. *Arch. Exp. Pathol. Pharmacol.* **237**:285-295.

Beck, H. (1959). Experimentelle Ermittlung von Geruchsschwellenn einiger wichtiger Reizgase (Chlor, Schwefeldioxyd, Ozon, Nitrose) und Erscheinungen bei Einwirkung geringer Konzentrationen auf den Menschen. PhD Thesis, Universitat Wurzburg, pp. 1-69.

Beebe, G. W. (1960). Lung cancer in World War I veterans: possible relation to mustard-gas injury and 1918 influenze epidemic. *U.S. National Cancer Inst. J.* **25**:1231-1252.

Berdine, G. G., Peel, H. H., and Johanson, W. G. (1983). Soman intoxication-baboon model. In *Proceedings of the Symposium on Respiratory Care of Chemical Casualties.* Edited by H. H. Newball. Aberdeen Proving Ground, Maryland, U.S. Army Medical Research Institute of Chemical Defense, pp. 131-140.

Bergdoll, M. S. (1966). Immunization of Rhesus monkeys with enterotoxoid. *Br. J. Infect. Dis.* **116**:191-196.

Beswick, F. W., Holland, P., and Kemp, K. H. (1972). Acute effects of exposure to orth-chlorobenzylidene malonitrile (CS) and the development of tolerance. *Br. J. Ind. Med.* **29**:298-306.

Blake, J. (1840a). Observations on the physiological effects of various agents introduced into the circulation as indicated by the hemodynamometer. *Edinb. Med. Surg. J.* **51**:330-345.

Blake, J. (1840b). Observations and Experiments on the mode in which various poisonous agents act on the animal body. *Edinb. Med. Surg. J.* **53**: 35-49.

Braker, W., Mossman, A. L., and Siegel, D. (1977). *Effects of Exposure to Toxic Gases–First Aid and Medical Treatment.* Lyndhurst, NJ, Matheson.

Bramwell, W. (1915). Poultices and venesection in gas poisoning. *Br. Med. J.* **2**:460.

Brand, P. (1971). Effect of a local inhalation dexamethasone isonicotinate therapy on toxic pulmonary edemas caused by phosgene poisoning. *Dissertation,* Institute of Pharmacology and Toxicology of the University of Wurzburg.

Brodie, D. A. (1959). The effect of thiopental and cyanide on the activity of inspiratory neurons. *J. Pharmacol. Exp. Ther.* **126**:264-269.

Bruner, H. D., and Coman, D. R. (1945). The pathologic anatomy of phosgene poisoning in relation to the pathologic physiology. In *Fasciculus on Chemical Warfare Medicine.* Vol. II. *Respiratory Tract.* Washington, D.C., Committee on Treatment of Gas Casualties, Division of Medical Services of the National Research Council.

Bulatove, T. I. (1964). The significance of type E botulinal activation in laboratory diagnosis of botulism. *Ahur. Mikrobiol. Epidemiol. Immunobiol.* **8**:97-101.

Bunting, H. (1945a). Changes in the oxygen saturation of the blood in phosgene poisoning. In *Fasciculus on Chemical Warfare Medicien.* Vol. II. *Respiratory Tract.* Washington, D.C., Committee on Treatment of Gas Casualties, Division of Medical Services of the National Research Council.

Bunting, H. (1945b). Clinical findings in acute chlorine poisoning. In *Fasciculus on Chemical Warfare Medicine.* Vol. II. *Respiratory Tract.* Washington, D.C., Committee on Treatment of Gas Casualties, Division of Medical Services of the National Research Council.

Bunting, H. (1945c). The pathology of chlorine poisoning. In *Fasciculus on Chemical Warfare Medicine.* Vol. II. *Respiratory Tract.* Washington, D.C., Committee on Treatment of Gas Casualties, Division of Medical Services of the National Research Council.

Burrows, G. E., and Wag. J. L. (1970). Antagonism of cyanide toxicity by phenoxybenzamine. *Fed. Proc.* **35**:533.

Burrows, G. E., Liu, D. H. W., and Way, J. L. (1973). Effect of oxygen on cyanide intoxication: V. Physiologic effects. *J. Pharmacol. Exp. Ther.* **184**: 739-748.

Burrows, G. E., King, L., Tarr, S., and Way, J. L. (1977). The protective effect of vasoactive compounds as cyanide antagonists. *Proc. Int. Congr. Toxicol.* **31**:250-252.

Buscher, H. (1931). *Green and Yellow Cross.* Translated by N. Conway (1944). Cincinnati, Kettering Laboratory of Applied Physiology, University of Cincinnati.

Callaway, J. L., Yeoman, M. A., Jenkins, D. E., and Flake, R. E. (1974). Chlorine gas inhalation: discriminative function testing (abstract). *Am. Rev. Respir. Dis.* **109**:721-722.

Case, R. A. M., and Lea, A. J. (1955). Mustard gas poisoning, chronic bronchitis, and lung cancer; an investigation into the possibility that poisoning by mustard gas in the 1914-18 war might be a factor in the production of neoplasia. *Br. J. Prev. Soc. Med.* **9**:62-72.

Casman, E. P., and Bennett, R. W. (1964). Production of antiserum for staphylococcal enterotoxin. *Appl. Microbiol.* **12**:363-367.

Castro, J. A. (1968). Effects of alkylating agents on human plasma cholinesterase: the role of sulfhydryl groups in its active center. *Biochem. Pharmacol.* **17**:295-303.

Chapman, A. J., and White, C. (1978). Death resulting from lacrimatory agents. *J. Forens. Sci.* **23**:527-530.

Chasis, H., Bannon, J. H., Lauson, H. D., Whittenberger, J. L., Galdston, M., and Goldring, W. (1944). Pressure breathing—effects on respiration and circulation in patients with pulmonary edema of cardiac origin, with bronchial asthma or with acute and chronic pulmonary disease, considered in relation to the therapy of phosgene intoxication. Contract: W-49-036-cws-1. New York, University College of Medicine, March, 1944.

Chasis, H., Zapp, J. A., Bannon, J. N., Whittenberger, J. L., Helm, J., Doheny, J. J., and MacLeod, C. M. (1947). Chlorine accident in Brooklyn. *Occup. Med.* **4**:152-176.

Chen, K. K., Rose, C. L., and Clowes, G. H. A. (1933). Amylnitrite and cyanide poisoning. *J.A.M.A.* **100**:1920-1922.

Chester, E. H., Gillespie, D. G., and Krause, F. D. (1969). The prevalence of chronic obstructive pulmonary disease in chlorine gas workers. *Am. Rev. Respir. Dis.* **99**:365-373.

Clay, J. R., and Rossing, R. G. (1964). Histopathology of exposure to phosgene. *Arch. Pathol.* **78**:544-551.

Clements, J. A., Moore, J. C., Johnson, R. P., and Lynott, J. (1952). Observations of airway resistance in men given low doses of GB by chamber exposure. *U.S. Army Chemical Corps Medical Laboratories Research Report No. 122.* Edgewood Arsenal, Maryland, Army Chemical Center.

Coman, D. R., Bruner, H. D., Horn, R. C., Friedman, M., Boche, R. D., McCarthy, M. D., Gibbon, M. H., and Schultz, J. (1947). Studies on experimental phosgene poisoning—I. The pathologic anatomy of phosgene poisoning, with special reference to the early and late phases. *Am. J. Pathol.* **23**: 1037-1061.

Cookson, J., and Nottingham, J. (1969). *A Survey of Chemical and Biological Warfare.* New York, Monthly Review Press, pp. 1-419.

Cope, A. C., Dec. J., Cannan, R. K., Renshaw, B., and Moore, S. (1946). Ricin. *Chemical Warfare Agents and Related Chemical Problems.* Washington, D.C., National Defense Research Committee, pp. 179-203.

Cotes, J. E., Dabbs, J. M., Evans, M. R., and Holland, P. (1972a). Effect of CS aerosol upon lung gas transfer and alveolar volume in healthy men. *Q. J. Exp. Physiol.* **57**:199-200.

Cotes, J. E., Evans, R. L., Johnson, G. R., Martin, H. deV, and Reed, J. W. (1972b). The effect of CS aerosol upon exercise ventilation and cardiac frequency in healthy men. *J. Physiol.* **222**:77-78.

Cowles, S. R. (1983). Cancer of the larynz: occupational and environmental associations. *South. Med. J.* **76**:894-898.

Cralley, L. V. (1942). The effect of irritant gases upon the rate of ciliary activity. *J. Ind. Hyg. Toxicol.* **24**:193-198.

Crawley, G. J., Gray, I., Lebland, W. A., and Blanchard, J. W. (1966). Blood binding, distribution and excretion of staphylococcal enterotoxin in monkeys. *J. Infect. Dis.* **116**:48-56.

Cucinell, S. A. (1974). Review of the toxicity of long-term phosgene exposure. *Arch. Environ. Health.* **28**:272-275.

Cucinell, S. A., Swentzel, K. C., Biskup, R., Snodgrass, H., Lovre, S., Stark, W., Feinsilver, L., and Vocci, F. (1971). Biochemical interactions and metabolic fate of riot control agents. *Fed. Proc.* **30**-86-91.

Davidson, D. E., Davis, D., and Canfield, C. J. (1984). Chemoprophylaxis of cyanide intoxidation. In *Proceeding of the Fourth Annual Chemical Defense Bioscience Review.* Aberdeen Proving Ground, MD, U.S. Army Medical Research Institute of Chemical Defense, pp. 513-524.

Davis, S. B., and Ross, W. F. (1947). The reaction of mustard gas with protein. *J. Am. Chem. Soc.* **69**:1177-1181.

deCandole, C. A., Douglas, W. W., Evans, C. L., Holmes, R., Spencer, K. E. V., Torrance, R. W., and Wilson, K. M. (1953). The failure of respiration in death by anticholinesterase poisoning. *Br. J. Pharmacol.* **8**:466-475.

De Jong, R. H. (1985). *ICD Technical Report No. 85-01.* Drug Therapy of Nerve Agent Poisoning. Edgewood, MD, U.S. Army Medical Research and Development Command, pp. 1-38.

Delepine, S. (1923). Summary of notes on two fatalities due to inhaling phosgene (COCL2). *J. Ind. Hyg.* **4**:433-440.

Departments of the Army, the Navy and the Air Force (1947). *Treatment of Chemical Agent Casualties and Conventional Military Chemical Injuries. TM 8-285, NAVMED P-5041, AFM 160-12.* Washington, D.C., pp. 1-1 - E-5.

DeReuck, J., and Willems, J. (1975). Acute parathion poisoning. Myopathic changes in the diaphragm. *J. Neurol.* **208**:309-314.

Dick, C. J. (1981). Soviet chemical warfare capabilities. *Int. Defens Rev.* **1**: 31-38.

Diller, W. F. (1978). Medical phosgene problems and their possible solution. *J. Occup. Med.* **20**:189-193.

Dolman, C. E., and Iida, H. (1963). Type E botulism: its epidemiology, prevention and specific treatment. *Can. J. Publ. Health* **54**:293-308.

Durham, W. F., and Hayes, W. J. (1962). Organic phosphorus poisoning and its therapy: with special reference to modes of action and compounds that reactivate inhibited cholinesterase. *Arch. Environ. Health* **5**:21-47.

Dutreau, C. W., McGrath, F. P., and Bray, E. H. (1950). Toxicity Studies on GD. *Medical Division Research Report No. 8*. Maryland, Army Chemical Center, pp. 1-16.

Elam, J. O., Clements, J. A., Brown, E. S., and Elton, N. W. (1956). Artificial respiration for the nerve gas casualty. *U.S. Armed Forces Med. J.* 7:797-810.

Everett, E. D., and Overholt, E. L. (1968). Phosgene poisoning. *J. A. M. A.* **205**:243-245.

Ferris, B. G., Burgess, W. A., and Worcester, J. (1967). Prevalence of chronic respiratory disease in a pulp mill and a paper mill in the United States. *Br. J. Ind. Med.* **24**:26-37.

Flock, M. A., Cardella, M. A., and Gearinger, N. F. (1963). Studies on immunity to toxins of clostridium botulinum IX. Immunologic response of man to purified pentavalent ABCDE botulinum toxoid. *J. Immunol.* **90**:697-702.

Foster, R. W., and Ramage, A. G. (1975). Observations on the effect of dibenzoxazepine (CR) and N-nonoyl-vanillylamide (VAN) on sensory nerves. *Br. J. Pharmacol.* **53**:437-438.

Fox, M., and Scott, D. (1980). The genetic toxicology of nitrogen and sulfur mustard. *Mutat. Res.* **75**:131-168.

Frederiksson, T., Hansson, C., and Holmstedt, B. (1960). Effects of sarin in the anaesthetized and unanaesthetized dog following inhalation, percutaneous absorption and intravenous infusion. *Arch. Int. Pharmacodyn.* **126**:288-302.

Freeman, G., Clements, J. A., Moore, J. C., Imbody, J. E., Clanton, B. R., Ludeman, H. H., Berman, B., Craig, A., Cornblath, M., and Johnson, R. P. (1952). Observations on the effects of low concentrations of GB on man in rest and exercise. *Medical Laboratories Research Report No. 148*. Edgewood Arsenal, Maryland, Army Chemical Center.

Freitag, (1940). Chlorgasgefrahren. *J. Gesamte Schiess Spreugstoffwes.* **35**: 159.

Friedberg, K. D. (1968). Antidote bei Blausaurevergiftungen. *Arch. Toxikol.* **24**:41-48.

Frosolono, M. F. (1974). Basic mechanisms involved in phosgene damage to lungs. *Final Report for the Period Jan. 15, 1973 Through Jan. 14, 1974*. Washington, D.C., Manufacturing Chemist's Association.

Funckes, A. J. (1960). Treatment of severe parathion poisoning with 2-pyridine aldoxine methiodide (2-PAM). *Arch. Environ. Health* **1**:404-406.

Galdston, M., Leutscher, J. A. Jr., Longcope, W. T., and Ballich, N. L. (1947a). A study of the residual effects of phosgene poisoning in human subjects. I. After acute exposure. *J. Clin. Invest.* **26**:145-168.

Galdston, M., Luetscher, J. A. Jr., Longcope, W. T., and Ballich, N. L. (1947b). A study of the residual effects of phosgene poisoning in human subjects. II. After chronic exposure. *J. Clin. Invest.* **26**:168-181.

Ganz, J. W., Poser, W., and Erdmann, W. D. (1974). Untersuchungen zur Leber-toxizitaet von Nitrostigmin (Parathion, E 605) an der Perfundierten Rattenleber. *Arch. Toxicol.* **33**:31-40.

Gates, M., and Renshaw, B. (1946). Fluorophosphates and other phosphorus-containing compounds. In *Chemical Warfare Agents and Related Chemical Problems–NDRC Tech. Report.* Washington, Office of Scientific Research and Development, pp. 131-155.

Gates, M., Williams, J. W., and Zapp, J. A. (1946). Arsenicals. In *Chemical Warfare Agents and Related Chemical Problems–NDRC Tech. Report.* Washington, Office of Scientific Research and Development, pp. 83-114.

Geiger, J. C., and Fellow, P. H. (1924). The possible danger of absorption of toxin of C. botulinus through fresh wounds and from mucous surfaces. *Am. J. Publ. Health* **14**:309-310.

Gerard, R. W. (1948). Recent research on respiratory irritants. In *Advances in Military Medicine.* Edited by E. C. Andrus. Boston, Little, Brown, pp. 564-587.

Gilchrist, H. L. (1928). *A Comparative Study of WWI Casualties from Gas and Other Weapons.* Edgewood Arsenal, Maryland, U.S. Chemical Warfare School, pp. 1-51.

Gilchrist, H. L., and Matz, P. B. (1933). The residual effects of warfare gases: the use of phosgene gas, with report of cases. *Med. Bull. Veterans' Admin.* **10**:1-37.

Glass, W. I., Harris, E. A., and Whitlock, R. M. C. (1971). Phosgene poisoning– case report. *N.Z. Med. J.* **74**:386-389.

Goldberg, A. M., and Hanin, I. (1976). *Biology of Cholinergic Function.* New York, Raven Press.

Gregory, A. R. (1970). Inhalation toxicology and lung edema receptor sites. *Am. Ind. Hygiene Assoc. J.* **3**:454-459.

Griffin, H. E. (Chairman) (1976). *Chlorine and Hydrogen Chloride.* Committee on Medical and Biological Effects of Environmental Pollutants. Washington, D.C., National Academy of Sciences.

Grob, D. (1956). Manifestations and treatment of nerve gas poisoning in man. *U.S. Armed Forces Med. J.* **7**:781-789.

Grob, D., and Harvey, J. C. (1958). Effects in man of the anticholinesterase compound sarin (isopropyl methyl phosphonofluoridate). *J. Clin. Invest.* **32**:350-368.

Grob, D., and Johns, R. J. (1958). Use of oximes in the treatment of intoxica-tion by anticholinesterase compounds in normal subjects. *Am. J. Med.* **24**: 497-511.

Grob, D., Harvey, J. C., and Harvey, A. M. (1950). Observations on the effects in man of methyl isopropyl flurophosphonite (GB). *Medical Division Research Report No. 18.* Edgewood Arsenal, Maryland, Army Chemical Center.

Gross, P., Rinehart, W. E., and Hatch, T. (1965). Chronic pneumonitis caused by phosgene—an experimental study. *Arch. Environ. Health* **10**:768-775.

Gross, P., Rinehart, W. E., and deTreville, R. T. P. (1967). The pulmonary reactions to toxic gases. *Am. J. Hygiene* **23**:315-321.

Guyton, A. C., and MacDonald, M. A. (1947). Physiology of bolulinum toxin. *Arch. Neurol. Psychiatry* **57**:578-592.

Hambright, P., Franz, D. R., and Newball, H. H. (1984). Mechanisms of cyanide inhibition by scavengers. In *Proceedings of the Fourth Annual Chemical Defense Bioscience Review.* Aberdeen Proving Ground, MD, U.S. Army Medical Research Institute of Chemical Defense, pp. 525-539.

Hardy, G. C., and Barach, A. L. (1946). Positive pressure respiration in the treatment of irritant pulmonary edema due to chlorine gas poisoning. *J.A.M.A.* **128**:359.

Harrison, H. E. (1944). Lewisite vapor. In *Fasciculus on Chemical Warfare Medicine. Vol. III. Respiratory Tract.* Washington, D.C., Committee on Treatment of Gas Casualties, Division of Medical Services of the National Research Council, pp. 365-374.

Hayes, W. J. (1982). *Pesticides Studied in Man.* Baltimore, William & Wilkins, pp. 75-80, 284-330.

Hill, O. W., and Chesney, J. (1966). Botulism—an ever present menace. A report of 3 simultaneous infections due to type E. Review of the pediatric aspects and treatment. *Clin. Pediatr.* **5**:554-559.

Himsworth, H. (Chairman) (1971a). *Report of the Enquiry into the Medical and Toxicological Aspects of CS (Orthochlorobenzylidene Malonitrile). Part I.* Enquiry into the Medical Situation Following the Use of CS in Londonderry on 13th and 14th August, 1969. London, Her Majesty's Stationery Office. Command 4775, pp. 1-82.

Himsworth, H. (Chairman) (1971b). *Report of the Enquiry into the Medical and Toxicological Aspects of CS (Orthochlorobenzylidene Malonitrile). Part II.* Enquiry into Toxicological Aspects of CS and Its Use for Civil Purposes. London, Her Majesty's Stationery Office. Command 4775, pp. 1-82.

Holmstedt, B. (1959). Pharmacology of organophosphorus cholinesterase inhibitors. *Pharmacol. Rev.* **11**:567-588.

Holzer, E. (1962). Botulism caused by inhalation. *Med. Klin.* **41**:1735-1740.

Hoveid, P. (1956). The chlorine accident in Mjondalen (Norway) 26 January 1940: an after investigation. *Nord. Hyg. Tid.* **37**:59-66.

International Agency for Research on Cancer (1975). *IARC Monographs on the Evaluation of Carcinogenic Risk of Chemicals to Man.* Lyon, France, International Agency for Research on Cancer, **9**:181-182.

International Labor Office (1971). *Encyclopedia of Occupational Health and Safety.* New York, McGraw-Hill.

Ison, G. E., Burrows, G. E., and Way, J. L. (1982). Effect of oxygen on the antagonism of cyanide intoxication. Cytochrome oxidase in vivo. *Toxicol. Appl. Pharmacol.* **65**:250-256.

Ivanhoe, F., and Meyers, F. H. (1964). Phosgene poisoning as an example of neuroparalytic acute pulmonary edema: the sympathetic vasomotor reflex involved. *Dis. Chest* **46**:211-218.

Jax, W., Eimermacher, H., Sturm, A., Eben, A. Jr., Hofmann, K., and Grabensee, B. (1977). Neue Gesichtspunkte in der Behandlung von Alkylphosphorvergiftungen. *Intensivmedizin* **14**:78-82.

Johns, R. J., Bales, P. D., and Himwich, H. E. (1951). The effects of DFP on the convulsant dose of theophylline, theophylline-ethylenediamine, and 8-chlorotheophylline. *J. Pharmacol. Exp. Ther.* **101**:237-242.

Johnson, R. D., Gold, A. J., and Freeman, G. (1958). Comparative lung-airway resistance and cardiovascular effects in dogs and monkeys following parathion and sarin intoxication. *Am. J. Physiol.* **192**:581-584.

Jones, D. E., Kaplovitz, I., Harrington, D. C., and Hilmas, D. E. (1984). Anticonvulsant therapy for OP-induced lethality. In *Proceedings of the Fourth Annual Chemical Defense Bioscience Review.* Edited by R. E. Lindstrom. Aberdeen Proving Ground, Maryland, U.S. Army Medical Research Institute of Chemical Defense, pp. 415-531.

Jules, D., and Popa, I. (1966). *Rev. Sanit. Milit.* **5**:845-850.

Kao, I., Drachman, D. B., and Price, D. L. (1976). Botulinum toxin: mechanism of presynaptic action. *Science* **193**:1256-1258.

Kiese, M., and Weger, N. (1969). Formation of ferrihaemoglobin with aminophenols in the human for treatment of cyanide poisoning. *Eur. J. Pharmacol.* **7**:97-105.

Klose, R., and Gutensohn, G. (1976). Behandlung Einer Alkylphosphatintoxikation mit Gereinigter Serum Cholinesterase. *Prakt. Anaesth.* **11**:1-7.

Knox, W. E., Stumpf, P. K., Green, D. E., and Auerbach, V. H. (1948). The inhibition of sulfhydryl enzymes as the basis of bactericidal action of chlorine. *J. Bacteriol.* **55**:451-458.

Kowitz, T. A., Reba, R. C., Parker, R. T., and Spicer, W. S. (1967). Effects of chlorine gas upon respiratory function. *Arch. Environ. Health* **14**:545-558.

Kurosumi, S., Harada, Y., Sugimoto, Y., and Sasaki, H. (1977). Airway malignancy in poisonous gas workers. *J. Laryngol. Otol.* **91**:217-225.

Laciak, J., and Sipa, K. (1958). The importance of the sense of smelling in workers of some branches of the chemical industry. *Med. Prac.* **9**:85-90.

Lamanna, C. (1961). Immunological aspects of air-borne infection: some general considerations of response to inhalation of toxins. *Bacteriol. Rev.* **25**: 323-330.

Lamanna, C., and Carr, C. J. (1967). The botulinal, tetanal, and enterostaphylococcal toxins: a review. *Clin. Pharmacol. Ther.* **8**:286-332.

Lapushkov, A. G. (1973). Treatment of trichlorfon poisoning in animals. *Veterinariia* **11**:96-97.

Laskowski, M. B., Olson, W. H., and Dettbarn, W. D. (1976). Motor end-plate degeneration coincident with cholinesterase inhibition and increased frequency of miniature end-plate potentials. *Fed. Proc.* **35**:294.

Leadbeater, L., and Maidment, M. P. (1973). The respiratory absorption of CR in the rat. *Chemical Defense Establishment Technical Paper No. 130.* Porton Down, Wiltshire, England, pp. 1-18.

Leith, D. E., Albuquerque, E. X., Johanson, W. G., Urbanetti, J. S., Franz, D. R., and Mosberg, A. T. (1983). Report of discussion group I: Pathophysiology of nerve agent intoxication. In *Proceedings of the Symposium on Respiratory Care of Chemical Casualties.* Edited by H. H. Newball. Aberdeen Proving Ground, Maryland, U.S. Army Medical Research Institute of Chemical Defense, pp. 213-220.

Levina, M. M., and Kurando, T. B. (1967). Problems of labour hygiene and of state of health of workers at the isopropylphenylcarbamate production. *Gig. Sanit.* **32**:25-28.

Levina, M. M., Kurando, T. B., Belyakov, A. A., Smirnova, V. G., and Odlyzhko, S. L. (1966). Industrial hygiene problems and worker health in the monuron industry. *Gig. Tr. Prof. Zabol.* **10**:54-56.

Levine, S. (1975). Non peripheral chemoreceptor stimulation of ventilation by cyanide. *J. Appl. Physiol.* **39**:199-204.

Loevenhart, A. S., Lorenz, W. F., Martin, A. G., and Malone, J. Y. (1918). Stimulation of the respiration by sodium cyanide and its clinical application. *Arch. Intern. Med.* **21**:109-114.

Long, J. E., and Hatch, T. F. (1961). A method for assessing the physiological impairment produced by low-level exposure to pulmonary irritants. *Am. Ind. Hygiene Assoc. J.* **22**:6-13.

Longcope, W. T., Wintrobe, M. M., and Luetscher, J. A. (1943). Report of a case of phosgene poisoning. *OEMcmr - 253.* August 1, 1943.

Lopez, C. (1970). Therapy with corticosteroid compounds in acute poisoning with carbamate and organophosphate pesticides. *Int. Arch. Arbeitsmed.* **26**:51-62.

Louvre, S. C., and Cucinell, S. A. (1970). Some biological reactions of riot control agents. Edgewood Arsenal, MD, U.S. Army Medical Research Laboratory. *Tech Report EATR 4399*, pp. 1-29.

Lundy, P. M., and McKay, D. H. (1975). Mechanism of the cardiovascular activity of dibenz[b.f] [1,4] oxazepine (CR) in cats. Suffield, Ralston, Alberta, Canada: Defense Research Establishment, *Suffield Technical Paper No. 438*, pp. 1-27.

Luzhnikov, E. A. (1966). Some problems of clinical picture and treatment in acute poisoning with organophosphorus insecticides. *Gig. Tr. Prof. Zabol.* 36-42.

Luzhnikov, E. A., and Pankov, A. G. (1969). Experience in the use of cholinesterase reactivators in acute poisoning with organophosphoric compounds. *Klin. Med.* **47**:134-136.

Luzhnikov, E. A., Yaroslavsky, A. A., Molodenkov, M. N., Shurkalin, B. K., Evseev, N. G., and Barsukov, U. F. (1977). Plasma perfusion through charcoal in methyl parathion poisoning. *Lancet* **1**:38-39.

Manning, K. P;. Skegg, D. C. G., Stell, P. M., and Doll, R. (1981). Cancer of the larynx and other occupational hazards of mustard gas workers. *Clin. Otolaryngol.* **6**:165-170.

Manufacturing Chemists Association—Special Supplement (1970). *Accident Case Histories—Phosgene Poisoning.* Washington, D.C., pp. 1-3.

May, A. J., and Whaler, B. C. (1958). The absorption of clostridium botulinum type A toxin from the alimentary canal. *Br. J. Exp. Pathol.* **39**:307-316.

May, J. (1966). Solvent odor thresholds for the evaluation of solvent odors in the atmosphere. *Staub Reinhalt* **26**:385-389.

McNamara, B. P., Owens, E. J., Weimer, J. T., Ballard, T. A., and Vocci, F. J. (1969). Toxicology of riot control chemicals—CS, CN, and DM. Edgewood Arsenal, Maryland, U.S. Army Medical Research Laboratory. *Tech Report EATR 4309*, pp. 1-79.

Moore, S., and Gates, M. (1946a). Phosgene. In *Chemical Warfare Agents and Related Chemical Problems.* Washington, D. C., National Defense Research Committee, pp. 17-29.

Moore, S., and Gates, M. (1946b). Hydrogen cyanide and cyanogen chloride. In *Chemical Warfare Agents and Related Chemical Problems.* Washington, D.C., National Defense Research Committee, pp. 7-16.

Morgenstern, P., Koss, F. R., and Alexander, W. W. (1947). Residual mustard gas bronchitis: effects of prolonged exposure to low concentrations of mustard gas. *Ann. Intern. Med.* **26**:27-40.

Nakamura, T. (1956). Studies on the warfare gas injury in Japan. Report I. On the general condition of the poison gas island. *Gencho Hiroshima Igaku* **4**:1141-1149.

Namba, T., and Hiraki, K. (1958). PAM (Pyridine-2-aldoxime methiodide) therapy for alkylphosphate poisoning. *J.A.M.A.* **166**:1834-1839.

National Research Council (1976). *Chlorine and Hydrogen Chloride.* Washington, D.C., National Academy of Sciences, pp. 92-144.

National Research Council (1982). *Possible Long-Term Health Effects of Short-Term Exposure to Chemical Agents. Vol. 1, Anticholinesterases and Anticholinergics.* Washington, National Academy Press, pp. 1-9.

National Research Council (1984). *Possible Long-Term Health Effects of Short-Term Exposure to Chemical Agents. Vol. 2, Cholinesterase Reactivators, Psychochemicals, and Irritants and Vesicants.* Washington, D.C., National Academy Press, pp. 1-330.

Naughton, M. (1974). Acute cyanide poisoning. *Anaesth. Intens. Care* **4**:351-356.

NIOSH (1981). Occupational Health Guidelines for Chemical Hazards. DHHS (NIOSH) Publication No. 81-123. Washington, D.C., U.S. Government Printing Office.

Norman, J. E. (1975). Lung cancer mortality in World War I veterans with mustard gas injury: 1919-1965. *J. Natl. Cancer Inst.* **54**:311-317.

Norris, G. W. (1919). Some medical impressions of the war. *Trans. Coll. Physicians Phila.* **41**:120-128.

Norris, J. C., Moore, S., Fontenot, H. J., Wilson, R. D., Ho, I. K., and Hume, A. S. (1984). Interaction of carbon monoxide and cyanide. In *Proceedings of the Fourth Annual Chemical Defense Bioscience Review.* Aberdeen Proving Ground, Maryland, U.S. Army Research Institute of Chemical Defense, pp. 513-524.

Okada, E., Takahasi, K., and Nakamura, H. (1970). A study of chloropicrin intoxication. *Nippon Naika Gakka Zasshi* **59**:1214-1221.

Olivier, V. P., Kruse, C. W., Hsu, Y. C., Griffiths, A. C., and Kawata, K. (1973). The comparative mode of action of chlorine, bromine and iodine on f2 bacterial virus (abstract #ENVT 044). In *Abstracts of Papers, 166th National Meeting American Chemical Society.* Chicago, Ill. Aug. 26-31.

Owens, E. J., and Punte, C. L. (1963). Human respiratory and ocular irritation studies utilizing O-chlorobenzilidene malonitrile aerosols. *Am. Ind. Hygiene Assoc. J.* **24**:262-264.

Owens, E. J., McNamara, B. P., Weimer, J. T., Ballard, T. A., Thomas, W. V., Hess, T. L., Farrand, R. L., Ryan, S. G., Merkey, R. P., Olson, J. S., and Vocci, F. J. (1967). The toxicology of DM. Edgewood Arsenal, Maryland, U.S. Army Medical Research Laboratory, Technical Report 4108, pp. 1-131.

Park, S., and Giammona, S. T. (1972). Toxic effects of tear gas on an infant following prolonged exposure. *Am. J. Dis. Child.* **123**:245-246.

Patil, L. R. S., Smith, R. G., Vorwald, A. J., and Mooney, T. F. (1970). The health of diaphragm cell workers exposed to chlorine. *Am. Ind. Hygiene Assoc. J.* **31**:678-686.

Paulet, G. (1957). Sur une nouvelle mise au point du traitement de l'intoxication cyanhydrique. *Press Med.* **65**:573-576.

Paulet, G. (1958). Intoxication cyanhidrique et chelates de cobalt. *J. Physiol. (Paris)* **50**:438-442.

Pearce, R. G. (1920). Note on some respiratory studies made on late stages of gas poisoning. *J. Lab. Clin. Med.* **5**:411-417.

Polley, E. H., Vick, J. A., Ciuchta, H. P., Fischetti, D. A., Macchitelli, F. J., and Moutanerelli, N. (1965). Botulinum toxin, type A: effects on central nervous system. *Science* **147**:1036-1037.

Poulton, J. E. (1983). Cyanogenic compounds in plants and their toxic effects. In *Handbook of Natural Toxins. Part 1, Toxins inducing Effects in the Cardiovascular or Pulmonary Systems.* Vol. I. Edited by R. F. Keeler and A. T. Tu. New York, Marcel Dekker.

Punte, C. L. (1962). Inhalation studies with chloroacetophenone, diphenylaminochlorarsine and pelargonic morpholide—II. Human exposures. *Am. Ind. Hygiene Assoc. J.* **23**:199-202.

Punte, C. L., Owens, E. J., and Gutentag, P. J. (1963). Exposures to orthochlorobenzylidene malonitrile. *Arch. Environ. Health* **6**:366-374.

Rozmiarek, H., Capizzi, R. L., Papirmeister, B., Fuhrman, W. H., and Smith, W. J. (1973). Mutagenic activity in somatic and germ cells following chronic inhalation of sulfur mustard. *Mutat. Res.* **21**:13-14 (abstract).

Rumack, B. H. (1973). Anticholinergic poisoning: treatment with physostigmine. *Pediatrics* **52**:449-451.

Schultz, J. (1945). The prophylactic action of hexamethylenetetramine in phosgene poisoning. In *Fasciculus on Chemical Warfare Medicine. Vol. II. Respiratory Tract.* Washington, D.C., Committee on Treatment of Gas Casualties, Division of Medical Services of the National Research Council.

Seeley, T. D., Nowicke, J. W., Meselson, M., Guillemin, J., and Akratanakul, P. (1985). *Yellow Rain. Sci. Am.* **253**:128-137.

Seigler, D. S. (1977). The naturally occurring cyanogenic glycosides. *Prog. Phytochem.* **4**:83-120.

Sheldon, J. M., and Lovell, R. G. (1949). Asthma due to halogens. *Am. Practitioner* **4**:43-44.

Shohl, A. T., and Deming, C. L. (1920). Hexamethylenamin: its quantitative factors in therapy. *J. Urol.* **4**:419-437.

Shultz, W. H. (1918a). The reaction of the heart toward chlorine. *J. Pharmacol. Exp. Ther.* **11**:179-180.

Shultz, W. H. (1918b). The reaction of the respiratory mechanism to chlorine. *J. Pharmacol. Exp. Ther.* **11**:180-181.

Sidell, F. R. (undated). A summary of the investigations in man with BZ conducted by the U.S. Army 1960-1969. *CSL 000-137.* Edgewood, Maryland, Edgewood Arsenal.

Sidell, F. R., and Groff, W. A. (1974). The reactivatibility of cholinesterase inhibited by VX and sarin in man. *Toxicol. Appl. Pharmacol.* **27**:241-252.

Simon, F. P., and Potts, A. M. (1945). Metabolic aspects of phosgene poisoning. In *Fasiculus on Chemical Warfare Medicine. Vol. II. Respiratory Tract.* Washington, D.C., Committee on Treatment of Gas Casualties, Division of Medical Sciences of the National Research Council, pp. 188-233.

Snyder, S. H., Chang, K. J., Kuhar, M. J., and Yamamura, H. I. (1975). Biochemical identification of mammalian muscarinic cholinergic receptor. *Fed. Proc.* **34**:1915-1921.

Solomonson, L. P. (1981). Cyanide as a metabolic inhibitor. In *Cyanide in Biology.* Edited by B. Vennesland, E. E. Conn, C. J. Knowles, J. Westley and F. Wissing. London, Academic Press, pp. 11-28.

Soto, P. M. Jr., and Roessler, W. G. (1965). Staphylococcal enterotoxemia: pathologic lesions in Rhesus monkeys exposed by aerosol. *U.S. Army Biol. Lab. Tech. Manuscript 226.* Frederick, Maryland, Fort Detrick.

Spero, L., Stefanye, D., Brecher, P. I., Jacoby, H. M., Dalidowicz, J. E., and Schantz, E. J. (1965). Amino acid composition and terminal amino acids of staphylococcal enterotoxin. *Biochemistry* **4**:1024-1030.

Stares, J. (1983). *Chemical Weapons and Chemical Dearmament,* Stockholm, Stockholm International Peace Research Institute.

Stavrakis, P. (1971). The use of hexamethylenetetramine (HMT) in treatment of acute phosgene poisoning. *Ind. Med.* **40**:30-31.

Stein, A. A., and Kirwan, W. E. (1964). Chloracetophenone (tear gas) poisoning: a clinico-pathologic report. *J. Forensic Sci.* **9**:374-382.

Striker, G. E. (1967). A clinicopathologic study of the effects of riot control agents on monkeys. IV. O-chlorobenzylidene malonitrile (CS) grenade. Edgewood Arsenal, Maryland, U.S. Army Medical Research Laboratory. *Tech Report* 4071, pp. 1-27.

Striker, G. E., Streett, C. S., Ford, D. F., Herman, L. H., and Helland, D. R. (1967a). A clinicopathologic study of the effects of riot control agents on monkeys. Edgewood Arsenal, Maryland, U.S. Army Medical Research Laboratory. *Tech Report EATR 4068,* pp. 1-19.

Striker, G. E., Streett, C. S., Ford, D. F., Herman, L. H., and Helland, D. R. (1967b). Clinicopathological study of the effects of riot control agents on monkeys. V. Low concentrations of diphenylamino chloroarsine (DM) or O-chlorobenzylidene malonitrile (CS) for extended periods. Edgewood Arsenal, Maryland, U.S. Army Medical Research Laboratory. *Tech Report* 4072, pp. 1-31.

Sugiyama, H., and Hayama, T. (1965). Abdominal viscera as site of emetic action for staphylococcal enterotoxin in the monkey. *J. Infect. Dis.* **115**: 330-336.

Thorburn, K. M. (1982). Injuries after use of the lacrimatory agent chloro-acetophenone in a confined space. *Arch. Environ. Health* **37**:182-186.

Tobias, J. M., Postel, S., Pratt, H. M., Lushbaugh, C. C., Swift, M. N., and Gerard, R. W. (1949). Localization of the site of action of a pulmonary irritant, diphosgene. *Am. J. Physiol.* **158**:173-183.

Towill, L. E., Drury, J. S., Whitfield, B. C., Lewis, E. B., Galyan, E. L., and Hammons, A. S. (1978). Reviews of the environmental effects of pollutants. V. Cyanide. *U.S. EPA Doc. EPA-600/1-78-027.* Cincinnati, Ohio, U.S. Environmental Protection Agency.

Tschanatschev, I. S. (1957). Experimental therapy in the case of phsogene oxime intoxications. *Trav. Inst. Med. Superieur Sofia* **4**:99-109.

Tschanatschev, I. S. (1958). A case of phosgene oxime poisoning. *Trav. Inst. Med. Superieur Sofia* **5**:173-183.

Tschanatschev, I. S., and Dronsin, T. D. (1964). *Experimental Therapy in the Case of Inhalation Intoxication With Phosgene Oxime: Preliminary Report,* pp. 1-6.

Tyler, H. R. (1963a). Botulinus toxin: effect on the central nervous system of man. *Science* **139**:847-848.

Tyler, H. R. (1963b). Pathology of the neuromuscular apparatus in botulism. *Arch. Pathol.* **76**:55-59.

U.S. Dept. of the Army (1968). Treatment of chemical agent casualties and conventional military chemical injuries. *Technical Manual TM8-285.* Washington, D.C., Department of the Army.

Underhill, F. P. (1920). *The Lethal War Gases: Physiology and Experimental Treatment.* New Haven, Yale University Press.

United Nations Report (1970). *Chemical and Bacteriological (Biological) Weapons and the Effects of Their Possible Use.* New York, Ballantine Books.

Vedder, B. (1925). *The Medical Aspects of Chemical Warfare.* Baltimore, Williams & Wilkins.

Velikanov, I. M. (1934). Experimental immunization of man against botulism. *Klin. Med.* **12**:1802-1806.

Vettorazzi, G. (1977). State of the art of the toxicological evaluation carried out by the joint FAO/WHO Expert Committee on Pesticide Residues. III. Miscellaneous pesticides used in agriculture and public health. *Residue Rev.* **66**:137-184.

Vick, J. A., and Froehlich, H. L. (1985). Studies of cyanide poisoning. *Arch. Int. Pharmacodyn. Ther.* **273**:314-322.

Wada, S., Miyanishi, M., Nishimoto, Y., Kambe, S., and Miller, R. W. (1968).

Mustard gas as a cause of respiratory neoplasia in man. *Lancet* **1**:1161-1163.

Wagman, J., Edwards, R. C., and Schantz, E. J. (1965). Molecular size, homogeneity, and hydrodynamic properties of purified staphylococcal enterotoxin B. *Biochemistry* **4**:1017-1023.

Wannarka, G. L. (1984). Status of the pyridostigmine development effort. In *Proceedings of the Fourth Annual Chemical Defense Bioscience Review.* Edited by R. E. Lindstrom. Aberdeen Proving Ground, Maryland, U.S. Army Medical Research Institute of Chemical Defense, pp. 107-120.

Ward, J. R. (1962). Case report: exposure to a nerve gas. In *Artificial Respiration, Theory and Applications.* Edited by J. L. Wittenberger. New York, Harper and Row, pp. 258-265.

Waser, P. G. (ed.) (1975). *Cholinergic Mechanisms.* Raven Press, New York.

Watson, S. H., and Kibler, C. S. (1933). Drinking water as a cause of asthma. *J. Allergy* **5**:197-198.

Way, J. L., Rumack, B. H., Westley, J. L., Baskin, S. I., and Newball, H. H. (1984). Report of discussion group IV: Cyanide intoxication prophylaxis and therapy. In *Proceedings of the Symposium on Respiratory Care of Chemical Casualties (November 28-30, 1983, McLean, Virginia).* Ft. Detrick, Maryland, U.S. Army Medical Research and Development Command, pp. 241-250.

Weger, N. (1975). Therapy in cases of poisoning with mustard gas (yellow cross). *Dtsch. Arzt.* **23**:1749-1750.

Weill, H. R., Schwarz, G. M., and Ziskind, M. (1969). Late evaluation of pulmonary function after acute exposure to chlorine gas. *Am. Rev. Respir. Dis.* **99**:374-379.

Wells, W. J. H. B., McFarlan, C. W., and Webster, R. E. (1938). The detection of phosgene by odor. *EATR 250.* Aberdeen Proving Ground, Maryland, Edgewood Arsenal.

Westley, J. (1984). Roles of divalent sulfur in the biological detoxication of cyanide. In *Proceedings of the Fourth Annual Chemical Defense Bioscience Review.* Aberdeen Proving Ground, Maryland, U.S. Army Medical Research Institute of Chemical Defense, pp. 525-539.

WHO Consultants (1970). Chemical agents. In *Health Aspects of Chemical and Biological Weapons.* Geneva, World Health Organization, pp. 23-59.

Williams, R. L., and Pearson, J. E. Jr. (1970). Functional study of the renal effect of the anticholinesterase paraoxon. *Arch. Int. Pharmacodyn.* **184**:195-208.

Wilson, I. B. (1951). Acetylcholinesterase. XI. Reversibility of tetraethyl-pyrophosphate inhibition. *J. Biol. Chem.* **190**:111-117.

Winternitz, M. C. (1919). Anatomical changes in the respiratory tract initiated by irritating gases. *Mil. Surg.* **44**:476-493.

Winternitz, M. C. (1920). *Collected Studies on the Pathology of War Gas Poisoning.* New Haven, Yale University Press, pp. 1-165.

Wood, J. R. (1950). Medical problems in chemical warfare. *J.A.M.A.* **144**:605-609.

Yamamura, H. I., Kuha, M. J., Greenberg, D., and Snyder, S. H. (1974). Muscarinic cholinergic receptor binding: regional distribution in the monkey brain. *Brain Res.* **66**:541-546.

Zielhius, R. L. (1970). Tentative emergency exposure limits for sulfur dioxide, sulfuric acid, chlorine and phosgene. *Ann. Occup. Hygiene* **13**:171-176.

9

Inhalational Drug Abuse

JACOB LOKE
and RICHARD ROWLEY

Yale University School of Medicine
New Haven, Connecticut

PETER JATLOW

Yale University School of Medicine
and Yale-New Haven Hospital
New Haven, Connecticut

HERBERT D. KLEBER

Yale University School of Medicine
and Connecticut Mental Health Center
New Haven, Connecticut

The abuse of drugs has been a part of society for millennia. The use of the opium poppy by the Sumerian civilization was recorded as early as 4000 B.C. (Maurer and Vogel, 1967). Also recorded is the chewing of coca leaves by the South American Indians for more than 2000 years (Grinspoon and Bakalar, 1976) and the drinking of tea made from Jimson weed (Jamestown weed), an hallucinogen by the British troops in Jamestown, Virginia as early as the 1600s (Hollister, 1968). Documentation of marijuana smoking dates back to texts from ancient China, Greece, India, and Assyria. The psychedelic drug (mescaline) from the peyote cactus was eaten by North American Indian tribes for their ecstatic visions (Slotkin, 1956). Over the centuries different civilizations have accepted certain drugs as medications, recreational substances and aspects of sacred rites. Other drugs have been forbidden by social consensus, taboo, or law.

The last 100 years have been a time of rapid change in western society and this change has extended to the role of drugs, and society's attitude toward the abuse of drugs. In the early 19th century the abuse of drugs, excluding tobacco and alcohol, was fairly restricted in western society as much due to lack of availability as due to intolerance by society. Many factors have conspired to change

349

Table 1 Common Features of Inhalational Dependence-Producing Drugs

Drugs	Pleasure reward	Neuropsychological toxicity	Reinforcement (self-administered)		Tolerance	Withdrawal symptoms	Long-term damage	
			Humans	Monkey			Mental	Physical
Opiates								
Opium	+	+	+	+	+	++	0	?
Heroin	+	+	+	+	+	++	0	?
Major psychostimulants								
Cocaine	+	+	++	++	+	+	+	+
Cannabis								
Hashish, marihuana-THC	+	+	+	0	+	+	+	?
Hallucinogens								
Phencyclidine	+	+	+	+	+	+	+	+
Solvents								
Benzene	+	+	+	?	+	?	0	+
Toluene	+	+	+	?	+	?	0	+
Acetone CCl$_4$	+	+	+	?	+	?	0	+
Trichloroethylene	+	+	+	?	+	?	0	+
Ether, N$_2$O, CHCl$_3$	+	+	+	?	+	?	0	+

Modified and adapted from Nahas, 1984.

this: the maturing of world trade, the development of the hypodermic syringe, the isolation of morphine and heroin from the opium poppy, the proliferation of chemical means for extracting, isolating, and synthesizing new compounds, the emergence of wealthy syndicates founded on drug trafficking, the emergence of an addict subculture, and changing social attitudes, mores, as well as pleasure rewards (Table 1).

Since the late 19th century, drug abuse and narcotic addiction have been significant problems in the United States. The last 40 years, in particular, have been a period of phenomenal rise in the prevalence of drug or chemical abuse. In the 1950s the intentional inhalation of gasoline for its euphoric state was reported (Clinger and Johnson, 1951) and in the 1960s young adults were abusing the volatile nitrites including amyl nitrite (Newell et al., 1985) as a form of getting high (Sigell et al., 1978) and as a sex stimulant. Other recreational inhaled chemicals include nitrous oxide, chloroform, and organic solvents (Cornish, 1980; Nicholi, 1983; Fortenberry, 1985). However, the four most important abused drugs are marijuana, cocaine, heroin, and phencyclidine. Except for heroin, which is typically administered in drug abuse by the intravenous route (a minority of cocaine abusers also use this drug intravenously), these drugs are usually inhaled or snorted. In England, over 1/3 of heroin addicts take in the drug via smoking. This is less common in the United States because of the lower heroin potency here (46% potency in England versus 7% in the United States) (Stimson, 1985).

Recently, this trend toward inhalation as the administrative route of choice for drug abuse has accelerated further. Because of the potential development of hepatitis B and the acquired immune deficiency syndrome associated with intravenous drug abuse (Selik et al., 1984), inhalational drug abuse of marijuana, and cocaine in particular has shown explosive growth. The abuse of "crack" a form of cocaine that can be smoked instead of snorted (the latter route is self-limiting because of vasoconstriction) has reached epidemic proportion (*Newsweek*, 1986). In New York City, the heroin epidemic of the late 1960s and early 1970s has reportedly been replaced by crack in the 1980s as the drug of choice for illicit drug use by young people and teenagers (*New York Times*, 1986).

Today, the scope of the problem, including its economic and social impact and the medical consequences, is unprecedented (*Time*, 1986). Profits from illicit drug traffic are estimated at $60 billion per year in the United States and rank in sales second to those of one of the nation's largest corporations, Exxon (Smith, 1982). The most widely used illegal drug is marijuana. It has been estimated that one quarter of the American population has tried the drug and 20 million people use it on any given day (Nicholi, 1983). Though heroin has decreased in popularity, there are still about 500,000 heroin addicts. There has been a surge in the number of people using cocaine, now estimated to be about 4 or 5 million (*Newsweek*, 1986).

The epidemiology of inhalation drug abuse, their pharmacology, toxicology, clinical recognition, and therapy are the subject of this chapter.

I. Opiate Abuse

A. History

Recorded history reveals as early as 4000 B.C. that the Sumerian civilization cultivated and used opium poppy (Maurer and Vogel, 1967). Since that time opium has been variably available and accepted in different societies. Opium smoking has a long history of popularity in Asia and in the Middle East. In Europe, acceptance has been traditionally more restrained. Over the last 100 years, however, the nature of opium abuse has undergone dramatic changes and the scope of abuse has shown explosive growth. This has been the result of technological advances and social changes. The refinement of morphine, the subsequent synthesis of more potent opiate derivatives including heroin, and the invention of the hypodermic needle, coupled with changing social mores and the development of an addict subculture have conspired to make opiate addiction a significant social problem in many western societies including the United States.

The opium poppy, *Papaver somniferum,* can be grown in most temperate climates. The plant blooms in the summer, at which time opium-containing latex can be collected. The raw opium has many natural alkaloids including morphine, codeine, papaverine, narcotine, and thebaine. Opium is prepared for smoking by boiling down the latex. It is smoked in an elaborate pipe. Morphine, a more refined opium product prepared by boiling the latex in a small quantity of water and adding small amounts of lime, was first isolated in 1803. The remaining opiates are either semisynthetic (e.g., heroin, codeine, and dilaudid), produced by chemical modification of the morphine molecule, or totally synthetic (e.g., Dolophine [methadone] and Demerol [meperidine]). Heroin or diacetylmorphine is one of the most potent of the semisynthetic products and is a white crystalline powder prepared by a multistep chemical modification of morphine. First produced in 1898 by a German pharmaceutical firm, Bayer, heroin was named for its "heroic" curative powers (Goode, 1984). Many forms of heroin which vary in color, purity, and potency are found in the illicit drug market. In order to increase the profit from illegal drug sale, street heroin is usually only 3-20% pure. The heroin is typically "cut" with milk sugar, lactose, or quinine, though occasionally confectioners' sugar, talcum powder, mannite, flour, aspirin, and tranquilizers are used. Heroin has even been adulterated with poisonous substances such as strychnine, cyanide, arsenic, or parathion (Froede, 1972).

Narcotic addiction in the United States has been a problem for the last century, although the nature of the addict has changed. In the latter half of the 19th century and early in the 20th century, opium and morphine were common ingredients in over-the-counter medications marketed for treatment of headaches, toothaches, nervousness, and many other illnesses (Musto, 1973). Consequently, many individuals with medical problems became narcotic addicts. In the early 1900s, there were an estimated 500,000 narcotic addicts in the United States. This changed with the Harrison Act of 1914, which banned sales of over-the-counter narcotics, and a subsequent Supreme Court decision outlawing the medical maintenance of narcotic addicts. Due to these severe restrictions on availability, and laws limiting opiate use, addiction problems diminished. By the end of World War II, there were only an estimated 20,000 narcotic abusers in the United States (Goode, 1984). Following 1945, however, a new addict subculture emerged characterized in large part by those seeking pleasure from drug use. In the United States, this subculture grew steadily in the 1950s and 1960s and explosively in the late 1970s and early 1980s.

Heroin is the most commonly used narcotic in the United States today (Drug Abuse Warning Network, 1983). Over 2 million Americans have used heroin (Fishburne et al., 1980). Estimates of the number of narcotic addicts vary widely, ranging between 200,000 and 800,000; 500,000 is probably a reasonable estimate (DuPont, 1978). While accurate figures on the total scope of narcotic addiction are difficult to gather, the increasing rate is clear. The number of reported deaths by heroin overdose increased from 474 to 771 from 1979 to 1982 (Drug Abuse Warning Network, 1983). Intravenous injection is the most prevalent route of administration, since this produces the most rapid and intense effects. Other routes of administration include subcutaneous ("skin popping") (Hirsch, 1972), nasal inhalation, and oral ingestion. These alternative routes are particularly prevalent among female addicts (Helpern, 1972), and increasingly popular with the growing awareness of the transmission of AIDS among intravenous abusers. Opium and heroin smoking, while present and prevalent in Asia, is quite rare in the United States.

B. Pharmacology and Toxicology

The opiates have fast and powerful neurologic, physical, and psychic effects. These effects appear to be mediated by drug interactions with several closely related receptors that share properties with peptide enkephalin and endorphin receptors. The intensity of opiate effects is dependent on a number of factors including potency of the particular derivative, and the dose and route of administration. In pharmacologic doses, opiates produce profound analgesia and striking changes in mood, characterized by tranquility and euphoria. Drowsiness, respiratory depression, and muscular rigidity are also common. In addition to these neurologic effects the other physical effects of the opiates are complex and clinically significant. These include decreased gastrointestinal motility, nausea and vomiting, peripheral arterial and venous dilatation, reduced hypothalamic response to stimuli and altered pituitary secretion (Jaffe and Martin, 1980).

Experience with opiate overdoses in humans is collected primarily from the setting of illicit use and is a tragically frequent occurrence in this setting. The overwhelming majority of addicts experience at least one overdose in their life, and an estimated 1% of opiate addicts die each year due to acute toxic reactions (Louria et al., 1967). Important factors that lead to narcotic overdose or death in addicts include potency of the heroin (a function of the purity of the street packets of the illicit drug), impurities, drug tolerance, length of abstinence, and synergistic effect with alcohol and other drugs. The latter include the street drug "speedball," a combination of heroin with cocaine or amphetamine. Such "drug mixing" was implicated in the death of comedian/actor John Belushi. Most narcotic overdoses are taken by the intravenous or "mainline" route, although it has been demonstrated that nasal inhalation ("sniffing" or "snorting") of codeine or heroin has resulted in death (Hirsch and Adelson, 1972). Shallow sniffing results in absorption primarily from the nasal and pharyngeal mucosa and deeper sniffing produces a combination of mucosal absorption, aspiration, and swallowing. In various series, 3-10% of heroin overdoses have been administered by the inhalational route, producing a clinical picture similar to intravenous overdose (Frand, 1972; Duberstein and Kaufman, 1971; Steinberg and Karliner, 1968).

C. Clinical and Pathophysiological Features

Depressed consciousness with stupor or coma, pinpoint pupils, and respiratory depression constitute the classic triad of opiate overdose. While these features are central to the recognition of opiate overdose, the pulmonary complications are the primary cause of morbidity and mortality. One of the most striking complications of opiate overdose is pulmonary edema (Rosenow, 1972). In a New York City series of 149 patients with acute heroin overdose who presented to an emergency room with stupor or coma and depressed respiration, pulmonary edema was present in 48% of cases (Duberstein and Kaufman, 1971). Symptoms were originally described in 1880 by Osler (Osler, 1880); there are numerous reports describing in detail opiate-related pulmonary edema (Morrison et al., 1970; Frand et al., 1972; Siegel, 1972; Light and Dunham, 1975; Stern and Subbarao, 1983). The clinical presentation is similar to that of other types of pulmonary edema, with profound hypoxemia and acidosis. In 16 cases of heroin pulmonary edema (Frand et al., 1972), severe arterial hypoxemia was noted with a mean arterial oxygen tension (PaO_2) of 36.5 mmHg; also present were hypercapnia with arterial carbon dioxide tension ($PaCO_2$) of 56 mmHg and a combined respiratory and metabolic acidosis (average pH 7.15). There was also a decrease in vital capacity (VC) and forced expiratory volume in 1 sec (FEV_1), although the FEV_1/FVC was preserved (average, 83.6%); furthermore the single breath diffusing capacity was reduced (54% of predicted) (Table 2). In another study of 39 patients with heroin-induced pulmonary edema (Duberstein and Kaufman, 1971), the mean PaO_2 was 50 mmHg, $PaCO_2$ 53 mmHg, pH 7.22, and arterial oxygen saturation (SaO_2) 78%; 16 patients in this study without pulmonary edema had a mean PaO_2 of 74 mmHg, $PaCO_2$ 49 mmHg, pH 7.26, and SaO_2 91%.

The manifestations of acute noncardiac pulmonary edema in heroin intoxication on chest radiographs classically consist of a bilateral diffuse alveolar filling process radiating from the central to the peripheral lung zones. This fluffy, "butterfly" distribution usually resolves in 24-72 hr (Stern and Subbarao, 1983), unless there is superimposed bacterial or aspiration pneumonia (Light and Dunham, 1975). Less commonly, the pulmonary edema may involve most of one lung or a single lobe. In 1880, Osler recorded a fatal case of unilateral left-sided pulmonary edema following morphine overdose with the patient lying on his left side. Coarse mottling of the lungs are observed in mild forms of pulmonary edema. There may also be a delay in the onset of pulmonary edema for 6-10 hr after the initial presentation to the hospital (Saba et al., 1974). In some patients abnormal radiographic findings are not seen but bilateral pulmonary edema develops in subsequent admissions for opiate intoxication (Morrison et al., 1970).

Pathologically, patients with acute opiate pulmonary edema have a severe acute pneumonitis called "narcotic lungs" (Siegel, 1972). In an autopsy series by Siegel, on gross examination the lungs were voluminous and heavy when examined within 3 hr of intravenous narcotism. Histologic study reveals congestion, edema, and varying numbers of large and small mononuclear cells in the alveolar space and alveolar walls. From 3 to 12 hr, whitish froth is seen in the upper and lower airways with progressive congestion, edema, and hemorrhage in multiple areas of the lung. Beyond 12 hr, there is a progressive pneumonitis with patchy involvement about the bronchial tree, and the predominant cell is the neutrophil. Aspirated material is noted in some patients on gross examination of the lung since aspiration pneumonitis is a frequent complication of heroin overdose.

The pathophysiological mechanism of opiate pulmonary edema remains unclear. In patients with heroin pulmonary edema, the concentration of protein in the pulmonary edema fluid (obtained immediately after endotracheal intubation) has been shown to be higher than in serum when compared with those patients who have congestive heart failure (98.3 versus 40.0%). This finding supports the concept of increased pulmonary capillary permeability (Katz et al., 1972). Proposed mechanisms leading to increased capillary permeability

Table 2 Pulmonary Function Studies in Acute Heroin Overdose and Heroin Addiction

	Group 1 (16 pts) Heroin pulmonary edema		Group 2 (9 pts) Heroin overdose		Group 3 (25 pts) "Control" addicts	
	Mean	S.D.	Mean	S.D.	Mean	S.D.
Vital capacity (VC; liters)	2.12	±1.11	4.05	±1.16	4.15	±1.15
Vital capacity/percent predicted ratio	46.74	±23.94	79.83	±20.39	89.38	±19.48
FEV_1 (liters)	1.78	±1.20	3.14	±1.14	2.99	±0.83
$FEV_1/FVC\%$	83.56	±9.38	80.11	±8.05	74.12	±10.12
Single breath diffusing capacity (ml/min mmHg; D_LCO)	16.05	±5.21	28.13	±8.29	22.3	±6.86
D_LCO (% pred.)	53.65	±14.58	92.60	±30.49	74.06	±19.86
Arterial PaO_2 (mmHg)	36.53	±5.92	70.14	±18.98	89.37	±11.67
Arterial $PaCO_2$ (mmHg)	56.11	±19.41	39	±7.95	35.62	±5.44
pH	7.15	±0.14	7.35	±0.071	7.41	±0.036

Adapted from Frand et al., 1972.

include hypoxia; hypersensitivity reaction; histamine mediated effect; neurogenic effect; or a direct toxic effect of heroin, diluents, or adulterants (Frand, 1972).

In addition to these pulmonary complications several other less common acute manifestations of inhaled opiate toxicity include hypotension due to vasodilatation, tachycardia, and rarely transient atrial fibrillation (Duberstein and Kaufman, 1971). Muscular rigidity, acute rhabdomyolysis and myoglobinuria, and seizure activity, particularly in association with meperdine or propoxyphene, are also reported (Schreiber et al., 1971; Greenwood, 1974; D'Agostino and Arnett, 1979; Firooznia et al., 1983). In intravenous abusers, a number of additional complications are seen, including several pulmonary complications: (a) infections such as septic embolism, bacterial pneumonia, and opportunistic infection; (b) Kaposi sarcoma; and (c) miscellaneous complications of foreign body granulomas, pulmonary hypertension, and pleural and mediastinal disease (Stern and Subbarao, 1983). Nonpulmonary complications include endocarditis, hepatitis, tetanus, malaria, colonic pseudo-obstruction, and acquired immune deficiency syndrome, which are beyond the scope of this chapter (Louria et al., 1967; Cherubin, 1967; Sternbach et al., 1980; Gottlieb et al., 1983; Gallo et al., 1984; Balthazar and Lefleur, 1983). While these complications are not related to inhalation abuse, many addicts have a history of intravenous injections and these entities should be considered in the evaluation of any heroin abuser.

The documented long-term consequences of opiate abuse are primarily pulmonary and related to previous pulmonary edema. These consequences include abnormalities in gas exchange, restrictive ventilatory defect, and reduction in single breath diffusing capacity (Karliner et al., 1969; Frand et al., 1972; Light and Dunham, 1975). The latter abnormality can be present for months after the initial pulmonary edema. Most studies have investigated primarily intravenous abusers in whom persistent abnormalities in vital capacity and diffusing capacity have been found. In one study of 25 patients with a history of heroin addiction but no known cardiorespiratory illness or history of hospitalization for drug overdose, a mild reduction in the single breath diffusing capacity (74% of predicted) was noted (Frand et al., 1972). In another study of the lung function of 512 intravenous drug abusers who were also chronic cigarette smokers, the investigators found 42% (214/512) (Table 3) to have a diffusing capacity below 75% of predicted (mean 65.7%). In addition, obstructive lung disease and interstitial lung disease was present in 6% and 7%, respectively (Overland et al., 1980). The investigators found no roentgenographic evidence of pulmonary hypertension in any of their patients and demonstrated that significant respiratory symptoms were unusual. Bronchiectasis as a consequence of opiate pulmonary edema or

Table 3 Relationship of Alterations in Pulmonary Function to Age and Duration of Intravenous Drug Abuse in 512 Heroin Addicts

Group	Pulmonary function test category	Subjects No.	Subjects %	Age ± SEM (yr)	Mean D_{LCO} ± SEM (% predicted)	Mean duration of intravenous drug abuse (yr ± SEM)
1	Normal	247	48	27.3 ± 0.4	89.9 ± 0.9	6.9 ± 0.5
1a	Low D_{LCO}	190	38	26.6 ± 0.4	65.8 ± 0.5[a]	5.8 ± 0.5
2	Obstructive	27	4	26.6 ± 1.1	89.0 ± 2.4	6.6 ± 1.3
2a	Obstructive and low D_{LCO}	8	2	37.0 ± 4.3[a]	65.9 ± 2.4[a]	15.4 ± 5.2[a]
3	Restrictive	24	4	24.7 ± 1.1	90.3 ± 4.4	5.0 ± 1.1
3a	Restrictive and low D_{LCO}	16	3	25.9 ±1.1	65.5 ± 1.7[a]	4.3 ± 0.9

[a]In comparison with the normal group, significant at $P < 0.001$.
From Overland et al., 1980.

addiction has also been the subject of several reports (Stern and Subbarao, 1983; Banner et al., 1979; Schachter and Basta, 1973; Warnock et al., 1972). Bilateral large upper lobe bullous disease has been observed in intravenous drug abusers (Goldstein et al., 1986). Other investigators have shown perfusion defects in the upper lobes with normal ventilation scans in these areas (Thomashow et al., 1977). Thus, microemboli leading to an occlusive disease at the apical pulmonary capillaries may produce microbullae that coalesce to form large bullae in the upper lobes. The cause of chronic lung disease, its exact relationship to pulmonary edema, and its incidence in the setting of inhalational abuse remain unclear. Concurrent tobacco abuse, other inhalational drug abuse (Tilles et al., 1986), granulomatous, vasculitic, and fibrotic effects on the pulmonary vasculature only seen with intravenous drug abuse (Overland et al., 1980; Pare et al., 1979), and the complications of aspiration may all play a role in these abnormalities.

Information on opium smoking comes primarily from Asia. The effect on lung function in a group of 40 opium smokers was studied by Poh (1972). He found airflow obstruction in one group and no evidence of airflow obstruction, but hyperinflation and decreased diffusing capacity in the other group. The effect of cigarette smoking complicating the effect of opium smoking could not be excluded. In another study, 54 opium smokers with chronic obstructive pulmonary disease were found to have moderate to severe airway obstruction with hyperinflation and airtrapping; in 32 patients, there was also a restrictive defect attributed to peribronchiolar fibrosis (Da Costa et al., 1971).

In addition to these various physiologic effects, one of the most important physical properties of chronic opiate abuse is that it produces an extremely powerful physical dependency. Physical addiction can occur in as short as 3 weeks of narcotic use. When physical addiction is present, abstinence for as few as 12 hours produces signs of withdrawal. These include diaphoresis, nausea, and anxiety, progressing to rhinorrhea, lacrimation, fever, and chills (Khantzian and McKenna, 1979). The fever is usually less than 100°F. If the temperature is higher, intercurrent infection, cocaine intoxication or sedative withdrawal, instead of opiate withdrawal may be present. (It is not unusual for one or more of these conditions to exist along with opiate withdrawal.) Subsequent severe withdrawal, which occurs if no opiates are taken is characterized by abdominal pain, nausea and vomiting, diarrhea, weakness, flushing, and low-back pain. Without treatment, these symptoms gradually disappear in 7-10 days. The intensity of withdrawal, however, precludes most individuals from withdrawing without medical assistance and methadone therapy.

D. Clinical Evaluation and Therapy

Recognition, administration of narcotic antagonists, respiratory support, and oxygen therapy are the fundamentals of treating narcotic overdose. Narcotic overdose should be considered in any patient with the triad of pinpoint pupils, depressed or labored respirations, and depressed consciousness, stupor, or coma. One of these signs may be absent and should not exclude the diagnosis. Stigmata of intravenous, subcutaneous, or intramuscular drug abuse may be evident on the skin in the upper arms and thighs, although these may not be present in addicts who abuse drugs by the intranasal route (Hirsch, 1972). In the initial assessment, the vital signs are measured and the level of consciousness is assessed (Nicholson, 1983). Any indication of upper airway compromise with impaired sensorium and severe respiratory depression necessitates endotracheal intubation and mechanical ventilation. Routine blood studies are performed in addition to examination of blood, urine, and gastric contents for toxicological analysis. A chest radiograph is obtained, and serial arterial blood gas determinations are performed to evaluate the degree of hypoventilation.

In general, hypotension and tachycardia are not reliably present. The temperature is normal in the majority of patients with heroin-induced pulmonary edema and, in one series, 56% of patients had clear lungs on auscultation (Duberstein and Kaufman, 1971). The chest radiograph may be normal or show evidence of pulmonary edema. Other non-specific findings include leukocytosis and an abnormal electrocardiogram with conduction disturbances or atrial fibrillation.

The cornerstones of treatment include administration of an opiate antagonist (Millman, 1985; Martin, 1976) and oxygen therapy (Senay et al., 1982). There are a number of opiate antagonists. Undesirable opiate agonist effects have been observed with nalorphine and cyclazocine. Naloxone (Narcan) with its short duration of action is the drug of choice for acute opiate overdose. Naloxone should be given to any comatose patient where overdose is suspected and when there is significant respiratory depression. The use of naloxone in patients with tachypnea is not recommended, to avoid precipitating withdrawal symptoms. The usual dose is 0.4 mg intravenously (Nicholson, 1983; Millman, 1985) which can be repeated every 3 to 5 min as needed. Therapy should be continued until the patient is aroused and has adequate alveolar ventilation. Because the duration of action of naloxone is short—60-90 min (Handal et al., 1983; Evans et al., 1974), naloxone may be administered again after 2-3 hr as necessary. If the overdose was from a long-acting narcotic such as methadone, naloxone may need to be given over a 24-hr period. Usually responses to naloxone are dramatic. If there is no response in the sensorium, pupillary status, or respiratory rate to the naloxone, causes other than opiates, such as additional concomitant drug ingestion (e.g., sedatives or other drug abuse) or head trauma, should be considered. Gastric lavage may be indicated in those who have ingested other oral drugs. Oxygen and endotracheal intubation with mechanical ventilation are indicated transiently for severe respiratory depression and coma. Intravenous fluids and dopamine may be needed for hypotension. Aspiration pneumonia or bacterial pneumonia may be frequent and should be managed with the appropriate antibiotics. Pneumonia was present in 30% of 149 patients with heroin overdose in one study (Duberstein and Kaufman, 1971). Recovery in uncomplicated cases is typically rapid, with many patients feeling well in minutes to hours.

Opiate overdose victims with complicating pulmonary edema appear more acutely ill. Patients are usually cyanotic and frequently have a frothy white edema exuding from nostrils and mouth. On physical examination, diffuse bilateral crackles are present. On x-rays, there are typically bilateral, diffuse, fluffy acinar infiltrates extending almost to the periphery, though radiographic asymmetry may be present. Severe arterial hypoxemia and hypercapnia are noted. Clinical suspicion of pulmonary edema in a setting of opiate overdose should always be high. Therapy similar to that for uncomplicated opiate overdose, with a narcotic antagonist and supportive measures, is fundamental. However, endotracheal intubation with mechanical ventilation may be required and, in cases of gastric aspiration, the institution of positive end-expiratory pressure is often beneficial (Light and Dunham, 1975). The use of corticosteroids and prophylactic antibiotics may be indicated in this setting, although no prospective studies have been completed to confirm their utility. Patients with uncomplicated pulmonary edema frequently recover within 2-3 days.

After the acute treatment, therapy for the narcotic addiction will depend on the severity of the drug dependence and the psychosocial aspects of the patient. Various detoxification programs have been advocated including methadone and clonidine (Catapres) substitution for the opiate addiction (Millman, 1985; Gold et al., 1980). Methadone is given in a dose of 20-40 mg per day or more depending on the drug tolerance of the patient. The mental and respiratory status of the patient is monitored on methadone therapy. Often, the patient wants a progressive increase in his methadone dose, and a short-acting sedative drug in the form of lorazepam (Ativan) may be added to reduce the withdrawal symptoms. The use of methadone can be continued for short- or long-term maintenance or gradually tapered over a 1-2 week period as a form of detoxification. Clonidine (Catapres), an alpha-adrenergic agonist approved as an antihypertensive medication, has also been demonstrated to relieve many of the symptoms of narcotic drug withdrawal (Gold et al., 1978; Charney et al., 1981). Initially, it can be given in divided doses of 0.1-0.2 mg and increased to a maximum of 1-1.5 mg daily in three divided doses in 4-10 days (Millman, 1985).

Finally, naltrexone, a new narcotic antagonist with the potential for blocking the effects of narcotics and thus preventing the physical dependence, has been approved by the Food and Drug Administration in 1984 for treatment of chronic narcotic addiction (Kleber and Kosten, 1984; Kleber, 1985; Kleber et al., 1985; Washton et al., 1984). It is a long-acting narcotic antagonist that is given orally and has few side effects. Several phases are needed in the naltrexone treatment program. In the induction phase, the patient is withdrawn from narcotics and then begins naltrexone after being off narcotics for 7-10 days. After a naloxone test dose to determine abstinence, a maintenance dose of 50 mg/day of naltrexone is administered for a few days. This is then switched to a maintenance regime of 100 mg on Monday and Wednesday and 150 mg on Friday. In the stabilization phase, which lasts for about 4 weeks, withdrawal symptoms may be ameliorated with antianxiety medications or low dose clonidine. Finally, in the maintenance phase, the drug should be continued for a number of months, and in some patients, indefinitely in combination with psychotherapy. Recently, in the treatment of opiate withdrawal symptoms, clonidine hydrochloride in combination with naltrexone has been shown to be rapid, safe, and effective therapy for abrupt withdrawal from methadone (Charney et al., 1986). Psychotherapy, counseling, and family support are other important factors that are needed beside detoxification drug therapy in the management of narcotic drug abuse. In addition to methadone and naltrexone maintenance, the residential therapeutic community (e.g., Daytop) and self-help groups (e.g., Narcotics Anonymous) are frequently used for treatment. Regardless of the method of treatment, relapse back to narcotics is frequent and the condition is best described as a chronic relapsing disease.

II. Marijuana

A. History

Marijuana is one of the oldest intoxicants known. Derived from the plant *Cannabis sativa,* which was cultivated in the past for the hemp fiber, marijuana has been eaten, cooked, smoked, and sniffed for thousands of years for its euphoric effect. It was grown in China nearly 5000 years ago for its fiber and medicinal properties (Camp, 1936) and the Chinese Emperor Shen Nung in 2723 B.C. documented the use of cannabis in herbal medicine (Rubin, 1975). Cannabis was unknown to the Western hemisphere until the 16th century (Ames, 1936). In the middle of the 19th century, marijuana was used in Western medicine in the treatment of pain, convulsion, insomnia, asthma, and other medical disorders. With the discovery of new synthetic drugs and better understanding of their pharmacologic actions, the medicinal use of marijuana waned in the early 20th century. In the 1920s there was significant recreational and social use of the drug as an intoxicant, and the United States Congress enacted in 1937 the Marijuana Tax Act, which declared illegal the use of marijuana. However, other countries continued to allow use of the drug and in 1956, the United Nations Commission on Narcotic Drugs estimated there were over 200 million regular users (Tashkin and Cohen, 1981). In the 1960s marijuana regained its popularity as an intoxicant in the United States. Recently, it has been estimated that 57 million Americans have used marijuana (Miller et al., 1983), and possession of small amounts has been decriminalized in 11 states. Today, marijuana, also known as pot, weed, grass, Acapulco gold, and Mary Jane, is one of the most widely used drugs in our society. Only tobacco, ethanol, and caffeine exceed it in usage (Khantzian and McKenna, 1979). The names for cannabis preparations vary in different countries; the pure resin is known as hashish in the United States and charas in India; flowering tops as ganja in India; dried mature leaves as bhang in India and the Middle East; and the smoking mixture as marijuana in America and Europe, kif in North Africa, dagga in South Africa, and macohna in Brazil (Pillard, 1970).

Cannibus sativa is a hardy plant that grows well in temperate and tropical climates. Formerly the plant was cultivated for natural hemp fiber from its stem, but with the production of synthetic fibers, the plant has been grown mainly for its intoxicants. From the seed of the plant, varnish or paint can also be manufactured. It is from the flowering tops, especially from the female plants, that the resin with the active intoxicants—cannabinoids—are found. In earlier years, marijuana sold on the street was a crude preparation of the whole plant including flowers, leaves, seeds, and stems. Inhalation of marijuana smoke is the most popular method for obtaining rapid absorption and the euphoric effect of the drug. The preparation is normally hand-rolled into a cigarette commonly called a joint and smoked down to a small butt ("roach"). Marijuana can also be ingested but has the disadvantage of slow absorption (Lemberger et al., 1972).

Hashish is a more refined preparation from the *Cannabis sativa* plant with 5-10 times more tetrahydrocannabinol (THC) per weight than marijuana (Pillard, 1970; Henderson et al., 1972). The active ingredients in the hemp plant are concentrated in the resin at the flowering top of the plant, and hashish is prepared by scraping this resin from the plant. This refined product is usually marketed in small compressed briquets and smoked with a pipe. The hashish is shaved from the briquet into the pipe bowl; a small piece of screen is placed in the bottom of the bowl to prevent the inhalation of burning and irritating particles (Tennant et al., 1971). Corrected for differences in potency, the physiological and psychological effects of hashish are essentially identical to those of marijuana.

B. Pharmacology and Toxicology

Extensive efforts have been made to analyze the chemical composition of marijuana. The crude preparation contains approximately 420 compounds (Turner, 1980; Turner et al., 1980) and with pyrolysis the chemical complexity is increased. In the 1940s tetrahydrocannabinol was suspected to be the active agent. Not until the early 1960s was the major psychoactive ingredient, delta-9-trans-tetrahydrocannabinol (delta-9-THC) isolated in its pure form (Gaoni and Mechoulam, 1964). Delta-9-THC ($C_{21} H_{28} O_2$) is a noncrystalline, highly lipophilic compound and its lack of water solubility precludes parenteral administration. Delta-9-THC is also rather unstable and is degraded by heat, light, acids, and atmospheric oxygen, which accounts for the fact that it tends to lose potency with storage. The concentration of delta-9-THC varies with different species and sources of marijuana. Cannabis contains, in addition to delta-9-THC, many other cannabinoids, esters, and alkaloids. The principal cannabinoids include delta-9-THC, delta-8-THC, and cannabidiol (CBD) (Mechoulam, 1970). Three main marijuana types can be classified according to their cannabinoid content: drug type (THC $>$ 1% and CBD$=$0; intermediate drug type (THC $>$ 0.50% and CBD $>$ 0.50%); and fiber type (THC $<$ 0.25% and CBD $>$ 0.50%) (Paris and Nahas, 1984). The chemical analyses were done with the technique described by Doorenbos and co-workers (1971). Cannabinoids are also present with decreasing concentration in the leaves and bracts of the plant. Over the past decade there has been a steady trend toward higher levels of THC as marijuana preparations are increasingly limited to the flowering tops of the plants and higher THC-producing species of *C. sativa* are cultivated. Thus, the potency of street marijuana has increased (NIDA, 1982).

There is a significant difference in the bioavailability of delta-9-THC when it is administered by the oral or inhalational routes (King et al., 1976). Oral administration of marijuana produces erratic and lower plasma levels compared with smoking. Smoking marijuana can achieve plasma kinetics of THC similar to that following intravenous administration (Ohlsson et al., 1980). The amount of marijuana absorbed depends on the degree of inhalation, user experience, and the potency or concentration of the drug in the cigarette. Therefore, when a marijuana cigarette is smoked, the amount of THC absorbed will vary; it has been estimated that less than 50% of the delta-9-THC is absorbed. Gas chromatography mass spectrometry has been used for measurement of delta-9-THC in blood and tissues (Fishbein, 1982; Harvey et al., 1980). In the blood, about 3% of the delta-9-THC is in the free state, with the remaining 97% bound to protein where lipoprotein seems to be the main binding site (Wahlqvist et al., 1970). Pharmacologic effects begin within minutes and peak in 10-20 min after the plasma concentrations have attained their peak at 7-8 min with the initial smoking (Perez-Reyes et al., 1982). The total effect lasts less than 3 hr. It has been estimated that subjects experience the "high" of marijuana at a blood level of above 2 ng/ml after smoking and above 0.2 ng/ml after oral use (Harvey, 1984). Thus there is a difficulty in interpreting the plasma THC level and evaluating the psychoactive effects (Cohen, 1986). Delta-9-THC is converted to an inactive metabolite mainly through biliary excretion and is excreted in the feces and urine.

Tolerance develops relatively rapidly to the behavioral and physiological effects of the drug but also decays rapidly. Physical dependency may develop following heavy usage but the withdrawal symptoms are mild (Jones and Benowitz, 1976).

C. Neuropsychological Effects

It is the intoxicating psychic effects of marijuana that have led to its widespread abuse. Most marijuana smokers experience an increased sense of relaxation and happiness. A subjective feeling of exhiliration, euphoria, and peacefulness is reported as characteristic of a marijuana high in the majority of 100 regular users (Table 4) (Halikas et al., 1971). Other commonly experienced sensations included increased hunger and thirst, an altered perception of space and time, increased auditory, smell, touch and taste effects and better sleep (Tart, 1970). While these psychological effects are common to frequent users, it is known that less experienced smokers have less of a subjective response (Stark-Adamec et al., 1981).

Associated with these relatively mild subjective psychological effects, there is a transient intellectual and psychomotor influence. Studies have demonstrated mild intellectual deficits in the setting of marijuana intoxication, including impaired short- and long-term memory and difficulty with simple computation, concepts, and oral communication (Nicholi, 1983). Psychomotor deficiencies with impairment of fine motor coordination have been observed. Sensory, perceptual, and tracking dysfunctions may be seen and present one of the more dangerous aspects of marijuana intoxication. The more affected individuals may be a potential danger to themselves or others when driving or flying, due to impaired ability to perform (Smiley et al., 1981; Janowsky et al., 1976). Because of these psychophysiological and psychomotor effects of marijuana some private industries and government institutions have implemented programs to detect marijuana or other drug abuse in their employees through urine tests (Dogoloff et al., 1985; Schwartz and Hawks, 1985). Urine testing, however, indicates only whether or not an individual has smoked or ingested marijuana, and does not measure impairment (Mason and McBay, 1985). Furthermore, passive inhalation of marijuana smoke resulted in detection of cannabinoids in the urine and blood of healthy volunteers (Morland et al., 1985). These adverse intellectual and psychomotor effects usually resolve in 8-12 hr.

Beyond these relatively mild intoxicating properties, in higher doses marijuana has significant acute adverse psychological effects. Feelings of depersonalization, derealization, despondency, anxiety, and frank sensory hallucinations become increasingly common especially when the drug is smoked by naive subjects (Isbell et al., 1967). Infrequently, frank acute psychosis (Hart, 1976) may develop. Studies from France (Moreau, 1845), India (Ewens, 1904; Chopra, 1971), United States (Mayor's Committee on Marihuana, 1944), Sweden (Bernhardson and Gunn, 1972; Tunving, 1985), England (Carney et al., 1984), and United States troops in Vietnam (Talbott and Teague, 1969) have reported multiple cases of marijuana-induced acute psychosis (Chopra and Smith, 1974; Kaplan, 1971). The symptoms include emotional instability, rapid mood swings,

Table 4   Effects During Marihuana Intoxication (No. = 100)

	Occurrence (%)		
	Usually (> 50%)	Occasionally	Once or never
Acute effects			
High feeling (exhilarated, euphoric)	82	17	1
Relaxation	79	21	0
Keener sound sense	76	21	3
Peaceful	74	25	1
Increased sensitivity	74	23	3
Increased hunger	72	24	4
Time slowed down	62	35	3
Increased thirst	62	32	6
Dry mouth and throat	61	38	1
Aftereffects			
Calm	60	32	8
Mind clear	56	39	5
More restful sleep	52 (10-50)	42	6
Awaken refreshed	44	46	10
Driving well	36	20	37
More sleep	29	51	20
Increased appetite	27	36	37
More dreams	24	37	36
Clearer thinking	18	53	29
More alert and sensitive	17	55	28
Happy or euphoric	16	62	22
Fewer dreams	13	32	52
Improved sexual performance	11	31	50

Adapted in part from Halikas et al., 1971.

mania, irresistible impulses, delusions, illusions, and hallucinations. The latter are rare except when related to use of potent marijuana resulting in very high blood levels (Brill and Nahas, 1984). Although it has been stated that cannabis use does not lead to violence (Abel, 1977; Mendelson et al., 1974), in some individuals placed in certain settings, destructive behavior and violence may occur (Talbott and Teague, 1969). While the subjects who experience acute psychosis from marijuana generally had no predating history of mental illness, it is clear that individuals with underlying psychiatric illness are particularly prone to the acute psychotoxic reaction. Many studies have demonstrated that patients with schizophrenia or other psychiatric illness are more likely to relapse following marijuana abuse (Brill and Nahas, 1984; Carney et al., 1984; Szymanski, 1981; Treffert, 1978; Thacore and Shukla, 1976; Harding and Knight, 1973).

Instead of the "high" and elevation of mood commonly associated with marijuana use, some individuals may experience the acute effects of cannabis intoxication, which vary from anxiety (Keeler, 1967) and panic states (Bromberg, 1934; Weil, 1970) to acute psychosis (Talbott and Teague, 1969; Chopra, 1971). Even in chronic marijuana users, 16% of this group of one hundred individuals had adverse effects including anxiety, fear, amnesia, confusion and hallucinations (Halikas et al., 1971). In an informal survey of Boston University Student Health Service with a student population of 20,000, about five to seven adverse anxiety reactions to marijuana were reported yearly, however, these figures are probably underestimated (Pillard, 1970). Other adverse effects include paranoia and "flashbacks," a delayed re-enactment or repeat of the original experience of marijuana several days or months after abstinence from cannabis use (Keeler et al., 1968; Smith, 1968; Pillard, 1970; Anderson, 1973), and dysphoric reactions consisting of disorientation, catatonia-like immobility, acute panic, and heavy sedation (Brill and Nahas, 1984; Ablon and Goodwin, 1974).

The chronic use of marijuana may have adverse neuropsychological effects compounding these acute effects. With habitual use, an amotivational syndrome consisting of apathy, loss of ambition, lethargy, difficulty in concentration, impaired judgment and memory, and social deterioration has been observed (Smith, 1968; Miras, 1969; Campbell, 1976; Cohen, 1986), even though the existence of this syndrome is questioned by some psychiatrists. Although acute cannabis intoxication may cause an acute psychosis in normal or subjects predisposed to mental illness, the role of chronic abuse in the causation of chronic psychiatric disease remains controversial (Brill and Nahas, 1984). After chronic and mild cannabis abuse, anxiety, anorexia, sweating, tremors, muscle spasms, and restlessness may occur with sudden discontinuation (Jones and Benowitz, 1976). These withdrawal symptoms seldom persist for more than 3 days and the dependency associated with marijuana is minimal compared to that with narcotic abuse. In a recent follow-up study of regular marijuana users, depression, alcohol abuse, and antisocial personality were further increased in chronic marijuana users. These diagnoses however, were present in the initial interview (Weller and Halikas, 1985). In general, evidence for long-term significant adverse psychological effects of marijuana are inconclusive. Chronic marijuana users do not show any signs of cerebral atrophy on computer-assisted tomography (Co et al., 1977; Kuehule et al., 1977) or significant abnormalities on electroencephalographic studies (Rodin et al., 1970; Fink, 1976), although others report adverse central nervous system development in neonates and adolescents (Fried, 1980; Nahas, 1984).

D. Pathophysiological Effects

Distinct from the neuropsychological effects, cannabis has significant pharmacologic effects on the pulmonary (Tashkin et al., 1973; Tashkin and Cohen, 1981; Tilles et al., 1986), and cardiovascular systems (Renault et al., 1971; Beaconsfield et al., 1972; Tashkin et al., 1977). There is evidence for effects on the reproductive system (Kolodny et al., 1974; Hembree et al., 1979; Smith et al., 1983) and chromosomal integrity in the immune system (Nahas et al., 1974; Cushman and Khurana, 1977) though the clinical significance of these observations is unclear (Rachelefsky et al., 1976).

When a marijuana cigarette is smoked, one of the most consistent effects is on the cardiovascular system. The heart rate, systemic blood pressure, peripheral blood flow and cardiac output are increased (Beaconsfield et al., 1972; Tashkin et al., 1977; Gash et al., 1978). These effects seem to be in part dose dependent (Renault et al., 1971). They may be mediated through the beta-adrenergic system since pretreatment with propranolol has been shown to block the increase in heart rate (Beaconsfield et al., 1972; Kanakis et al., 1976). Increases in heart rate of 15-65 beats/min have been observed and occasionally tachycardia of 140 beats/min may result. Exercise performance appears to be slightly reduced (Shapiro et al., 1976). Electrocardiographic and arrhythmias have been noted (Johnson and Domino, 1971; Kochar and Hosko, 1973), although others have failed to show these changes (Benowitz and Jones, 1975). In young healthy individuals, these consequences on the cardiovascular system of marijuana smoking are of little clinical significance. However, in elderly patients or those with coronary artery disease, cerebrovascular disease, or hypertension, these effects can be harmful and at times life-threatening. One study showed a significant increase in angina in older patients who smoke marijuana (Aronow and Cassidy, 1974). In addition, in patients with coronary artery disease a decrease in stroke index, cardiac index, and ejection fraction after marijuana smoking may occur due to delta-9-tetrahydrocannabinol with an increase in carboxyhemoglobin level (Prakash et al., 1975).

The pulmonary effects of cannabis smoking have been well described (Vachon et al., 1973; Tashkin et al., 1973, 1980). Controlled studies have established that marijuana, either inhaled or ingested orally is a bronchodilator. In one study, 32 healthy experienced male marijuana smokers were found to have an immediate significant increase in specific airway conductance, achieving peak levels at 15 min that lasted as long as 60 min following use of a single marijuana cigarette (Tashkin et al., 1973). These findings indicate dilatation of airways. Bronchodilator effect are prolonged (up to 6 hr) with oral ingestion of marijuana. An increase in flow rates and normal ventilatory response to carbon dioxide inhalation has been shown (Vachon et al., 1973). In contrast, Zwillich et al., (1978) showed that marijuana is both a respiratory and metabolic stimulant, causing a significant increase in the ventilatory response to hypercapnia and no change in the ventilatory response to hypoxia.

Although marijuana is a potent bronchodilator when smoked, other compounds in the marijuana smoke may be irritating to the respiratory tract and cause bronchitis (Waldman, 1970; Henderson et al., 1972), as well as a mild airway obstruction in very heavy marijuana users who smoked for 6-8 weeks (Tashkin et al., 1976).

When used on a chronic basis, the bronchodilator properties of delta-9-tetrahydrocannabinol of marijuana become clinically insignificant and are overshadowed by the inflammatory responses in the tracheobronchial tree. Symptomatically heavy cannabis smokers, particularly those smoking hashish, may have pharyngitis, rhinitis, and bronchitis. Bronchoscopy with biopsies of tracheal mucosa in six hashish smokers who smoked 50 g or more of hashish a month showed abnormal respiratory mucosae with atypical cells, epithelial cell hyperplasia, and loss of cilia (Henderson et al., 1972). Using the technique of bronchoalveolar lavage in marijuana smokers, there is an increase in the cell count of the respiratory cells similar to that in cigarette smokers, with an increase in differential cell count of polymorphonuclear cells compared to nonsmokers (Reynolds and Chretien, 1984).

In a study of 74 regular marijuana smokers, there were no differences in spirometric indices of FVC, FEV_1, or $FEF_{25-75\%}$, or tests of small airways, but there were significant differences in the airway resistance and specific airway conductance between the marijuana smokers and matched control nonsmokers of marijuana (Tashkin et al., 1980). Abnormalities involving the large airways are therefore suggested. Recently it has shown that there was a reduction in single breath carbon monoxide diffusing capacity (65% of predicted) in nine healthy females who smoked marijuana heavily, even when cigarette smoking was taken into account (Tilles et al., 1986). These subjects had normal total lung capacity and spirometry. However, in a series of 279 young habitual smokers of marijuana (with or without concomitant cigarette smoking in 35 and 144, respectively), the diffusing capacity of marijuana smokers without tobacco was comparable to the diffusing capacity of nonsmoking control subjects. Even

Table 5 Adjusted Means for Lung Function Measures by Sex and Marijuana and Tobacco-Smoking Status

Men (n = 259)

Lung function measure	Marijuana smokers		Control subjects	
	Current tobacco	Never or former tobacco	Current tobacco	Never or former tobacco
	(n=82)	(n=94)	(n=27)	(n=56)
FVC (liters)	5.42	5.52	5.51	5.35
FEV_1 (liters)	4.38	4.50	4.54	4.38
FEV_1/FVC (%)	81.15	81.57	82.59	82.03
FEF_{25-75} (liters/sec)	4.29	4.45	4.70	4.30
$\dot{V}max_{25}$ (liters/sec)	9.12	8.99	9.14	8.56
$\dot{V}max_{50}$ (liters/sec)	5.06	5.15	5.47	4.92
$\dot{V}max_{75}$ (liters/sec)	2.14	2.25	2.22	2.19
$\Delta\dot{V}max_{50}$ (%)	35.30	42.98	40.17	34.93
$Viso\dot{V}$ (%)	23.1	19.6	19.1	18.6
$\Delta N_2/L$ (%)	0.88	0.74	0.79	0.70
CV/VC (%)	10.05	9.06	11.98	8.79
CC/TLC (%)	32.49	30.86	35.29	33.01
DLCO (ml/min/mmHg)	28.68	31.03	29.88	32.13
TLC (liters)	7.23	7.25	7.49	7.27
FRC (liters)	3.55	3.53	3.82	3.75
RV (liters)	1.83	1.74	2.00	1.95
Raw (cmH_2O/liter/sec)	1.79	1.87	1.48	1.49
SGaw (L/cmH_2O/liter/sec)	0.19	0.19	0.21	0.22

	Women (n = 128)			
	(n=31)	(n=32)	(n=29)	(n=36)
FVC (liters)	3.94	3.70	3.65	3.88
FEV_1 (liters)	3.24	3.10	3.02	3.30
FEV_1/FVC (%)	82.49	83.74	82.94	85.44
FEF_{25-75} (liters/sec)	3.31	3.30	3.41	3.69
$\dot{V}max_{25}$ (liters/sec)	6.67	6.48	6.48	6.62
$\dot{V}max_{50}$ (liters/sec)	3.91	3.85	3.91	4.29
$\dot{V}max_{75}$ (liters/sec)	1.69	1.72	1.65	1.92
$\Delta \dot{V}max_{50}$ (%)	32.94	41.41	28.52	41.63
Viso$\dot{V}$ (%)	26.4	22.0	24.5	19.7
$\Delta N_2/L$ (%)	1.28	1.11	1.52	0.92
CV/VC (%)	10.67	10.32	12.12	9.34
CC/TLC (%)	37.01	36.84	41.63	36.50
DLCO (ml/min/mmHg)	22.04	24.04	21.05	26.05
TLC (liters)	5.61	5.24	5.36	5.47
FRC (liters)	2.88	2.74	2.94	2.83
RV (liters)	1.66	1.55	1.72	1.60
Raw (cmH_2O/liter/sec)	1.91	2.30	1.77	1.96
SGaw (L/cmH_2O/liter/sec)	0.22	0.20	0.23	0.22

$\dot{V}max_{25}$, $\dot{V}max_{50}$, $\dot{V}max_{75}$, flow rates 25, 50, and 75% of FVC, respectively; $\Delta \dot{V}max_{50}$, change in maximal expiratory flow between curves obtained breathing 80% helium–20% oxygen and breathing air at 50% of the vital capacity; Viso$\dot{V}$, volume of isoflow; $\Delta N_2/L$, change in nitrogen concentration per liter in phase III of single-breath nitrogen washout curve; CV, closing volume; CC, closing capacity; Raw, airway resistance; SGaw, specific airway conductance.

(From Tashkin et al., 1987.)

when cigarette smoking was taken into account, the diffusing capacity was little affected (diffusing capacity in male marijuana smokers with tobacco smoke was 28.68 ml/min/mmHg versus 29.88 ml/min/mmHg in control male cigarette smokers) (Tashkin, personal communications; Tashkin et al., 1987) (Table 5). Furthermore, the marijuana smoker has normal spirometric and lung volume studies including tests for small airway functions, but lower values for airway resistance and specific airway conductance compared to control smokers and nonsmokers, thus confirming the investigators earlier study (Tashkin et al., 1980). While heavy marijuana smoking appears to have an irritating and inflammatory effect on the tracheobronchial tree and alveoli, these effects seem to be generally mild on lung function.

Another pulmonary consideration is the carcinogenic potential of cannabis smoke (Cohen, 1981). Experimental evidence appears to indicate carcinogenicity comparable to that of tobacco smoke (Hoffman et al., 1975). Comparable concentrations of the volatile nitrosamines are found in tobacco and marijuana smokes and the "tar" yield is similar. Also, marijuana smoke has a higher concentration of polynuclear aromatic hydrocarbons, which are known carcinogens. The carcinogens benzopyrene and benzanthracene have been shown to be much higher in marijuana tar than in tobacco tar (Hoffman et al., 1975; Novotny et al., 1976). When marijuana smoke condensate is painted on mouse skin, metaplasia of sebaceous glands (Magus and Harris, 1971; Cottrell et al., 1973) and carcinogenicity have been shown, although marijuana tar had less tumorigenicity than tobacco tar (Hoffman et al., 1975). Similarly to tobacco smoke, marijuana also results in abnormalities in growth, DNA synthesis, and mitosis in animal and human lung cultures (Leuchtenberger and Leuchtenberger, 1976). While these experimental findings suggest the carcinogenicity of marijuana, the clinical significance of these observations remains to be elucidated. No clinical study has correlated an increase in incidence of lung carcinoma with marijuana smoking. While it appears that a carcinogenic risk exists with marijuana smoking, the magnitude of this risk remains to be determined (Nahas, 1984).

A pulmonary consequence occasionally seen with marijuana smoking is the result of marijuana contaminants rather than an intrinsic property of cannabis itself. *Aspergillus*, paraquat, *Salmonella*, and other pathogenic bacterial contamination has been documented (Taylor et al., 1982; Kagen, 1981; Marijuana and Health, 1980; Ungerleider et al., 1982). Bacterial contamination of marijuana with *Salmonella muenchen* caused outbreaks of gastroenteritis in Ohio and Michigan (Taylor et al., 1982) as a result of ingestion of the *Salmonella* organism by hand-to-mouth or cigarette-to-mouth contamination. These investigators postulated that the marijuana contamination may be due to fertilization of marijuana plants with untreated animal manure, contamination during drying or storage, or adulteration with dried animal manure to increase the weight. Other pathogenic gram-negative bacteria (*Klebsiella pneumoniae, Enterobacter agglomerans, Enterococcus, Bacillus* species, and *Enterobacter cloacae*) have been incriminated as contaminants in marijuana intended for therapeutic use in cancer patients (Ungerleider et al., 1982). The fungus *Aspergillus* is frequently found in old and moldy marijuana, and there are case reports of *Aspergillus*-contaminated marijuana causing pulmonary disease, including allergic bronchopulmonary aspergillosis (Llamas et al., 1978), fungal sensitization (Kagen, 1981; Kagen et al., 1983), and invasive pneumonitis in a 17-year-old boy with granulomatous disease (Chusid et al., 1975). In the latter case, there was an associated defect in phagocytic function, which may be the reason for the susceptibility to the *Aspergillus* pneumonitis. Therefore for cancer patients who are to smoke marijuana to control nausea and vomiting, the marijuana should be prepared in a sterile condition either with ethylene oxide or radiation (Ungerleider et al., 1982).

In the marijuana eradication programs in the 1970s, particularly in Mexico, paraquat which was used as a defoliant, was sprayed onto the marijuana fields. Initially paraquat was thought to be quickly deactivated biologically, however, it was subsequently suggested that continuous heavy use of paraquat-sprayed marijuana may be hazardous (Smith et al., 1978b) and cause lung fibrosis (Thurlbeck et al., 1976). Taken by mouth, paraquat has been shown to cause pulmonary fibrosis (Copland et al., 1974), and in experimental animals given paraquat by the intrabronchial route, the lung shows focal hemorrhage, congestion of capillaries, and moderate thickening of the alveolar septa (Zavala and Rhodes, 1978). Motivated by these findings, paraquat spraying was discontinued. However, there are no reported cases of lung damage or fibrosis due to paraquat sprayed marijuana in humans (Tashkin and Cohen, 1981; Tilles et al., 1986). Furthermore, when paraquat, which is highly water soluble, is pyrolyzed, the major portion is destroyed by pyrolysis, and it is changed to bipyridine, a respiratory irritant present also in tobacco smoke. These factors may account for the minimal effect, if any, of paraquat-sprayed marijuana on the lung.

In addition to these cardiovascular and pulmonary effects, other medical consequences of marijuana have been suggested. Prominent among these are observations that marijuana has adverse effect on reproductive function (Kolodny et al., 1974; Bauman, 1980), and fetal growth during prenatal exposure (Hingson et al., 1983); and appears to impair some indices of immune functions (Nahas et al., 1974). In a group of 20 chronic marijuana smokers, a dose-related oligospermia was found, which was associated with a decrease in plasma testosterone levels with no alteration in luteinizing hormone, follicle-stimulating hormone, or prolactin levels (Kolodny et al., 1974). Other authors have not noted a reduction in plasma testosterone levels in marijuana smokers

(Mendelson et al., 1974; Coggins et al., 1976). Pubertal arrest has been reported in a 16-year-old who smoked marijuana for a few years (Copeland et al., 1980). In females, chronic anovulatory ovarian cycles have been observed in marijuana smokers (Bauman, 1980). However, minimal alteration in the menstrual cycles has been noted in another study (Smith et al., 1983). Fetal growth and retardation were shown to occur in mothers who smoked marijuana during pregnancy (Hingson et al., 1983), as well as the neonatal abstinence syndrome noted in babies exposed to marijuana in utero (Fried, 1980).

Several studies have shown an effect of marijuana on the immune system (Gupta et al., 1974; Cushman et al., 1976; Nahas et al., 1979). Changes in function and structure of the pulmonary macrophages in marijuana smokers have been demonstrated (Mann et al., 1971; Huber et al., 1975). Other studies have however failed to demonstrate changes in humoral or cell-mediated immunity in chronic marijuana smoking (Rachelefsky, 1976; White et al., 1976) or ability of the alveolar macrophages to phagocytize viable bacteria (Drath et al., 1979). Further studies are needed to evaluate the effects of chronic marijuana smoking on the immune system in patients who are immunosuppressed, since the drug has antiemetic effect and is useful in the treatment of nausea and vomiting in cancer patients (Chang et al., 1979; Poster et al., 1981).

E. Clinical Evaluation and Therapy

Considering that more than 50 million Americans have used marijuana (Nicholi, 1983) and that 20 million Americans use marijuana daily, remarkably few seek medical attention. Even in a large city, emergency room visits related strictly to marijuana smoking are a rarity. Acute fatal toxicity of cannabis is extremely rare (Heyndrickx, 1970). The adverse acute psychological reactions occasionally bring marijuana smokers to the health care system. Patients with anxiety reactions and panic attacks associated with acute intoxication occasionally seek medical attention. These reactions are usually self limited resolving within several hours, and are best treated conservatively with reassurance (Cohen, 1986), a quiet setting, and occasionally a benzodiazepine. Acute toxic reactions with delirium or organic psychosis are comparatively rare. Reactions of this severity may indicate the presence of other abused drugs, particularly phencyclidine in the smoked substance. While these reactions are self-limited, they can require hospitalization and observation. Rarely, symptoms may last for months to years; there is a report of chronic cannabis psychosis lasting for more than 1 year (Tunving, 1985). It may be difficult to attribute the chronic psychosis to marijuana, as opposed to underlying mental disorder and attempts should be made to distinguish the chronic cannabis syndrome from other psychopathology. A trial of abstinence from marijuana use in patients with the chronic cannabis syndrome can lead to an increase in alertness and physical ability (Cohen, 1986) when coupled with psychotherapy.

III. Phencyclidine

A. History

Phencyclidine (1-[1-phenylcyclohexyl] piperidine hydrochloride) was synthesized about 30 years ago for surgical anesthesia (Greifenstein, 1958; Chen et al., 1959), and the drug was marketed in the United States in 1963 as a nonnarcotic dissociative anesthetic agent, Sernyl, with its chemical structure similar to ketamine. However, in 1965, the drug was quickly withdrawn because of a large number of postoperative adverse reactions including delirium, agitation, hallucination, psychosis and seizures (Burns and Lerner, 1976; Smith et al., 1978). It was used later as a veterinary agent (Sernylan) before its subsequent total removal from the market. Phencyclidine (PCP) first appeared as a street drug in 1967 in the Haight-Ashbury District in San Francisco (Meyers et al., 1968). It soon fell into disfavor however due to its reputation for frequent bad trips (Stein, 1973; Fauman et al., 1976). In the 1970s, the drug began to appear on the illicit drug market but was misrepresented as other psychoactive drugs including marijuana, mescaline, cocaine, and LSD because of its unpleasant effects. The sale of phencyclidine was attractive to drug traffickers, since PCP is easily manufactured illegally, with a production cost of approximately 5 cents for a street dose (Giannini and Price, 1985). As a result, PCP became a common ingredient in illicit street preparations (Lundberg et al., 1976; Rainey and Crowder, 1974). One survey showed 78% of street preparations to be adulterated with PCP (Hart et al., 1972), though most analyses showed a lower range of 10-26% (Lundberg et al., 1976). In the late 1970s and early 1980s phencyclidine had become increasingly accepted on the drug scene and is often sold without adulteration. It is a powerful, satisfying, mind-altering drug that is inexpensive and widely available. Recent national surveys estimate that 8 million Americans have used the drug including 5-1/2 million young people between the ages of 12 and 25 years (Nicholi, 1983). In one study of 981 patients with PCP intoxication, the median age was 23 years (McCarron et al., 1981). PCP's widespread use has been called an epidemic (Davis, 1982) though it clearly is used far less than marijuana and cocaine (Fishburne et al., 1980).

PCP has scores of exotic street names including angel dust, hog, animal tranquilizer, cadillac, crystal joints, cyclone, goon, killer joints, mist, peace, pig, killer, rocket fuel, and supergrass (Perry, 1976; Beede, 1980). It is most commonly sold on the street in combination with parsley leaves or other herbs that can be rolled into a cigarette and smoked as a "joint." PCP can also be bought in tablet form, often in combination with other illicit drugs. Occasionally PCI is taken orally or snorted and only rarely is it injected intravenously (McCarron, 1986).

B. Pharmacology and Toxicology

When PCP is smoked, the onset of action may be within a few minutes; peak
activity is normally reached in 15-30 min and the effects may last from 4 to 6
hr or even longer, dependent on the dose (Burns and Lerner, 1976; Petersen and
Stillman, 1978). With oral administration of PCP, the onset of effects is within
45 min, peak effect is achieved by 1.5 hr and lasts for 1 to 3 hr. Immediate effects are obtained with intravenous PCP, which has a duration of prominent symptoms of 1 to 2 hr (Cook et al., 1982a). The half-life of PCP is estimated from 11
to 89 hr (Giannini and Price, 1985). The drug is metabolized by hydroxylation
in the liver into weakly active components and significant quantities of PCP are
excreted unchanged in the urine (Cook et al., 1982a,b). The neurophysiologic
mechanism of action of PCP is not well defined. PCP acts primarily on the central nervous system with stimulatory, depressant, hallucinogenic, and analgesic
effects. It inhibits the metabolism of multiple neurotransmitters including dopamine, acetylcholine, gamma-aminobutyric acid (Giannini and Price, 1985), serotonin (Smith et al., 1977), and norepinephrine. The effects on the dopaminergic
system may be the most important neurochemical activity, though nonadrenergic,
serotonenergic, and cholinergic disturbances also play a role. The opiate receptors and endorphins are also affected. The drug is nonaddicting and has no withdrawal potential, though some degree of tolerance may develop.

C. Neuropsychological Effects

The clinical effects of the drug on the central nervous system are complex, variable, and dose dependent (Giannini and Price, 1985; Burns and Lerner, 1976).
However, classification of PCP intoxication with reference to the dosage may
be difficult (Khantzian and McKenna, 1979) since the clinical findings may be
variable and compounded by polydrug abuse and inability to determine the
dose of PCP taken. A clinical classification according to patients' sensorium
and behavior has been used (McCarron et al., 1981b). The major clinical patterns include acute brain syndrome, toxic psychosis, catatonic syndrome, and
coma, while the behavioral toxicity of euphoria, agitation, bizarre and violent
behavior, and lethargy and stupor are considered as the minor patterns (Table
6). Acute brain syndrome is defined as disorientation with confusion, and
catatonic syndrome consists of posturing, rigidity, negativism, mutism, and
staring.

When the drug is taken by the inhalational route, there are acute behavioral and neurophysiological effects. A PCP high is characterized by a sensation of oblivion, fantasy, and euphoria. Less desirable sensations include dis-
tortions in body image, perceptual disturbances including auditory and visual
hallucinations, paranoia, and feelings of indifference, social isolation, and de-

Table 6 Clinical Patterns of Acute PCP Intoxication

	Total cases	PCP only (N = 597) (%)	PCP + other (N = 403) (%)
Major patterns			
Coma	106	9.2	12.7
Catatonic syndrome	117	14.6	7.4
Toxic psychosis	166	16.8	16.4
Acute brain syndrome	248	26.6	22.1
Minor patterns			
Lethargy/stupor	38	2.3	6.0
Bizarre behavior	98	10.6	8.7
Violent behavior	115	9.7	14.1
Agitation	51	3.5	7.4
Euphoria	26	3.0	2.0
Asymptomatic	35	3.7	3.2

From McCarron et al., 1981b.

spair. The individual on a PCP high usually appears agitated and or belligerent. Irrational, hostile, combative, aggressive, and bizarre behavior are seen (Petersen and Stillman, 1978) and have been termed behavioral toxicity. Occasionally, however, the patient may be drowsy, lethargic, mute, stare blankly, and does not respond to painful stimuli since phencyclidine has depressant as well as stimulatory effects. In a study of 1000 cases of PCP intoxication, combinations of bizarre behavior, violence, agitation, and euphoria were present in 32.5% of cases in patients who were conscious and alert, toxic psychosis was present in 16.6% of cases, and acute brain syndrome and catatonic syndrome were present in 24.8% and 11.7% of cases, respectively (McCarron et al., 1981b).

The undesirable effects of PCP are unpredictable and include frank psychosis (Yesavage and Freman, 1978; Luisada, 1978; McCarron et al., 1981b) PCP psychosis is similar in presentation to schizophrenia (Luby et al., 1959; Allen and Young, 1978). The clinical findings vary with the different categories of schizophrenia. The patient may exhibit a blunted or vacant affect associated with frank incoherence of speech, suspicion, hostility, bizarre paranoid delusions, hallucinations and tendency toward violence. The initial phase of psychosis with violent psychotic manifestations usually lasts for 5 days followed by gradual

Table 7 Characteristics of PCP-Induced Coma (N = 55, PCP only)

Characteristic	% Occurrence		
	Severe (N = 12)	Moderate (N = 17)	Mild (N = 26)
No response to deep pain	83	35	15
Nystagmus	67	53	69
Hypertension	50	59	46
Tachycardia	58	35	31
Generalized rigidity	50	24	0
Grand mal seizures	42	12	11
Tremor/twitching	42	12	0
Absent DTRs	42	12	0
Localized dystonias	25	0	0
Hypersalivation	25	6	0
Temperature $< 36.67°C$	25	12	4
Respirations $< 12/min$	17	12	0
Hyperactive DTRs	17	29	8
Pupils $\leqslant 1$ mm	17	6	4
Profuse diaphoresis	8	6	0
Athetosis	8	6	0
Facial grimacing	9	0	0
Respirations $> 30/min$	8	0	0
Temperature $> 38.89°C$	8	6	0
Pupils > 4 mm	0	6	4
Urinary retention	0	12	0

From McCarron et al., 1981b.

resolution with restlessness and confusion over the next five days and finally personality reintegration and improvement of thought disorders and paranoia within one week (Luisada and Brown, 1976). It is during the acute psychotic phase that many of the deaths associated with PCP may occur. The affected individual often feels invulnerable and commits bizarre acts of violence with disregard for his or her own well being and alteration of the mental state. Accidents and suicide in this setting account for the majority of PCP-related deaths (Bruns et al., 1975; Noguchi and Nakamura, 1978; Crider, 1986).

One of the important neurologic/pharmacologic actions of PCP is the vestibulocerebellar syndrome. Typically the patient has horizontal or vertical nystagmus, muscle incoordination, dysarthria, and ataxia. This reaction is induced by minimal doses of PCP and is useful in identifying the PCP-intoxicated individual. Other neurologic findings include increased deep-tendon reflexes and muscular hypertonia. Sensory examination reveals decreased pinprick sense, termed dissociative anesthesia, and other sensory alterations involving hearing, vision, taste, and smell. Muscular hypertonia may precipitate tonic or clonic seizures. In conscious patients the size of the pupils are normal, equal, and reactive to light, but in some individuals the pupils may be mydriatic, and in comatose patients, miotic pupils may be seen. Prolonged coma and general seizure activity have been reported with PCP but appear to be due to high doses taken by the oral or intravenous route. Coma was present in 10.6% of 1000 cases of PCP intoxication and the duration of coma was classified as mild (less than 2 hr duration), moderate (lasting from 2 to 24 hr), and severe (coma more than 24 hr) (McCarron et al., 1981b). The clinical features of PCP-induced coma are shown in Table 7. The minor neurologic alterations associated with PCP intoxication are usually brief. Full recovery usually occurs within 8 hr and in the majority at 72 hr, although in severe cases or coma the recovery may take longer (Burns and Lerner, 1976; McCarron et al., 1981b).

Evidence that chronic use of phencyclidine may produce long-term neurologic, cognitive, and behavioral dysfunction is suggested. Studies of chronic PCP users have shown some tolerance to the drug, as well as anxiety, fatigue, irritability, depression, paranoid psychosis, and memory loss (Stillman and Petersen, 1979) and a chronic dementia (Millman, 1985).

D. Pathophysiological Effects

The other effects of PCP intoxications are on the cardiovascular, pulmonary, thermoregulatory, and renal systems. A hyperadrenergic state with hypertension and tachycardia may be present and may progress to hypertensive encephalopathy (Eastman and Cohen, 1975) and intracerebral hemorrhage. Cerebrovasospasm has been documented with PCP in laboratory animals (Altura and Altura, 1981). Altered autonomic function with diaphoresis, hypersalivation and bronchorrhea may be present, and there may be hyperpyrexia (Jan et al., 1978) or hypothermia and urinary retention (McCarron et al., 1981b). Involuntary muscular activity with muscle injury can lead to acute rhabdomyolysis, myoglobinuria and renal failure (Cogen et al., 1978; Barton et al., 1980; McCarron, 1986). There may be bronchospasm, and laryngospasm on attempted intubation for respiratory failure. Respirations are not depressed except in massive oral doses or when PCP is abused with ethanol, opiates, sedatives, or hypnotics. Abnormal neonatal neurobehavior has been shown in infants delivered to women who used phencyclidine during pregnancy (Chasnoff et al., 1983).

E. Clinical Evaluation and Therapy

Acute PCP intoxication should be suspected in the emergency room when the clinical constellation of unexplained bizarre behavior, horizontal and vertical nystagmus, and mild hypertension is evident, especially in a patient with poly-drug abuse of smoking or snorting drugs. In severe cases, there may be psychosis, seizures, and coma. In patients who are not comatose or need mechanical ventilation, the treatment is primarily supportive. The patient should be admitted to the intensive care unit and placed in a quiet room with minimal sensory input. Efforts to talk down the patient often intensify the agitation and other symptoms and are to be avoided. Serum should be sent for toxicologic screen including PCP, sedative-hypnotics, ethyl alcohol, and opiates. In addition, urine is sent for toxicologic and drug abuse screen including PCP (Reynolds, 1976; Barton et al., 1981), cocaine, and marijuana: the three most commonly inhaled drugs. The mental and respiratory status as well as blood pressure are monitored. The patient may need to be restrained to protect him or her from self-harm. Diazepam (Valium) in small doses (2-3 mg given intravenously) needed is often helpful to reduce excitement and agitation. Adequate hydration is necessary, and to hasten the drug excretion of PCP, the urine is acidified, which can increase PCP clearance by 25-fold (Beede, 1980). This can be accomplished by giving ascorbic acid 2 g in 500 ml 5% dextrose in water intravenously every 6 hr until the urine pH is below 5. Furosemide 20-40 mg may be given intravenously for additional diuresis. In mild intoxication, the urinary excretion can be increased by giving cranberry juice and ascorbic acid 1-2 g/day. With these simple supportive measures, most patients with inhalational PCP intoxication are discharged from the emergency room within 8-12 hr and have full resolution of symptoms within 24 hr. Drug counseling should be recommended prior to discharge.

PCP intoxication complicated by stupor or coma requires more careful monitoring. The fact that the patient is stuporous or comatose implies at least a moderate dose and is associated with high doses of oral or intravenous PCP. If the route of administration was inhalational, except in cases where the PCP was snorted, severe intoxication with coma are uncommon. With oral ingestion of PCP either unintentionally or through abuse, gastric lavage is indicated (McCarron, 1986) and is usually performed within 6 hr of oral overdose. Sodium sulfate 0.3 g/kg given through the gastric tube may enhance fecal excretion (Beede, 1980). In a comatose patient with severe respiratory depression or upper airway compromise due to secretions, endotracheal intubation is indicated. Intubation may pre-cipitate laryngospasm; succinylcholine chloride has been given prior to endotra-cheal intubation (Burns and Lerner, 1976; Thompson et al., 1982). In these pa-tients with severe intoxication, acidification of urine to a pH of less than 5 can be achieved with ascorbic acid (2 gm/500 ml 5% dextrose intravenously) or am-monium chloride (2.75 mEq/kg in 60 ml 0.9% saline solution) given through the gastric tube (Beede, 1980). For the hypertensive crises, diazoxide (Hyperstat) (1-3 mg/kg up to 150 mg in a 10-30 sec intravenous infusion) and nitroprusside (Nipride) (0.5-10 µg/kg/min as an intravenous infusion) can be given. Since PCP causes an increase in heart rate, the potential for cardiac arrhythmia is present, and 1 mg of propranolol (Inderal) can be given intravenously for cardiac arrhyth-mia (Giannini and Price, 1985) and also to decrease the adrenergic effects. Neu-romuscular blockage with pancuronium bromide (Pavulon) may be used to de-crease the muscle motor activity. Seizures can be treated with diazepam (Valium) in 2-3 mg increments given intravenously (Senay et al., 1982).

Phencyclidine psychosis is one of the severe complications of PCP intoxi-cation and constitutes a psychiatric emergency (Luisada and Brown, 1976). The goals of hospitalization are to prevent self-injury and injury to others due to patients' bizarre and combative behavior, decrease the external stimuli and agitation, and ameliorate the psychosis. To treat the psychosis and reduce agi-tation, several pharmacologic interventions have been used. Diazepam (Valium) or lorazepam (Ativan) often may be helpful in reducing anxiety but has no role in the treatment of psychosis. Earlier, the use of chlorpromazine (Thorazine) was advocated as the ideal antipsychotic agent (Luisada and Brown, 1976). How-ever, other investigators have not recommended the use of phenothiazines be-cause of the anticholinergic properties of PCP and the hypotension that can be observed with phenothiazines (Perry, 1976; Burns and Lerner, 1976; Showalter and Thornton, 1977). In one study, chlorpromazine was given to 66 patients with PCP psychotoxicity; 5 (7.6%) became hypotensive and 4 of these patients had normal or mild systolic hypertension (McCarron et al., 1981b). In contrast, haloperidol was given to 168 patients and 1 (0.6%) had hypotension. Halo-peridol (Haldol) has been recommended as the drug of choice for ameliorating psychosis (Showalter and Thornton, 1977; Giannini and Price, 1985). The drug can be given intramuscularly 5 mg every 20 min for two to three doses. Other drugs that are under investigation for modifying the behavioral changes due to PCP include physostigmine (Castellani et al., 1982) (2 mg intramuscularly every 20 min) meperidine (Demerol) (50 mg intramuscularly every 20 min) (Giannini and Price, 1985; Giannini et al., 1985), and reserpine (Serpasil) (Berlant, 1985), but their clinical utility remains to be further elucidated. Even with antipsy-chotic medication (haloperidol) for the PCP-induced psychosis, the psychotic symptoms have persisted for more than 30 days in one study (Allen and Young,

1978) and some patients have exhibited schizophrenic symptoms about a year later without PCP abuse (Luisada and Brown, 1976). It is of note that schizophrenics or those with underlying psychiatric disease who received PCP have relapses of their mental illness (Luby et al., 1959; Fauman et al., 1976). Electroconvulsive therapy may be useful in PCP-induced psychosis that fails to respond to antipsychotic medications (Rosen et al., 1984). Chronic abusers of PCP may show a chronic psychiatric illness with paranoia, depression, memory loss, and a chronic dementia (Millman, 1985).

IV. Cocaine

A. History

The use of cocaine in the form of coca leaves chewed by South American Indians has been known since pre-Incan times. Cocaine alkaloid was extracted from coca leaves (which has 1-2% cocaine) about 1860 in Europe. It was used briefly for the treatment of depression before application as a local anesthetic agent was noted. In the late 19th and early 20th centuries, cocaine was included in many over the counter medications, tonics, and soft drinks. The ingredients of coca leaves were included in Coca-Cola until 1903, although it has been reported that coca leaves are still part of the ingredients of Coca-Cola but the cocaine has been removed (Goode, 1984). William Stewart Halsted, the famous surgeon at The Johns Hopkins Medical School in the early 1890s, was a cocaine addict. Sigmund Freud did extensive research on cocaine, used it himself, (Byck, 1974) and recommended it as a general tonic. Because of widespread narcotic and cocaine abuse, the Harrison Narcotic Act in 1914 and the Narcotic Drugs Import and Export Act in 1922 were enacted and the abuse of cocaine waned. Between the 1930s and the late 1960s, the abuse of cocaine had almost disappeared from the drug scene (Adams and Durell, 1984). In the mid-1970s cocaine began to regain its popularity (Wetli and Wright, 1979; Grabowski, 1984) and has shown an explosive growth in the past few years, especially with "crack," the freebase and highly potent smoked form of cocaine, which most likely originated in the Bahamas (Jekel et al., 1986). Earlier, cocaine, known as the "champagne of drugs," was limited in its availability because of its high cost and limited in its administration by snorting. However, due to an increase in acreage for the growth of the coca bush, and easy preparation of crack, which is administered through smoking, the illicit street drug has become much cheaper. The term "crack" comes from the sound produced when the material is heated. Crack is manufactured by mixing cocaine with baking soda and water to precipitate the free base. During the process of freebasing, the potency of the cocaine may be increased up to 90% purity. The retail value of sales of cocaine as an illegal recreational drug was reported to be $29 billion in 1980, higher than marijuana or other dangerous drugs (Smith, 1982). Fifteen million Americans used cocaine on a nonmedical basis in 1979, and it ranked only behind alcohol, cigarettes, and marijuana as the most abused drug (Fishburne et al., 1980). In 1986, the number of people who used cocaine at least once will be approximately 25 million. It is estimated that about 6 million people use the drug on a regular basis and about 3 million are addicted to it (Miller, 1985). Because of the inherent risk that intravenous drug abuse may lead to the development of the acquired immune deficiency syndrome, hepatitis, and other factors, crack, with its easy availability and smoking as the route of administration, has become the drug of choice for many drug abusers (*New York Times,* 1986; *Newsweek,* 1986). The abuse of crack has become a major and growing public health problem, especially in the northeast and far west.

B. Pharmacology and Toxicology

Cocaine is a potent central nervous system stimulant that also affects the respiratory centers, cardiovascular/pulmonary, and other systems (Cregler and Mark, 1986). It increases cardiac contraction, blood pressure, and heart rate as well as the pulmonary arterial pressure (Petersen and Stillman, 1977; Millman, 1985). The sympathomimetic effects of the drug may cause hypertension, coronary artery spasm, myocardial infarction, arrhythmias, and sudden cardiac death (Isner, 1986; Schachne, 1984; Kossowsky and Lyon, 1984; Coleman et al., 1982). There is relaxation of the bronchial muscle, dilated pupils, and an increase in body temperature. The psychophysiological effects on the central nervous system include euphoria, a state of well-being, and an increase in alertness and physical ability especially when the individual's performance is affected by fatigue or lack of sleep. It is also a local anesthetic agent (Ritchie and Greene, 1980) with properties of vasoconstriction of mucous membranes and it has applications in otorhinolaryngologic surgery. The drug can be given intravenously, intranasally, topically, and orally. The usual route of administration is intranasal. However, with the conversion of cocaine hydrochloride, is "snorted," to a free base (crack) (Siegel, 1982), smoking has become an increasingly common route of administration. The onset of action of cocaine depends on the route of administration and the dose. High blood levels are achieved after intravenous cocaine, with the peak effect occurring after 3-5 min (Javaid, 1978). Intranasal human application results in peak plasma levels at 25-60 min. Residual cocaine can be present on the nasal mucosa for 3 hr after intranasal administration, and the vasoconstrictive properties of cocaine may be the cause of the prolonged and rate-limited absorption of cocaine (Van Dyke et al., 1976). The peak "high" is felt 60-90 min after oral ingestion (Van Dyke et al., 1978). The effects of intranasal cocaine occur about 90 sec after intake compared to about 12-15 sec when taken via the smoked route. Since cocaine euphoria is a function of not just blood level but speed and degree of change of blood level, the crack form is highly addicting. The repetitive use of the drug is further increased by the rapid onset of dysphoria as the blood level of the cocaine decreases. The use of cocaine every 15-30 min is not uncommon to avoid this dysphoria, and binge use may go on from 8 to 48 hr before the "crash" occurs.

Chemically, cocaine is methylbenzoylecgonine and is an alkaloid extracted from the South American plant *Erythroxylon coca*. After purification to its hydrochloride salt, cocaine is a white crystalline powder and is water soluble. Pure cocaine (base or freebase) is almost insoluble in water. It is metabolized by esterases in liver (Jones, 1984), cholinesterases in plasma, and by nonenzymatic hydrolysis. The major urinary cocaine metabolites are benzoylecgonine (Fish and Wilson, 1969) and ecgonine methyl ester (Inaba et al., 1978). In samples from patients with a pseudocholinesterase deficiency, there was a marked decrease in the in vitro rate of cocaine degradation, indicating the probable role of plasma cholinesterase in cocaine metabolism (Inaba et al., 1978; Jatlow et al., 1979). The plasma half-life of cocaine is about 1.5 hr. About 80% of the drug is excreted in the urine as ecgonine methyl ester and benzoylecgonine, both of which can be detected in the urine by drug abuse screening.

Cocaine rapidly produces acute tolerance to its psychological and cardiovascular effects (Fischman et al., 1985). In addition, it is a powerful reinforcer and acute withdrawal can produce an abstinence syndrome different from that seen typically with opiates (Gawin and Kleber, 1986).

The acute toxic reaction of cocaine has been described as acute cocainism (Wetli and Wright, 1979), or cocaine reaction (Gay, 1982), characterized as an adrenergic storm affecting the central nervous system, respiratory and cardiovascular systems, and progressing to respiratory distress, accelerated ventricular rhythm (Benchimol et al., 1978), acute myocardial infarction (Isner et al., 1986; Howard et al., 1985), hyperpyrexia (Cregler and Mark, 1986), generalized seizures, coma, and death (Mittleman and Wetli, 1984; Nakamura and Noguchi, 1981). There has been a steady increase in cocaine-related overdose deaths since the 1970s. In 1985, the Drug Abuse Warning Network (DAWN) reported a 91% increase in cocaine-related deaths. Cocaine has been recognized as one of the most dangerous illicit drugs in common use (Pollin, 1985).

C. Neuropsychological Effects

Cocaine exerts a complex action on the central nervous system. With cortical stimulation, there is euphoria or "high," relief of fatigue and boredom, diminished appetite, and increased mental ability and sociability. The acute stimulant and euphoriant effects include excitement, emotional lability, and restlessness followed by depression, irritability, and apprehension.

Pseudohallucinations may be present with tactile ("cocaine bugs"), visual ("snow lights"), auditory, gustatory, and olfactory changes (Gay, 1982). The behavioral pattern due to cocaine will depend on the route of administration and its dose. Learning and verbal report were affected after intravenous and intranasal cocaine; however, the behavioral effects of the drug may not be evident on mild recreational use of cocaine (Fischman, 1984). In addition, it has been shown in volunteers with a history of cocaine abuse that there is a reduction in physiological and subjective effects of cocaine when it is given repeatedly (Fischman et al., 1985). Thus, pretreatment of subjects with an intranasal administration of cocaine caused a decrease in the subjective effects determined by the Addiction Research Center Inventory, the Profile of Mood States, and the subjective effects questionnaire when the cocaine was subsequently given intravenously. The development of acute tolerance resolved within 24 hr.

There is a belief among current cocaine users and Andean Indians who chew coca that the drug improves working ability or performance, and professional athletes have been known to use the drug for this effect besides the "high." Cocaine given intravenously or intranasally (10 or 25 mg) had no effect on hand grip strength (Resnick et al., 1980). In contrast, in subjects deprived of sleep for 24-48 hr, inhalation of 96 mg cocaine partially reversed the fatigue-induced decrement in performance (Fischman and Schuster, 1980).

Cocaine alters the interneural communications of neurotransmitters—catecholamines, norepinephrine, and dopamine (Ritchie and Green, 1980)—resulting in an excess of norepinephrine and dopamine, and blockade of serotonin synthesis. Norepinephrine release leads to stimulation of the sympathetic nervous system, hypothalamus, and the reticular-activating system, accounting for the sympathomimetic effects, the effects on thirst, hunger, body temperature, emotions, arousal, and sleep. Receptor supersensitivity (beta-adrenergic or dopaminergic) may be a neurochemical substrate for postcocaine dysphoria or craving, and human cocaine abusers have been noted to have elevated levels of plasma growth hormone and decreased plasma prolactin, which confirms the adrenergic and dopaminergic receptor effects seen in animals (Kleber and Gawin, 1984a,b). The alteration in dopaminergic receptors and the dopaminergic reward pathway may have pharmacologic implications for the treatment of the craving that often leads to cocaine relapse.

One of the most severe forms of psychopathologic reactions to cocaine is the cocaine-induced psychosis, manifested by perceptual disturbances, visual, olfactory, and auditory hallucinations with delusions, violent loss of impulse control, depression, and paranoia (Siegel, 1978, 1982; Kleber and Gawin, 1984a). This is usually associated with high doses of cocaine and individuals with psychiatric disorders may have their illness exacerbated or precipitated with cocaine use (Aronson and Craig, 1986). Because of its stimulant effect on the central nervous system, cocaine has been given intravenously to depressed patients, and there was an increase in heart rate, blood pressure and respiratory rate associated with a tearful emotional catharsis (Post et al., 1974; Grinspoon and Bakalar, 1981).

The long-term chronic effect of cocaine on a recreational basis of no more than two or three times a week was earlier thought to pose no serious problems (Siegel, 1977), but such use is now believed to be the forerunner of more intensive use. When cocaine is used daily in significant amount or on a binge basis, patients experience anorexia, insomnia, irritability, difficulty in concentration, perceptual disturbance, depression, and psychological dependence (Washton et al., 1985; Grinspoon and Bakalar, 1981). It should be noted that with crack the chronic effect may be similar to the continued high-dose abuse of cocaine in the earlier years (Siegel, 1977). Recently it has been shown in laboratory animals given free access to heroin or cocaine that the mortality rate for 30 days of continuous testing was 36% for animals self-administering heroin, and 90% for those self-administering cocaine, suggesting that cocaine was several times as lethal to the rats as heroin (Bozarth and Wise, 1985).

D. Pathophysiological Effects

The effects on the cardiovascular system will depend on the dose and route of administration of cocaine. A small dose (25 mg) absorbed systemically causes an increase in pulse rate and blood pressure of 30-50% above normal and 15-20% above normal, respectively (Gay, 1982). In another study after intravenous cocaine administration of 16 mg, the mean heart rate in nine male volunteer subjects with a long history of intravenous cocaine abuse increased from a baseline of 74 beats/min to 100 beats/min and it further increased to 112 beats/min after 32 mg cocaine intravenously (Fischman et al., 1976). The peak increase in systolic blood pressure was 10-15% at 10 min after the intravenous administration of 16 and 32 mg of cocaine. An intranasal dose of 10 mg had no physiological effect, but at 25 mg there was an increase in blood pressure and the presence of euphoria. In contrast, intravenous cocaine caused alterations in psychophysiological effects even when the dose was 10 mg, and the authors noted that the average street dose of cocaine was 20-50 mg intranasally (Grinspoon and Bakalar, 1981).

Although there is a dose-related response in heart rate when cocaine is given intravenously, the increase in heart rate and blood pressure (the latter is more variable) is decreased when the subjects are pretreated with an intranasal dose of cocaine (Fischman et al., 1985). With placebo pretreatment and 32 mg cocaine given intravenously, the mean peak heart rate of eight subjects was 112 beats/min. In contrast when the same dose of cocaine was administered intravenously in subjects who had inhaled 96 mg cocaine intranasally 1 hr earlier, the peak heart rate was significantly lower: 101 beats/min. There was no effect of cocaine on the respiratory rate in the above study.

The skin may be pale due to peripheral vasoconstriction. Dilated pupils and hyperpyrexia may be present. Cocaine may lead to arrhythmias (Cregler and Mark, 1986; Benchimol et al., 1978), and thus to life-threatening cardiovascular events. Cardiac arrhythmias including ventricular premature beats, ventricular tachycardia and fibrillation, myocarditis, acute myocardial infarction, and sudden death have been observed, and there may not be underlying heart disease in precipitating the cardiac events (Isner et al., 1986). The subject may complain of chest pain and dyspnea, and coronary artery spasm with acute myocardial infarction have been documented in multiple case reports and studies (Coleman et al., 1982; Kossowsky and Lyon, 1984; Howard et al., 1985; Simpson and Edwards, 1986). Cocaine may induce coronary vasoconstriction (Schachne et al., 1984). Although there is the potential onset of cardiac dysfunction related to cocaine abuse, in a controlled medical environment the sympathomimetic effects of topical cocaine on cardiovascular function were not evident when patients with coronary artery disease were anesthetized (Barash et al., 1980).

Fatalities have occurred following as little as 25 mg cocaine applied to mucous membranes (Gay, 1982) and there is a wide variation in toxic and fatal doses of cocaine. In a study of 60 cocaine-related overdose deaths in the Dade County Medical Examiner's Department in Miami from 1978 to 1982, the average blood cocaine concentration at the time of death was 6.2 mg/liter, with a wide range of 0.1 mg/liter to 20.9 mg/liter. Thus the evaluation of toxicological data at the time of death has to be interpreted with caution (Mittleman and Wetli, 1984). In this study the mean blood cocaine concentration was 5.5 mg/liter with the nasal route for cocaine deaths and 6.6 mg/liter for the intravenous route; the latter route of administration was responsible for at least half the deaths. Oral ingestion of cocaine as the cause of death was related in all cases in one study to massive oral ingestion of cocaine or breakage of cocaine-filled condoms in the gastrointestinal tract (Wetli and Wright, 1979). Death can be quite sudden, with the patient presenting to the emergency room agitated or delirious and then dying of cardiopulmonary arrest. Autopsy findings in the cocaine-related deaths were nonspecific with pulmonary edema, visceral congestion, and occasionally visceral petechiae (Mittleman and Wetli, 1984). A 21-year-old man with a history of intravenous cocaine abuse developed chest pain within 1 min and cardiopulmonary arrest within 1 hr after the intravenous ingestion. At autopsy he was noted to have severe coronary obstructive lesions and acute platelet thrombosis (Simpson and Edwards, 1986). Cocaine-induced coronary artery spasm was suggested; also there was a lymphocytic myocarditis that may have been related to his 5 years of cocaine abuse. In a study of cocaine-related fatalities (111 cases in 27 study sites in Canada and the United States) the onset of the lethal effects of cocaine were rapid: two-thirds of the victims died in less than 5 hr and one-third within the first

hour after administration of the drug (Finkle and McCloskey, 1978). The
terminal events were seizures followed by respiratory arrest. Deaths from
drug combinations (e.g., speed-balling-heroin and cocaine) are more common
than deaths from cocaine alone (Grinspoon and Bakalar, 1981; Finkle and
McCloskey, 1978).

Nasal perforation has been reported (Gay, 1982) with the intranasal route
of administration of cocaine but its frequency is not clear. In 111 cocaine-related deaths in which 7.2% of the cases used cocaine intranasally, although 54%
were not available for evaluation, there was not a single case of nasal perforation
(Finkle and McCloskey, 1978). Intranasal cocaine and its adulterants have resulted in acute and chronic rhinitis and, in some rare cases, septal necrosis due
to the powerful vasoconstriction of the mucous membranes. Also, in a group of
intranasal cocaine abusers the nasal mucous membranes were erythematous with
occasionally hemorrhagic membranes, but septal perforations were not noted
(Snyder and Snyder, 1985). Thus there seems to be more concern about nasal perforation than actual occurrence, at least as documented in the medical literature.

In a preliminary study of lung function in two cocaine smokers, the
arterial blood gases were normal at rest and after exercise, but there was
abnormal single-breath diffusing capacity. One subject had a history of intravenous drug abuse that could explain the above findings. The other subject, a cigarette smoker and abuser of marijuana, had a single-breath diffusing
capacity of 62% of predicted and had been freebasing cocaine for 2 months.
Both the cigarette smoking and especially the chronic marijuana use could account for the patient's abnormal diffusing capacity (Tilles, et al., 1986).

In 19 consecutive chronic smokers of free-base cocaine, lung function tests
were performed and abnormalities in single-breath diffusing capacity were seen
in 10 (53%) (Itkonen et al., 1984). Similar reduction in single-breath diffusing
capacity was not observed in seven cocaine snorters. There was no evidence of
airway obstruction (Table 8). Also, five subjects had progressive multistage exercise test on a treadmill, and except for a lower maximum oxygen uptake and
a mild increase in maximum alveolar-arterial oxygen difference, the exercise response was normal (Table 9). The abnormality in the pulmonary gas exchange
manifested by a decrease in single-breath diffusing capacity was postulated to be
due to cocaine-induced vasoconstriction resulting in a decrease in pulmonary
blood flow and pulmonary hypertension (Itkonen et al., 1984). Further studies
are needed to evaluate the acute effects of freebase cocaine smoking or crack on
lung function tests, including the single-breath diffusing capacity. Besides the
abnormal findings in pulmonary gas exchange, the patient may have dry lips
and a wispy voice (probably due to the local anesthetic effect of cocaine smoke),
sore throat, and black or bloody sputum as a result of chronic cocaine smoking
(Siegel, 1982). The very potent vasoconstrictive property of cocaine when it is

Table 8 Comparison Between "Freebase" Cocaine Users With Normal or Reduced Carbon Monoxide Diffusing Capacity (DLCO)

Variable	DLCO $\leqslant 70\%$ of predicted (n=10)	DLCO $\geqslant 70\%$ of predicted (n=9)
DLCO (% predicted)	59.0 ± 2.3	87.5 ± 4.2
TLC (% predicted)	85.3 ± 3.2	93.2 ± 4.9
FEV_1 (% predicted)	83.8 ± 1.6	82.8 ± 2.3
FEF_{75-25} (% predicted)	101.5 ± 8.1	103.1 ± 12.0
Age (yr)	29.1 ± 1.3	30.1 ± 2.2
Duration of freebase use (months)	22.0 ± 5.0	26.7 ± 6.2
No. (%) dyspneic	7 (70)	3 (33)

TLC, indicates total lung capacity; FEV_1, forced expiratory volume in 1 sec; FEF_{75-25}, flow during middle portion of vital capacity.
From Itkonen et al., 1984.

Table 9 Response to Exercise in Five Freebase Cocaine Abusers With Abnormal Single-Breath Diffusing Capacity ($DLCO_{SB}$)

Variable	Mean	SEM
Age (yr)	29.6	1.4
Duration of abuse (yr)	1.5	0.3
$DLCO_{SB}$ (% predicted)	61.6	2.4
% Maximum predicted heart rate attained	77.2	3.5
$\dot{V}O_2$ max (mL/kg/min)	25.9	1.6
% Maximum predicted VO_2 attained	68.0	3.7
(A-a) O_2 max	20.2	1.9
Δ VD/VT rest-exercise (%)	-3.5	1.4

$\dot{V}O_2$ max, maximum oxygen uptake; A-a O_2 max, maximum alveolar-arterial oxygen gradient; VD/VT ratio of dead space to tidal volume.
From Itkonen et al., 1984.

inhaled through freebase crack smoking with a pipe may result in subcutaneous emphysema (Khouzam, 1986) and pneumomediastinum (Morris and Shuck, 1985).

Other medical effects of cocaine include the central nervous system complications of subarachnoid hemorrhage, cerebral infarction and seizures, and intestinal ischemia (Cregler and Mark, 1986). Cocaine can also have harmful effects on the immune system, especially the primary immune response in laboratory animals (Watson et al., 1983), and can cause hyperprolactinemia and sexual dysfunction (Cocores et al., 1986), higher rate of spontaneous abortion in pregnant cocaine abusers, and abnormal neonatal neurobehavior in cocaine-exposed infants (Chasnoff et al., 1985).

E. Clinical Evaluation and Therapy

Cocaine is a potent central nervous system stimulant and also causes a significant increase in heart rate, respiratory rate, and blood pressure. The severity of the neuropsychophysiological changes and the sympathomimetic effects will depend on the dose and route of administration of cocaine. Minor neuropsychophysiological changes are usually not seen in the emergency room. Difficulty in breathing, dilated pupils, palpitation, chest pain, cardiac disease, hypertension, and seizures in a person with no prior history of cardiac hisease or seizures should make one suspect cocaine overdose, especially if there are history or stigmata of drug abuse. The patient who presents with chest pain and dyspnea may have cardiac arrhythmia or ischemia in addition to tachycardia and hypertension. The primary concern is to support the cardiopulmonary system (Senay et al., 1982) with maintenance of a patent airway and assessment of the vital signs, level of consciousness, and status of arterial oxygenation. In the advent of significant tachycardia, hypertension, or ventricular ectopy, propranolol (Inderal) 1 mg intravenously may be administered (Gay, 1982; Rappolt et al., 1976). The dose can be repeated. If there is further ventricular ectopy on cardiovascular monitoring, lidocaine can be given in a 50-100 mg bolus intravenously and repeated as needed, or an infusion drip of lidocaine can be started. Acute hypertensive crises with encephalopathy may need aggressive therapy with diazoxide (Hyperstat) or nitroprusside (Nipride).

Cocaine is a potent convulsant (Jones, 1984) and when there is convulsion and the patient is not responsive, ultra-short-acting barbiturate (thiopental 50-100 mg) may be given intravenously (Gay, 1982; Grinspoon and Bakalar, 1981), while attempts are made to maintain a patent airway and endotracheal intubation may be indicated. The tonic and clonic convulsions may proceed to status epilepticus. The deep tendon reflexes are increased. Diazepam (Valium) has been recommended as the drug of choice for treatment of status epilepticus; if the seizures are not controlled with diazepam, pancuronium

(Pavulon) may be given in addition to endotracheal intubation and mechanical ventilation (Haddad, 1986). The control of seizures and correction of metabolic acidosis are important in the maintenance of cardiovascular function (Jonsson, 1983). Cardiovascular collapse and severe hypoxia with respiratory depression also require mechanical ventilation. Cases have been reported in which the cardiopulmonary arrest of several minutes' duration has resulted in permanent cerebral damage (Gay, 1982).

In the treatment of hyperpyrexia, the core temperature is monitored by rectal thermometer after the application of cooling blanket and ice water for sponging. In patients who are stuporous or comatose, there may be aspiration pneumonia as the cause of the fever, and chest x-rays and appropriate cultures should be performed before antibiotic therapy is instituted.

Diazepam given intravenously or orally has been recommended for the anxiety, restlessness, and agitation. An oral dose of diazepam (Valium) of 10-20 mg every 6-8 hr may be given. For cocaine psychosis, the therapy is haloperidol (Haldol). The psychosis can persist for 3-5 days after stopping the use of cocaine (Washton et al., 1985). Beside the psychosis, other acute psychiatric complications include dysphoric agitation and acute postuse depression (the postcocaine "crash") (Kleber and Gawin, 1984a,b). For the transient agitation as described above, diazepam can be used and, in more persistent cases. propranolol can be added (Gay, 1982; Miller, 1985). Suicidal ideation and depressive symptoms are present during the postcocaine crash and are usually transient, requiring no acute treatment other than close observation; they abate after sleep normalization (Kleber and Gawin, 1984a,b, 1986).

The chronic effects of cocaine lead to psychological dependence and addiction. It is difficult to treat the drug's dependence because cocaine is a powerful reinforcing agent. In a survey of crack users who called the "800-COCAINE" national hotline, psychiatric complaints include severe depression (85%), irritability (78%), paranoia (65%), loss of sexual desire (58%), memory lapses (40%), violent behavior (31%), and suicide attempts (18%) (Washton et al., 1986). The psychotherapeutic modalities for the addictive behaviors consist of behavioral, supportive, and psychodynamic treatments (Kleber and Gawin, 1984 a,b). Pharmacotherapy is useful and may control the psychiatric symptoms when used in addition to psychotherapy without the need for hospitalization. Severe depression or psychotic symptoms that last beyond 1-3 days after the postcocaine crash warrant hospitalization for in-patient therapy. In severe abusers of cocaine, the pharmacologic agents used for cocaine abstinence are mainly tricyclic antidepressants such as desipramine (Kleber and Gawin, 1984a,b). Lithium carbonate can be used when a diagnosis of bipolar disorder is present and methylphenidate if a diagnosis of attention deficit disorder is made; otherwise, these two drugs are not useful in these patients. Bromocriptine has been used for the treatment of postcocaine craving (Dackis and Gold, 1985), but the number of cases are too small to allow one to draw conclusions yet.

Finally, the documentation of abuse of cocaine or other drugs in the urine and blood is discussed at the end of this chapter.

V. Inhalants

A. History

The recreational inhalation of gases for their euphoric and intoxicating effects dates back approximately 200 years. The anesthetic gas-nitrous oxide was used by H. Davy for the control of his toothache, and he experienced pain relief and pleasure (Davy, 1800) long before it was available as a gas for surgical anesthesia. The inhalants play a minor role in the epidemiologic survey of inhalation drug abuse, but their potential for causing medical and psychiatric morbidity and mortality (Sharp and Brehm, 1977; Garriott and Petty, 1980) is always there. The inhalants discussed here include anesthetic gas (nitrous oxide), organic solvents (toluene), hydrocarbon mixtures (gasoline), aerosol propellants (trichloro-monofluoromethane), and volatile nitrites (amyl nitrite).

B. Anesthetic Gases: Nitrous Oxide

Pharmacology, Pathophysiology, and Toxicology

Nitrous oxide is a colorless gas with a sweetish odor. It is a weak anesthetic agent but a potent analgesic, with a 50% concentration in the inspired air equivalent to 10 mg of morphine given intramuscularly. After inhalation of the gas, there is euphoria, relaxation, lightheadedness, and a "detached" attitude toward pain and the surroundings (Steward, 1985). Nitrous oxide increases the respiratory depression caused by opiates and other anesthetic gases, and results in mild cardiovascular depression.

Nitrous oxide is knowl also as "laughing gas" and "whippets." It has been abused because of its ability to produce a "high" effect when it is inhaled. Case reports have shown numbness of the hands and feet—a toxic polyneuropathy (Sahenk et al., 1978; Nevins, 1980)—from inhalation of nitrous oxide (N_2O) delivered from cartridges through a whipped cream dispenser. The latter was commonly used in N_2O abuse in the mid-1970s (Drug Poll, 1976). The peripheral neuropathy was postulated to be due to contaminants in the N_2O cartridges of trichloroethylene, toluene, and phenol, which are known neurotoxins (Sahenk et al., 1978). The abuse of homemade nitrous oxide has caused transient acute pulmonary toxicity in a 20-year-old man (Messina and Wynne, 1982) due to the inhalation of other toxic byproducts in the homemade N_2O (nitric oxide and nitrogen dioxide) that are usually removed through commercial purification of the anesthetic gas. When the nitrous oxide is obtained from dental offices and hospitals and abused on a chronic basis, a disabling peripheral neuropathy in two dentists and a health worker have been demonstrated (Layzer et al., 1978). Partial improvement in the numbness of the hands and feet was noted after stopping the N_2O abuse. Barotrauma in the form of pneumomediastinum has been observed when nitrous oxide was inhaled under high pressures orally (LiPuma et al., 1982). Death has resulted from abuse of nitrous oxide and it can be quantitated in blood by gas chromatographic analysis in toxicologic examinations (Garriott and Petty, 1980).

Therapy

Therapy is supportive depending on the symptoms. The patient is also warned against future use of the inhalation of nitrous oxide.

C. Organic Solvents: Toluene

Pharmacology, Pathophysiology, and Toxicology

The organic solvents are present in many workplaces and households. Methylene chloride is used for stripping paint and trichloroethane for cleaning upholstery. Toluene (methyl benzene) is present in glue, paint, and lacquers, and degreasing agents or cleaning fluids contain carbon tetrachloride or trichloroethylene. The abuse of these organic solvents is mainly for their hallucinogenic and intoxicating effects (Crites and Schuckit, 1979). However, the toxic effects with inhalation are not on the pulmonary system but on the renal, hepatic, hematologic, and neurologic systems (Hayden, et al., 1976).

Hepatorenal damage has been reported in a glue sniffer (O'Brien et al., 1971) and similar findings are seen in sniffers of trichloroethylene solvent (Baerg and Kimberg, 1970). Inhalation of toluene can produce euphoria, headache, nausea and dizziness, and, at higher concentrations, there are signs of ataxia and intention tremor (Benignus, 1981). In monkeys, brief inhalation of toluene resulted in impairment of cognitive and motor abilities (Taylor and Evans, 1985). Cerebellar, cortical, and functional impairment have been shown in toluene abusers (Fornazzari et al., 1983) and schizophreniform psychosis has been associated with chronic industrial toluene exposure (Goldbloom and Chouinard, 1985). Volatile substances of toluene or methylene chloride can be identified in blood samples by flame ionization gas chromatography (Garriott and Petty, 1980).

Therapy

Discussion of the therapy for hepatorenal (Hayden et al., 1976) or other systems involved with organic solvents is beyond the scope of this chapter.

D. Hydrocarbon Mixtures: Gasoline

Pharmacology, Pathophysiology, and Toxicology

The intentional inhalation of gasoline vapors for its hallucinogenic effect was reported in the 1950s (Clinger and Johnson, 1951). Since then, much has been
learned about the pathophysiology of gasoline sniffing and its therapy (Fortenberry, 1985). Gasoline is a mixture of hydrocarbons and also contains aromatic
hydrocarbon such as xylene, toluene, benzene, and tetraethyl lead. The latter is
added to gasoline for its antiknock property. It has been suggested that tetraethyl lead may be responsible for the behavioral changes and hallucinations (Valpey et al., 1978) resulting from gasoline sniffing. Acute encephalopathy due to
gasoline sniffing may produce euphoria, visual and auditory hallucinations, ataxia,
and irritability. Chronic gasoline sniffing can produce a chronic encephalopathy
manifested by dementia, ataxia, chorea, tremor, and myoclonus (Fortenberry,
1985). The acute and chronic encephalopathy is probably from intoxication due
to organic lead in the gasoline (Valpey et al., 1978). Peripheral neuropathy, acute
myopathy, and myoglobinuria have been demonstrated with gasoline sniffing. In
severe cases, there may be seizures, coma, and death. The diagnostic test in a patient who is suspected of gasoline sniffing abuse is measurement of the blood
lead level (Fortenberry, 1985).

Therapy

Chelation therapy has been used for the treatment of the tetraethyl lead toxicity
and may decrease the blood lead level and improve some of the neurologic symptoms. Dimercaprol, calcium disodium edetate, and penicillamine are some of the
chelating agents used (Fortenberry, 1985).

E. Aerosol Propellants: Trichloromonofluoromethane

Pharmacology, Pathophysiology, and Toxicology

In order to dispense the contents of aerosol household products, gases are
used as pressurizers (freon). The fluorocarbons are the major aerosol propellants. Subjects have sniffed the aerosol propellants for the high effect. In a review of 34 "inhalant" deaths in Dallas County from 1971 to 1977, the leading
cause of fatality (16 of 34 cases or 47%) was due to freon abuse, whether from
spray cooking lubricant, air freshener, or deodorant (Garriott and Petty, 1980).
The fluorocarbon propellants (trichloromonofluoromethane [F-11] or dichloro-
difluoromethane [F-12]) have been shown to induce fatal cardiac arrhythmia
when they are inhaled, especially at high concentrations (Hayden et al., 1976;
Garriott and Petty, 1980). They are also neurotoxic. Death is usually sudden

as the result of the cardiac arrhythmia and at autopsy there is no specific pathologic change aside from the acute pulmonary congestion.

The aerosol propellants used in hair sprays have been shown to cause a transient increase in pulmonary airway resistance (Zuskin and Bouhuys, 1974) and small airways dysfunction (Zuskin et al., 1981). However, the effects on lung function are mild and not clinically significant. Acute exposure to isobutane, propane and fluorocarbons (F-12 and F-11) in concentrations of 250, 500, or 1,000 ppm for periods of 1 min-8 hr did not result in any decrease in lung function or cardiac arrhythmia, except in one subject in whom the arrhythmia was not reproducible with further exposure (Stewart et al., 1978). The degree of exposure to the aerosol propellants for the volunteers in the above study was more than the customary exposure with proper use of the aerosol products. The cardiac toxicity of the aerosol propellants when they are abused may depend on their different chemical types. Because of the effect of freon on the ozone layer of the atmosphere, nonfreon aerosol propellants (isobutane, n-butane, and isopropane), considered to be less toxic, have replaced freon. Recently it has been shown that even nonfreon aerosol propellants can be associated with seizures and ventricular tachycardia when they are accidentally abused by a child (Wason et al., 1986). The levels of isobutane and n-butane from the aerosol propellants can be measured in the patient's serum. The medical overuse of aerosolized sympathomimetic drugs in patients with asthma, leading at times to the development of cardiac arrhythmia and death will not be discussed here.

Therapy

Therapy for the adverse effects on the cardiovascular and neurologic systems will depend on the clinical presentation.

F. Volatile Nitrites: Amyl Nitrite

Pharmacology, Pathophysiology, and Toxicology

Amyl nitrite has been used for the medical treatment of angina pectoris for more than 100 years. It has been abused as an intoxicant and as a sex stimulant (Sigell et al., 1978). The street names for amyl nitrite include snappers, poppers, and pearls. Butyl and isobutyl nitrites used as room odorizers are also inhaled for their "high" effect. The effects of the volatile nitrites are on the central nervous system, the cardiovascular, and hematologic systems (Newell et al., 1985; Haley, 1980). There is hypotension with peripheral vasodilatation and tachycardia. Toxic effects consist of flushing of the face, headache, eye orbital pain, increase in intraocular pressure (Pearlman and Adams, 1970), cyanosis, syncope, and cardiovascular collapse. There is also formation of methemoglobinemia with nitrites, which can be fatal (Shesser et al., 1982). Clues to the diagnosis of significant levels of methemoglobinemia include central and peripheral cyanosis, a dark blue color of the arterial blood gas sample, and the methemoglobin value. Volatile nitrites can be nitrosation reagents, which can lead to formation of N-nitrosamines and N-nitrosamides. These are mutagenic and carcinogenic compounds. The abuse of amyl nitrite among male homosexuals may be related to the current epidemic of the acquired immune deficiency syndrome and to Kaposi's sarcoma (Newell et al., 1985; Jorgensen and Lawesson, 1982).

Therapy

Therapy in patients with syncope and cardiovascular collapse should be directed to relief of the hypotension and support of the cardiovascular system. In patients with history of volatile nitrites abuse leading to mental status alteration and significant methemoglobinemia, the administration of intravenous methylene blue can be life-saving (Shesser et al., 1981).

G.   Documentation of Drug Use Through Analyses of Biological Fluid

Evidence for the abuse of drugs is generally accomplished by identification of the drug and/or its metabolite(s) in urine. Detection of a drug in urine only establishes exposure. It does not indicate the amount of drug consumed, and, most importantly, it provides no information about the patient's clinical condition or degree of impairment at the time the sample was taken. The length of time during which a urine screen will remain positive following drug use depends on the particular drug, the quantity used, as well as interindividual differences in drug disposition. Thus, the time of administration cannot be estimated with any degree of accuracy on the basis of a urinalysis. As a consequence, most drug abuse screening procedures on urine are generally qualitative. Little, if any, useful clinical information can be obtained by determining the actual concentrations of drugs in urine. A quantitative analysis of the parent or active form of the drug in blood or plasma is required for correlation with clinical condition or behavioral effects. Some drugs, such as the long-acting barbiturates and the major cannabinoid metabolite, may persist in the urine for days to weeks after drug use.

Methodology

Immunoassays are the most widely used techniques for the first-step screening of urine for the presence of abused drugs (Spector and Parker, 1970; Leute et al., 1971; Schneider et al., 1973; Godolphin, 1982; Sunshine, 1982). Radioimmunoassay (Roche) and various nonisotopic immunoassays are commercially available in kit form for most of the major drugs of abuse including those administered by inhalation. One of the most widely used nonisotopic immunoassays is the EMIT technique (Syva, Palo Alto, CA), which is a competitive binding immunoassay that uses an enzyme-labeled ligand. More recently, other nonisotopic immunoassays including fluorescence polarization (Abbott) have become available or are about to be released. Most of these techniques allow one to analyze a single urine specimen in a matter of minutes with minimal manipulations and are amenable to automation. Antibodies are often directed toward the predominant compound in urine, which may be a metabolite rather than the parent drug. The immunoassays are often exquisitely sensitive, but, as with many other immunoassays, most available antibodies demonstrate some degree of cross-reactivity, which can result in false-positive findings. Thus when urine drug abuse screening is performed for purposes that are not entirely clinical, it is considered axiomatic to confirm positive results using a procedure that is based on a different principle and is more specific. The most specific and sensitive procedure used for confirmation is gas chromatography/mass spectrometry (Foltz et al., 1980). This technique, however, is quite laborious and expensive and some laboratories prefer to use simpler procedures such as conventional gas chromatography for confirmation. Thin-layer chromatography is widely used for drug abuse screening and has the benefit of detecting multiple drugs concurrently (Dole et al., 1966; Davidow et al., 1968; Mule, 1969). As with the immunoassays, it is essential to confirm any positives when the test is used as part of a drug abuse screening program. Also, immunoassay and chromatography are used to evaluate drug overdose in the emergency room. In this instance, where the clinical and laboratory findings are being coordinated, and the purpose of the assay is to facilitate acute clinical management, clinical judgment can be used as to the need for confirmation.

A negative urine test, regardless of the method used, does not unequivocally rule out past exposure to the drug in question. A negative test only indicates that the quantity present is less than the detection limit of the analytical method used. It is customary for laboratories to set cutoff limits or thresholds that are somewhat higher than the detection limit in order to reduce the risk of false-positive results. If a confirmatory test is to be used, greater latitude can be taken in setting a low threshold or cutoff limit for the screening test.

The drugs that appear to be most commonly abused by the inhalational route, aside from nicotine, are marijuana, cocaine, PCP, and, on occasion, heroin. As with other routes of administration, each is detected by analysis of urine for the drug or its predominant metabolite, although the drug smoker is also exposed to other pyrolytic products, some of which may be toxic or pharmacologically active. As a consequence of the large absorptive area in the lung, smoked drugs are very rapidly absorbed, and their effects can be comparable to that following administration of an intravenous bolus.

Individual Drugs

Cocaine

Cocaine may be taken by the intravenous, oral, intranasal, buccal, and pulmonary routes (Paly et al., 1982). The effective yield of cocaine when smoked as the free base is greater than when the hydrochloride salt is used. More efficient and less dangerous methods for preparing the freebase from the salt, and its easier availability on the streets, have resulted in a considerable escalation in the use of this route.

Cocaine has a plasma half-life of about 1 hr (Wilkinson et al., 1980; Barnett et al., 1981). Its major metabolites, which arise via the hydrolytic route, are benzoylecgonine and ecgonine methyl ester. Cholinesterase appears to play a major role in the hydrolysis of cocaine in serum (Stewart et al., 1979; Jatlow et al., 1979). Cocaine disappears from serum rapidly in vitro if an enzyme inhibitor such as fluoride ion is not added to the sample. Identification of cocaine abuse by analysis of urine generally depends upon detection of benzoylecgonine. While this metabolite may persist in urine for several days after cocaine use, the parent drug itself may only be detectable for a few hours. Radioimmunoassay and enzyme immunoassay kits are available that use antibodies directed toward benzoylecgonine. Confirmatory procedures ideally are based upon gas chromatography/mass spectrometry, although the metabolite can also be detected using thin layer or high pressure liquid chromatography. Benzoylecgonine is sufficiently polar that appropriately optimized extraction techniques are essential. The half-lives of benzoylecgonine (6-8 hr) and of ecgonine methyl ester (5 hr) are longer than that of cocaine, allowing their persistence in urine for considerably longer periods of time (Ambre, 1985). The finding of these metabolites in urine only indicates prior use and does not document intoxication with cocaine at the time of sample collection.

Cocaine concentrations in plasma can be determined using gas chromatography coupled to nitrogen-sensitive detectors (Jatlow and Bailey, 1975) or, even more specifically, coupled to a mass spectrometer. Peak plasma concentrations following recreational doses generally have been in the range of 100-1000 μg/ml (Wilkinson et al., 1980; Van Dyke et al., 1978). Higher concentrations has occurred with current cocaine abuse patterns. After an overdose, a wide range of concentrations have been found, often greater than 1 μg/ml (Wetli and Wright, 1979).

Marijuana (Hawks, 1982)

The active ingredient of marijuana is tetrahydrocannabinol. Quantitation of the parent compound in serum is essential for establishing intoxication or impairment. Concentrations of the parent drug in serum are low, generally in the few nanograms per milliliter range, and, with the use of currently available methodology, are detectable only for a short time after use. Drug abuse screening generally relies on the detection of the major metabolite 11-nor-delta-9-THC-9-carboxylic acid (THC-acid). Exquisitively sensitive immunoassays are available, which can detect as little as 25 ng/ml of the predominant metabolite in urine. THC-acid can be detected in urine for days or even weeks after marijuana use, especially in chronic users. Thus, conclusions regarding behavior cannot be drawn from a positive urine assay. There are some data to suggeat that low levels of the metabolite may be detected transiently in urine following passive exposure to marijuana smoke, although this risk can be reduced by setting the cutoff limit for the assay sufficiently high (Cone and Rolley, 1986). Confirmation of positive immunoassay results for cannabinoids is considered essential, and is accomplished most specifically with gas chromatography/mass spectrometry, although other gas chromatographic detectors have been used.

Phencyclidine (Petersen and Stillman, 1978)

While drug abuse screening programs often include phencyclidine in their protocols, the clinician is most often concerned about this drug with the acutely psychotic patient, often in the emergency room, for whom differentiation between schizophrenia and a drug-induced psychoses is a major question. A nonisotopic immunoassay is available that permits detection of phencyclidine in urine with adequate sensitivity for clinical care. As with other drugs, confirmation is required when the analysis is performed for purposes other than acute clinical management. Chromatographic techniques reveal characteristic patterns of both PCP and its hydroxylated metabolites. Potentially toxic pyrolytic products of PCP have been suggested, although existing procedures for detection of PCP use are not directed at such compounds.

Heroin

Heroin is rapidly deacetylated to morphine in the body, and the latter is excreted in the urine as unchanged morphine, and, to a much larger extent, as the glucouronide conjugate of morphine. Thus detection of heroin use is accomplished by identification of morphine in the urine. This does not, however, permit a determination of whether the opiate was used in the form of heroin or as morphine. Codeine is metabolically demethylated to morphine, although in such instances both codeine and morphine can usually be found in the urine if a chromatographic procedure is used. Immunoassay is the mainstay of screening for opiate use and both radioimmunoassay and homogeneous nonisotopic immunoassays are available. The antibodies that detect morphine cross-react to varying degrees with some other opiates including heroin, morphine and its glucouronide conjugate, and codeine. However, they do not react with adequate sensitivity to such other compounds as meperidine and propoxyphene, which share similar actions but not structure with morphine. Immunoassays are particularly useful because the antibody reacts with the glucouronide metabolite as well as the parent compound. Chromatographic confirmatory procedures, if they are to detect heroin or morphine use more than 12-24 hr after its use, or are to be used to confirm sensitive immunoassays, require hydrolysis of the conjugates to morphine prior to the extraction step. With use of an adequately sensitive immunoassay for morphine or opiates in conjunction with an appropriately sensitive confirmatory procedure, heroin use can be detected for up to 24 hr to several days after its administration.

In summary, current technologies, both immunologic and physical, are sufficiently sensitive and, in conjunction with appropriate confirmation, sufficiently accurate to identify drugs of abuse reliably. These assays are often directed at inactive metabolites, and in general urinary screens only document use and not effect. While this chapter has been concerned with drug abuse via the inhalation route, current approaches do not permit identification of the route of administration, although the possibility of detecting distinctive pyrolytic products exists.

References

Abel, E. L. (1977). The relationship between cannabis and violence. A review. *Psychol. Bull.* **84**:193-211.

Ablon, S. L., and Goodwin, F. K. (1974). High frequency of dysphoric reactions to tetrahydrocannabinol among depressed patients. *Am. J. Psychiatry* **131**: 448-453.

Adams, E. H., and Durell, J. (1984). Cocaine: a growing public health problem. In *Cocaine: Pharmacology, Effects and Treatment of Abuse.* Edited by J. Grabowski. NIDA Research Monograph 50. Rockville, Md., U.S. Department of Health and Human Resources, National Institute on Drug Abuse, pp. 9-14.

Allen, R. M., and Young, S. J. (1978). Phencyclidine-induced psychosis. *Am. J. Psychiatry* **135**:1081-1084.

Altura, B. T., and Altura, B. M. (1981). Phencyclidine, lysergic acid diethylamide, and mescaline: cerebral artery spasms and hallucinogenic activity. *Science* **212**:1051-1052.

Ambre, J. (1985). The urinary excretion of cocaine and metabolites in humans: a kinetic analysis of published data. *J. Anal. Toxicol.* **9**:241-245.

Ames, O. (1936). *Economic Annuals and Human Culture.* Cambridge, MA. Botanical Museum of Harvard University.

Anderson, F. E. (1973). Marijuana flashbacks. *Am. J. Psychiatry* **130**:1399.

Aronow, W. S., and Cassidy, J. (1974). Effect of marihuana and placebo-mari huana smoking on angina pectoris. *N. Engl. J. Med.* **291**:65-67.

Aronson, T. A., and Craig, T. J. (1986). Cocaine precipitation of panic disorder. *Am. J. Psychiatry* **143**:643-645.

Baerg, R. D., and Kimberg, D. V. (1970). Centrilobular hepatic necrosis and acute renal failure in "solvent sniffers." *Ann. Intern. Med.* **73**:713-720.

Balthazar, E. J., and Lefleur, R. (1983). Abdominal complications of drug addiction: radiologic features. *Semin Roentgenol.* **18**:213-220.

Banner, A. S., Rodriguez, J., Sunderrajan, E. V., Argarwal, M. K., and Addington, W. W. (1979). Bronchiectasis: a cause of pulmonary symptoms in heroin addicts. *Respiration* **37**:232-237.

Barash, P. G., Kopriva, C. J., Langou, R., Van Dyke, C., Jatlow, P., Stahl, A., and Byck, R. (1980). Is cocaine a sympathetic stimulant during general anesthesia? *JAMA* **243**:1437-1439.

Barnett, G., Hawks, R., and Resnick, R. (1981). Cocaine pharmacokinetics in humans. *J. Ethnopharm.* **3**:353-366.

Barton, C. H., Sterling, M. L., and Vaziri, N. D. (1980). Rhabdomyolysis and acute renal failure associated with phencyclidine intoxication. *Arch. Intern. Med.* **140**:568-569.

Barton, C. H., Sterling, M. L., and Vaziri, N. D. (1981). Phencyclidine intoxication: clinical experience in 27 cases confirmed by urine assay. *Ann. Emerg. Med.* **10**:243-246.

Bauman, J. (1980). Marijuana and the female reproductive system. Testimony before the Subcommittee on Criminal Justice of the Committee on the Judiciary, U.S. Senate, Health Consequences of Marihuana Use, Jan. 16-17, 1980. Washington, D.C., U.S. Government printing Office, pp. 85-88.

Beaconsfield, P., Ginsburg, J., and Rainsburg, R. (1972). Marihuana smoking: cardiovascular effects in man and possible mechanisms. *N. Engl. J. Med.* **287**:209-212.

Beede, M. S. (1980). Phencyclidine intoxication. Insights into a growing problem of drug abuse. *Postgrad. Med.* **68**:201-209.

Benchimol, A., Bartall, H., and Desser, K. B. (1978). Accelerated ventricular rhythm and cocaine abuse. *Ann. Intern. Med.* **88**:519-520.

Benignus, V. (1981). Neurobehavioral effects of toluene: a review. *Neurobehav. Toxicol. Teratol.* **3**:407-415.

Benowitz, N. L., and Jones, R. T. (1975). Cardiovascular effects of prolonged delta-9-tetrahydrocannabinol ingestion. *Clin. Pharmacol. Ther.* **18**:287-297.

Bernhardson, G., and Gunne, L. M. (1972). Forty-six cases of psychosis in cannabis abusers. *Int. J. Addict.* **7**:9-16.

Berlant, J. L. (1985). Reserpine and phencyclidine-associated psychosis: three case reports. *J. Clin. Psychiatry* **46**:542-544.

Bozarth, M. A., and Wise, R. A. (1985). Toxicity associated with long-term intravenous heroin and cocaine self-administration in the rat. *JAMA* **254**: 81-83.

Brill, H., and Nahas, G. G. (1984). Cannabis intoxication and mental illness. In *Marihuana in Science and Medicine*. Edited by G. G. Nahas. New York, Raven Press, pp. 263-305.

Bromberg, W. (1934). Marihuana intoxication. A clinical study of *Cannabis sativa* intoxication. *Am. J. Psychiatry* **91**:303-330.

Burns, R. S., and Lerner, S. E. (1976). Perspectives: acute phencyclidine intoxication. *Clin. Toxicol.* **9**:477-501.

Burns, R. S., Lerner, S. E., Corrado, R., James, S. H., Schnoll, S. H. (1975). Phencyclidine-states of acute intoxication and fatalities. *West J. Med.* **123**:345-349.

Byck, R. (1974). *Cocaine Papers: Sigmund Freud.* New York, Stonehill Publishing.

Camp, W. H. (1936). The antiquity of hemp as an economic plant. *J. N.Y. Bot. Gard.* **37**:110-114.

Campbell, I. (1976). The amotivational syndrome and cannabis use with emphasis on the Canadian scene. *Ann. N.Y. Acad. Sci.* **282**:33-36.

Carney, M. W. P., Bacelle, L., and Robinson, B. (1984). Psychosis after cannabis abuse. *Br. Med. J.* **288**:1047.

Castellani, S., Adams, P. M., and Giannini, A. J. (1982). Physostigmine treatment of acute phencyclidine intoxication. *J. Clin. Psychiatry* **43**:10-12.

Chang, A. E., Shiling, D. J., Stillman, R. C., Goldberg, N. H., Seipp, C. A., Barofsky, I., Simon, R. M., and Rosenberg, S. A. (1979). Delta-9-tetrahydrocannabinol as an antiemetic in cancer patients receiving high dose methotrexate. A prospective, randomized evaluation. *Ann. Intern. Med.* **91**: 819-824.

Charney, D. S., Sternberg, D. E., Kleber, H. D., et al. (1981). The clinical use of clonidine in abrupt withdrawal from methadone. *Arch. Gen. Psychiatry* **38**:1273-1277.

Charney, D. S., Heninger, G. R., and Kleber, H. D. (1986). The combined use of clonidine and naltrexone as a rapid, safe, and effective treatment of abrupt withdrawal from methadone. *Am. J. Psychiatry* **143**:831-837.

Chasnoff, I. J., Burns, W. J., Hatcher, R. P., and Burns, K. A. (1983). Phencyclidine: effects on the fetus and neonate. *Dev. Pharmacol. Ther.* **6**:404-408.

Chasnoff, I. J., Burns, W. J., Schnoll, S. H., and Burns, K. A. (1985). Cocaine use in pregnancy. *N. Engl. J. Med.* **313**:666-669.

Chen, G., Ensor, C. R., Russell, D., and Bohner, B. (1959). The pharmacology of 1-(1-phencyclohexyl) piperidine HCl. *J. Pharmacol. Exp. Ther.* **127**: 241-250.

Cherubin, C. E. (1967). The medical sequelae of narcotic addiction. *Ann. Intern. Med.* **67**:23-33.

Chopra, G. S. (1971). Marihuana and adverse psychotic reactions. *Bull. Narcotics* **28**:15-22.

Chopra, G. S., and Smith, J. W. (1974). Psychotic reactions following cannabis use in East Indians. *Arch. Gen. Psychiatry* **30**:24-27.

Chusid, M. J., Gelfand, J. A., Nutter, C., and Fauci, A. S. (1975). Pulmonary aspergillosis, inhalation of contaminated marijuana smoke, chronic granulomatous disease. *Ann. Intern. Med.* **82**:682-683.

Clinger, O. W., and Johnson, N. A. (1951). Purposeful inhalation of gasoline vapors. *Psychiatr. Q.* **25**:557-567.

Co, B. T., Goodwin, D. N., Gado, M., Mikhoul, M., and Hill, S. Y. (1977). Absence of cerebral atrophy in chronic cannabis users. *JAMA* **237**:1229-1230.

Cocores, J. A., Dackis, C. A., and Gold, M. S. (1986). Sexual dysfunction secondary to cocaine abuse in two patients. *J. Clin. Psychiatry* **47**:384-385.

Cogen, F. C., Rigg, G., Simmons, J. L., and Domino, E. F. (1978). Phencyclidine-associated acute rhabdomyolysis. *Ann. Intern. Med.* **88**:210-212.

Coggins, W. J., Swenson, E. W., Dawson, W. W., Fernandez-Salas, A. Hernandez-Bolanos, J., Jiminez-Autillon, C. F., Solano, J. R., Vinocour, R., and Faerrou-Valdez, F. (1976). Health status of chronic heavy cannabis users. *Ann. N.Y. Acad. Sci.* **282**:148-161.

Cohen, S. (1981). Adverse effects of marijuana: selected issues. *Ann. N.Y. Acad. Sci.* **362**:119-124.

Cohen, S. (1986). Marijuana. In American Psychiatric Association. Ann. Rev. Vol. 5. Edited by A. J. Frances, R. E. Hales. American Psychiatric Press, Washington, D.C., pp. 200-211.

Coleman, D. L., Ross, T. F., and Naughton, J. L. (1982). Myocardial ischemia and infarction related to recreational cocaine use. *West. J. Med.* **136**:444-446.

Cone, E. J., and Rolley, E. J. (1986). Contact highs and urinary cannabinoid excretion after passive exposure to marijuana smoke. *Clin. Pharmacol. Ther.* **40**:247-256.

Cook, C. E., Brine, D. R., Jeffcoat, A. R., Hill, J. M., Wall, M. E., Perez-Reyes, M., and DiGuiseppi, S. R. (1982a). Phencyclidine disposition after intravenous and oral doses. *Clin. Pharmacol. Ther.* **31**:625-634.

Cook, C. E., Brine, D. R., Quin, G. D., Perez-Reyes, M., and DiGuiseppi, S. R. (1982b). Phencyclidine and phenylcyclohexene disposition after smoking phencyclidine. *Clin. Pharmacol. Ther.* **31**:635-641.

Copeland, K. C., Underwood, L. E., and Van Wyck, J. J. (1980). Marihuana smoking and pubertal arrest. *J. Pediatr.* **96**:1079-1080.

Copland, G. M., Kolin, A., and Shulman, H. S. (1974). Fatal pulmonary intraalveolar fibrosis after paraquat ingestion. *N. Engl. J. Med.* **291**:290-292.

Cornish, H. H. (1980). Solvents and vapors. In *Toxicology: The Basic Science of Poisons,* 2nd ed. Edited by Casarett and Doull. New York, Macmillan, pp. 468-496.

Cottrell, J. S., Sohn, S. S., and Vogel, W. H. (1973). Toxic effects of marihuana tar on mouse skin. *Arch. Environ. Health* **26**:277-278.

Cregler, L. L., and Mark, H. (1986). Medical complications of cocaine abuse. *N. Engl. J. Med.* **315**:1495-1500.

Crider, R. (1986). Phencyclidine: changing abuse patterns. In *Phencyclidine: An Update.* Edited by D. H. Clouet, Rockville, MD, National Institute on Drug Abuse. (NIDA Research Monograph 64) (DHEW Publication No. (ADM)86-1443, pp. 163-173.

Crites, J., and Schuckit, M. A. (1979). Solvent misuse in adolescents at a community alcohol center. *J. Clin. Psychiatry* **40**:63-67.

Cushman, P., and Khurana, R. (1977). A controlled cycle of tetrahydrocannabinol smoking: T and B cell rosette formation. *Life Sci.* **20**:971-979.

Cushman, P., Khurana, R., and Hashim, G. (1976). THC: evidence for reduced rosette formation by normal T lymphocytes. In *Pharmacology of Marihuana.* Edited by M. Braude and S. Szara. New York, Raven Press. p. 207.

Dackis, C. A., and Gold, M. S. (1985). Bromocriptine as treatment of cocaine abuse. *Lancet* **1**:1151-1152.

DaCosta, J. L., Tock, E. P. C., and Boey, H. K. (1971). Lung disease with chronic obstruction in opium smokers in Singapore. *Thorax* **26**:555-571.

D'Agostino, R. S., and Arnett, E. N. (1979). Acute myoglobinuria and heroin snorting. *JAMA* **241**:277.

Davidow, B., Petri, N., and Quame, B. (1968). A thin-layer chromatographic screening procedure for detecting drug abuse. *Am. J. Clin. Pathol.* **50**: 714-719.

Davis, B. L. (1982). The PCP epidemic: a critical review. *Int. J. Addict.* **17**: 1137-1155.

Davy, H. (1800). *Researches, Chemical and Philosophical: Chiefly Concerning Nitrous Oxide.* London, Johnson.

Dogoloff, L. I., Angarola, R. T., and Price, S. C. (1985). Urine Testing in the Workplace. Rockville, Md., American Council for Drug Education.

Dole, V. P., Kim, W. K., and Eglitis, I. (1966). Detection of narcotic drugs, tranquilizers, amphetamines and barbiturates in urine. *JAMA* **198**:349-352.

Doorenbos, N. J., Fetterman, P. S., Quimby, M. W., and Turner, C. E. (1971). Cultivation, extraction and analysis of *Cannabis sativa L. Ann. N.Y. Acad. Sci.* **191**:3-15.

Drath, D. B., Shorey, J. M., Price, L., and Huber, G. L. (1979). Metabolic and functional characteristics of alveolar macrophages recovered from rats exposed to marijuana smoke. *Infect. Immunity* **25**:268-272.

Drug Abuse Warning Network (1983). Data from the Drug Abuse Warning Network (DAWN) Statistical Series. Quarterly Report, Provisional Data, Series G, No. 12 (July-September). Rockville, Md., National Institute on Drug Abuse.

Drug Abuse Warning Network (DAWN) (1985). Drug by SMSA 12-month totals for 60 months ending September 1984 for Heroin/Morphine, Cocaine and PCP/PCP combination. Rockville, Md., National Institute on Drug Abuse.

Drug Poll (1976). *Yale Daily News,* March 29, p. 27.

Duberstein, J. L., and Kaufman, D. M. (1971). A clinical study of an epidemic of heroin intoxication and heroin-induced pulmonary edema. *Am. J. Med.* **51**:704-714.

DuPont, R. L. (1978). International challenge of drug abuse. A perspective from the United States. NIDA monograph #19, Washington, D.C.

Eastman, J. W., and Cohen, S. N. (1975). Hypertensive crisis and death associated with phencyclidine poisoning. *JAMA* **231**:1270-1271.

Evans, J. M., Hogg, M. I. J., Lynn, J. N., and Rosen, M. (1974). Degree and duration of reversal by naloxone of effects of morphine in conscious subjects. *Br. Med. J.* **2**:589-591.

Ewens, G. F. W. (1904). Insanity following the use of Indian hemp. *Indian Med. Gazette* **39**:401-413.

Fauman, B., Aldinger, G., Fauman, M., and Rosen, P. (1976). Psychiatric sequelae of phencyclidine abuse. *Clin. Toxicol.* **9**(4):529-538.

Fink, M. (1976). Effects of acute and chronic inhalation of hashish, marijuana, and delta-9-tetrahydrocannabinol on brain electrical activity in man: evidence for tissue tolerance. *Ann. N.Y. Acad. Sci.* **282**:387-398.

Finkle, B. S., and McCloskey, K. L. (1978). The forensic toxicology of cocaine (1971-1976). *J. Forensic Sci.* **23**:173-189.

Firooznia, H., Golimbu, C., Rafii, M., and Lichtman, E. A. (1983). Radiology of musculoskeletal complications of drug addiction. *Semin Roentgenol.* **18**: 198-206.

Fischman, M. W. (1984). The behavioral pharmacology of cocaine in humans. In *Cocaine: Pharmacology, Effects and Treatment of Abuse.* Edited by J. Grabowski. NIDA Research Monograph 50. Rockville, Md., U.S. Department of Health and Human Services, National Institute on Drug Abuse, pp. 72-91.

Fischman, M. W., and Schuster, C. R. (1980). Cocaine effects in sleep-deprived humans. *Psychopharmacology* **72**:1-8.

Fischman, M. W., Schuster, C. R., Resnekov, L., Shick, F. E., Krasnegor, N. A., Fennell, W., and Freedman, D. X. (1976). Cardiovascular and subjective effects on intravenous cocaine administration in humans. *Arch. Gen. Psychiatry* **33**:983-989.

Fischman, M. W., Schuster, C. R., Javaid, J., Hatano, Y., and Davis, J. (1985). Acute tolerance development to the cardiovascular and subjective effects of cocaine. *J. Pharmacol. Exp. Ther.* **235**:677-682.

Fish, F., and Wilson, W. D. C. (1969). Excretion of cocaine and its metabolites in man. *J. Pharmacol.* **21**:1355-1385.

Fishbein, L. (1982). Chromatography of environmental hazards. In *Drugs of Abuse,* Vol. 4. Amsterdam, Elsevier, pp. 394-423.

Fishburne, P. M., Abelson, H. I., and Cisin, I. (1980). National Survey on Drug Abuse: Main Findings: 1979. Washington, D.C., Department of Health and Human Services (DHHS publication no. (ADM) 80-976).

Foltz, R. L., Fentiman, A. F., and Foltz, R. B. (eds.) (1980). GC/MS Assays for Abused Drugs in Body Fluid. NIDA Research Monograph 32. Washington, D.C., U.S. Government Printing Office.

Fornazzari, L., Wilkinson, D. A., Kapur, B. M., and Carlen, P. L. (1983). Cerebellar, cortical and functional impairment in toluene abusers. *Acta Neurol. Scand.* **67**:319-329.

Fortenberry, J. D. (1985). Gasoline sniffing. *Am. J. Med.* **79**:740-744.

Frand. U. I., Shim, C. S., and Williams, M. H. Jr. (1972). Heroin-induced pulmonary edema. *Ann. Intern. Med.* **77**:29-35.

Fried, P. A. (1980). Marihuana use by pregnant women: Neurobehavioral effects in neonates. *Drug Alcohol Depend.* **6**:415-424.

Froede, R. (1972). Drugs of abuse: legal and illegal. *Human Pathol.* **3**:23-36.

Gallo, R. C., Salahuddin, S. Z., Popovic, M., et al. (1984). Frequent detection and isolation of cytopathic retroviruses (HTLV-III) from patients with AIDS and at risk for AIDS. *Science* **224**:500-503.

Gaoni, Y, and Mechoulam, R. (1964). Isolation, structure and partial synthesis of an active constituent of hashish. *J. Am. Chem. Soc.* **86**:1646-1647.

Garriott, J., and Petty, C. S. (1980). Death from inhalant abuse: Toxicological and pathological evaluation of 34 cases. *Clin. Toxicol.* **16**:305-315.

Gash, A., Karliner, J. S., Janowsky, D., and Lake, C. R. (1978). Effects of smoking marihuana on left ventricular performance and plasma norepinephrine. Studies in normal men. *Ann. Intern. Med.* **89**:448-452.

Gawin, F. H., and Kleber, H. D. (1986). Abstinence symptomatology and psychiatric diagnosis in cocaine abusers. *Arch. Gen. Psychiatry* **43**:107-113.

Gay, G. R. (1982). Clinical management of acute and chronic cocaine poisoning. *Ann. Emerg. Med.* **11**:562-572.

Giannini, A. J., and Price, W. A. (1985). PCP: management of acute intoxication. *Resident Staff Physician* **31**(Nov):23PC-31PC.

Giannini, A. J., Loiselle, R. H., Price, W. A., and Giannini, M. C. (1985). Chlorpromazine vs meperidine in the treatment of phencyclidine psychosis. *J. Clin. Psychiatry* **46**:52-54.

Godolphin, W. (1982). Enzyme multiplied immunoassay technique. In *Methodology for Analytical Toxicology*, Vol. II. Edited by I. Sunchine and P. Jatlow. Boca Raton, FL, CRC Press, pp. 189-203.

Gold, M. S., Redmond, D. E. Jr., and Kleber, H. D. (1978). Clonidine blocks acute opiate withdrawal symptoms. *Lancet* **2**:599-602.

Gold, M. S., Pottash, A. C., Sweeney, D. R., and Kleber, H. D. (1980). Opiate withdrawal using clonidine. *JAMA* **243**:343-346.

Goldbloom, D., and Chouinard, G. (1985). Schizophreniform psychosis associated with chronic industrial toluene exposure: case report. *J. Clin. Psychiatry* **46**:350-351.

Goldstein, D. S., Karpel, J. P., Appel, D., and Williams, M. H. Jr. (1986). Bullous pulmonary damage in users of intravenous drugs. *Chest* **89**:266-269.

Goode, E. (1984). *Drugs in American Society,* 2nd ed. New York, Alfred A. Knopf.

Gottlieb, M. S., Groopman, J. E., Weinstein, W. M., Fahey, J. L., and Detels, R. (1983). The acquired immunodeficiency syndrome. *Ann. Intern. Med.* **99**:208-220.

Grabowski, J. (1984). Cocaine 1984: introduction and overview. In *Cocaine: Pharmacology, Effects and Treatment of Abuse.* Edited by J. Grabowski. NIDA Research Monograph 50. Rockville, Md., U.S. Department of Health and Human Services, National Institute on Drug Abuse, pp. 1-8.

Greenwood, R. J. (1974). Lumbar plexitis and rhabdomyolysis following abuse of heroin. *Postgrad. Med. J.* **50**:772-773.

Greifenstein, F. E., Yoshitake, J., DeVault, M., and Gajewski, J. E. (1958). A study of 1-aryl cyclohexylamine for anesthesia. *Anesth. Analg. Curr. Res.* **37**(5):283-294.

Grinspoon, L., and Bakalar, J. B. (1976). *Cocaine: A Drug and Social Evolution.* New York, Basic Books, pp. 9-10.

Grinspoon, L., and Bakalar, J. B. (1981). Adverse effects of cocaine: selected issues. *Ann. N.Y. Acad. Sci.* **362**:125-131.

Gupta, S., Grieco, M. H., and Cushman, P. (1974). Impairment of rosette-forming T-lymphocytes in chronic marihuana smokers. *N. Engl. J. Med.* **291**:874-877.

Haddad, L. M. (1986). Cocaine abuse: background, clinical presentation and emergency treatment. *IM. Intern. Med. Specialist* **7**:67-75.

Haley, T. J. (1980). Review of the physiological effects of amyl, butyl, and isobutyl nitrite. *Clin. Toxicol.* **16**:317-329.

Halikas, J. A., Goodwin, D. W., and Guze, S. B. (1971). Marihuana effects: a survey of regular users. *JAMA* **217**:692-694.

Handal, K. A., Schauben, J. L., and Salmone, F. R. (1983). Naloxone. *Ann. Emerg. Med.* **12**:438-445.

Harding, T., and Knight, F. (1973). Marihuana-modified mania. *Arch. Gen. Psychiatry* **29**:635-637.

Hart, J. B., McChesney, J. C., Grief, M. et al. (1972). Composition of illicit drugs and the use of drug analysis and abuse abatement. *J. Psychedelic Drugs* **5**:83-88.

Hart. R. H. (1976). A psychiatric classification of cannabis intoxication. *J. Am. Acad. Psychiatry Neurology* **1**(4):83-95.

Harvey, D. J. (1984). Chemistry, metabolism, and pharmacokinetics of the cannabinoids. In *Marihuana in Science and Medicine*. Edited by G. G. Nahas. New York, Raven Press, pp. 37-107.

Harvey, D. J., Leuschner, J. T. A., and Paton, W. D. M. (1980). Measurement of delta tetrahydrocannabinol in plasma to the low picogram range by gas chromatography-mass spectrometry using metastable ion detection. *J. Chromatogr.* **202**:83-92.

Hawks, R. L. (Ed.) (1982). The analysis of cannabinoids in biological fluids. NIDA Research Monograph 42. Washington, D.C., U.S. Government Printing Office.

Hayden, J. W., Comstock, E. G., and Comstock, B. S. (1976). The clinical toxicology of solvent abuse. *Clin. Toxicol.* **9**:169-184.

Helpern, M. (1972). Fatalities from narcotic addiction in New York City—incidence, circumstances and pathologic findings. *Human Pathol.* **3**:13-21.

Hembree, W. C., Nahas, G. G., Zeidenberg, P., and Huang, H. F. S. (1979). Changes in human spermatozoa associated with high dose marihuana smoking. In *Marihuana: Biological Effects, Analysis, Metabolism, Cellular Responses, Reproduction and Brain*. Edited by G. G. Nahas and W. D. M. Paton. New York, Pergamon Press, pp. 429-439.

Henderson, R. L., Tennant, F. S., and Guerry, R. (1972). Respiratory manifestations of hashish smoking. *Arch. Otolaryngol.* **95**:248-251.

Heyndrickx, A., Scheiris, C., and Schepens, P. (1970). Toxicological study of a fatal intoxication in man due to cannabis smoking. *J. Pharm. Belg.* **24**: 371-376.

Hingson, R., Alpert, J. J., Day, N., Dooling, E., Kayn, H., Morelock, S., Oppenheimer, E., and Zuckerman, B. (1982). Effects of maternal drinking and marijuana use on fetal growth and development. *Pediatrics* **70**:539-546.

Hirsch, C. S. (1972). Dermatopathology of narcotic addiction. *Human Pathol.* **3**:37-53.

Hirsch, C. S., and Adelson, L. (1972). Acute fatal intranasal narcotism. Report of two fatalities following narcotic "snorting." *Human Pathol.* **3**: 71-73.

Hoffman, D., Brunnemann, K. D., Gori, G. B., and Wynder, E. L. (1975). On the carcinogenicity of marijuana smoke. *Recent Adv. Phytochem.* **9**: 63-81.

Hollister, L. E. (1968). Chemical psychoses. *LSD and Related Drugs*. American Lecture Series. Springfield, Illinois, Charles C Thomas.

Howard, R. E., Hueter, D. C., and Davis, G. J. (1985). Acute myocardial infarction following cocaine abuse in a young woman with normal coronary arteries. *JAMA* **254**:95-96.

Huber, G. L., Simmons, G. A., McCarthy, C. R., Cutting, M. B., Laguarda, R., and Pereira, W. (1975). Depressant effect of marihuana smoke on antibacterial activity of pulmonary alveolar macrophages. *Chest* **68**:769-773.

Inaba, T., Stewart, D. J., and Kalow, W. (1978). Metabolism of cocaine in man. *Clin. Pharmacol. Ther.* **23**:547-552.

Isbell, H., Gorodetsky, G. W., Jasinski, D., Claussen, U., Spulak, F., and Korte, F. (1967). Effect of delta-9-transtetrahydrocannabinol in man. *Psychopharmacologia* **11**:184-188.

Isner, J., Mark Estes, N. A. III, Thompson, P. D., Costanzo-Nordin, M. R., Subramanian, R., Miller, G., Katsas, G., Sweeney, K., and Sturner, W. Q. (1986). Acute cardiac events temporally related to cocaine abuse. *N. Engl. J. Med.* **315**:1438-1443.

Itkonen, J., Schnoll, S., and Glassroth, J. (1984). Pulmonary dysfunction in "freebase" cocaine users. *Arch. Intern. Med.* **144**:2195-2197.

Jaffe, J. H., and Martin, W. R. (1980). Opioid analgesics and antagonists. In *The Pharmacological Basis of Therapeutics*, 6th ed. Edited by A. G. Gilman, L. S. Goodman, and A. Gilman. New York, Macmillan.

Jan. K. M., Dorsey, S., and Bornstein, A. (1978). Hog hog: hyperthermia from phencyclidine (letter). *N. Engl. J. Med.* **299**:722.

Janowsky, D. S., Meacham, M. P., Blaine, J. D., Schoor, M., and Bozzetti, L. P. (1976). Marijuana affects on simulated flying ability. *Am. J. Psychiatry* **133**:384-388.

Jatlow, P. L., and Bailey, D. N. (1975). Gas chromatographic analysis for cocaine in human plasma with the use of a nitrogen detector. *Clin. Chem.* **21**:1918-1921.

Jatlow, P., Barach, P. G., Van Dyke, C., Radding, J., and Byck, R. (1979). Cocaine and succinylcholine sensitivity: a new caution. *Anesth. Analg.* **58**:235-238.

Javaid, J. I. (1978). Cocaine plasma concentration; relation to physiological and subjective effects in humans. *Science* **202**:227-228.

Jekel, J. F., Podlewski, H., Dean-Patterson, S., Allen, D. F., Clarke, N., and Cartwright, P. (1986). Epidemic free-base cocaine abuse. Case study from the Bahamas. *Lancet* **1**:459-462.

Johnson, S., and Domino, E. F. (1971). Some cardiovascular effects of marihuana smoking in normal volunteers. *Clin. Pharmacol. Ther.* **12**:762-768.

Jones, R. T. (1984). The pharmacology of cocaine. In *Cocaine: Pharmacology, Effects and Treatment of Abuse*. Edited by J. Grabowski. NIDA Research Monograph 50. Rockville, Md., National Institute on Drug Abuse, pp. 34-53.

Jones, R. T., and Benowitz, N. (1976). The 30-day-trip—clinical studies of cannabis tolerance and dependence. In *Pharmacology of Marihuana*. Edited by M. C. Braude and S. Szara. New York, Raven Press, pp. 627-642.

Johnsson, S., O'Meara, M., and Young, J. B. (1983). Acute cocaine poisoning: Importance of treating seizures and acidosis. *Am. J. Med.* **75**:1061-1064.

Jorgensen, K. A., and Lawesson, S. O. (1982). Amyl nitrite and Kaposi's sarcoma in homosexual men. *N. Engl. J. Med.* **307**:893-894.

Kagen, S. L. (1981). Aspergillus: an inhalable contaminant of marijuana. *N. Engl. J. Med.* **304**:483-484.

Kagen, S. L., Kurup, V. P., Sohnle, P. G., and Fink, J. N. (1983). Marijuana smoking and fungal sensitization. *J. Allergy Clin. Immunol.* **71**:389-393.

Kanakis, C. Jr., Pouget, J. M., and Rosen, K. M. (1976). The effects of delta-9-tetrahydrocannabinol (cannabis) on cardiac performance with and without beta blockade. *Circulation* **53**:703-707.

Kaplan, H. S. (1971). Psychosis associated with marijuana. *N.Y. State J. Med.* **71**:433-435.

Karliner, J. S., Steinberg, A. D., and Williams, M. H. Jr. (1969). Lung function after pulmonary edema associated with heroin overdoses. *Arch. Intern. Med.* **124**:350-353.

Katz, S., Aberman, A., Frand, U. I., Stein, I. M., and Fulop, M. (1972). Heroin pulmonary edema evidence for increased pulmonary capillary permeability. *Am. Rev. Respir. Dis.* **106**:472-474.

Keeler, M. H. (1967). Adverse reactions to marihuana. *Am. J. Psychiatry* **124**: 674-677.

Keeler, M. H., Reifler, C. B., and Liptzin, M. B. (1968). Spontaneous recurrence of marihuana effect. *Am. J. Psychiatry* **125**:384-386.

Khantzian, E. J., and McKenna, G. J. (1979). Acute toxic and withdrawal reactions associated with drug use and abuse. *Ann. Intern. Med.* **90**:361-372.

Khouzam, N. (1986). The cocaine user who looked like a bullfrog. *Hosp. Practice,* September 15, pp. 157-158.

King, L. J., Teale, J. D., and Macks, V. (1976). Biochemical aspects of cannabis. In *Cannabis and Health.* Edited by J. D. P. Graham. London, Academic Press, pp. 77-107.

Kleber, H. D. (1985). Naltrexone. *J. Subst. Abuse Treat.* **2**:117-122.

Kleber, H. D., and Gawan, F. H. (1984a). The spectrum of cocaine abuse and its treatment. *J. Clin. Psychiatry* **45** (12, Sec. 2):18-23.

Kleber, H. D., and Gawin, F. H. (1984b). Cocaine abuse: a review of current and experimental treatments. In *Cocaine: Pharmacology, Effects and Treatment of Abuse.* NIDA Research Monograph 50. Rockville, Md., U.S. Department of Health and Human Services, National Institute on Drug Abuse, pp. 111-129.

Kleber, H. D., and Gawin, F. H. (1986). Cocaine. In *Annual Review. Drug Abuse and Drug Dependence.* Edited by A. J. Frances and R. E. Hales. Washington, D.C., American Psychiatric Press Inc., pp. 160-185.

Kleber, H. D., and Kosten, T. R. (1984). Naltrexone induction: psychologic and pharmacologic strategies. *J. Clin. Psychiatry* **45** (9, Sec. 2):29-38.

Kleber, H. D., Kosten, T. R., Gaspari, J., et al. (1985). Nontolerance to the opioid antagonism of naltrexone. *Biol. Psychiatry* **20**:66-72.

Kochar, M. S., and Hosko, M. J. (1973). Electrocardiographic effects of marihuana. *JAMA* **225**:25-27.

Kolodny, R. C., Masters, W. H., Kolodner, R. M., and Toro, G. (1974). Depression of plasma testosterone levels after chronic intensive marihuana use. *N. Engl. J. Med.* **290**:872-874.

Kossowsky, W. A., and Lyon, A. F. (1984). Cocaine and acute myocardial infarction. A probable connection. *Chest* **86**:729-731.

Kuehule, J., Mendelson, J. H., Davis, K. R., and New, P. F. J. (1977). Computed tomographic examination of heavy marijuana smokers. *JAMA* **237**:1231-1232.

Layzer, R. B., Fishman, R. A., and Schafer, J. A. (1978). Neuropathy following abuse of nitrous oxide. *Neurology* **28**:504-506.

Lemberger, L., Weiss, J. L., Watanabe, A. M., Galanter, I. M., Wyatt, R. J., and Cardon, P. V. (1972). Delta-9-tetrahydrocannabinol. Temporal correlation of the psychologic effects and blood levels after various routes of administration. *N. Engl. J. Med.* **286**:685-688.

Leuchtenberger, C., and Leuchtenberger, R. (1976). Cytological and cytochemical studies of the effects of fresh marijuana cigarette smoke on growth and DNA metabolism of animal and human lung cultures. In *Pharmacology of Marihuana.* Edited by M. C. Braude and S. Szara. New York, Raven Press, pp. 595-612.

Leute, R. K., Ullman, E. F., Goldstein, A., and Herzenberg, L. A. (1972). Spin immunoassay technique for determination of morphine. *Nature New Biol.* **236**:93-94.

Light, R. W., and Dunham, T. R. (1975). Severe slowly resolving heroin-induced pulmonary edema. *Chest* **67**:61-64.

LiPuma, J. P., Wellman, J., and Stern, H. P. (1982). Nitrous oxide abuse: a new cause for pneumomediastinum. *Radiology* **145**:602.

Llamas, R., Hart, D. R., and Schneider, N. S. (1978). Allergic broncho-pulmonary aspergillosis associated with smoking moldy marihuana. *Chest* **73**:871-872.

Louria, D. B., Hensle, T., and Rose, J. (1967). The major medical complications of heroin addiction. *Ann. Intern. Med.* **67**:1-22.

Luby, E. D., Cohen, B. D., Rosenbaum, G., Gottlieb, J., and Kelley, R. (1959). Study of a new schizophrenomimetic drug—Sernyl. *Arch. Neurol. Psychiatry* **81**:363-369.

Luisada, P. V., and Brown, B. I. (1976). Clinical management of the phencyclidine psychosis. *Clin. Toxicol.* **9**:539-545.

Luisada, P. V. (1978). The phencyclidine psychosis, phenomenology and treat-
    ment. In *Phencyclidine (PCP) Abuse: An Appraisal.* Edited by R. C.
    Petersen and R. C. Stillman. Washington, D.C., National Institute of Drug
    Abuse, (Res. Monogr. Series No. 21), pp. 241-254.

Lundberg, G. D., Gupta, R. C., and Montgomery, S. H. (1976). Phencyclidine:
    patterns seen in street drug analysis. *Clin. Toxicol.* **9**:503-511.

Magus, R. D., and Harris, L. S. (1971). Carcinogenic potential of marihuana smoke
    condensate. *Fed. Proc.* **30**:279.

Mann, P. E. G., Cohen, A. B., Finley, T. N., and Ladman, A. J. (1971). Alveolar
    macrophages: structural and functional differences between nonsmokers and
    smokers of marijuana and tobacco. *Lab. Invest.* **25**:111-119.

Martin, W. R. (1976). Naloxone. *Ann. Intern. Med.* **85**:765-768.

Mason, A. P., and McBay, A. J. (1985). Cannabis: pharmacology and interpreta-
    tion of effects. *J. Forensic Sci.* **30**:615-631.

Maurer, D. W., and Vogel, V. H. (1967). *Narcotics and Narcotic Addiction,* 3rd
    ed. Springfield, IL, Charles C Thomas.

Mayor's Committee on Marihuana (1944). *The Marijuana Problem in the City of
    New York—Sociological, Medical, Psychological and Pharmacological Studies.*
    Lancaster, PA, Cattell Press.

McCarron, M. M. (1986). Phencyclidine intoxication. In *Phencyclidine: An Up-
    date.* Edited by D. H. Clouet. Rockville, MD, National Institute on Drug
    Abuse (NIDA Research Monograph 64) (DHEW Publication No. (ADM)
    86-1443, pp. 209-217.

McCarron, M. M., Schulze, B. W., Thompson, G. A., Conder, M. C., and Goetz, W.
    A. (1981a). Acute phencyclidine intoxication: incidence of clinical find-
    ings in 1000 cases. *Ann. Emerg. Med.* **10**:237-242.

McCarron, M. M., Schulze, B. W., Thompson, G. A., Conder, M. C., and Goetz, W.
    A. (1981b). Acute phencyclidine intoxication: clinical patterns, compli-
    cations and treatment. *Ann. Emerg. Med.* **10**:290-297.

Mechoulam, R. (1970). Marihuana chemistry. *Science* **168**:1159-1166.

Mendelson, J. H., Kuehule, J., Ellingboe, J., and Babor, T. F. (1974). Plasma
    testosterone levels before, during and after chronic marihuana smoking.
    N. Engl. J. Med. **291**:1051-1055.

Messina, F. V., and Wynne, J. W. (1982). Homemade nitrous oxide: no laughing
    matter. *Ann. Intern. Med.* **96**:333-334.

Meyers, F. H., Rose, A. J., and Smith, D. E. (1968). Incidents involving the
    Haight-Ashbury population and some uncommonly used drugs. *J. Psyche-
    delic Drugs* **1**:139-146.

Miller, G. W. (1985). The cocaine habit. *Am. Family Physician* **31**(No. 2):173-
    176.

Miller, J. D. et al. (1983). National survey on drug abuse. Main Findings, 1982.
    Washington, D.C., U.S. Government Printing Office.

Millman, R., (1985). Drug abuse and dependence. In *Cecil Textbook of Medi-*

cine, 17th ed. Edited by J. B. Wyngaarden and L. H. Smith, Jr. Philadelphia, W. B. Saunders, pp. 2015-2024.

Miras, C. J. (1969). Experience with chronic hashish smokers. In *Drugs and Youth.* Edited by J. R. Wittenborn, H. Brill, J. P. Smith, and S. A. Wittenborn. Springfield, Charles C Thomas, pp. 191-198.

Mittleman, R. E., and Wetli, C. V. (1984). Death caused by recreational cocaine use, an update. *JAMA* **252**:1889-1893.

Moreau, J. J. (1845). *Du Hachisch et de l'Alienation Mentale: Etudes Psychologiques.* Paris Librarie de Fortin, Masson, (English edition: *Hashish and Mental Illness.* Edited by H. Peters and G. G. Nahas. New York, Raven Press, 1973).

Morland, J., Bugge, A., Skuterud, B., Steen, A., Wethe, G. H., and Kjeldsen, T. (1985). Cannabinoids in blood and urine after passive inhalation of cannabis smoke. *J. Forensic Sci.* **30**:997-1002.

Morris, J. B., and Shuck, J. M. (1985). Pneumomediastinum in a young male cocaine user. *Ann. Emerg. Med.* **14**:194-196.

Morrison, W. J., Wetherill, S., and Zyroff, J. (1970). The acute pulmonary edema of heroin intoxication. *Radiology* **97**:347-351.

Mule, S. J. (1969). Identification of narcotics, barbiturates, amphetamines, tranquilizers, and psychotomimetics in human urine. *J. Chromatogr.* **39**:302-311.

Musto, D. F. (1973). *The American Disease: Origins of Narcotic Control.* New Haven, Yale University Press.

Nahas, G. G. (1984). Toxicology and Pharmacology. In *Marihuana in Science and Medicine.* Edited by G. G. Nahas. New York, Raven Press, pp. 109-246.

Nahas, G. G., Suciu-Foca, N., Armand, J. P., and Morishima, A. (1974). Inhibition of cellular mediated immunity in marihuana smokers. *Science* **183**:419-420.

Nahas, G. G., Davies, M., and Osserman, F. F. (1979). Serum immunoglobulin concentration in chronic marihuana smokers. *Fed. Proc.* **38**:591.

Nakamura, G. R., and Noguchi, T. T. (1981). Fatalities from cocaine overdoses in Los Angeles County. *Clin. Toxicol.* **18**:895-905.

National Institute on Drug Abuse (NIDA) (1982). Marijuana and health: Ninth annual report to the United States Congress from the Secretary of Health and Human Services. Rockville, Md., NIDA, DHHS Publ. No. (ADM) 82:1216.

Nevins, M. A. (1980). Neuropathy after nitrous oxide abuse. *JAMA* **244**:2264 (letter).

Newell, G. R., Mansell, P. W. A., Spitz, M. R., Reuben, J. M., and Hersh, E. M. (1985). Volatile nitrites. Use and adverse effects related to the current epidemic of the acquired immune deficiency syndrome. *Am. J. Med.* **78**:811-816.

New York Times. (1986). Growth in heroin use ending as city users turn to
crack. Vol. CXXXV No. 46896 September 13, pp. 1, 8.

Newsweek (1986). The drug crisis, crack and crime. June 16, pp. 15-22.

Nicholi, A. M. Jr. (1983). The nontherapeutic use of psychoactive drugs: a
modern epidemic. *N. Engl. J. Med.* **308**:925-933.

Nicholson, D. P. (1983). The immediate management of overdose. *Med. Clin.
North Am.* **67**:1279-1293.

Noguchi, T. T., and Nakamura, G. R. (1978). Phencyclidine-related deaths in
Los Angeles County 1976. *J. Forensic Sci.* **23**:503-507.

Novotny, M., Lee, M. L., and Bartle, K. D. (1976). A possible chemical base
for the higher mutagenicity of marijuana smoke as compared to tobacco
smoke. *Experientia* **32**:280-282.

O'Brien, E. T., Yeoman, W. B., and Hobby, J. A. E. (1971). Hepatorenal
damage from toluene in a "glue sniffer." *Br. Med. J.* **2**:29-30.

Ohlsson, A., Lindgren, J. E., Wahlen, A., Agurell, S., Hollister, L. E., and Gillespie, H. K. (1980). Plasma delta-9-tetrahydrocannabinol concentrations
and clinical effects after oral and intravenous administration and smoking.
Clin. Pharmacol. Ther. **28**:409-416.

Osler, W. (1880). Oedema of left lung morphia poisoning. *Montreal Gen.
Hosp. Reports* **1**:291-292.

Overland, E. S., Nolan, A. J., and Hopewell, P. C. (1980). Alteration of pulmonary function in intravenous drug abusers. Prevalence, severity, and
characterization of gas exchange abnormalities. *Am. J. Med.* **68**:231-
237.

Paly, D., Jatlow, P., Van Dyke, C., Jeri, R., and Byck, R. (1982). Plasma cocaine concentrations during cocaine paste smoking. *Life Sci.* **30**(9):731-
738.

Pare, J. A., Fraser, R. G., Hogg, J. C., Howlett, J. G., and Murphy, S. B. (1979).
Pulmonary "mainline" granulomatosis. Talcosis of intravenous methadone abuse. *Medicine* **58**:229-239.

Paris, M., and Nahas, G. G. (1984). Botany: the unstabilized species. In *Marihuana in Science and Medicine.* Edited by G. G. Nahas. New York,
Raven Press, pp. 3-36.

Pearlman, J. T., and Adams, G. L. (1970). Amyl nitrite inhalation fad. *JAMA*
212:160.

Perez-Reyes, M., DiGuiseppi, S., Davis, K. H., Schindler, V. H., and Cook, C. E.
(1982a). Comparison of effects of marihuana cigarettes of 3 different
potencies. *Clin. Pharmacol. Ther.* **31**:617-624.

Perez Reyes, M., DiGuiseppi, S., and Ondrosek, G. (1982b). Free-base cocaine
smoking. *Clin. Pharmacol. Ther.* **4**:459-465.

Perry, D. C. (1976). PCP revisited. *Clin. Toxicol.* **9**:339-348.

Petersen, R. C., and Stillman, R. C. (Ed.) (1977). Cocaine 1977. Washington, D.C., National Institutes on Drug Abuse, Research Monograph Series No. 13.

Petersen, R. C., and Stillman, R. C. (Eds.) (1978). Phencyclidine (PCP) abuse: an appraisal. Rockville, Md., National Institute on Drug Abuse. (NIDA Research Monograph 21) (DHEW Publication No. (ADM) 78-728).

Pillard, R. C. (1970). Marihuana. *N. Engl. J. Med.* **283**:294-303.

Poh, S. C. (1972). The effects of opium smoking in cigarette smokers. *Am. Rev. Respir. Dis.* **106**:239-245.

Pollin, W. (1985). The danger of cocaine. *JAMA* **254**:98 (editorial).

Post, R. M., Kotlin, J., and Goodwin, F. M. (1974). The effects of cocaine on depressed patients. *Am. J. Psychiatry* **131**:511-517.

Poster, D. S., Penta, J. S., Bruno, S., and MacDonald, J. S. (1981). Delta-9-tetrahydrocannabinol in clinical oncology. *JAMA* **245**:2047-2051.

Prakash, R., Aronow, W. S., Warren, M., Laverty, W., and Gottschalk, L. A. (1975). Effects of marihuana and placebo marihuana smoking on hemodynamics in coronary disease. *Clin. Pharmacol. Ther.* **18**:90-95.

Rachelefsky, G. S., Opelz, G., Mickey, M. R., Lessin, P., Kiuchi, M., Silverstein, M. J., and Stiehm, E. R. (1976). Intact humoral and cell-mediated immunity in chronic marijuana smoking. *J. Allergy Alin. Immunol.* **58**:483-490.

Rainey, J. M. Jr., and Crowder, M. K. (1974). Prevalence of phencyclidine in street drug preparations (letter). *N. Engl. J. Med.* **290**:466-467.

Rappolt, R. T. Sr., Gay, G. R., and Inaba, D. S. (1976). Propranolol in the treatment of cardiopressor effects of cocaine. *N. Engl. J. Med.* **295**:448.

Renault, P. F., Schuster, C. R., Heinrich, R., and Freeman, C. X. (1971). Marihuana: standardized smoke administration and dose effect curves on heart rate in humans. *Science* **174**:589-591.

Resnick, R. B., Kestenbaum, R. S., and Schwartz, L. K. (1980). Acute systemic effects of cocaine in man: a controlled study by intranasal and intravenous routes. In *Cocaine.* Edited by F. R. Jeri. Lima, Pacific Press, pp. 17-20.

Reynolds, H. Y., and Chretien, J. (1984). Respiratory tract fluids: analysis of content and contemporary use in understanding lung diseases. *DM* **30**:46-67.

Reynolds, P. C. (1976). Clinical and forensic experiences with phencyclidine. *Clin. Toxicol.* **9**(4):547-552.

Ritchie, J. M., and Greene, N. M. (1980). Local anesthetics. In *The Pharmacological Basis of Therapeutics,* 6th ed. Edited by L. S. Goodman and A. Gilman. New York, Macmillan, pp. 300-320.

Rodin, E. A., Domino, E. F., and Porzak, J. P. (1970). The marihuana-induced "social high." Neurological and electroencephalographic concomitants. *JAMA* **213**:1300-1302.

Rosen, A. M., Mukherjee, S., and Shinbach K. (1984). The efficacy of ECT in phencyclidine-induced psychosis. *J. Clin. Psychiatry* **45**:220-222.

Rosenow, E. C. III (1972). The spectrum of drug-induced pulmonary disease. *Ann. Intern. Med.* **77**:977-991.

Rubin, V. (Ed.) (1975). Cannabis and culture. The Hague, Mouton.

Saba, G. P., James, A. E., Johnson, B. A., et al. (1974). Pulmonary complications of narcotic abuse. *Am. J. Roentgenol.* **122**:733-739.

Sahenk, Z., Mendell, J. R., Couri, D., and Nachtman, J. (1978). Polyneuropathy from inhalation of N_2O cartridges through a whipped cream dispenser. *Neurology* **28**:485-487.

Schachne, J. S., Roberts, B. H., and Thompson, P. D. (1984). Coronary-artery spasm and myocardial infarction associated with cocaine use. *N. Engl. J. Med.* **310**:1665-1666.

Schachter, E. N., and Basta, W. (1973). Bronchiectasis following heroin overdose: a report of two cases. *Chest* **63**:363-366.

Schneider, R. S., Lindquist, P., Wong, E. T., Rubenstein, K. E., and Ullman, E. F. (1973). Homogeneous enzyme immunoassay for opiates in urine. *Clin. Chem.* **19**:821-825.

Schreiber, S. N., Liebowitz, M. R., Bernstein, L. H. et al. (1971). Limb compression and renal impairment (crush syndrome) complicating narcotic overdose. *N. Engl. J. Med.* **284**:368-369.

Schwartz, R. H., and Hawks, R. L. (1985). Laboratory testing of marijuana use. *JAMA* **254**:788-792.

Selik, R. M., Haverkos, H. W., and Curran, J. W. (1984). Acquired immune deficiency syndrome (AIDS) trends in the United States 1978-1982. *Am. J. Med.* **76**:493-500.

Senay, E. C., Raynes, A. E., Becker, C. E., and Schnoll, S. H. (1982). The primary physician's guide to drug abuse treatment. (NMTS Medical Monograph Series Vol. 1, No. 7). Rockville, Md., National Institute on Drug Abuse, U.S. Department of Health and Human Services (DHHS) Publication No. (ADM) 82-1194).

Shapiro, B. J., Reiss, S., Sullivan, S. F., Tashkin, D. P., Simmons, M. S., and Smith, R. T. (1976). Cardiopulmonary effects of marihuana smoking during exercise. *Chest* **70**:441 (abstract).

Sharp, C. W., and Brehm, M. L. (Eds.) (1977). Review of inhalants: Eupohria to dysfunction. Rockville, MD, National Institute on Drug Abuse (NIDA Research Monograph 15) (DHEW Publication No. (ADM 77-553).

Shesser, R., Mitchell, J., and Edelstein, S. (1981). Methemoglobinemia from isobutyl nitrite preparations. *Ann. Emerg. Med.* **10**:262-264.

Showalter, C. V., and Thornton, W. E. (1977). Clinical pharmacology of phencyclidine toxicity. *Am. J. Psychiatry* **134**:1234-1238.

Siegel, H. (1972). Human pulmonary pathology associated with narcotic and other addictive drugs. *Human Pathol.* **3**:55-66.

Siegel, R. K. (1977). Cocaine: recreational use and intoxication. In *Cocaine 1977.* Edited by R. C. Petersen and R. C. Stillman. Washington, D.C., United States Government Printing Office.

Siegel, R. K. (1978). Cocaine hallucinations. *Am. J. Psychiatry* **135**:309-314.

Siegel, R. K. (1982). Cocaine smoking. *J. Psychoactive Drugs* **4**:277-359.

Sigell, L. T., Kapp, F. T., Fusaro, G. A., Nelson, E. D., and Falck, R. S. (1978). Popping and snorting volatile nitrites: a current fad for getting high. *Am. J. Psychiatry* **135**:1216-1218.

Simpson, R. W., and Edwards, W. D. (1986). Pathogenesis of cocaine induced ischemic heart disease. *Arch. Pathol. Lab. Med.* **110**:479-484.

Slotkin, J. S. (1956). *The Peyote Religion.* New York, Free Press.

Smiley, A., Ziedman, K., and Moskowitz, H. (1981). Pharmacokinetics of drug effects on driving performance: driving simulator tests of marihuana alone and in combination with alcohol. Report to the National Institute on Drug Abuse. Los Angeles, Southern California Research Insititue.

Smith, C. G., Almirez, R. G., and Berenberg, J. (1983). Tolerance develops to the disruptive effects of delta-9-tetrahydrocannabinol on primate menstrual cycle. *Science* **219**:1453-1455.

Smith, D. E. (1968). The acute and chronic toxicity of marijuana. *J. Psychedelic Drugs* **2**:37-47.

Smith, D. E., et al. (1978). The diagnosis and treatment of the PCP abuse syndrome. In *Phencyclidine (PCP) Abuse: An Appraisal.* Edited by R. C. Petersen and R. C. Stillman. Rockville, Md., National Institute on Drug Abuse (NIDA Research Monograph 21) (DHEW Publication No. (ADM) 79-728).

Smith, R. C., Meltzer, H. Y., Arora, R. C., et al. (1977). Effects of phencyclidine on [^{3}H] catecholamine and [^{3}H] serotonin uptake in synaptosomal preparations from rat brain. *Biochem. Pharmacol.* **26**:1435-1439.

Smith, R. J. (1978). Spraying of herbicides on Mexican marijuana backfires on U.S. *Science* **199**:861-864.

Smith, W. F. (1982). Drug traffic today—challenge and response. *Drug Enforcement* (Summer):2-6.

Snyder, R. D., and Snyder, L. B. (1985). Intranasal cocaine abuse in an allergists office. *Ann. Allergy* **54**:489-492.

Spector, S., and Parker, C. W. (1970). Morphine radioimmunoassay. *Science* **168**:1347-1348.

Stark-Adamec, C., Adamec, R. E., and Pihl, R. O. (1981). The subjective marijuana experience: great expectations. *Int. J. Addictions* **16**:1169-1181.

Stein, J. I. (1973). Phencyclidine induced psychosis–the need to avoid unnecessary sensory influx. *Milit. Med.* **138**:590-591.

Steinberg, A. D., and Karliner, J. S. (1968). The clinical spectrum of heroin pulmonary edema. *Arch. Intern. Med.* **122**:122-127.

Stern, W. Z., and Subbarao, K. (1983). Pulmonary complications of drug addiction. *Semin. Roentgenol.* **18**:183-197.

Sternbach, G., Moran, J., and Eliastam, M. (1980). Heroin addiction. Acute presentation of medical complications. *Ann. Emerg. Med.* **9**(3):161-169.

Stewart, D. J., Inaba, T., Lucassen, M., and Kalow, W. (1979). Cocaine metabolism: cocaine and norcocaine hydrolysis by liver and serum esterases. *Clin. Pharmacol. Ther.* **25**:464-468.

Stewart, R. D. (1985). Nitrous oxide sedation/analgesia in emergency medicine. *Ann. Emerg. Med.* **14**:139-148.

Stewart, R. D., Newton, P. E., Baretta, E. D., Herrmann, A. A., Forster, H. V., and Soto, R. J. (1978). Physiological response to aerosol propellants. *Environ. Health Perspect.* **26**:275-285.

Stillman, R., and Petersen, R. C. (1979). The paradox of phencyclidine (PCP) abuse (editorial). *Ann. Intern. Med.* **90**:428-430.

Stimson, G. (1985). Can a war on drugs succeed? *New Soc.* November 15, pp. 275-278.

Sunshine, I. (1982). Radioimmunoassay. In *Methodology for Analytical Toxicology,* Vol. II. Edited by I. Sunshine and P. Jatlow. Boca Raton, FL., CRC Press, pp. 205-214.

Szymanski, H. V. (1981). Prolonged depersonalisation after marijuana use. *Am. J. Psychiatry* **138**:231-233.

Talbott, J., and Teague, J. (1969). Marihuana psychosis. Acute toxic psychosis associated with the use of cannabis derivatives. *JAMA* **210**:299-302.

Tart, C. T. (1970). Marihuana intoxication: common experiences. *Nature* **226**: 701-704.

Tashkin, D. P., and Cohen, S. (1981). *Marijuana Smoking and Its Effects on the Lungs.* New York, The American Council on Marijuana and other Psychoactive Drugs.

Tashkin, D. P., Shapiro, B. J., and Frank, I. M. (1973). Acute pulmonary physiologic effects of smoked marijuana and oral delta-9-tetrahydrocannabinol in healthy young men. *N. Engl. J. Med.* **289**:336-341.

Tashkin, D. P., Shapiro, B. J., Lee, Y. E., and Harper, C. E. (1976). Subacute effects of heavy marihuana smoking on pulmonary function in healthy men. *N. Engl. J. Med.* **294**:125-129.

Tashkin, D. P., Levisman, J. A., and Abbasi, A. S. (1977). Short term effects of smoked marihuana on left ventricular function in man. *Chest* **72**:20-26.

Tashkin, D. P., Calvarese, B. M., Simmons, M. S., and Shapiro, B. J. (1980).

Respiratory status of seventy-four habitual marijuana smokers. *Chest* **78**: 699-706.

Tashkin, D. P., Coulson, A. H., Clark, V. A., Simmons, M., Bourque, L. B., Duann, S., Spivey, G. H., and Gong, H. (1987). Respiratory symptoms and lung function in habitual heavy smokers of marijuana alone, smokers of marijuana and tobacco, smokers of tabacco alone and nonsmokers. *Am. Rev. Respir. Dis.* **135**:209-216.

Taylor, D. N., Wachsmuth, I. K., Shangkuan, Y., et al. (1982). Salmonellosis associated with marijuana. *N. Engl. J. Med.* **306**(21):1249.

Taylor, J. D., and Evans, H. L. (1985). Effects of toluene inhalation on behavior and expired carbon dioxide in macaque monkeys. *Toxicol. Appl. Pharmacol.* **80**:487-495.

Tennant, F. S., Preble, M., Prendergast, T. J., and Ventry, P. (1971). Medical manifestations associated with hashish. *JAMA* **216**:1965-1969.

Thacore, V. R., and Shukla, S. R. P. (1976). Cannabis psychosis and paranoid schizophrenia. *Arch. Gen. Psychiatry* **33**:383-386.

Thomashow, D., Summer, W. R., Soin, J., Wagner, H. N., and Brown, T. C. (1977). Lung disease in reformed drug addicts: diagnostic and physiologic correlations. *Johns Hopkins Med. J.* **141**:1-8.

Thompson, J. D., Fish, S., and Ruiz, E. (1982). Succinylcholine for endotracheal intubation. *Ann. Emerg. Med.* **11**:526-529.

Thurlbeck, W. M., and Thurlbeck, S. M. (1976). Pulmonary effects of paraquat poisoning. *Chest* **69**:276-280.

Tilles, D. S., Goldenheim, P. D., Johnson, D. C., Mendelson, J. H., Mello, N. K., and Hales, C. A. (1986). Marijuana smoking as cause of reduction in singlebreath carbon monoxide diffusing capacity. *Am. J. Med.* **80**:601-606.

Time (1986). America's crusade. What is behind the latest war on drugs? Vol. 128 No. 11, September 15, pp. 60-68.

Treffert, D. A. (1978). Marijuana use in schizophrenia: a clear hazard. *Am. J. Psychiatry* **135**:1213-1215.

Tunving, K. (1985). Psychiatric effects of cannabis use. *Acta Psychiatry Scand.* **72**:209-217.

Turner, C. E. (1980). Chemistry and metabolism. In *Marijuana Research Findings 1980*. Edited by R. C. Petersen. NIDA Research Monograph 31. DHHS Publication No. (ADM) 80-1001 Washington D.C., U.S. Government Printing Office, pp. 81-97.

Turner, C. E., Elsohly, M. A., and Boeren, E. G. (1980). Constituents of *Cannabis sativa L.* A review of the natural constituents. *J. Nat. Proc.* **43**:169-234.

Ungerleider, J. T., Andrysiak, T., Tashkin, D. P., and Gale, R. P. (1982). Contamination of marihuana cigarettes with pathogenic bacteria. Possible source of infection in cancer patients. *Cancer Treat Rep.* **66**:589-591.

Vachon, L., Fitzgerald, M. X., Solliday, N. H., Gould, I. A., and Gaensler, E. A. (1973). Single dose effect of marihuana smoke: bronchial dynamics and respiratory center sensitivity in normal subjects. *N. Engl. J. Med.* **288**: 985-989.

Valpey, R., Sumi, S. M., Copass, M. K., and Goble, G. J. (1978). Acute and chronic progressive encephalopathy due to gasoline sniffing. *Neurology* **28**:507-510.

Van Dyke, C., Barash, P. G., Jatlow, P., and Byck, R. (1976). Cocaine: plasma concentrations after intranasal application in man. *Science* **191**:859-861.

Van Dyke, C., Jatlow, P., Ungerer, J., Barash, P. G., and Byck, R. (1978). Oral cocaine: plasma concentrations and central effects. *Science* **200**:211-213.

Wahlqvist, M., Nilsson, I. M., Sandberg, F., Agurell, S., and Grandstrand, B. (1970). Binding of delta-tetrahydrocannabinol to human plasma proteins. *Biochem. Pharmacol.* **19**:2579-2584.

Waldman, M. M. (1970). Marijuana bronchitis. *JAMA* **211**:501.

Warnock, M. L., Ghahremani, G. G., Rattenborg, C., Ginsberg, M., and Valenzuela, J. (1972). Pulmonary complication of heroin intoxication. Aspiration pneumonia and diffuse bronchiectasis. *JAMA* **219**:1051-1053.

Washton, A. M., Pottash, A. C., and Gold, M. S. (1984). Naltrexone in addicted business executives and physicians. *J. Clin. Psychiatry* **45** (9, Sec. 2):39-41.

Washton, A. M., Gold, M. S., Pottash, A. C. (1985). Opiate and cocaine dependencies. Techniques to help counter the rising tide. *Postgrad. Med.* **77**: 293-300.

Washton, A. M., Gold, M. S., and Pottash, A. C. (1986). Crack. *JAMA* **256**:711 (letter).

Wason, S., Gibler, W. B., and Hassan, M. (1986). Ventricular tachycardia associated with non-freon aerosol propellants. *JAMA* **256**:78-80.

Watson, E. S., Murphy, J. C., Elsohly, H. N., Elsohly, M. A., and Turner, C. E. (1983). Effects of the administration of coca alkaloids on the primary immune responses of mice: interaction with delta-9-tetrahydrocannibinol and Ethanol. *Toxicol. Appl. Pharmacol.* **71**:1-13.

Weil, A. T. (1970). Adverse reactions to marihuana: classification and suggested treatment. *N. Engl. J. Med.* **282**:997-1000.

Weiss, R. D., Goldenheim, P. D., Mirin, S. M., Hales, C. A., and Mendelson, J. H. (1981). Pulmonary dysfunction in cocaine smokers. *Am. J. Psychiatry* **138**:1110-1112.

Weller, R. A., and Halikas, J. A. (1985). Marijuana use and psychiatric illness: a follow-up study. *Am. J. Psychiatry* **142**:848-850.

Wetli, C. V., and Wright, R. K. (1979). Death caused by recreational cocaine use. *JAMA* **241**:2519-2522.

White, S. C., Brin, S. C., and Janicki, B. W. (1975). Mitogen-induced blastogenic responses of lymphocytes from marihuana smokers. *Science* **188**: 71-72.

Wilkinson, P., Van Dyke, C., Jatlow, P., Barash, P., and Byck, R. (1980). Intranasal and oral cocaine kinetics. *Clin. Pharmacol. Ther.* **27**(3):386-394.

Yesavage, J. A., and Freman, A. M. III (1978). Acute phencyclidine (PCP) intoxication: psychopathology and prognosis. *J. Clin. Psychiatry* **39**:664-666.

Zavala, D. C., and Rhodes, M. L. (1978). An effect of paraquat on the lungs of rabbits. *Chest* **74**:418-420.

Zuskin, E., and Bouhuys, A. (1974). Acute airway responses to hair spray preparations. *N. Engl. J. Med.* **290**:660-663.

Zuskin, E., Loke, J., and Bouhuys, A. (1981). Helium-oxygen flow-volume curves in detecting acute response to hairspray. *Int. Arch. Occup. Environ. Health* **49**:41-44.

Zwillich, C. W., Doekel, R., Hammill, S., and Weil, J. V. (1978). The effects of smoked marijuana on metabolism and respiratory control. *Am. Rev. Respir. Dis.* **118**:885-891.

10

Environmental Inhaled Agents and Their Relation to Lung Cancer

W. K. LAM

University of Hong Kong
and Queen Mary Hospital
Hong Kong

Y. X. DU

Guangzhou Medical College
and Guangzhou Research Center for
     Lung Cancer
Guangzhou, China

I. Introduction

Lung cancer is a major health problem worldwide, and its incidence is highest in the industrialized countries, particularly in Western Europe and North America, where it accounts for more deaths than any other cancer (Silverberg, 1985). In the United States, lung cancer mortality has risen sharply from 18,300 in 1950 to 61,800 in 1969, 98,400 in 1979, and 139,000 in 1984 (Silverberg, 1985). These deaths accounted for 35% of all cancer deaths among men, and 18% of those among women, and 5% of all deaths in the United States. It is the leading cause of cancer death in men above the age of 35, and its incidence is now increasing faster among American women than among men. From 1969 to 1979, there was a 44% rise in lung cancer in men but a 120% rise in women, and lung cancer is now replacing breast cancer as the leading cause of cancer mortality among American women (American Thoracic Society, 1985; Harris, 1983; Silverberg, 1985). The high incidence of lung cancer in Chinese women, particularly Cantonese, has been noted in China (Du et al., 1984), Hong Kong (Chan et al., 1979; Kung et al., 1984; Lam et al., 1983), Singapore (MacLennan et al., 1977), and the United States (Fraumeni and Mason, 1974).

It has been suggested that up to 80-90% of all cancers are related to environmental factors (Alderson, 1982; Higginson, 1976; WHO, 1964). For lung cancer, the main causative agent is known, namely inhaled tobacco smoke, but other carcinogenic substances are also being identified both in the ambient environment and the workplace. In this chapter, some environmental inhaled carcinogens, confirmed or suspected, will be reviewed and salient generalizations of chemical carcinogenesis will also be presented because an understanding of this is essential for a preventive approach.

Active cigarette smoking and asbestos exposure are not subjects of discussion in this chapter.

II. Chemical Carcinogenesis

Carcinogenesis requires a long time for its full expression, and its biology is extremely complex. It is now recognized that chemical carcinogenesis is a multistage process, consisting of at least two steps: initiation and promotion (Boutwell, 1985; Harris, 1983; Hecker et al., 1982; Slaga, 1983; Yuspa and Harris, 1982).

A. Initiation

Initiation is a rapid and irreversible process whereby a heritable but unexpressed change in the cell is accomplished. It is thought to involve permanent, mutation-like alteration in DNA. The initiated cells are not manifest tumor cells, but will develop into tumor cells that replicate to produce gross tumors when another promoting stimulus (promoter) is applied.

B. Promotion

The second step, promotion, is a longer process that is reversible in the early phases. It is thought to be mediated through effects on the cell membrane (Miller, 1979). While initiating agents are carcinogenic by themselves, the promoting agents are not, and must be given after initiating agents to exert their effect (Yuspa and Harris, 1982). Promoters cause a pleiotropic change in initiated cells (Boutwell, 1985), with alterations in enzyme activity and other transformed cell characteristics (Klein-Szanto, 1984).

Agents exhibiting both initiating and promoting activities are termed complete carcinogens, while incomplete carcinogens are those capable only of initiation. It is important to appreciate that promoting agents may give the appearance of complete carcinogens by promoting cells initiated by ambient environmental agents (Pitot, 1982). Humans are exposed inevitably to low, initiating doses of carcinogens such as cosmic and terrestrial ionizing radiation and polycyclic hydrocarbon emissions from all sources. The determining factor for ultimate carcinogenesis in many cases may be the level of the promoting agent (Boutwell, 1985). Promoting agents may be present in the environment, for example, cigarette smoke, which is a complete carcinogen with many promoting agents (Hoffmann and Wynder, 1971; Pitot, 1982), or produced endogenously, such as some hormones (Boutwell, 1985). The importance of molecular mechanisms of tumor promotion as a basis for cancer prevention cannot be overemphasized, and interested readers are referred to several reviews of this rapidly changing field (Fujiki et al., 1984; Slaga, 1983).

C. Metabolic Activation

While some chemical carcinogens are direct-acting, many have to be metabolically activated before exerting their carcinogenic actions (Cohen, 1981; Miller, 1981). The metabolites that are active initiators of carcinogenesis have the special property of being strong electrophilic reactants (positively charged) that readily bind to negatively charged cellular macromolecules, including DNA (Harris, 1983; Miller, 1981; Miller and Miller, 1981; Upton, 1982). Reaction of electrophiles with DNA, which can result in mutation, is probably the essential component of initiation (Miller, 1981; Miller and Miller, 1981). The promotion stage of carcinogenesis, on the other hand, does not depend on alteration of DNA.

The metabolic activation of the carcinogen benzo(a)pyrene is one of the best studied. Human bronchus has been shown to metabolize benzo(a)pyrene into various metabolites, in particular the reactive diolepoxide 7, 8-dihydro-7, 8-dihydroxybenzo(a)pyrene 9, 10-oxide, which can bind to DNA of bronchus by covalent bonds and possibly initiate tumor formation (Cohen, 1981).

A multitude of factors, exogenous or endogenous, interact throughout the stages of initiation (including metabolic activation), promotion, and tumor progression to determine ultimate carcinogenesis and tumor growth (Alderson, 1982; Miller, 1979; Upton, 1982; Yuspa and Harris, 1982; Weisburger and Williams, 1982). Among the factors related to the stimuli are the dose, concentration, and the presence of other chemicals in the environment, and among the factors related to the host are age, sex, nutritional, immunologic, and hormonal status, and metabolic conversion of chemicals in the body. This myriad of factors would explain the differences in susceptibility to the carcinogenic effects of a given chemical.

D. Identification of Chemical Carcinogens

The identification of chemicals with carcinogenic activity requires epidemiologic and laboratory methods.

Epidemiologic Methods

These include case observations, which are rarely conclusive but are simple and may provide valuable leads for further investigations, case-control studies, and cohort studies.

Case-Control Studies

In case-control studies, the frequency of a suspected causative factor is compared in a group of persons with a cancer (cases) and a group without (controls). The main difficulty lies in the selection of a control group that is validly matched in all relevant variables, but can be conducted more quickly and less expensively than cohort studies.

Cohort Studies

In cohort studies, a group of persons exposed to a suspected causative factor before disease is followed over time, and the frequency of the disease is measured. The control group consists of persons similar to the cohort group, but without exposure to the suspected factor. Occupational groups provide an important source of cohorts with heavy exposures to various chemicals. Cohort studies yield incidence rates as well as relative risk but require a large study population and a long follow-up period.

The method of logistic regression is now widely used as a means of adjusting for confounding variables when analyzing both case-control and cohort studies.

For more detailed discussions on epidemiologic methods, readers are referred to several excellent sources (Breslow and Day, 1980; MacMahon and Pugh, 1979; Newell et al., 1982).

Laboratory Methods

These include assays in laboratory animals and short-term tests in microorganisms, cultured cells, and other in vitro systems.

In Vivo Assays

Animal studies are used to identify individual carcinogens and to explore the interaction among the effects of carcinogens in cancer induction. Animal models for exposure of the lungs to respiratory carcinogens through inhalation have been developed (Nettesheim and Griesemer, 1978), and are especially suitable for testing volatile chemicals, for example, benzo(a) pyrene inhalation by hamsters and bis(chloromethyl)ethyl inhalation by rats and hamsters (Harris, 1983). The extrapolations of animal data to human, are however, fraught with problems and uncertainties (Alderson, 1982; Samuels and Adamson, 1985; Upton, 1982), particularly extrapolations across species and across differences in dose and conditions of exposure. Arsenic, for instance, has not been shown to be carcinogenic in animal models (Frank, 1982) despite its well known effect in humans.

In Vitro Assays

These are short-term tests, and are more rapid and economical than animal studies to meet the rapidly increasing demands for chemical carcinogen screening. They include mutagenicity tests in various assay systems, morphologic transformation of human tissue and cells (including bronchus) in culture, binding of chemicals to DNA, and DNA damage and repair (Ames, 1979; Harris et al., 1980; Heidleberger and Mondal, 1979; Tomatis et al., 1982; Weisburger and Williams, 1982). Of these, transformation of human epithelial cells in culture is of particular relevance, since most neoplasms in humans are epithelial. Whether these in vitro tests will prove to be more validly applicable to humans remains to be determined, but their rapidity, economy, and sensitivity would make them valuable for prescreening suspect chemicals.

III. Nonoccupational Environmental Inhalation Exposures

As stated, most human cancers are thought to be caused by environmental factors both in the general environment and in the workplace. The lung, with its 60-90 m^2 of epithelial surface directly exposed to inhaled air, is an immediate target for airborne carcinogens. In this section, the role of air pollution (including fossil fuel combustion products), natural background ionizing radiation, and environmental tobacco smoke in the development of human lung cancer will be reviewed.

A. Ambient Air Pollution

General Considerations

A number of particulate and vapor phase organic compounds, particularly the polycyclic aromatic hydrocarbons, are present in ambient air. They are produced by combustion of fossil fuels and other organic hydrocarbons, by various industrial sources, and from secondary reactions in the air.

The role of ambient air pollution in human lung cancer continues to be controversial (Doll, 1978; Friberg and Cederlof, 1978; Shy and Struba, 1982; Speizer, 1983). The argument for its being a risk factor is based on animal data and several lines of epidemiologic evidence.

Animal Data

Animal studies have demonstrated the carcinogenicity of particulate phase organic matter including benzo(a)pyrene in polluted air (Hoffmann and Wynder,

1977; National Research Council, 1972). Inhalation studies have also shown that common gaseous air pollutants such as sulfur dioxide (Laskin et al., 1970) and particulate pollutant such as ferric oxide (Nettesheim et al., 1975) can enhance or promote tumorigenicity of respiratory carcinogens such as benzo(a)-pyrene. Extrapolating data from animal experiments to human beings has a number of limitations, and the role of these pollutants in human lung cancer has yet to be demonstrated.

Epidemiologic Data

Urban/rural gradients of mortality. Lung cancer is consistently more commonly seen in urban areas than in rural areas (Doll, 1978; Haenszel et al., 1962). People in urban areas are known to smoke more than those in rural areas and, after controlling for smoking habit, a comparison of the rates of lung cancer in urban and rural areas shows only small differences, ranging from a 1.26 to a 2.33-fold increase of the disease in urban residents (Doll, 1978; Harris, 1983; Report of Task Group, 1978).

 Migrant studies. Studies of emigrants from England to the United States (Friberg and Cederlof, 1978; Reid et al., 1966) have shown that the incidence of lung cancer among emigrants is lower than among Englishmen in England but higher than among those born in the United States. This is interpreted as showing the long-term effects of air pollution in the native country, the so-called "British urban factor." These studies are, however, deficient in that smoking was not satisfactorily assessed, and the possibilities that emigrants may not be representative samples of their native countrymen, and that they are exposed to more hazardous occupations in their new countries, cannot be excluded (Speizer, 1983).

 Quantitative studies. Quantitative relationships between indices of ambient air carcinogens and lung cancer in population groups have been studied. Using benzo(a)pyrene (BaP) concentration as an index of air pollution, quantitative studies have been carried out to relate it to regional differences (Carnow and Meier, 1973) or occupational group/general population differences (Pike et al., 1975) in lung cancer rates. These studies have been criticized as fraught with pitfalls (Friberg and Cederlof, 1978; Higgins, 1977; Shy and Struba, 1982). Not only is cigarette smoking not controlled and data collection and assumptions in analysis unsatisfactory, but the use of BaP as the index for air carcinogenicity is open to question. BaP is only one of the more than 100 polycyclic aromatic hydrocarbons among the organic particulates in polluted air (Lee et al., 1976; Shy and Struba, 1982). There is no good correlation between ambient level of BaP and other polycyclic aromatic hydrocarbons. Moreover, in view of the 20-30-year latency for cancer, it is inappropriate to associate lung cancer rates with BaP measurements taken at the same time.

Occupation cohorts. Occupational exposure to tar, coal gas, and combustion products from coke ovens is associated with a two- to threefold excess of lung cancer (Shy and Struba, 1982). Extrapolating these occupational risks to the general population is untenable, yet when one considers that even though these workers experience concentrations of these substances (using BaP as an index) 10-100 times those found in ambient air and their risk factor was only two- to threefold, the extremely low risk for ambient air is apparent. An increase in lung cancer may, however, occur in the special situation where residential area is in close proximity to heavy industrial pollution (Lloyd et al., 1985).

Urbanization and industrial sources of air pollution (BaP) correspond chronologically with the increase in cigarette smoking (Friberg and Cederlof, 1978). Occupational exposures are also different for urban dwellers compared to their rural counterparts. Cigarette smoking and, to a lesser extent, occupational exposures are such major determinants that, after controlling for their effects, air pollution is estimated to cause no more than 2% of all lung cancers or 5 cases per 100,000 persons per year (Doll, 1978; Higgins, 1984; Speizer, 1983).

The components of "urban excess" are multifactorial, smoking and occupational exposures apart, and may be related to myriad outdoor and indoor pollutants and other lifestyle factors, and measurement of BaP alone as an index is inadequate. It is suggested (Shy and Struba, 1982) that to advance our knowledge in this area, individual exposure to specific sources of ambient air carcinogen should be defined, and well-designed analytic studies of air pollution as a human carcinogen should be carried out.

Air pollution may be related to cancer in ways other than causation. Richters and Richters (1983) have, for instance, demonstrated that nitrogen dioxide can facilitate blood-borne cancer cell metastasis in animal models, which may be relevant to the well-known increased cancer mortality associated with polluted urban environment.

Several specific ambient air pollutants, indoors and outdoors, will now be considered.

Diesel Exhaust Emissions

Diesel powered vehicles, a potent source of polycyclic hydrocarbon exposure, are increasingly important modes of transportation. It is estimated that in the United States 18% of all vehicles on the roads were diesel powered in 1985 (Speizer, 1983), and there is a growing concern about the resulting deterioration in air quality, with its possible effect on the incidence of lung cancer. There is no doubt that diesel exhaust contains polycyclic hydrocarbons with carcinogenic potential in animal models. The Royal College of Physicians (1970) noted, however, that the increase in the use of diesel fuel in Britain has followed rather than preceded the sharp rise in lung cancer incidence and hence could not have been a major etiologic factor. Epidemiologic studies of human lung cancer relating to diesel exhaust, usually in occupational groups (Kaplan, 1959; Leupker and Smith, 1978), suffered from numerous deficiencies in design (Higgins, 1984; National Research Council, 1981) including the lack of data on smoking and the relatively short exposure period, and no definite conclusion on the potential cancer hazards of exposure to diesel emission can be drawn. A more recent Canadian study (Howe et al., 1983) has also been confounded by asbestos exposure as the dose-response relationship shown disappeared after correction for asbestos exposure. Similarly, recent studies from Britain (Rushton et al., 1983) and Sweden (Damber and Larsson, 1985) were inconclusive, although a synergistic effect between smoking and occupational exposure was suggested. Further studies allowing for cigarette smoking and other known risk factors are needed to define better the risk of diesel exhaust emission.

Indoor Coal Combustion

Coal combustion releases a multitude of chemicals among which are aromatic amines and metal compounds such as arsenic and nickel (Friberg and Cederlof, 1978), which are known carcinogens. Excess risks of lung cancer have been reported for coke oven workers (Redmond et al., 1972) and gas workers (Doll et al., 1972) who were heavily exposed to products of coal carbonization. There is a high incidence of lung cancer in females in Guangzhou (Canton), China (Du et al., 1984), with a low male to female ratio (1.87 to 1). In a study relating cigarette consumption, household coal consumption (for cooking), industrial coal consumption, and concentration of air pollutants (SO_2, NO_2, sedimentary dust, benzo(a)pyrene) to lung cancer mortality rate, the correlation coefficient for household coal consumption was the highest ($r = 0.911$, $p < 0.01$) (Du et al., 1985), and was considered the predominant factor for females. Coal has been the main cooking fuel in Guangzhou since 1960, and housewives are exposed in a situation where the stove is without a chimney and the kitchen is always near to the bedroom or living room. Another interesting epidemic of lung cancer has been noted in Xuanwei county in Yunnan Province, China (Du et al., 1985), where the male to female ratio is 1:1, cigarette smoking is a minor factor, and a high mortality rate is seen in coal burning areas (152/100,000) compared with a low rate of 0.7/100,000 in non-coal-burning areas. This is related to the rich coal resources in Xuanwei and use of improper coal stoves that cause severe indoor air pollution. A recent study by Wu et al. (1985) also suggested that childhood exposure to coal burning for heating or cooking may account for 22% of the bronchial adenocarcinoma in women who do not smoke. Coal combustion in the home as a risk factor for lung cancer warrants further investigation.

Kerosene Cooking Stoves

Exposure to fumes from the kerosene stove as a risk factor for lung cancer in Chinese women was first suggested by Leung in Hong Kong (1977). This observation is of particular interest because lung cancer is the leading cause of cancer deaths among women in Hong Kong (98% of the population being Chinese) who have one of the highest lung cancer mortality rates in the world (28.5/100,000 or 26% of all female cancer deaths in 1984) (Hong Kong Government, 1985). Previous reports (Chan et al., 1979; Lam et al., 1983) have shown that about half of the patients were nonsmokers. Kerosene was the main cooking fuel in Hong Kong in the 1950s and 1960s, being replaced by cleaner fuels such as liquid petroleum gas and piped coal gas in the last 10 years or so. Electricity has not been popular because its heat is more difficult to control and thus not favorable for the Chinese style of cooking. In two subsequent case-control studies (Koo et al., 1984; Lam et al., 1985), the association between kerosene fuel use and lung cancer was found to be weak and not significant ($p > 0.01$), with no clearly defined dose-response relationship. The numbers of patients however were small, 200 and 163 only; further studies in larger number of patients are indicated.

Chinese Incense Smoke

Burning of Chinese incense at home, either for ancestor worship or deity worship, is common among the large non-Christian population in Hong Kong, especially older women. Chinese incense smoke has been shown to contain several polycyclic aromatic hydrocarbons, including 3,4-benzopyrene (Schoental and Gibbard, 1967), and the free radical content of the tar condensates was estimated to be comparable with that obtained for cigarette tar. A small case-control study involving 163 female patients and 180 female controls (Lam et al., 1985) did not, however, demonstrate an association between indoor incense burning and lung cancer. It is interesting to note that as many as 72% of the controls and 67% of the cases had been exposed to incense smoke regularly.

B. Natural Background Ionizing Radiation

General Considerations

Ionizing radiation is radiation that removes electrons from atoms, and includes energetic particles such as alpha-(α) and beta-(β) particles and protons, and electromagnetic rays such as x- and gamma-rays (Boice and Land, 1982). Human beings have always been exposed to natural background radiation from cosmic rays and terrestrial radiations due to natural occurrence of radioisotopes (Klement et al., 1972; NCRP, 1975). Uranium and thorium are abundant in the earth's crust, and they give rise to a series of decay products that emit radioactive particles including α-particles and β-particles (Parkes, 1982a). α-Particles are positively charged helium nuclei with great mass and ionizing power but only weak penetrating capacity. They are therefore radiations of high linear energy transfer that release energy in short tracks of dense ionization (Boice and Land, 1982). When applied to the airways, they cause ionization maximally when they have passed through the bronchial mucosa and reached the basal cells (Parkes, 1982a). The double-strand DNA molecule is thought to be the critical target for radiation-induced cellular damage (Boice and Land, 1982). β-Particles are electrons with great penetrating capacity but less ionizing power. Since ionization is thought to be the cause of malignant transformation in living cells, inhaled α-particles are considered more important than β-particles in the development of lung cancer.

Uranium in the earth's crust gives rise to decay chain products through radium 226 to the gas radon 222, which in turn gives rise to other isotopes collectively termed radon daughters (Parkes, 1982a). Radon 222 and the three radon daughters, polonium 218, polonium 214, and polonium 210, are important α-particles emitters. Thorium likewise decays into decay chain products of which thorium B (lead 212) and thorium C (bismuth 212) are α-particles emitters. All these products are emitted by soil, rocks, and building materials and are dispersed in the atmosphere to attach to water vapor, dust, or cigarette smoke particles, attaining aerosol sizes of 0.25-0.4 μm (Davies, 1967). In this state, they can, on inhalation, penetrate well to the trachea, bronchi, and beyond (Parkes, 1982b) and exert their ionizing effect.

Risk of Lung Cancer

The carcinogenic potential of ionizing radiation has been known since the turn of the century and the association between lung cancer and mining of uranium has long been documented. Earlier studies (Frigerio and Stowe, 1976; Jacobson et al., 1976) to find the link between cancer and natural background radiation have been negative. These studies have the drawback of uncertainties of dose levels, migration patterns, and selection factors for place of residence (Boice and Land, 1982). To overcome some of these problems, the High Background Radiation Research Group in China (1980) studied a large stable population in Guangdong province; 90% of the families have lived in the areas for six or more generations. This stable population of 73,000 persons had received three times the amount of natural background radiation (from monazite particles washed down by rain from granite surface rock to the basin region where they lived) as 77,000 inhabitants in a comparison region. No difference in cancer mortality was demonstrated.

Similarly, a recent study in Guangzhou, China, (Wu ZH, personal communication) has shown no difference between the degree of indoor radioactive pollutants (radon, thoron, and their daughters) in lung cancer patients' houses and in the controls' houses. The possibility that the dose-effect curve had a zero slope at these low doses of radiation cannot, however, be excluded. More recently, a Swedish study (Edling et al., 1984) has found high concentrations of radon and its daughters in indoor air in about 35,000 houses, and a lung cancer hazard was thought likely to be present.

In the United States, calculations based on measurement of average activity concentration of radon indoors have given a maximum lifetime risk of lung cancer of 0.12% (Evans et al., 1981). This has assumed linear extrapolation and neglected latency and accumulation interval, but would not change the general conclusion that this is a relatively small fraction of the 4% lifetime risk of lung cancer in Americans, which is largely due to cigarette smoking. Other workers have put estimates of lung cancer in the general population due to radon daughter exposure as varying from 1-5% to over 10% (Edling, 1985). Radon daughter exposure, however, is important for nonsmokers since it has been estimated to account for more than 20% of lung cancers seen in nonsmokers (Harley and Pasternack, 1981). In fact, based on the use of a linear nonthreshold extrapolation model, it has been suggested that exposure to natural background radiation would account for about 1.3% of the total cancer incidence in the United States (Jablon and Bailar, 1980; Upton, 1982).

Conversely, there are reports that low levels of ionizing radiation may be beneficial to many life forms including human life (Henry, 1961; Hickey et al., 1981; Hickey and Clelland, 1982; Luckey, 1981). Mean background radiation levels and some cancer mortalities including those of the respiratory organs may be negatively correlated (Frigerio and Stowe, 1976; Hickey et al., 1981). This is thought to be due to beneficial stimulation—perhaps of toxoids or vaccines—by low levels of ionizing radiation, a phenomenon termed hormesis (Luckey, 1981).

C. Environmental Tobacco Smoke (Passive Smoking)

General Considerations

Active cigarette smoking is now firmly established to be the dominant factor for the present epidemic of lung cancer worldwide, as is well summarized in a series of no less than 14 U.S. Surgeon General's Reports from 1964 to 1982 and four reports (one being a follow-up report) of the Royal College of Physician of London from 1962 to 1983 on smoking and health. The subject is not within the scope of discussion in this chapter. Passive smoking or involuntary smoking is the exposure of nonsmokers to tobacco combustion products in the indoor environment, and has aroused interest and concern in recent years because of fears concerning possible serious health hazards, particularly lung cancer.

Tobacco smoke is a complex mixture of more than 2000 chemicals many of which have been shown to be carcinogens, both in the gas phase (e.g., N-nitrosocompounds) and particulate phase (e.g., benzo(a)pyrene and 5-methylchrysene as tumor initiators, volatile phenols as tumor promoters, and lung-specific carcinogens such as polonium 210 and nickel compounds) (Harris, 1983; Wynder and Hoffmann, 1982). Polonium 210 (^{210}Po) is of particular interest as there has been recent renewed interest implicating radiation from cigarette smoking as a major causative factor in lung cancer (Martell, 1983; Winters and DiFrenza, 1983). α-Emitting radioisotopes from soils, particularly the long-living ^{210}Po, are concentrated on tobacco trichomes, which persist when tobacco is dried and processed. They would appear in cigarette smoke (Martell, 1974) and on inhalation would deposit at the bronchus to irradiate the tissues there. The passive smoker is exposed to the same radioelements in the tobacco as the active smoker. A second source of radiation exposure relates to radon and its daughters emanating from soils and building materials, which occur in much higher concentrations indoor than outdoors. Smoke particles act as condensation nuclei for radon daughters to keep them airborne, and hence the exposure of the passive smoker to naturally occurring radon daughters is increased in a smoky environment (Winters and DiFrenza, 1983).

It is known that chemical compositions of mainstream and sidestream smoke (constituting 15% and 85% of smoke, respectively, created by smokers in a room) are different (Correa et al., 1983; Fielding, 1985; Royal College of Physicians, 1983; Weiss et al., 1983). Mainstream smoke emerges into the environment after having been drawn through the cigarette, filtered by the smokers' own lungs, and then exhaled. Sidestream smoke comes directly from the burning end of the cigarette. The two differ in composition, and many potentially carcinogenic constituents such as nitrosamine and ^{210}Po are in higher concentration in sidestream smoke (Weiss et al., 1983; Winters and DiFrenza, 1983). The biological significance of this is unclear, and as sidestream smoke is rapidly diluted in room air, this difference between main and sidestream would become less important. Wynder and Goodman (1983) did raise the possibility that because sidestream smoke with its appreciable amount of gaseous components would penetrate into the peripheral parts of the lung better, passive smoking might cause an increase in peripheral lung tumors, such as adenocarcinoma, which is common among non-smokers.

Epidemiologic Studies

The first major epidemiologic study on passive smoking and lung cancer was reported by Hirayama (1981). In a cohort study of 91,540 nonsmoking married women aged 40 or above, he found that age-adjusted lung cancer mortality rates were lowest for wives of nonsmokers, intermediate for wives of light or exsmokers and highest for wives of heavy smokers. The author estimated that lung cancer risk associated with passive smoking was about one-third to one-half that associated with active smoking. Altogether there have now been no less than 15 studies examining the association between passive smoking and lung cancer and they are summarized in Table 1. Most of the studies show a positive association, although the association is generally weak with odd ratios of 1.2:3.5 for exposed relative to nonexposed (Blot and Fraumeni, 1986; Weiss, 1986). Lam et al. (1985) stratified nonsmoking female patients into a centrally located tumor group and a peripherally located tumor group according to whether the tumor could be visualized by flexible fiberoptic bronchoscopy or not, and found that passive smoking might contribute to adenocarcinoma of the peripheral type (p = 0.01) but not of the central type. This result is interesting; it appears to be in line with Wynder and Goodman's suggestion (1983) that passive smoking may act on more peripheral sites in the lung.

These studies (Table 1) have generated much discussion and commentary in the literature (Blot and Fraumeni, 1986; Lee, 1982; Rylander, 1984; Weiss, 1986; Wynder and Goodman, 1983), and, aside from the small number of cases in some studies and the variable statistical methods employed, some other deficiencies and methodologic issues have been emphasized.

First, the proportion of histologically or cytologically confirmed diagnosis varied greatly. In Trichopoulos's study (1981), 35% of cases were not histologically confirmed, and cases of adenocarcinoma and alveolar cell carcinoma were excluded. Also, no definition of histologic type was given by Hirayama (1981), and histologic type was obtained only during the first 6-12 years of Garfinkle's cohort study (1981).

Second, degree of exposure to passive smoking was not quantified in most studies. The information that one is married to a smoker is not a precise description of the degree of exposure to environmental tobacco smoke. Quantitation of passive smoke has been recognized as extremely difficult (Royal College of Physicians, 1983; Weiss et al., 1983). Sidestream smoke is diluted by room air to a variable extent. The room air itself also contains smoke that has been inhaled and then exhaled into the air. The duration of smoke exposure, the number and smoking habits of the smokers, the proximity to smokers, the characteristics of the room including size and ventilation, and the presence and nature of absorptive surfaces are all important variables. The amount of the various components of tobacco smoke breathed by the nonsmoker from a smoky atmosphere are therefore extremely variable, and there are no agreed standards for expressing environmental tobacco smoke exposure. Also, many of the studies defined passive smoking narrowly as that resulting from the spouses' smoking habits only.

Table 1 Studies of Passive Smoking and Lung Cancer

Author	Study design	Country	Results	Statistical significance
Chan et al. (1979)	Case-control	Hong Kong	No association for females	No
Garfinkle (1981)	Cohort	U.S.	+ Association in females	No
Hirayama (1981)	Cohort	Japan	+ Association in nonsmoking females	Yes
Trichopoulos et al. (1981)	Case-control	Greece	+ Association in nonsmoking females	Yes
Correa et al., (1983)	Case-control	U.S.	+ Association in both males and females	Yes
Knoth et al. (1983)	Cases	Germany	+ Association when compared to German population	Not tested
Koo et al., (1983)	Case-control	Hong Kong	No associatiation for females	No
Gillis et al. (1984)	Cohort	Scotland	+ Association in males but not females	Not tested

Kabat and Wynder (1984)	Case-control	U.S.	+ Association in males but not females	Males: yes; females: no
Garfinkle et al. (1985)	Case-control	U.S.	+ Association in nonsmoking females	Yes
Lam et al. (1985)	Case-control	Hong Kong	+ Association only in non-smoking females with peripheral-type adenocarcinoma	Yes for defined group
Sandler et al. (1985)	Case-control	U.S.	+ Association between overall cancer risk and cumulative lifetime exposure	Yes for linear trend for overall cancer risk, but not for lung cancer
Wu et al. (1985)	Case-control	U.S.	+ Association for adeno-carcinoma in females	No
Akiba et al. (1986)	Case-control	Japan	+ Association in nonsmoking females	$p = 0.07$
Lee et al. (1986)	Case-control	England	+ Association in nonsmoking females	No

(Adapted from Weiss, 1986, with permission.)

It did not take into account other sources of exposure—cohabiting relatives including parents during childhood, workplace, public transportation, movie theaters, restaurants etc.—which could be substantial. There have been attempts at quantitation: Koo et al. (1983) tried to quantify passive smoking by summating the total hours and years of exposure from regular sources in the home or workplace, and Sandler et al. (1985) calculated the cumulative effects of lifetime household exposure to cigarette smoke on cancer risk. Valid and practical dose description or quantitation methods and cumulative exposure indices should be devised and standardized. They can be done either by measurements as in the direct measurement by urinary cotinine (Wald et al., 1984), or by extensive questionnaires evaluating all possible sources of environmental tobacco smoke exposure. There are, however, no data available on the validity of passive smoke exposure information obtained by questionnaires (Pershagen, 1984).

The third issue is the potential problem of incorrect categorization of exposure status (Weiss, 1986). Garfinkle et al. (1985), for instance, found that 40% of the women classified as nonsmokers in hospital records were in fact smokers at some time on verification, compared with only 8.5% of the controls who were similarly misclassified. Also, in case-control studies, patients with lung cancer would tend to interpret their disease as related to passive smoking, thus giving rise to recall bias (Rylander, 1984).

The causative link between passive smoking and lung cancer has remained controversial. The 1986 Surgeon General's report (U.S. Department of Health & Human Services, 1986) concluded that involuntary smoking is a cause of lung cancer in healthy nonsmokers. While Repace and Lowrey (1985) and the National Research Council (1986) have estimated that 20-30% of the annual lung cancer deaths among nonsmokers are due to passive smoking, the American Thoracic Society (1985) and Blot and Fraumeni (1986) are of the view that the body of epidemiologic data pointing to a causative role for passive smoking in the development of lung cancer is growing but not yet conclusive. Given the biological plausibility of the association (because cigarette smoke is a known carcinogen) and the ubiquitous nature of environmental tobacco smoke exposure, further epidemiologic and other studies need to be carried out to resolve this issue.

IV. Occupational Inhalation Exposures

Occupational exposure to many agents is known to increase the incidence of lung cancers, particularly in smokers. Tobacco smoke is such a dominant respiratory carcinogen in humans that by comparison industrial carcinogens are responsible for only a small proportion of lung cancers (Parkes, 1982a). The importance of identifying these industrial carcinogens lies in the fact that the cancer is

potentially preventable by appropriate control measures. Also, industrial exposures have been the primary means for identifying carcinogenic agents in humans.

Asbestos is probably the most widely studied of all occupational respiratory carcinogens, and it has been shown that about 20% of deaths in asbestos-
exposed workers are from lung cancer (Selikoff et al., 1964). The subject will
not be further discussed in this review; interested readers are referred to some
excellent sources (Becklake, 1976; Casey et al., 1981; Parkes, 1982c; Selikoff
and Lee, 1978).

A. Polycyclic Aromatic Hydrocarbons

Carbon-containing products that originate from coal or petroleum include coal
gas, coke, gasoline, kerosene, and tar. The risk of developing lung cancer has
been clearly demonstrated in British gas house workers (Doll et al., 1972) and
U.S. coke oven workers in the carbonization of steel (Redmond et al., 1972), all
of whom were exposed to coal carbonization volatiles; the risk factor is approximately two- to threefold (Shy and Struba, 1982). The risk for roofers, oil refinery workers, and carbon black (over 99% carbon with traces of polycyclic
aromatic hydrocarbons) workers is less certain (Hodgson and Jones, 1985;
Parkes, 1982a).

The measurement of benzo(a)pyrene, one of the polycyclic aromatic
hydrocarbons and a well-known carcinogen in laboratory animals, is commonly
used as an index of risk, but it is uncertain whether this is a good representative
index. Another important question is whether a linear extrapolation to low
level exposures is appropriate.

B. Ionizing Radiation

Uranium and thorium, which usually occur together in the earth's crust, give rise
to a series of decay products that emit carcinogenic particles, including radon 222
and the radon daughters. Lung cancer patients among miners exposed to radioactive ores in the mines of Schneeberg and Joachimstahl in central Europe were
among the earliest occupationally related cases. In the United States, an increased
risk of lung cancer has been established among uranium miners in the Colorado
Plateau region (Archer et al., 1976; Samet et al., 1984). Because uranium and
thorium are present in rocks, significant airborne radioactivity due to their decay
products occurs in all types of mines, and it is thought to be the cause of increased
incidence of lung cancer among the fluorspar (fluorite) miners of Newfoundland
and the hematite miners of England (Fraumeni, 1974).

The risk of lung cancer in miners is increased by cigarette smoking, and it has
been estimated that overall there is an excess of approximately 30-40 cases/10^6
person-years and working level month (WLM) on a lifetime basis in both smoking
and nonsmoking miners aged over 50 (Edling and Axelson, 1983).

C. Arsenic

Arsenic has so far not succeeded in producing tumors in laboratory animals, and epidemiologic studies of workers exposed to arsenicals provide the primary sources of evidence suggesting that they are respiratory carcinogens. A three- to eightfold increase in the expected incidence of lung cancer was observed among exposed workers (Lee and Fraumeni, 1969; Mabuchi et al., 1980) and a positive dose-response relationship was shown. It is estimated (Frank, 1982) that in the United States about 1.5 million workers in over 100 job categories including alloy or smelter workers and workers involved in the manufacturing of pesticides, glass, paints, and pigments, are occupationally exposed to arsenic.

D. Nickel

Reports of the development of lung cancer following exposure in nickel processing plants have appeared since 1930s in South Wales (Doll et al., 1970) and Norway (Pedersen et al., 1973). It is not known whether it is the dust form from crude ore, the gaseous nickel carbonyl, or the resulting pure nickel in the processing that is the specific causative agents, although studies from Norway showed that the risk was mainly confined to the early stage of refining, involving heavy exposure to dust from relatively crude ore (Pedersen et al., 1973). In a follow-up of 967 workers in a nickel processing plant in South Wales, Doll et al. (1977) found that the increased risk was primarily seen in workers employed before 1925, indicating that implementation of measures to decrease exposure to dust and fumes since then has significantly reduced the hazard.

E. Chromium

Chromate workers have long been reported to have an increased incidence of lung cancer (Frank, 1982). Chromium is mainly used in the production of pigments and alloys, and the risk is mainly evident in chromate workers including chromate pigment workers, and less definite with ferrochromium alloy workers (Langard et al., 1980; Langard and Vigander, 1983). The hexavalent compounds appear to be the most frequently implicated for carcinogenicity (Frank, 1982).

F. α-Halogen Ethers

These are volatile electrophilic reactants used in industry in the synthesis and preparation of bactericides, fungicides, ion-exchange resins, and polymers (Harris, 1983). Two forms are important: chloromethyl methyl ether and the more potent bis-(chloromethyl)ether. Their carcinogenicity has been described in laboratory animals (Drew et al., 1975), and exposed workers have shown an increased risk of lung cancer (Nelson, 1976; Weiss et al., 1979; McCallum et al., 1983), which was related more to the degree than to the duration of exposure.

G. Miscellaneous

Many other inhalable industrial chemicals have been implicated as respiratory carcinogens (Frank, 1982; Parkes, 1982a). Some are mainly of historical interest (e.g., mustard gas) while others are either products of small industries (e.g., manufacture of isopropyl alcohol from crude isopropyl oil) or are only suspected respiratory carcinogens (e.g., vinyl chloride, beryllium, cadmium, and chloroprene). They will not be further discussed here.

Many studies have reported specific histopathologic lung cancer associations with various environmental exposures (Frank, 1978, 1982; Harris, 1983), including squamous cell cancer with arsenic, nickel, and chromium; small cell cancer with radiation and α-halogen ethers; and large cell cancer and adenocarcinoma with vinyl chloride. Often, however, an increased incidence of all cell types is seen (Edling, 1985). Ives et al. (1983), after reviewing studies reporting specific histopathologic associations, concluded that there is at present no unequivocal evidence demonstrating that a specific lung cancer cell type is uniquely associated with a specific occupational exposure.

V. Prevention

A preventive approach to a disease requires an understanding of its causes and pathogenesis, a rational preventive scheme, and public education. For human lung cancer, it is generally accepted that approximately 80% or more of all cases are due to environmental factors, so that it is a largely preventable disease. Active cigarette smoking is undoubtedly the most important factor, but it is in the prevention of occupational lung cancers that most comprehensive control measures have been formulated and implemented.

Prevention of occupational lung cancers follows several steps (Davies, 1982). First, industrial carcinogens should be identified by epidemiologic and laboratory methods. The current knowledge of chemical carcinogenesis, even though incomplete, provides exciting opportunities for cancer prevention. That strong electrophilic reactivity is a basic requirement for initiation of carcinogenesis permits some predictions of possible carcinogenicity from examination of chemical structures of substances proposed for industrial use. After identification of carcinogens, the second step is enactment of legislation to prohibit or control their use, followed by enforcement of this legislation. Legislation for compensation, public education, and medical surveillance are all parts of the mechanisms of prevention. In the United States, the Occupational Safety and Health Act was passed in 1970, giving workers stong legal rights and imposing on employers the responsibility for providing a safe work environment. Two important agencies were established: the National Institute for Occupational Safety and Health (NIOSH), which carries out research on work hazards and recommends new health and safety standards to the Occupational Safety and Health Administration (OSHA), which in turn prescribes and enforces health and safety standards. In the United Kingdom, the Health and Safety Act of 1974 similarly lays on employers the duty of ensuring the health and safety of their employees as far as is reasonably practicable and of conducting their undertakings so that those outside are not harmed (neighborhood risks).

To control radiation levels in mines, the U.S. Public Health Service introduced the working level (WL) unit, which is defined as any combination of radon daughters in 1 liter of air that will result in emission of 1.3×10^5 million electron volts/liter of potential alpha energy. The measure of total radiation exposure of miners is expressed as a working level month (WLM), which is inhalation for 1 working month (170 hr) of air with a radon daughter concentration of 1 WL. Most authorities accept that no workers should have an exposure of more than 4 WLM a year (Parkes, 1982a). Efficient ventilation of the mine is essential, and radon daughter concentration in mine air should be monitored. At the iron mine in Malmberget, Sweden, (Radford and Renard, 1984), for instance, an extensive new ventilation system has resulted in annual exposures of less than 1 WLM, which represents a great improvement over past standards.

These industrial control measures, as well as monitoring and minimizing radon daughters and other respiratory carcinogens in ambient air both indoor and outdoor, are all very important, but one must not lose sight of the fact that active cigarette smoking remains the single most important causative factor for the majority of lung cancer patients. Large scale antismoking campaigns are being launched by health organization and authorities in many countries. The total problem of cigarette smoking is both socioeconomic and medicopsychological. Change of attitude toward smoking in a community requires major educational, organizational, and legislative measures, and the medical profession has the responsibility to lead the way in this area of health education. The World Health Theme should be remembered by all: "smoking or health, the choice is yours."

References

Akiba, S., Kato, H., and Blot, W. J. (1986). Passive smoking and lung cancer among Japanese women. *Cancer Res.* **46**:4804-4807.

Alderson, M. (1982). The causes of cancer. In *The Prevention of Cancer.* Edited by M. Alderson. London, Edward Arnold, pp. 20-79.

American Thoracic Society. (1985). Cigarette smoking and health. *Am. Rev. Respir. Dis.* **132**:1133-1138.

Ames, B. N. (1979). Identifying environmental chemicals causing mutation and cancer. *Science* **204**:587-592.

Archer, V. E., Gillam, J. D., and Wagoner, J. K. (1976). Respiratory disease mortality among uranium miners. *Ann. N.Y. Acad. Sci.* **271**:280-293.

Becklake, M. R. (1976). Asbestos-related diseases of the lung and other organs: their epidemiology and implications for clinical practice. *Am. Rev. Respir. Dis.* **114**:187-227.

Blot, W. J., and Fraumeni, J. F., Jr. (1986). Passive smoking and lung cancer. *JNCI* **77**:993-1000.

Boice, J. D., and Land, C. E. (1982). Ionizing radiation. In *Cancer: Epidemiology and Prevention.* Edited by D. Schottenfeld, and I. F. Fraumeni. Philadelphia, Saunders, pp. 231-253.

Boutwell, R. K. (1985). Tumor promoters in human carcinogenesis. In *Important Advances in Oncology 1985.* Edited by V. T. deVita, S. Hellman, and S. A. Rosenberg. Philadelphia, Lippincott, pp. 16-27.

Breslow, N. E., and Day, N. E. (1980). *Statistical Methods in Cancer Research: 1: The Analysis of Case-Control Studies.* Lyon, International Association for Research in Cancer Press.

Carnow, B. W., and Meier, P. (1973). Air pollution and pulmonary cancer. *Arch. Environ. Health* **27**:207-218.

Casey, K. R., Rom, W. N., and Moatamed, F. (1981). Asbestos related diseases. *Clin. Chest Med.* **2**:179-202.

Chan, W. C., Colbourne, M. J., Fung, S. C., and Ho, H. C. (1979). Bronchial cancer in Hong Kong 1976-1977. *Br. J. Cancer* **39**:182-192.

Cohen, G. M. (1981). Pulmonary metabolism of inhaled chemicals and irritants. In *Scientific Foundations of Respiratory Medicine.* Edited by J. G. Scadding and G. Cumming. London, Heinemann, pp. 286-296.

Correa, P., Pickle, L. W., Fontham, E., Lin, Y., and Haenszel, W. (1983). Passive smoking and lung cancer. *Lancet* **2**:595-597.

Damber, L., and Larsson, L. G. (1985). Professional driving, smoking, and lung cancer: a case referent study. *Br. J. Ind. Med.* **42**:246-252.

Davies, C. N. (1967). *Assessment of Airborne Radioactivity.* Vienna, International Atomic Energy Agency, pp. 3-20.

Davies, J. M. (1982). The prevention of industrial cancer. In *The Prevention of Cancer.* Edited by M. Alderson. London, Edward Arnold, pp. 184-209.

Doll, R. (1978). Atmospheric pollution and lung cancer. *Environ. Health Perspect.* **22**:23-31.

Doll, R., Morgan, L. G., and Speizer, F. E. (1970). Cancers of the lung and nasal sinuses in nickel workers. *Br. J. Cancer* **24**:623-632.

Doll, R., Vessey, M. P., Beasley, R. W., Buckley, A. R., Fears, E. C., Fisher, R. E. W., Gammon, E. J., Gunn, W., Hughes, G. O., Lee, K., and Norman-Smith, B. (1972). Mortality of gas-workers—final report of a prospective study. *Br. J. Ind. Med.* **29**:394-406.

Doll, R., Mathews, J. D., and Morgan, L. G. (1977). Cancer of the lung and nasal sinuses in nickel workers: a reassessment of the period of risk. *Br. J. Ind. Med.* **34**:102-105.

Drew, R. T., Laskin, S., Kuschner, M., and Nelson, N. (1975). Inhalation carcinogenicity of alpha halo ethers. *Arch. Environ. Health* **30**:61-69.

Du, Y. S., Hu, M. J., Feng, J. W., Huang, L. F., and Wu, X. F. (1984). A preliminary analysis of trends of lung cancer death rate in Guangzhou (Canton), China. *Proceedings of the International Seminar on Environmental Impact Assessment.* Scotland, United Kingdom. WHO and University of Aberdeen.

Du, Y. X., Chen, X. W., Liang, Z. Q., Feng, J. W., Huang, L. F., Wu, X. F., and Feng, Z. Z. (1985). Lung cancer and air pollution in Guangzhou (Canton), China. *Proceedings of the 78th Annual Meeting of the Air Pollution Control Association.* Detroit, Air Pollution Control Association, pp. 96, 85-59B.5.

Edling, C. (1985). Radon daughter exposure and lung cancer. *Br. J. Ind. Med.* **42**:721-722.

Edling, C. and Axelson, O. (1983). Quantitative aspects of radon daughter exposure and lung cancer in underground miners. *Br. J. Ind. Med.* **40**:182-187.

Edling, C., Kling, H., and Axelson, O. (1984). Radon in homes—a possible cause of lung cancer. *Scand. J. Work Environ. Health* **10**:25-34.

Evans, R. D., Harley, J. H., Jacobi, W., McLean, A. S., Mills, W. A., and Stewart, C. G. (1981). Estimate of risk from environmental exposure to radon-222 and its decay products. *Nature* **290**:98-100.

Fielding, J. E. (1985). Smoking: health effects and control (First of two parts). *N. Engl. J. Med.* **313**:491-498.

Frank, A. (1978). Occupational lung cancer. In *Pathogenesis and Therapy of Lung Cancer.* Edited by C. C. Harris. New York, Marcel Dekker, pp. 25-52.

Frank, A. (1982). The epidemiology and etiology of lung cancer. *Clin. Chest Med.* **3**:219-228.

Fraumeni, J. (1974). Chemicals in the induction of respiratory tract cancer. *Proceedings of the 11th International Cancer Congress.* Excerpta Medica International Congress, Series 351, Vol. 3. Florence, New York, Excerpta Medica, pp. 327-335.

Fraumeni, J. F., and Mason, T. J. (1974). Cancer mortality among Chinese Americans 1950-1969. *J. Natl. Cancer Inst.* **52**:659-665.

Friberg, L., and Cederlof, R. (1978). Late effects of air pollution with special reference to lung cancer. *Environ. Health Perspect.* **22**:45-66.

Frigerio, N. A., and Stowe, R. S. (1976). Carcinogenic and genetic hazard from background radiation. In *Biological and Environmental Effects of Low-Level Radiation.* Vol. 2. Vienna, International Atomic Energy Agency, pp. 385-393.

Fujiki, H., Hecker, E., Moore, R. E., Sugimura, T., and Weinstein, I. B. (1984). *Cellular Interactions by Environmental Tumour Promoters,* Princess Takamatsu Symposium, Vol. 14. Tokyo, Japan Scientific Societies Press.

Garfinkle, L. (1981). Time trends in lung cancer mortality among nonsmokers and a note on passive smoking. *J. Natl. Cancer Inst.* **66**:1061-1066.

Garfinkle, L., Auerbach, O., and Joubert, L. (1985). Involuntary smoking and lung cancer: a case-control study. *J. Natl. Cancer Inst.* **75**:463-469.

Gillis, C. R., Hale, D. J., Hawthorne, V. M., and Boyle, P. (1984). The effect of environmental tobacco smoke in two urban communities in the west of Scotland. *Eur. J. Respir. Dis.* **65**(suppl):121-126.

Haenszel, W., Loveland, D., and Sirken, M. (1962). Lung cancer mortality as related to residence and smoking histories I. White males. *J. Natl. Cancer Inst.* **28**:947-1001.

Harley, N. H., and Pasternack, B. S. (1981). A model for predicting lung cancer risks induced by environmental levels of radon daughters. *Health Phys.* **40**: 307-316.

Harris, C. C. (1983). Respiratory carcinogenesis and cancer epidemiology. In *Lung Cancer: Clinical Diagnosis and Treatment.* Edited by M. J. Straus. New York, Grune & Stratton, pp. 1-20.

Harris, C. C., Trump, B. F., and Stone, G. D. (1980). *Methods in Cell Biology,* Vols. 21A & 21B. New York, Academic Press.

Hecker, E., Fusenig, N. E., Kunz, W., Marks, F., and Thielmann, H. W. (eds.) (1982). Cocarcinogenesis and biological effects of tumor promoters. In *Carcinogenesis. A Comprehensive Survey,* Vol. 7. New York, Raven Press.

Heidleberger, C., and Mondal, S. (1979). In vitro chemical carcinogenesis. In *Carcinogens: Identification and Mechanisms of Action.* Edited by A. C. Griffin, and C. R. Shaw. New York, Raven Press, pp. 85-92.

Henry, H. F. (1961). Is all nuclear radiation harmful? *J.A.M.A.* **176**:671-675.

Hickey, R. J., Bowers, E. J., Spence, D. E., Zemel, B. S., Clelland, A. B., and Clelland, R. C. (1981). Low level ionizing radiation and human mortality: multi-regional epidemiological studies: a preliminary report. *Health Phys.* **40**:625-641.

Hickey, R. J., and Clelland, R. C. (1982). Radioactivity in cigarette smoke (letter to editors). *N. Engl. J. Med.* **307**:1450.

Higgins, I. T. T. (1977). Epidemiology of lung cancer in the United States. In *Air Pollution and Cancer in Man.* Edited by V. Morf, D. Schmahl, and L. Tomatis. IARC Scientific Publications, No. 16. Lyon, International Agency for Research on Cancer, pp. 191-203.

Higgins, I. T. T. (1984). Air pollution and lung cancer: diesel exhaust, coal combustion. *Prev. Med.* **13**:207-218.

Higginson, J. (1976). Importance of environmental factors in cancer. In *Environmental Pollution and Carcinogenic Risks.* Edited by C. Rosenfeld and W. Davies. INSERM Symposium series 52:15. Lyon, IARC Scientific Publications, No. 13.

High Background Radiation Research Group, China (1980). Health Survey in high background radiation areas in China. *Science* **209**:877-880.

Hirayama, T. (1981). Nonsmoking wives of heavy smokers have a higher risk of lung cancer: a study from Japan. *Br. Med. J.* **282**:183-185.

Hodgson, J. T., and Jones, R. D. (1985). A mortality study of carbon black workers employed at five United Kingdom factories between 1947 & 1980. *Arch. Environ. Health* **40**:261-268.

Hoffman, D., and Wynder, E. L. (1971). A study of tobacco carcinogenesis XI. Tumor initiators, tumor accelerators, and tumor promoting activity of condensate fractions. *Cancer* **27**:848-864.

Hoffman, D., and Wynder, E. L. (1977). Organic particulate pollutants. In *Air Pollution.* Vol. 11, 3rd ed. Edited by A. C. Stein. New York, Academic Press, pp. 361-455.

Hong Kong Government (1985). Main causes of death from cancer in Hong Kong 1975-1984. Table 18. *1984-1985 Departmental Report, Director of Medical and Health Services.* Hong Kong Government Printer.

Howe, G. R., Fraser, D., Lindsay, J., Presnal, B., and Yu, S. Z. (1983). Cancer mortality (1965-1977) in relation to diesel fumes & coal exposure in a cohort of retired railroad workers. *J. Natl. Cancer Inst.* **70**:1015-1019.

Ives, J. C., Buffler, P. A., and Greenberg, S. D. (1983). Environmental associations and histopathologic patterns of carcinoma of the lung: the challenge and dilemma in epidemiologic studies. *Am. Rev. Respir. Dis.* **128**:195-209.

Jablon, S., and Bailar, J. A. (1980). The contribution of ionizing radiation to cancer mortality in the United States. *Prev. Med.* **9**:212-226.

Jacobson, A. P., Plato, P. A., and Frigerio, N. A. (1976). The role of natural radiations in human leukemogenesis. *Am. J. Publ. Health* **66**:31-37.

Kabat, G. C., and Wynder, E. L. (1984). Lung cancer in non-smokers. *Cancer* **53**:1214-1221.

Kaplan, I. (1959). Relationship of noxious gases to carcinoma of the lung in railroad workers. *J.A.M.A.* **171**:2039-2043.

Klein-Szanto, A. J. P. (1984). Morphological evaluation of tumor promoter effects on mammalian skin. In *Mechanism of Tumor Promotion,* vol. 2, *Tumor Promotion and Skin Carcinogenesis.* Edited by T. J. Slaga. Boca Raton, FL, CRC Press, pp. 42-72.

Klement, A. W., Miller, C. R., Minx, R. P., and Shleien, B. (1972). *Estimate of Ionizing Radiation Doses in the US 1960-2000.* Washington, D.C., U.S. Environmental Protection Agency, ORP/CSD, 72-1.

Knoth, A., Bohn, W., and Schmidt, F. (1983). Passive smoking as a causal factor for bronchial carcinoma in female nonsmokers. *Med. Klin.* **78**:66-69.

Koo, L. C., Ho, H. C., and Saw, D. (1983). Active and passive smoking among female lung cancer patients and controls in Hong Kong. *J. Exp. Clin. Cancer Res.* **4**:367-375.

Koo, L. C., Lee, N., and Ho, J. H. C. (1984). Do cooking fuels pose a risk for lung cancer? A case-control study of women in Hong Kong. *Ecol. Dis.* 2:255-265.

Kung, I. T. M., So, K. F., and Lam, T. H. (1984). Lung cancer in Hong Kong Chinese: mortality and histological types 1973-1982. *Br. J. Cancer* 50: 381-388.

Lam, W. K., So, S. Y., and Yu, D. Y. C. (1983). Clinical features of bronchogenic carcinoma in Hong Kong—Review of 480 patients. *Cancer* 52:369-376.

Lam, W. K., Kung, T. M., So, S. Y., and Bacon-shone, J. H. (1985). Active and passive smoking, kerosene stove usage and home incense burning among female lung cancer patients: a case-control study. *Proceedings of the XV World Congress on Diseases of the Chest.* Sydney, Australia, American College of Chest Physicians and Thoracic Society of Australia, p. 33.

Langard, S., Andersen, A., and Gylseth, B. (1980). Incidence of cancer among ferrochromium and ferrosilicon workers. *Br. J. Ind. Med.* 37:114-120.

Langard, S., and Vigander, T. (1983). Occurrence of lung cancer in workers producing chromium pigments. *Br. J. Ind. Med.* 40:71-74.

Laskin, S., Kuschner, M., and Drew, R. T. (1970). Studies in pulmonary carcinogenesis. In *Inhalation Carcinogenesis,* AEC Symposium Series 18. Edited by M. G. Hanna, P. Nettesheim, and J. Gilbert. Tennessee, Atomic Energy Commission, pp. 321-352.

Lee, A. M., and Fraumeni, J. F. (1969). Arsenic and respiratory cancer in man: an occupational study. *J. Natl. Cancer Inst.* 42:1045-1052.

Lee, M. L., Novotny, M., and Bartle, K. D. (1976). Gas chromatography/ mass spectrometric and nuclear magnetic resonance determination of polynuclear aromatic hydrocarbons in airborne particulates. *Anal. Chem.* 48:1566-1572.

Lee, P. N. (1982). Passive smoking. *Food Chem. Toxicol.* 20:223-229.

Lee, P. N. (1986). Relationship of passive smoking to risk of lung cancer and other smoking-associated diseases. *Br. J. Cancer* 54:97-105.

Leung, J. S. M. (1977). Cigarette smoking, the kerosene stove and lung cancer in Hong Kong. *Br. J. Dis Chest* 71:273-276.

Leupker, R. V., and Smith, M. L. (1978). Mortality in unionized truck drivers. *J. Occup. Med.* 20:677-682.

Lloyd, O. L., Smith, G., Lloyd, M. M., Holland, Y., and Gailey, F. (1985). Raised mortality from lung cancer and high sex ratios of births associated with industrial pollution. *Br. J. Ind. Med.* 42:475-480.

Luckey, T. D. (1981). Ionizing radiation hormesis of non-specific immunity. *Microecol. Ther.* 11:113-123.

Mabuchi, K., Lilienfeld, A. M., and Snell, L. M. (1980). Cancer and occupational exposure to arsenic—a study of pesticide workers. *Prev. Med.* 9: 51-77.

MacLennan, R., Da Costa, J., Day, N. E., Law, C. H., Ng, Y. K., and Shanmu-garatnam, K. (1977). Risk factors for lung cancer in Singapore Chinese: a population with high female incidence rates. *Int. J. Cancer* **20**:854-860.

MacMahon, B., and Pugh, T. F. (1979). *Epidemiology: Principles and Methods.* Boston, Little, Brown.

Martell, E. A. (1974). Radioactivity of tobacco trichomes and insoluble cigarette smoke particles. *Nature* **249**:215-217.

Martell, E. A. (1983). Radiation at bronchial bifurcations of smokers from indoor exposure to radon progency. *Proc. Natl. Acad. Sci.* **80**:1285-1289.

McCallum, R. I., Woolley, V., and Petrie, A. (1983). Lung cancer associated with chloromethyl methyl ether manufacture: an investigation at two factories in the United Kingdom. *Br. J. Ind. Med.* **40**:384-389.

Miller, E. C. (1981). The metabolic activation of chemical carcinogens. In *Cancer: Achievements, Challenges and Prospects for the 1980s.* Vol. 1. Edited by J. H. Burchenal, and H. R. Oettgen. New York, Grune & Stratton, pp. 269-279.

Miller, E. C., and Miller, J. A. (1981). Searches for ultimate chemical carcinogens and their reactions with cellular macromolecules. *Cancer* **47**:2327-2345.

Miller, J. A. (1979). Concluding remarks on chemicals and chemical carcinogenesis. In *Carcinogens: Identification and Mechanism of Action.* Edited by A. C. Griffin and C. R. Shaw. New York, Raven Press, pp. 455-469.

National Research Council (1972). *Particulate Polycyclic Organic Matter.* Committee on Medical and Biological Effects of Environmental Pollutants, National Academy of Sciences. Washington, D.C., National Academy of Sciences.

National Research Council (1981). *Health Effects of Exposure to Diesel Exhaust.* Washington, D.C., National Academy Press.

National Research Council (1986). Environmental tobacco smoking: measuring exposures and assessing health effects. Washington, D.C., National Academy Press.

NCRP (National Council on Radiation Protection and Measurements) (1975). *Background Radiation in the United States,* Report No. 45. Washington, D.C.

Nelson, N. (1976). The chloroethers—occupational carcinogens: a summary of laboratory and epidemiology studies. *Ann. N.Y. Acad. Sci.* **271**:81-90.

Nettesheim, P., Creasia, D., and Mitchell, T. (1975). Studies on the carcinogenic and cocarcinogenic effects of inhaled synthetic smog and ferric oxide particles. *J. Natl. Cancer Inst.* **55**:159-169.

Nettesheim, P., and Griesemer, R. A. (1978). Experimental models for studies of respiratory tract carcinogenesis. In *Pathogenesis and Therapy of Lung Cancer.* Edited by C. Harris. New York, Marcel Dekker, pp. 75-188.

Newell, G. R., Boutwell, W. R., Morris, D. L., Tilley, B. C., and Branyon, E. S. (1982). Epidemiology of cancer. In *Cancer: Principles and Practice of Oncology*. Edited by V. T. DeVita, S. Hellman, and S. A. Rosenberg. Philadelphia, Lippincott, pp. 3-32.

Parkes, W. R. (1982a). Lung cancer and occupation. In *Occupational Lung Disorders*. London, Butterworth, pp. 499-507.

Parkes, W. R. (1982b). Inhaled particles and their fate in the lungs. In *Occupational Lung Disorders*. London, Butterworth, pp. 45-53.

Parkes, W. R. (1982c). Asbestos-related disorders. In *Occupational Lung Disorders*. London, Butterworth, pp. 233-296.

Pedersen, E., Hogetveit, A. C., and Anderson, A. (1973). Cancer of respiratory organs among workers at a nickel refinery in Norway. *Int. J. Cancer* **12**: 32-41.

Pershagen, G. (1984). Validity of questionnaire data on smoking and other exposures, with special reference to environmental tobacco smoke. *Eur. J. Respir. Dis.* **133**(suppl):76-80.

Pike, M. C., Gordon, R. J., Henderson, B. E., Menck, H. R., and Soo Hoo J. (1975). Air pollution. In *Persons at High Risk of Cancer*. Edited by J. F. Fraumeni. Academic Press, New York, pp. 225-239.

Pitot, H. C. (1982). The natural history of neoplastic development: the relation of experimental models to human cancer. *Cancer* **49**:1206-1211.

Radford, E. P., and Renard, K. G. (1984). Lung cancer in Swedish iron miners exposed to low dose of radon daughters. *N. Engl. J. Med.* **310**:1485-1494.

Redmond, C. K., Ciocco, A., Lloyd, J. W., and Rush, H. W. (1972). Long-term mortality study of steel workers. VI. Mortality from malignant neoplasms among coke oven workers. *J. Occup. Med.* **14**:621-629.

Reid, D. D., Cornfield, J., Markush, R. E., Siegel, D., Pederson, E., and Haenszel, W. (1966). Studies of disease among migrants and native population in Great Britain, Norway and the United States III. Prevalence of cardio-respiratory symptoms among migrants and native born in the U.S. In *Epidemiological Study of Cancer and Other Chronic Diseases*. Edited by W. Haenszel. National Cancer Institute. Monograph 19, pp. 321-346.

Repace, J. L., and Lowrey, A. H. (1985). A quantitative estimate of nonsmokers' lung cancer risk from passive smoking. *Environ. Int.* **1**:3-22.

Report of a Task Group (1978). Air pollution and cancer: risk assessment and methodology and epidemiological evidence. *Environ. Health Perspect.* **22**: 1-12.

Richters, A., and Richters, V. (1983). A new relationship between air pollutant inhalation and cancer. *Arch. Environ. Health* **38**:69-75.

Royal College of Physicians (1970). *Air Pollution and Lung Cancer. Air Pollution and Health*. London, Pitman, pp. 48-57.

Royal College of Physicians (1983). *Health or Smoking–Follow-Up Report*. London, Pitman, pp. 72-81.

Rushton, L., Alderson, M. R., and Nagarajah, C. R. (1983). Epidemiological survey of maintenance workers in London Transport Executive bus garages and Chiswick Works. *Br. J. Ind. Med.* **40**:340-345.

Rylander, R. (1984). Environmental tobacco smoke and lung cancer. *Eur. J. Respir. Dis.* **113**(suppl):127-133.

Samet, J. M., Kutvirt, D. M., Waxweiler, R. J., and Key, C. R. (1984). Uranium mining and lung cancer in Navajo men. *N. Engl. J. Med.,* **310**:1481-1484.

Samuels, S. W., and Adamson, R. H. (1985). Quantitative risk assessment: report of the Subcommittee on Environmental Carcinogenesis, National Cancer Advisory Board. *J. Natl. Cancer. Inst.* **74**:945-951.

Sandler, D. P., Wilcox, A. J., and Everson, R. B. (1985). Cumulative effects of lifetime passive smoking on cancer risk. *Lancet* **1**:312-314.

Schoental, R., and Gibbard, S. (1967). Carcinogens in Chinese incense smoke. *Nature* **216**:612.

Selikoff, I. J., Chung, J., and Hammond, E. C. (1964). Asbestos exposure and neoplasia. *J.A.M.A.* **188**:22-26.

Selikoff, I. J., and Lee, D. H. K. (1978). *Asbestos and Disease.* New York, Academic Press.

Shy, C. M., and Struba, R. J. (1982). Air and water pollution. In *Cancer: Epidemiology and Prevention.* Edited by D. Schottenfeld and J. F. Fraumeni. Philadelphia, Saunders, pp. 336-363.

Silverberg, E. (1985). Cancer statistics 1985. CA **35**:19-35.

Slaga, T. J. (ed.) (1983). Tumour promotion in internal organs. In *Mechanisms of Tumor Promotion,* Vol. 1. Boca Raton, FL, CRC Press.

Speizer, F. E. (1983). Assessment of the epidemiological data relating lung cancer to air pollution. *Environ. Health Perspect.* **47**:33-42.

Tomatis, L., Breslow, N. E., and Bartsch, H. (1982). Experimental studies in the assessment of human risk. In *Cancer: Epidemiology and Prevention.* Edited by D. Schottenfeld and J. F. Fraumeni. Philadelphia, Saunders, pp. 44-73.

Trichopoulos, D., Kalandidi, A., Sparros, L., and MacMahon, B. (1981). Lung cancer and passive smoking. *Int. J. Cancer* **27**:1-4.

Upton, A. C. (1982). Principles of cancer biology: etiology and prevention of cancer. In *Cancer: Principles and Practice of Oncology.* Edited by V. T. DeVita, S. Hellman, and S. A. Rosenberg. Philadelphia, Lippincott, pp. 33-58.

U.S. Department of Health and Human Services (1986). *The Health Consequences of Involuntary Smoking: A Report of the Surgeon General.* Rockville, MD, Public Health Service.

Wald, N. J., Boreham, J., Bailey, A., Ritchie, C., Haddow, J. E., and Knight G. (1984). Urinary cotinine as marker of breathing other peoples's tobacco smoke. *Lancet* **1**:230-231.

Weisburger, J. H., and Williams, G. M. (1982). Chemical carcinogenesis. In *Cancer Medicine.* Edited by J. F. Holland and E. Frei III. Philadelphia, Lea & Febiger, pp. 42-95.

Weiss, S. T. (1986). Passive smoking and lung cancer—what is the risk? *Am. Rev. Respir. Dis.* **133**:1-3.

Weiss, S. T., Tager, I. B., Schenker, M., and Speizer, F. E. (1983). The health effects of involuntary smoking. *Am. Rev. Respir. Dis.* **128**:933-942.

Weiss, W., Moser, R. L., and Auerbach, O. (1979). Lung cancer in chloroethyl ethers. *Am. Rev. Respir. Dis.* **120**:1031-1037.

WHO (1964). *Prevention of Cancer.* Technical Report Series No. 276. Geneva.

Winters, T. H., and DiFrenza, J. (1983). Radioactivity and lung cancer in active and passive smokers. *Chest* **84**:653-654.

Wu, A. H., Henderson, B. E., Pike, M. C., and Yu, M. C. (1985). Smoking and other risk factors for lung cancer in women. *J. Natl. Cancer Inst.* **74**:747-751.

Wynder, E. L., and Goodman, M. C. (1983). Smoking and lung cancer: some unresolved issues. *Epidemiol. Rev.* **5**:177-207.

Wynder, E. L., and Hoffmann, D. (1982). Tobacco. In *Cancer: Epidemiology and Prevention.* Edited by D. Schottenfeld and J. F. Fraumeni. Philadelphia, W. B. Saunders, pp. 277-292.

Yuspa, S. H., and Harris, C. C. (1982). Molecular and cellular basis of chemical carcinogenesis. In *Cancer: Epidemiology and Prevention.* Edited by D. Schottenfeld and J. F. Fraumeni. Philadelphia, W. B. Saunders, pp. 23-43.

11

The Toxic Environment and Its Medical Implications with Special Emphasis on Smoke Inhalation

JACOB LOKE, RICHARD A. MATTHAY, and G. J. WALKER SMITH

Yale University School of Medicine
New Haven, Connecticut

The environment we live in has the potential to release toxic gases, fumes, and hazardous chemicals which can have detrimental effects on the pulmonary or other systems of the body (Hartnett, 1986; Kizer, 1984). This has been devastatingly demonstrated by several environmental disasters such as the volcanic gas eruption in 1986 in Cameroon, Africa, that released a poisonous gas killing 1500 people; the industrial pesticide plant accident in Bhopal, India, in 1984, where the lethal gas, methyl isocyanate, leaked into the air (Ferguson, et al., 1986; Nemery et al., 1985; Salmon et al., 1985), killing 2500 people (Zaidi, 1986), and left many more victims with chronic respiratory disease (Meier, 1986; Kamat et al., 1985), and the explosion of a tank containing a commercial solvent resulting in acute chemical injury of the airways and lungs in six people three of whom later died from exposure (Conner et al., 1962). Lung injuries have been caused by industrial accidents involving mixtures of toxic gases, including hydrogen chloride (Rosenthal et al., 1978) and sulfur dioxide (Charan et al., 1979); chlorine gas inhalation (Adelson and Kaufman, 1971; Jones et al., 1986); aerial pesticide spraying (Ratner and Eshel, 1986); and zinc chloride (smoke bomb) inhalation (Matarese and Matthews, 1986). The meltdown of the nuclear plant reactor at Chernobyl in the Soviet Union in 1986 resulted in deaths due to an acute radiation syndrome (Saenger,

1986; Milroy, 1984) and probably will lead to increased cancer incidence in the population of Chernobyl and throughout Europe in future years.

We are surrounded by chemicals, various materials, and physical agents in the work place (Chan-Yeung and Lam, 1986; Himmelstein and Frumkin, 1985; Wegman, et al., 1982) or home (Reisz and Gammon, 1986; Caplan et al., 1986; Alarie, 1985; Leaderer, 1982; Breysse, 1981; Alarie and Ancerson, 1979; Stewart and Hake, 1976; Murphy et al., 1976; Stone, 1974) which have the potential of becoming toxic if safety procedures are not adhered to. Every year, fires occur in homes or buildings (Terrill et al., 1978; Fein et al., 1980; Hartzell et al., 1983; Levin et al., 1983b; Cahalane and Demling, 1984; Committee on Fire Toxicology, 1986) as a result of careless accidents which could have been avoided if proper safety procedures were followed. In addition, substances harmful to the lungs are present in cigarette smoke and in inhaled substance abuse (Glassroth et al., 1987). The health consequences of a toxic agent, which may lead to cancer (Vena and Fiedler, 1987; Olsen and Asnaes, 1986; Steenland, 1986; Woods, 1979; Wiadana et al., 1976) or radiation health hazard (Rall, 1984), may not be evident for some time (Schottenfeld, 1984). For example, the release of radon gas from the natural breakdown of uranium found in the earth or rocks of surrounding homes (Eckholm, 1986), may go unnoticed by victims and may account for the subsequent increase in cases of lung cancer (Radford and Renard, 1984).

In this chapter, it is impossible to cover all aspects of inhalation toxicology which range from passive cigarette smoke exposure to the most severe type of chemical warfare inhalation lung injury (Winternitz, 1920). Accordingly, we discuss smoke inhalation as a prototype for acute and chronic lung injury with emphasis on: (1) the fire environment, (2) the evaluation of products of pyrolysis and combustion in laboratory animals and its correlation in humans, and (3) the diagnostic workup and management of acute and chronic inhalation lung injury.

I. The Toxic Fire Environment

According to the National Fire Protection Association, there were about 2.4 million fires in the United States in 1985, of which 859,500 were structure fires, 72.4 percent being residential fires resulting in a property loss of over $7 billion (Karter, 1986). In residential fires, an ignition source is usually attributed to such items as a lighted cigarette or matches, a wood stove or kerosene space heater, an electrical or heating equipment malfunction, fuel-lighted material from appliances in the kitchen, or arson. In addition, 4885 people died from fires in homes (Karter, 1986). Cigarette-ignited fires were the major cause of house fire deaths in a study by Mierley and Baker (1983). In the home, there are many forms of combustible materials including wood furniture, carpets, wall paper, plastic paneling on walls and ceilings, upholstery, plywood and particle board paneling,

Table 1 Toxic Products of Combustion

Material	Use	Major toxic chemical products of combustion
Polyvinylchloride	Wall and floor covering; telephone cable insulation	Hydrogen chloride (P); carbon monoxide
Polyurethane	Upholstery	Isocyanates (P) (toluene 2,4-diisocyanate); hydrogen cyanide
Lacquered wood veneer; wallpaper	Wall covering	Acetaldehyde (P); formaldehyde (P); oxides of nitrogen (P); acetic acid
Acrylic	Light diffusers	Acrolein (P)
Nylon	Carpet	Hydrogen cyanide; ammonia (P)
Acrilan	Carpet	Hydrogen cyanide; acrolein (P)
Polystyrene	Miscellaneous	Styrene; carbon monoxide

P - Pulmonary irritant.
Source: Reproduced with permission from Genovesi et al., 1977.

cellulose fiber, polyurethane material, papers, and clothing. Many of these materials release toxic products of combustion (Table 1).

The toxic fire environment depends not only on the materials that are available at the time of the fires, but also on the flammability of these products and the thermal decomposition modes of these materials. Different materials have varied ignition temperatures and varying degrees of flammability. Also, products can be degraded in the flaming (combustion) condition, or nonflaming (smoldering or pyrolysis) condition, or both. Under field conditions, pyrolysis is defined as thermal decomposition of materials in an area without sufficient oxygen, and combustion represents thermal degradation of material where there is an adequate supply of oxygen. In the laboratory, differentiating between pyrolysis and combustion has important implications since toxic gases may be increased when substances are decomposed in the pyrolysis state rather than in the combustion state, and the degree of emission of toxic gases (e.g., from combusion of plastic polymers) can be different under flaming or nonflaming conditions (Levin et al., 1985b). Other factors that may contribute to the spread of a fire and smoke include the quantity of material that is available, the presence of other combustibles, ventilation conditions, the volume in which the combustion products may spread, the ignition sources, and the fire protection systems (Levin et al., 1983b).

In general, there are several major parameters that need to be considered in the morbidity and mortality of fire victims: (1) smoke and its toxic gases— which will depend on the materials that are undergoing pyrolysis and combustion; (2) high temperatures, or heat; (3) direct consumption by the flames of the fire; (4) oxygen deficiency; (5) secondary effects due to mechanical factors or structural damage related to the fires; and (6) development of fear and panic (Kimmerle, 1974). The majority of deaths from fires are due to the inhalation of smoke or toxic gases, not due to high temperatures or burns (Coleman, 1981; Trunkey, 1978; Birky, 1976).

II. Smoke and Its Toxic Gases

Smoke is a suspension of visible small particulate matter in hot air and toxic gases. The toxic gases can be present as the invisible component. Pyrolysis and combustion of carbonaceous material leads to the formation of black smoke due to the particulate component of carbon or soot which can be adhered with organic acids and aldehydes (Zikria, 1972). White smoke or fumes may be seen with the thermal decomposition of plastic polymers (Dyer and Esch, 1976). The upper respiratory tract is usually able to filter out the inhaled larger particles while allowing the invisible toxic gases and particles of 5 to 10 μm or less in diameter to enter the central or peripheral airways (Hogg, 1985).

A. Carbon Monoxide

Carbon-containing material is ubiquitous in the environment. During the incomplete combustion of these materials and in the presence of a limited supply of air or ventilation, carbon monoxide is produced. Studies have shown that the most dangerous toxic gas produced in fires is carbon monoxide (Kimmerle, 1974; Gold et al., 1978; Pitt et al., 1979; Mierley and Baker, 1983; Lowry et al., 1985a) (Table 2). It is the predominant cause of death among fire victims at the scene of the fire or during the first 24 hours after the fire (Levine and Radford, 1977).

Carbon monoxide is an odorless, colorless, tasteless, but poisonous gas. It competes with oxygen for the binding sites on hemoglobin molecules, since the affinity of carbon monoxide for human hemoglobin is 210 times greater than that of oxygen (Lawther, 1975). Also, carbon monoxide causes a shift of the oxygen hemoglobin dissociation curve to the left and impairs oxygen release at the tissue level (Ayres et al., 1973; Winter and Miller, 1976). The ultimate result of carbon monoxide poisoning is tissue hypoxia (Brody and Coburn, 1969). Since there is a greater amount of oxygen consumption in the brain and myo-

Table 2 Toxic Gases Produced During Structural Fires

Gas	Maximum, ppm	Range, ppm	Average, ppm	STEL, %[a]	IDLH, %[a]	STLC, %[a]
Carbon monoxide (CO)	15,000	0-15,000	1,450	28.5	10.5	10.5
Hydrochloric acid (HCl)	40	0-40	1.1	2.6	0	0
Hydrocyanic acid	40	0-40	3.7	10.5	0	0
Aldehydes (formaldehyde and acetaldehyde)	15	1-15	5	2.5	—	—
Total hydrocarbons	1,200	500-1,200	800	—	—	—

[a]Levels observed in percent of samples analyzed.

Abbreviations: ppm, parts per million; STEL, short-term exposure limits; IDLH, immediate danger to life or health; STLC, short-term lethal concentration.

Source: Reproduced with permission from Lowry et al., 1985.

Table 3 Symptoms Associated with Varying Levels of Carbon Monoxide Poisoning

CO in atmosphere, %	COHb in blood, %	Physiological and subjective symptoms
0.007	10	No appreciable effect, except shortness of breath on vigorous exertion; possible tightness across the forehead; dilation of cutaneous blood vessels
0.012	20	Shortness of breath on moderate exertion; occasional headache with throbbing in temples
0.022	30	Decided headache, irritable, easily fatigued, judgment disturbed, possible dizziness, dimness of vision
0.035-0.052	40-50	Headache, confusion, collapse, fainting on exertion
0.080-0.122	60-70	Unconsciousness, intermittent convulsions, respiratory failure, death if exposure persists
0.195	80	Rapidly fatal
0.195	over 80	Immediately fatal

Abbreviations: CO, carbon monoxide; COHb, carboxyhemoglobin.
Source: Reproduced with permission from Winter et al., 1976.

cardium, signs and symptoms of tissue hypoxia due to carbon monoxide poisoning are reflected in the central nervous system and the cardiovascular system (Aronow et al., 1977; Winter and Miller, 1976; Kuller et al., 1975; Zikria et al., 1975; Anderson et al., 1967, 1973; Ayres et al., 1970). The acute central nervous system findings depend on the level of carbon monoxide poisoning (Henderson and Haggard, 1943; Winter and Miller, 1976) (Table 3). There may be headache, dizziness, impairment in the performance of certain psychomotor tests (Beard and Grandstaff, 1970), behavioral incapacitation (Purser and Berrill, 1983), reduced visual discrimination, confusion, ataxia, convulsions, and coma (Stewart, 1975). A cherry red color of the skin and mucous membranes may be present with carbon monoxide poisoning but this is not a reliable sign (Mellins and Park, 1975) and an uncommon finding (Grace and Platt, 1981). In fact, none of the above mentioned findings are specific. Accordingly, direct determination of the blood carboxyhemoglobin (COHb) level is important for establishing the diagnosis of carbon monoxide poisoning (Zikria et al., 1975).

Cutaneous skin blisters (Myers et al., 1985a) and retinal hemorrhages (Kelly and Sophocleus, 1978; Eckfeldt, 1978) are other clinical manifestations of carbon monoxide poisoning. Central nervous system sequelae, as a result of central nervous system anoxia due to carbon monoxide, include memory impairment, deterioration of personality and neuropsychiatric abnormalities (Smith and Brandon, 1973), movement disorders, cerebellar ataxia, and postanoxic encephalopathy.

Increases in pulse rate and cardiac output have been observed with acute carbon monoxide poisoning with no significant increase in ventilation (Chiodi et al., 1941). Studies of the systemic hemodynamic and respiratory effects of acute elevation of carboxyhemoglobin to 10% in humans showed an increase in cardiac output from 5.01 to 5.56 liters/min, an increase in minute ventilation from 6.86 to 8.64 liters/min with a decrease in arterial oxygen tension and arterial carbon dioxide tension from 81 to 76 mmHg and 40 to 38 mmHg, respectively, and a decrease in mixed venous oxygen tension from 39 to 31 mmHg (Ayres, 1973). Myocardial tissue oxygen tension from coronary sinus measurements also decreased. Elevated blood concentrations of carboxyhemoglobin result in: (1) decreased exercise tolerance and myocardial ischemia in patients with coronary artery disease with COHb levels of 4.5 percent (Anderson et al., 1973), (2) a significant decrease in exercise time from onset of angina pectoris in patients with coronary heart disease and a COHb level of 2.68 percent (Aronow and Isbell, 1973), and (3) a significant reduction in exercise performance in patients with chronic obstructive pulmonary disease (Aronow et al., 1977). However, in a recent study of 30 patients with ischemic heart disease who were exposed to carbon monoxide and developed an acute elevation of COHb levels to 3.8%, there was no effect on exercise left ventricular ejection fraction or on time to onset of angina, duration of angina, or development of ST-segment depression during exercise (Sheps et al., 1987). Case reports of transmural myocardial infarction (Scharf et al., 1974) and myocardial toxicity (Anderson et al., 1967) have been reported in individuals with carbon monoxide exposure. Myocardial cytopathic effects have been demonstrated in animals (rats) exposed to high concentrations of carbon monoxide (Thomas and O'Flaherty, 1982). Other acute effects of significant carboxyhemoglobinemia include lactic acidosis (Buehler et al., 1975), diabetes insipidus (Halebian et al., 1985), pulmonary edema, central hearing loss, disseminated intravascular coagulation, myonecrosis, and hyperglycemia (Goldfrank et al., 1986). Polycythemia has been observed with chronic carbon monoxide exposure (Smith and Landaw, 1978).

Although carbon monoxide has been thought to have no effect on the lungs per se, an ultrastural study of the lungs of carbon monoxide exposed rabbits showed epithelial and endothelial cell swelling, interstitial edema, and depletion of lamellar bodies in alveolar type II cells (Fein, 1980a), suggesting that carbon monoxide poisoning may induce noncardiogenic, permeability-type pulmonary edema in humans.

The chronic long-term effects of low-level carbon monoxide exposure on atherosclerosis also have been shown (Astrup, 1972). In humans, the breakdown of hemoglobin leads to formation of carbon monoxide which is the explanation for a carboxyhemoglobin level of 0.5% even in nonsmoking individuals. Depending on the methodology for the determination of the carboxyhemoglobin level in blood, in cigarette smokers the carboxyhemoglobin level varies from 5% to 10% and in nonsmokers from 2% to 3% (Lawther and Commins, 1970; Loke et al., 1976). Heavy cigar smokers may have peak carboxyhemoglobin levels of 20% or higher (Stewart, 1975; Freedman, 1975). The measurement of the carboxyhemoglobin level in a fire victim provides a measure of the degree of smoke inhalation (Clark et al., 1981), and also has been used as an indirect indicator of lung injury due to inhalation of toxic gases other than carbon monoxide (Dyer and Each, 1976), which are usually not determined in the blood. In industrial societies, carbon monoxide is the most common air pollutant, and the petrol engine of motor vehicles is an important source of carbon monoxide pollution (Stewart, 1975; Lawther, 1975). Therefore, ambient carbon monoxide should be taken into consideration in determining carboxyhemoglobin levels, in addition to active or passive cigarette smoking, oxygen therapy, and the half life of carboxyhemoglobin (Clark et al., 1981). It should be noted that the half life of carboxyhemoglobin in healthy sedentary adults at sea level is about 4-5 hours (Stewart, 1975).

There are different methodologies for determining carboxyhemoglobin (COHb) levels in the blood (Small et al., 1975; Ranieri et al., 1974; Collison et al., 1968). Commercially available instruments for the measurement of COHb include the IL 282 CO-Oximeter, (Instrumentation Laboratories, Lexington, MA) and the OSM-3 Hemoximeter (Radiometer, Copenhagen, Denmark). Expired alveolar carbon monoxide can be estimated with an infrared carbon monoxide analyzer (Ecolyzer-Energetics Science, Elmsford, NY), and can provide a practical field and bloodless method for the estimation of COHb (Stewart, 1976; Rees et al., 1980). It has been suggested (U.S. National Air Pollution Control Administration, 1970) that there are adaptations to carbon monoxide with regard to symptoms after repeated exposures to this gas, and this is certainly observed in cigarette smokers when compared to nonsmokers. Cigarette smokers may tolerate higher levels of carboxyhemoglobin in the blood and remain asymptomatic in contrast to nonsmokers (Hebbel et al., 1978). However, this may not be the case in subjects with ischemic heart disease when exposed to low concentrations of carbon monoxide (Anderson et al., 1973; Aronow and Isbell, 1973). Finally, it should be noted that significant and occult carbon monoxide poisoning (Kirkpatrick, 1987;

Leaderer, 1982; Grace and Platt, 1981) and even fatalities due to carbon monoxide can occur at home from malfunction of portable kerosene space heaters (Fisher and Rubin, 1982), or from other heating systems, such as a furnace (Caplan et al., 1986).

In a study of wood and upholstery fires in a nonventilated room, the maximum carbon monoxide concentration (recorded by a portable carbon monoxide sampler) was 12,000 parts per million (ppm) (Sidor et al., 1973). In a fire situation, there may be a wide range of carbon monoxide concentrations in the ambient air depending on the amount of air supply and ventilation. Poorly ventilated, closed space buildings can have carbon monoxide levels of 3000 ppm (Barnard and Weber, 1979) (Table 4). In experimental fire studies of aircraft interiors to simulate postcrash fires, 90 seconds after ignition of the full-scale fire test, carbon monoxide concentration reached 10,000 ppm in the cabin; in another test, the carbon monoxide levels attained 26,000 ppm in 180 seconds (a fatal level for a 2.5 min exposure) (Mohler, 1975). In a study of the fire environments in the Dallas area, only 10.5% of the fires had carbon monoxide levels that exceeded immediate danger to life or health (1500 ppm) and the short-term lethal concentration (5000 ppm) (Table 2). Firefighters as well as fire victims can be exposed to lethal carbon monoxide levels in fires. For this reason, and due to the presence of other toxic gases in a fire, firefighters should always wear a compressed air breathing apparatus during fire fighting and rescue operations. It has been shown that wearing this apparatus results in a reduced blood carboxyhemoglobin levels after fires (Radford and Levine, 1976; Loke et al., 1976).

B. Hydrogen Cyanide

Analysis of toxic gases produced during structural fires in the Dallas area showed that carbon monoxide, hydrogen cyanide, hydrogen chloride, aldehydes (formaldehyde and acetaldehyde), and total hydrocarbons and free radicals of gases are released (Lowry, 1985a). In this study, carbon monoxide levels exceeded the short-term exposure limit (400 ppm) in an average of 28.5% of the fires. Hydrogen cyanide was present in only 12% of the fires, while hydrogen chloride was found in only 9%. Levels of hydrogen cyanide and hydrogen chloride posing immediate danger to life or health were not detected in the fires in the above study (Table 2). In another study, hydrogen cyanide was rarely documented as the primary toxic gas in fire victims (Hartzell et al., 1983). Frequently, it was detected at low levels in a study by Gold and co-workers, and was not significant in fire victims who died in Terrill's study (1978). However, there is a group of fire fatality victims and survivors in which significant cyanide blood levels (>25 μmol/L) have been measured (Symington et al., 1978; Clark, 1981) (Table 5). Also, lethal cyanide blood levels have been found in air-crash fatality victims (Mohler, 1975).

Table 4 Carbon Monoxide Levels in the Fire-Fighting Environment

Incident description	CO (ppm)	Comments
Foam rubber pillows burning in bathroom	150	Front part of apartment, light smoke
	1,600	Closed bathroom, dense black smoke
Greater alarm structure	200	1st Floor
	600	Mezzanine, light smoke
	2,000+	2nd Floor, fire area
2-Story dwelling fire on first floor living room	900	Immediately involved area, light smoke
	1,600	2nd Floor uninvolved but heavy smoke
	2,000+	1st Floor closet
2-Story dwelling fire on first floor and spread to second floor	300	1st Floor involved area
	800	2nd Floor uninvolved area
Dwelling area under house involved, rags soaked with flammable liquids	1,000	Inside house, no fire but heavy smoke
Dwelling service porch involved, carburetor cleaner fluid	1,800	Partially ventilated room
	3,000	Unventilated uninvolved bedroom

Source: Reproduced with permission from Barnard and Weber, 1979.

Table 5 Whole Blood Cyanide and Carboxyhemoglobin Concentrations in 53 House-Fire Survivors

	Cyanide (μmol/L)	Carboxyhemoglobin (%)
No smoke inhalation (n = 17)	5.0 (0.5-13)	3.8 (0.8-9.6)
Smokers (n = 11)	6.6 (2.2-13)	4.7 (2.9-9.6)
Nonsmokers (n = 6)	2.1 (0.5-3.9)	2.1 (0.8-3.2)
Smoke inhalation (n = 36)	25.8 (2.0-126)	14.5 (0.3-45)

Results are given as mean and range. The upper ranges of normal cyanide in smokers and nonsmokers are 20 μmol/L and 10 μmol/L, respectively. Those for carboxyhemoglobin are 10% and 5%, respectively.

Source: Reproduced with permission from Clark et al., 1981.

The toxic effects of thermodecomposition products of nitrocellulose roentgenographic film and plastics were recognized at the Clevelend Clinic Radiology Department fire in 1929 (Nichols, 1930) and at the Boston-Cocoanut Grove night club fire in 1942 (Mallory and Brickley, 1943). Toxic gases liberated with the combustion of nitrocellulose film include carbon monoxide, nitrogen dioxide, carbon dioxide, nitrous oxide, and hydrogen cyanide (Nichols, 1930). Since World War II, there has been a tremendous increase in the production and use of synthetic plastics and resins over natural materials. The toxic gases produced depend on the types of plastic polymers being pyrolyzed or burned (Zapp, 1962; MacFarland and Leong, 1962). Critical are the thermochemistry and kinetics of the particular plastic polymer. With the pyrolysis and combustion of polyurethane, for example, hydrogen cyanide will be produced (Mohler, 1975; Terrill et al., 1978; Levin et al., 1985b), while the combustion of polyvinyl chloride causes the release of hydrogen chloride (Dyer and Esch, 1976).

Hydrogen cyanide is produced during pyrolysis and combustion of nitrogen containing compounds such as flexible polyurethane foam used in upholstered furniture, seat cushions and bedding materials, wool, silk, and polyacrylonitrile fibers. Large-scale studies at the National Bureau of Standards using polyurethane foam slabs or padded chairs showed that larger quantities of hydrogen cyanide are generated when the slabs or chairs were in the flaming combustion mode after undergoing a smoldering mode (two-step thermal decomposition process), than if the same material was decomposed under strictly smoldering or flaming conditions alone (Levin, 1985b). Hydrogen cyanide is a colorless gas with a characteristic odor of bitter almonds and is probably not noted in fire situations. It is a histotoxic hypoxic poison which interferes with utilization of oxygen at the cellular level and inhibits cytochrome c oxidase in the mitochondria (Vogel et al., 1981; Hall and Rumack, 1986). As a result, anaerobic metabolism ensues and lactic acidosis develops. Also, hydrogen cyanide is a potent respiratory stimulant (Henderson and Haggard, 1943). It stimulates respiration in the initial phase of intoxication until the depressant effects on the central nervous system set in (Purser et al., 1984). Hydrogen cyanide acts rapidly. Symptoms can be noted in seconds followed by death within minutes of inhalation. The clinical manifestations depend on the blood cyanide levels (Stewart, 1974). A cyanide blood level of 0.5-1.0 mg/L is associated with a conscious but flushed patient with a rapid pulse. The patient who is tachypneic and stuporous and not responding to stimuli has a cyanide blood level of 1.0-2.5 mg/L. A blood cyanide level of 2.5 mg/L or more is considered severe poisoning. The patient is comatose and hypotensive with slow, gasping respirations and dilated pupils. The patient may present with a pink face and nailbeds in spite of inadequate respiration. In addition, the venous blood may be bright red in color as a result of poor oxygen utilization (Henderson and Haggard, 1943), and a severe metabolic lactic acidosis with an anion gap is present (Vogel et al., 1981). Because of cellular hypoxia, there is hyperpnea followed by dyspnea. Tachycardia is present initially followed by bradycardia, hypotension, apnea, coma, and death (Lee-Jones et al., 1970). Pulmonary edema has been observed (Graham et al., 1977).

The fire environment has the potential of releasing hydrogen cyanide depending on the products of pyrolysis and combustion (Levine and Radford, 1978). In combination with the carbon monoxide present in fires, the two gases can have an additive or synergistic adverse effect on cerebral metabolism (Pitt et al., 1979), producing a narcotized state in fire victims and rendering them incapable of escape from the scene of a fire, even when there is a sublethal concentration of hydrogen cyanide in the atmosphere. The incapacitating effects of hydrogen cyanide alone were confirmed in animal study in which monkeys were exposed to low levels of hydrogen cyanide gas due to pyrolysis products of polyacrylonitrile. The animals exhibited hyperventilation, followed by loss of consciousness after 1-5 min, a decrease in respirations, bradycardia, and a rapid recovery after exposure (Purser et al., 1984). Bradycardia, arrhythmias, and T-wave changes in the electrocardiogram have been shown in laboratory animals and in humans (Purser et al., 1984; Wexler et al., 1947). However, the association of myocardial pathology with hydrogen cyanide is much less than with carbon monoxide in laboratory animals (O'Flaherty and Thomas, 1982).

Although hydrogen cyanide may be present in fires associated with plastic polymers, the chemical diagnosis of cyanide poisoning is difficult, and there is no rapid method for determination of cyanide blood levels in most hospital clinical laboratories. Furthermore, hydrogen cyanide acts quickly at the cellular level, and the half life for cyanide is approximately 1 hr (Clark et al., 1981). Also, cyanide is metabolized in the body to a less toxic thiocyanate compound and excreted in the urine. Serum thiocyanate levels have been used as an indication of cyanide exposure (Levine and Radford, 1978), but because of the long half life of thiocyanate (4-8 days), a serum thiocyanate level evaluates previous cyanide exposure and may not reflect a particular acute cyanide exposure.

For a cyanide antidote to be effective, it must be given promptly to patients suspected of having cyanide poisoning. It has been suggested that patients with a high carboxyhemoglobin level also may have high cyanide levels, and accordingly these patients warrant empiric use of cyanide antidote therapy (Clark et al., 1981).

C. Hydrogen Chloride

Although carbon monoxide plays an important role in morbidity and mortality of fire victims, the increasing hazard and toxicity from the fumes and gases due to plastic fires on the lungs have been recognized (Cornish and Abar, 1969; Dyer and Esch, 1976; Alarie, 1985; Lowry et al. 1985a). Mortality has been observed in smoke inhalation fire victims without burns, in which there is severe chemical lung injury, but the carboxyhemoglobin level is within the sublethal range (Lowry et al., 1985b). Similar findings were observed in laboratory animals (Kishitani, 1971). This is the result of toxic gases and fumes such as hydrogen chloride, hydrogen cyanide, and other toxic gases. Thermal degradation of polyvinyl chloride, which is present in many plastic polymers, releases hydrogen chloride, a hydroscopic substance, which in combination with water vapor, hydrochloric acid forms an aerosol. Hydrochloric acid also has corrosive properties capable of causing significant irritation and a damaging effect on the mucous membranes of the eyes, nose, and respiratory tract. It should be noted that in the thermal degradation of polyvinyl chloride, neither chlorine gas or phosgene is produced (Sorenson, 1976). In a recent study of low-energy controlled fires of combined wood, paper, clothing, polyvinyl chloride, and other synthetic materials, free radicals (yet to be identified) were formed, and investigators suggested that these free radicals had the equivalent oxidative power of chlorine gas (Lowry et al., 1985b). The signs and symptoms of chlorine gas inhalation depend on the different levels of chlorine gas exposure (Table 6). Whether these free radicals produce similar signs and symptoms induced by chlorine gas remains to be elucidated.

In addition to the toxic gases and fumes from plastic polymers, intense heat is produced from the conflagration of plastic polymers, especially polyurethane. The heat energy release from combustion of cotton is 7122 BTU/lb, polyvinyl chloride 7720 BTU/lb, wood 8825 BTU/lb, polyurethane 16,000 BTU/lb, and

Table 6 Chlorine Exposure Thresholds and Limits

Cl_2 concentration, ppm	Effect of limit
0.03-3.5	Range of reported odor thresholds
1	Threshold limit value, OSHA time-weighted average (TWA); permissible level, 8-hr workday
1-3	Slight irritation; work possible without interruption
3	Permissible level for 15 min; 60-min emergency exposure limit (EEL)
3-6	Stinging or burning of eyes, nose, throat; lacrimation, sneezing, coughing
4	Suggested 30-min EEL
5	Severe irritation of eyes, nose, respiratory tract, intolerable after a few minutes; suggested 15-min EEL
7	Suggested 5-min EEL
14-21	Dangerous for 30 to 60 min, respiratory distress after 30 min
35-50	Lethal in 60 to 90 min
430	Lethal after 30 min
1000	Immediate incapacitation followed shortly by death

Source: Reproduced with permission from Lowry et al., 1985b.

polyethylene 20,050 BTU/lb (Sorenson, 1976). Iron, steel, and resistant structures are melted when exposed to tremendous heat generated as a result of combustion of plastic polymers, ultimately causing the structural collapse of homes and buildings.

D. Aldehydes

Several aldehydes including formaldehyde, acetaldehyde, and acrolein are among the noxious and irritant gases generated from pyrolysis and combustion in a fire. Aldehydes are irritants to the skin, the eyes, and the mucous membranes, and they cause denaturation of proteins and injury to the lung resulting in pulmonary edema and death. In an analysis of wood smoke and smoke from kerosene, greater amounts of carbon monoxide and aldehydes were present in wood smoke than in kerosene smoke (Zikria et al., 1972). Furthermore, Zikria et al. (1972) showed that animals exposed to wood smoke died with significant pathological findings in the lungs at autopsy. The kerosene smoke-exposed animals survived with less pulmonary injury.

Acrolein is present in cigarette smoke, photochemical smog, and fires involving polyethylene, polypropylene, and vinylon materials (Terrill et al., 1978). Because of the irritant effects of acrolein, the Occupational Safety and Health Administration (OSHA) sets the threshold limit value for an 8 hr exposure period at 0.1 ppm. The lungs of animals (rats) exposed for 62 days to an acrolein concentration of 4.0 ppm showed decreased flow-volume curves, a leftward shift of pressure volume curves, and an increase in lung volumes, suggesting airway obstruction of both small and large airways (Costa et al., 1986).

E. Additional Toxic Gases

Other toxic gases that can be produced in fires are nitrogen dioxide, oxides of nitrogen, metallic oxides, ammonia, isocyanates, sulfur dioxide, and organic compounds of hydrocarbon (Martin and Witschi, 1985; Lowry et al., 1985a; Holmberg and Lundberg, 1985; Kizer, 1984; Mullin et al., 1983; Henderson et al., 1979; Terrill et al., 1978).

III. Thermal Injury

Toxic gases are the leading causes of morbidity and mortality from fires. Flame, heat, or thermal factors are the other basic lethal factors in fires. When fire victims are in close proximity to the source of the fire, death can result from direct consumption of the victims by the flames. Flash fires can result in death because of the incineration of the victims without an elevation of the carboxyhemoglobin level (Hirsch et al., 1977). When fire victims survive the flame and heat insults, there are burns to the body surface and thermal injury to the upper airways and respiratory tract (Shirani et al., 1987; Colice et al., 1986; Demling, 1985; Panke and McLeod, 1985; Rapaport et al., 1982; Whitener et al., 1980; Head, 1980; Trunkey, 1978; Hunt et al., 1975; Wanner and Cutchavaree, 1973; DiVincenti et al., 1971; Beal et al., 1968). Specialized burn units have been established in the United States for the treatment of significant burns with and without inhalational lung injury, and survival from massive burn injury has been improved in recent years (Demling, 1983; Halebian et al., 1986; Pruitt, 1987).

Evaluation of thermal inhalation injury in dogs has shown that inhalation of hot air (350°C and 500°C) caused a thermal tracheitis of the upper trachea without injury to the lower trachea (Moritz et al., 1945). However, when the dogs inhaled flame from a blast burner, severe inflammation with mucosal edema, ulceration, and necrosis was observed in the upper and lower trachea. Furthermore, this study showed that inhalation of steam caused thermal injury in the dog extending from the trachea to the lung parenchyma (Moritz et al., 1945). Three fire victims were hospitalized with burns involving the face and other areas at the Cocoanut Grove night club fire in Boston in 1942. At autopsy in two of the three victims, the larynx was completely occluded by black charred material extending into the trachea (Mallory and Brickley, 1943). Also, diffuse bronchostenosis was noted in one patient, and in all patients there was a diffuse hemorrhagic and necrotizing membranous inflammatory process in the lower trachea and airways.

In an earlier study of 2297 burn patients at the Brooke Army Medical Center in Fort Sam Houston, San Antonio, thermal inhalation injury was present in 66 patients (2.9%) (DiVincenti et al., 1971). Characteristics of these thermal inhalation patients included: (1) burns occurring in a closed environment, (2) burns on the face and oropharyngeal area, (3) hoarseness, (4) wheezing, (5) shortness of breath, and (6) production of carbonaceous sputum. Thirty-two of the 66 patients (48.5%) received burns to more than 50% of the total body surface, 95% of the 66 had facial burns, 55% had upper airway edema in the oropharynx, and hemoptysis was noted in 6%. Forty-eight patients (72%) had tracheostomy, and 34 of 38 patients (90%) had laryngotracheobronchitis at autopsy. Overall mortality in the above study was 58%.

One of the physiological consequences of thermal inhalation injury is upper airway obstruction due to laryngeal edema and/or laryngospasm (Whitener et al., 1980; Crapo, 1981; Haponik et al., 1987). In patients with facial and pharyngeal burns, the presence of carbonaceous sputum and hoarseness in addition to surface burns should raise suspicion of upper airway obstruction. It has been demonstrated that patients with smoke inhalation, but without burns or other surface burns, can have acute laryngitis without edema. Most patients who have laryngeal edema have surface burns and are both tachypneic and hoarse (Wanner and Cutchavaree, 1973). Furthermore, laryngeal edema can occur in patients without surface burns due to inhalation of irritant gases. In a recent study, patients who had progressive upper airway edema had an average body surface area burn of 28% in contrast to those with stable airways who had a cutaneous surface burn area of only 8.0%. Also, 93% of patients with progressive upper airway edema had facial and or neck burns, while only 59% of patients with stable upper airways had these findings (Haponik et al., 1987). Moreover, when the follow-up serial studies of flow-volume curves showed a significant decrease in inspiratory and expiratory flow rates, the patients required endotracheal intubation for management of upper airway obstruction. Although upper airway obstruction may not be present initially, when the patient is first seen in the emergency room following smoke inhalation or thermal inhalation injury, it usually occurs within the first 24-48 hr. Therefore, clinical assessment with nasopharyngoscopy and flow-volume curve studies are important diagnostic tools in these patients. Severe tracheal and bronchial stenosis can occur as a late finding in patients with cutaneous burns and thermal inhalation injury (Colice et al., 1986; Beal, 1968; Mallory and Brinkley, 1943). Endobronchial polyposis may occur in patients several months after acute thermal inhalation injury and smoke inhalation, and the polyps can resolve spontaneously without specific treatment (Williams et al., 1983; Adams et al., 1979). Bronchiectasis may result as a complication of severe inhalation injury (Panke and McLeod, 1985).

With the same degree of smoke inhalation, the respiratory tract damage is more severe in burned than in nonburned patients. In dog experiments described by Zikria et al. (1968), there are three major phases of respiratory tract injury induced by steam burns. In the first phase (within the first hour), there is coagulation necrosis and an early reactive stage with edema in the tracheobronchial tree and early pulmonary parenchymal edema. In the next phase (up to 24 hours), there is a second reactive stage with development of interstitial and perivascular edema, further sloughing of mucosa, atelectasis, and hemorrhagic consolidation. Finally, in the third phase (more than 24 hours), known as the infection stage, bronchopneumonia develops behind respiratory tract obstruction secondary to a mechanical or a functional block. Necrotizing tracheobronchitis also occurs in this third phase. In the same report by Zikria et al. (1968), similar findings were found in 27 respiratory tract burn victims, all of whom died. The trachea in these individuals showed sloughed mucosa and ulcers, and there was severe pulmonary infection.

In burn patients, wound sepsis used to be the major cause of death. But with the advent of procedures for wound debridement and application of topical and intravenous antibiotics, wound sepsis has been controlled. Instead, respiratory complications of inhalation injury and pulmonary sepsis have replaced burn wound sepsis as the major cause of death in patients with thermal injury. Between 1981 and 1984, at the Shriners' Burn Institute in Galveston, Texas, inhalation injury was noted in 88 of 1018 patients (8.6%) with cutaneous burns. The mortality of patients with inhalation injury (documented by bronchoscopic findings of airway edema and inflammation, mucosal necrosis, and the presence of soot and charring in the airway) was 56% in contrast to a mortality rate of 4.1% in patients without inhalation injury (Thompson et al., 1986). In another 1058 burn patients at the U.S. Army Institute of Surgical Research in Fort Sam Houston, San Antonio, 373 burn patients had inhalation injury (diagnosed by bronchoscopy and/or ventilation perfusion lung scan) and 141 (38%) subsequently developed pneumonia, while only 60 of 685 burn patients (8.8%) without inhalation injury developed pneumonia (Shirani et al., 1987). Major pulmonary complications of burned patients include not only pneumonia but also laryngitis, tracheobronchitis, atelectasis, pulmonary edema and bronchiectasis (Phillips et al., 1963; DiVincenti et al., 1971). Opportunistic infections are the most frequent cause of morbidity and mortality in severely burned patients (Pruitt and McManus, 1984;

Spebar and Pruitt, 1981). Other complications of burned patients include acute renal failure (Planas et al., 1982), acute gastrointestinal disease (Czaja et al., 1974; McAlhany et al., 1976), and alteration in the immune system (Neilan et al., 1977; Demling, 1985). Thus, the clinical course (morbidity and mortality of patients who sustain smoke inhalation as well as thermal burn injury is significantly worse than patients with only smoke inhalation (Chu, 1981; Whitener et al., 1980; Pierson, 1976).

IV. Oxygen Deficiency in the Fire Environment

In a fire environment, pyrolysis and combustion of material, consumed oxygen and produced both carbon monoxide and carbon dioxide. Levels of oxygen and carbon dioxide in the ambient air of a fire depend on the supply of air and ventilation. In a confined-space wood fire, an inspired oxygen concentration as low as 17.5% has been detected (Sidor et al., 1973). The oxygen and carbon dioxide concentrations in a fire atmosphere monitored by a personal sampling apparatus did not exceed the lowest detectable limit of 0.26% while oxygen levels below 20% were not measured in any fire. Arterial hypoxemia can be aggravated by a low inspired oxygen concentration in the fire situation which can decrease from an oxygen concentration of 21 percent to 10-15 percent (Crapo, 1981). When the ambient air oxygen concentration decreases from 21% to about 17%, there is an impairment of motor coordination; when the inspired oxygen concentration is only 10% to 14%, the individual is conscious but has faulty judgment and fatigues easily; and when the oxygen concentration is in the range of 6-10%, the person is unconscious and death ensues (Hartzell et al., 1983; Kimmerle, 1974).

V. Pathophysiological Consequences of Acute Smoke Inhalation

There are several pulmonary pathophysiological consequences of acute smoke inhalation and its accompanying toxic gases, fumes, and particulate matter. In the absence of thermal injury, these consequences include: (1) impairment of the mucociliary function, (2) mucous hypersecretion and an inflammatory response in the tracheobronchial tree, tracheobronchitis and bronchiolitis, (3) alteration in biochemical factors in the lung, (4) cellular and immunological changes which may cause an increase in vascular permeability leading to pulmonary edema and alveolar hemorrhage, and (5) bronchoconstriction (Dressler, 1976; Said, 1978; Widdicombe, 1982; Fick et al., 1984; Loke et al., 1984; Sturgess, 1985; Rooney, 1985). The mucociliary blanket, a physical-chemical barrier to noxious substances (Frost et al., 1973), can transport particulate matter from the lungs by ciliary transport or expel mucus by reflexes such as coughing (Widdicombe, 1982). In animal studies, acute inhalation of wood smoke causes disruption of the mucociliary blanket of the tracheobronchial tree (Loke et al., 1984). To remove particulate matter from the conducting airways, mucociliary clearance and cough are required in the presence of intact ciliated epithelium and a mucous covering (Richardson, 1982). Acute irritation of the airways leads to an increase in secretion of airway mucus and impairs mucociliary transport.

The above findings may in part explain the clinical picture of tracheobronchitis seen in patients with smoke inhalation (Beal et al., 1968). As is discussed separately in this volume by Young and Reynolds, bronchoalveolar lavage (BAL) has been used to evaluate the cellular, immunological, and biochemical functions of the lungs in response to injury (Hunninghake et al., 1979). In inhalational lung injury a spectrum of inflammatory responses with mobilization of inflammatory cells has been demonstrated using BAL techniques. The pulmonary alveolar macrophage acts as the primary defense cell of the lung (Hocking and Golde, 1979), and this is the predominant cell lavaged from the lungs of acute smoke inhalation victims (Demarest et al., 1979) and laboratory animals (Fick et al., 1984; Loke et al., 1981). In patients with acute smoke inhalation studied by Demarest et al. (1979), the cellular yield of alveolar macrophages was 51.2 million versus 15.7 million in nonsmoking controls. Similar results have been reported in laboratory animals. However, the timing of the lavage procedure in relation to the acute inhalational insult may cause a variance in the BAL cellular yield. For instance, the overall cellular yield obtained by BAL decreased after 24 hours, contrasted with the yield immediately after smoke inhalation (Loke et al., 1984).

Alteration in alveolar macrophage chemotactic function also has been demonstrated (Demarest et al., 1979). In laboratory animals, alveolar macrophage chemotactic function may actually be *increased* after minimal inhalation of pyrolysis products of Douglas fir wood. However, with higher levels of inhalational exposure (reflected by a carboxyhemoglobin level of about 20 percent), there is impairment in alveolar macrophage chemotactic function (Loke et al., 1981a). In addition, after exposure to wood smoke, alveolar macrophage show surface characteristics change and these cells are smaller by scanning electron microscopy. Moreover, these cells show altered cytoplasmic morphology, display decreased surface adherence, and exhibit diminished phagocytic and bactericidal function (Loke et al., 1984; Fick et al., 1984). These alterations in pulmonary alveolar macrophage structure and function decrease lung defense barriers, and may explain in part the increased susceptibility of patients with smoke inhalation to pulmonary infection.

The biochemical changes in the lung after inhalation injury can be assessed by measuring lactate dehydrogenase, acid phosphatase, alkaline phosphatase, sialic acid, soluble protein, and surfactant in bronchoalveolar lavage supernatant fluid (Henderson et al., 1981; Beck et al., 1983; Finley and Ladman, 1972; Nieman et al., 1980; Blank et al., 1978; Rooney, 1985). Not only are the changes in BAL lactate dehydrogenase useful in assessing lung injury from different toxic agents, but they may be used in identifying sites of upper and lower airway injury as well (Beck et al., 1983). Type II alveolar cells, the site of surfactant synthesis and metabolism, proliferate in different toxic inhalational lung injury (Witschi, 1976). In cigarette smokers a low yield of pulmonary surfactant has been reported in BAL fluid (Finley and Ladman, 1972), while increased phospholipid concentrations have been noted in the lungs after nitrogen dioxide exposure (Blank et al., 1978). This latter finding is due to increased biosynthesis of phospholipids by an augmented number of type II alveolar cells and a decrease in removal of surfactant lipids. Moreover, in dogs exposed to wood and kerosene smoke in a chamber with an inspired oxygen concentration of 17% and a carbon monoxide concentration of 17,000 ppm, there was a significant decrease in surfactant function as demonstrated by an increase in surface tension forces from 7 to 22 dyn/cm using the modified Wilhelmy technique (Nieman et al., 1980). Alterations in lung phospholipid concentrations may have induced these changes; however, these concentrations were not measured. A qualitative loss in function of the pulmonary surfactant may also have been important. In our laboratory, no change in lung surfactant phospholipid content has been noted after wood smoke inhalation by rabbits (Loke et al., 1981a). However, lung phospholipid levels may depend upon the severity of inhalational lung injury.

In inhalation pulmonary injury, there may be an increase in neutrophils in the lungs, as well as development of a vascular permeability type pulmonary edema and the adult respiratory distress syndrome. There may also be release of multiple mediators of inflammation, activation of the complement system, and changes in immunoglobulins (Horovitz, 1981).

Bronchoconstriction may occur from inhalation of irritant, toxic gases or fumes and particulate matter, or there may or be vagus-mediated reflex bronchoconstriction (Pierson, 1976). Thermal, chemical, or mechanical factors that cause irritation of the nasal mucosa can produce other reflex responses in the form of hypersecretion of mucus in the trachea, inhibition of spinal reflexes, and alterations in bronchomotor tone. Also, there may be a reflex closure of the larynx in an attempt to prevent chemical or mechanical stimulants from entering the tracheobronchial tree (Widdicombe, 1982). The above changes together with the inhalation of carbon monoxide and other toxic gases cause arterial hypoxemia and bronchospasm (Webster et al., 1967; Landa et al., 1972; Winter and Miller, 1976; Genovesi et al., 1977; Loke and Matthay, 1981; Crapo, 1981). The major causes of arterial hypoxemia are carbon monoxide poisoning and ventilation-perfusion inequalities, and other factors such as cyanide poisoning or a low inspired oxygen concentration in the fire environment. Pulmonary function studies have shown evidence of both upper and lower airway obstruction after acute inhalation (Wanner and Cutchavaree, 1973; Loke et al., 1980; Whitener et al., 1980; Sheppard et al., 1986; Haponik et al., 1987). In the acute phase of lung injury from smoke inhalation, large airway obstruction predominates (Landa et al., 1972), and subsequently there may be large and/or small airway dysfunction depending on the severity of the inhalational injury and the toxic gases inhaled (Kirkpatrick and Bass, 1979; Murphy et al., Fleming et al., 1979).

VI. Pulmonary Pathology Following Smoke Inhalation

Autopsy findings in fire victims with reference to pulmonary lesions have been discussed in part in the section on thermal lung injury. Classic lung lesions in fire fatalities and war gas poisonings have been described by Mallory and Brickley (1943) and Winternitz (1920). The severity of pulmonary lesions at autopsy depends upon the degree of acute smoke inhalation, with and without burns. Gross examination of the trachea may reveal severe edema of mucous membranes which exhibit a fibropurulent exudate, carbonaceous material, and petechial hemorrhages. Microscopically, the epithelium of the trachea may be desquamated with an edematous mucosa and foci of hemorrhage, with or without leukocytic infiltration. A fibrinous hyaline membrane also may be present. The lumen of a bronchus may be plugged by desquamated cells, fibrin and leukocytes, and the alveoli may show focal areas of collapse, bronchopneumonia or hemorrhagic membranous bronchitis (Mallory and Brinkley, 1943). Severe pulmonary edema with superimposed pneumonia, hyaline membrane formation, multiple recent pulmonary thromboses, and ulcerative tracheobronchitis has been described in victims of fatal chlorine poisoning (Adelson and Kaufman, 1971). In patients that survive the acute inhalation insult, bronchiolitis obliterans may be demonstrated on lung biopsy (Gosink et al., 1973; Arora and Aldrich, 1980; Epler et al., 1985; Panke and McLeod, 1985).

In rabbits exposed to smoke from pyrolysis of Douglas fir wood or soft polyurethane foam, the histopathology of the trachea reveals a broad spectrum of injury ranging from coagulation necrosis of the entire epithelium with areas of pseudomembrane formation to intact epithelium with infiltration of polymorphonuclear cells (Loke et al., 1981a). In addition, acute bronchitis and atelectasis of the lungs have been described. The tracheal injury in some animals displayed marked epithelial sloughing and leukocyte infiltration, and a diffuse pattern of injury involving the entire trachea (Niederman et al., 1981). In vitro cultured tracheal epithelium from these animals with epithelial sloughing (but intact basal cells) showed regeneration. By 48 hours, basal cells were noted to form a covering over the epithelial surface and by 7 days there was a thin multicell covering of the epithelium. These same investigators exposed animals to the smoke from burning soft polyurethane. The animals died and severe tracheal injury was noted at autopsy. No in vitro tracheal regeneration was observed at 72 hours, suggesting the possibility of irreversible tracheal injury in these animals. In laboratory animals (rats) that died following acute smoke inhalation to white pine smoke, increased endothelial and alveolar membrane permeability and edema of the lung have been demonstrated (Dressler et al., 1976).

VII. Chronic Effects of Fire Fighting on Pulmonary Function

Firefighters are exposed on a chronic basis to different kinds of irritants and toxic gases, organic vapors, metal fumes, and particulates whether generated at building or residential fires or at the scene of industrial toxic gas accidents. Therefore, fire fighting is a hazardous and dangerous occupation (Evanoff and Rosenstock, 1986; Barnard and Duncan, 1975; Dyer and Esch, 1976; Peters et al., 1974; Abrams, 1984). Firefighters inhale toxic substances that can affect not only the pulmonary system but other systems as well. There are conflicting data in the literature with regard to whether firefighters have an increased morbidity and mortality from cardiovascular, pulmonary, or neoplastic disease, or from accidental causes (Mastromatteo, 1959a,b; Sidor and Peters, 1974; Barnard et al., 1975; Peters et al., 1974; Musk et al., 1977a,b, 1978, 1982; Loke et al., 1980; Sparrow et al., 1982; Unger et al., 1980; Young et al., 1980; Vena and Fiedler, 1987; Feuer and Rosenman, 1986; Lefcoe and Wonnacott, 1974; Niederman et al., 1983). We shall discuss only the chronic effects of firefighting on pulmonary function.

In a pulmonary function study of 1768 Boston firefighters performed in 1970-1971, a reduced forced expiratory volume in one-second (FEV_1) and forced vital capacity (FVC) were noted in cigarette smokers compared to non-smokers (Sidors and Peters, 1974). Cigarette smoking itself was important in the abnormal pulmonary function. The pulmonary function tests were repeated a year later on 1430 of the 1768 (81%) Boston firefighters that were surveyed in 1970-1971. This study showed that the annual rate of decline in FEV_1 and FVC was more than twice the expected rate (68 vs. 25 ml for FEV_1 and 77 vs. 30 ml for FVC). Also, the 64 firefighters who were hospitalized for smoke inhalation had a greater annual decline in FEV_1 and FVC than the fire fighters who were not hospitalized (Peters et al., 1974). However, in a three year follow-up study of 1146 active firefighters from the initial cohort of 1768 firefighters, no accelerated annual decline of FEV_1 or FVC was noted (Musk et al., 1977a).

Severely impaired pulmonary function was not demonstrated in a study of retired Boston fire fighters tested between 1970 to 1975. The FEV_1 was 3.19 liters (97% of predicted) in 1970, and 2.98 liters (95% of predicted) in 1975, while the FVC was 4.04 liters (97% of predicted) in 1970, and 4.01 liters (99% of predicted) in 1975 (Musk et al., 1977b). Finally, in a 6-year follow-up of 951 Boston firefighters there was no accelerated annual loss of FEV_1 or FVC. The increased use of a protective respiratory device or a self-contained air-breathing apparatus, may have protected these firefighters from exposure to the toxic fire environment (Musk et al., 1982), and selection factors may have played a role in the results (Sidor and Peters, 1974). The mean FEV_1, FVC. and FEV_1/FVC were all within normal limits in the study by Musk et al. (1982).

Normal pulmonary function tests including FEV_1, FVC, airway resistance, thoracic gas volume, and single-breath diffusing capacity were observed in 21 firefighters (with an average of 16 years of fire fighting) studied one month after exposure to dense smoke from combustion products of polyvinyl chloride (Tashkin et al., 1977). A study by our group of 51 firefighters in West Haven, Connecticut, showed a normal mean FEV_1 and FVC in addition to normal results of tests for small airway function, such as the maximum expiratory flow at 50% of FVC on air ($\dot{V}max_{50}$) and $\Delta\dot{V}max_{50}$—the percentage flow-rate response to breathing helium compared to air at 50% of FVC utilizing the maximum expiratory flow-volume curve (Loke et al., 1980). In a subsequent study of 49 firefighters in New Haven, normal lung function tests (FEV_1, FVC, and $\dot{V}max_{50}$) were again demonstrated (Abrams, 1984).

Twenty firefighters were studied with pulmonary function tests immediately after a fire and 18 months later in Houston, Texas, and there was a decrease in mean FEV_1 and FVC of 122 ml and 62 ml, respectively (Unger et al., 1980). In a group of 193 firefighters from Australia, there were no abnormalities in FEV_1, FVC, maximum midexpiratory flow rate, single breath diffusing capacity, or closing volume (Young et al., 1980). As part of the Normative Aging Study in Boston, 168 firefighters were evaluated every five years with pulmonary function tests. This study showed that during an initial period between 1963 and 1968 and a subsequent evaluation between 1968 and 1973, firefighters had a greater decline in FEV_1 and FVC of 12 ml/year and 18 ml/year, respectively, compared to non-firefighters, even after adjusting for smoking status (Sparrow et al., 1982). Excellent lung function was shown in 1006 firefighters studied in London using a Vitalograph spirometer to measure FEV_1 and FVC in 1976. In a subsequent evaluation of these firefighters a year later, the annual decline in FEV_1 and FVC was 92 ml and 107 ml, respectively, and the investigators suggested that this unexpected loss of lung function was related to instrumental variation and technique in performing the pulmonary function tests (Douglas et al., 1985).

Overall, the majority of the studies on the *chronic* effects of firefighting on pulmonary function have not shown a deleterious effect on FEV_1, FVC and maximum expiratory midflow rates (Table 7). However, there are case reports of

Table 7 Multiple Studies of the Chronic Effects of Firefighting on Lung Function

Pulmonary function abnormalities	No. of firefighters studied	Place of study	Authors
1. Lower FEV_1 and FVC compared to nonsmokers (not statistically significant)	1768	Boston, MA (1970-1971)	Sidor and Peters (1974)
2. Annual loss of FEV_1 and FVC more than twice the expected rate	1430	Boston, MA (1970-1972)	Peters et al. (1974)
3. No accelerated annual decline in FEV_1 or FVC over three years	1146	Boston, MA 1974	Musk et al. 1977
4. No accelerated annual decline in FEV_1 or FVC during a 6-year follow-up	951	Boston, MA 1976	Musk et al. 1982
5. Normal FEV_1, FVC, airway resistance, thoracic gas volume, and single-breath diffusing capacity	21	Los Angeles, CA 1974	Tashkin et al. 1977
6. Normal FEV_1, FVC, and small airway function ($\dot{V}max_{50}$ and $\Delta\dot{V}max_{50}$)	51	West Haven, CT 1975-1976	Loke et al. 1980

7. Normal FEV_1, FVC, and $\dot{V}max_{50}$	New Haven, CT 1982-1983	49	Abrams 1984
8. A decline in FEV_1 (122 ml) and FVC (62 ml) 18 months following smoke inhalation	Houston, TX 1978	20	Unger er al. 1980
9. Normal FEV_1, FVC, maximum midexpiratory flow rate, and single breath diffusing capacity	New South Wales, Australia	193	Young et al. 1980
10. A greater decline in FEV_1 (12 ml/yr) and FVC (18 ml/yr) than nonfirefighters after adjustment for smoking status	Boston, MA 1963-1973	168	Sparrow et al. 1982
11. Normal FEV_1 and FVC in 1976 but an annual decline in FEV_1 (92 ml) and FVC (107 ml) in 1977 which may be due to instrumental variation and technique	London, England 1976-1977	1006	Douglas et al. 1985

Abbreviations: FEV_1, forced expiratory volume in one-second; FVC, forced vital capacity; $\dot{V}max_{50}$, maximal midexpiratory flow rate at 50% of forced vital capacity, $\Delta\dot{V}max_{50}$, see text.

firefighters and fire victims who have severe obstructive airway disease several months and years after *acute* smoke inhalation (Loke et al., 1980; Kirkpatrick and Bass, 1979). Thus, even though in most chronic studies firefighters have normal lung function, there may be a selection factor involved whereby only the fit and healthy can fight fires, and those who develop respiratory problems may be unavailable for testing.

Constant exposure to irritant and toxic products of combustion may lead to an increase in airway hyperreactivity as seen in patients with occupational asthma (Chan-Yeung and Lam, 1986). Furthermore, airway hyperreactivity may serve as an early marker for those at risk to develop chronic obstructive airway disease. The methacholine inhalation challenge test (Wiedemann et al., 1986; Yeung and Lam, 1986) has been used by us on firefighters at their New Haven fire station to evaluate airway reactivity. No firefighter was accepted into our study if he had less than three years of firefighting experience or had been exposed to a fire within the past 24 hours. A methacholine responder was defined as a subject with a $PD_{20}FEV_1$ of 10 mg/ml or less (i.e., a 20% or greater decrease in FEV_1 with inhaled methacholine dose of 10 mg/ml or less (Abrams, 1984). In this study, 11 of 37 firefighters who had the bronchoprovocation test with methacholine were responders and showed a wide range of airway responsiveness (Fig. 1). Thus, in this group of firefighters with normal lung function, there was evidence of an increase in nonspecific airway responsiveness at the higher doses of methacholine concentration in some fire fighters. Asthmatics have a low PD_{20} FEV_1. (Niederman et al., 1983). Sheppard et al. (1986) demonstrated an acute increase in methacholine responsiveness in two firefighters after fire exposure. This increase in airway responsiveness returned to baseline values after 3 to 5 weeks, suggesting that acute fire exposure may lead to airway injury sufficient to cause a transient increase in airway responsiveness.

Although firefighters are not at an increased risk for developing chronic obstructive airway disease or severe impairment in lung function, they do have an increased incidence of cardiovascular disease and on-duty physical injuries. Physical fitness programs should be implemented for firefighters to decrease the morbidity and mortality of cardiovascular disease and on-duty physical injuries (Barnard and Anthony, 1980). In addition, we believe it should be mandatory for firefighters to wear a protective respiratory device (self-contained air breathing apparatus) during firefighting.

VIII.   Toxicity of Pyrolysis and Combustion Products: Evaluation in Laboratory Animals

A.   Use of Laboratory Animals to Study Injury from Pyrolysis and Combustion Products

Laboratory animals have been used to evaluate the pathophysiology of the three main combustion products of fire: smoke, heat, and toxic gases (Moritz et al., 1945; Zikria et al., 1972; Kimmerle, 1974; Zawacki et al., 1977; Walker et al.,

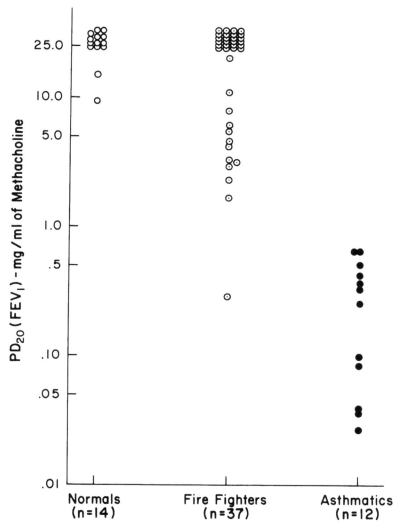

Figure 1 Airway responsiveness to methacholine in normals, asthmatics and firefighters. Asthmatics have a low PD_{20} (FEV_1), and fire fighters with normal lung function have a wide range of airway reactivity to methacholine inhalation but at higher doses of methacholine concentration.

1981; Herndon et al., 1984). Specifically, animals have been utilized to assess the toxic and lethal effects of both war gas poisoning (Winternitz, 1920) and the pyrolysis and combustion of new products, such as plastic polymers or flame-retardant materials (Kimmerle, 1974; Dressler et al., 1975; Petajan et al., 1975; Levin et al., 1983b; Purser et al., 1984). They have also been used to determine the potential carcinogenicity and mutagenicity of various chemicals and gases (Upton, 1986; Holmberg and Lundberg, 1985).

Several physiological tests or biological responses elicited from the laboratory animals have been used to evaluate the toxicity of products of combustion or pyrolysis. Among these are sensory and pulmonary irritation, and incapacitation studies (Alarie and Anderson, 1979; Dilley et al., 1979; Hartzell et al., 1983; Levin et al., 1983a; Purser and Berrill, 1983; Ferguson et al., 1986). Behavioral assessment, such as observation of the animals as to time of: (1) loss of equilibrium, (2) development of convulsions, (3) collapse and (4) death, has also been applied (Hilado, 1978). Toxicological end-point studies of acute mortality include: (1) the LD_{50}, the lethal dose that will cause death in 50% of the laboratory animals tested in a defined period; (2) the LC_{50}, the lethal concentration that will cause death in 50% of the animals tested in a defined period; and (3) the LT_{50}, the lethal time that will cause death in 50% of the animals tested under certain conditions (Kimmerle, 1974; Alarie and Anderson, 1979; Hilado, 1981; Klimisch et al., 1980) LC_{50} has been used as the biological end point in most studies and is used at the National Bureau of Standards for toxicological evaluations (Levin et al., 1983a,b).

Conditioned avoidance response (Dilley et al., 1979) and hind-leg flexion avoidance response (Hartzell et al., 1983) are techniques used for animal incapacitation studies. The EC_{50} is the concentration of smoke or other gas that effects a 50% hind-leg flexion avoidance response within a defined test time frame, while the ET_{50} is the time required to effect a 50% hind leg flexion avoidance response for a particular concentration of gas (Hartzell et al., 1983). Histopathology and bronchoalveolar lavage studies of the respiratory system, and biological assays of blood of the laboratory animals are other important studies use for evaluation of the toxic environment (Herndon et al., 1984; Fick et al., 1984; Henderson et al., 1981; Loke et al., 1981). The above studies can be used in either acute or chronic exposure experiments.

Various physiological and pulmonary responses have been used to correlate these data from laboratory animals with those of human victims at the industrial plant methyl isocyanate accident in Bhopal, India. In Chapter 3, Alarie and Schaper correlate the obstructive ventilatory pattern in animals with the obstructive airway disease noted among surviving victims in Bhopal. Thus, besides establishing that methyl isocyanate is a potent sensory and pulmonary irritant, these animal studies are valuable in extrapolating "safe" amounts of exposure for humans (Ferguson et al., 1986).

It may be difficult to correlate laboratory animal findings with those of humans in a fire situation by measuring only acute mortality as a toxicological end point (Birky, 1976). Accordingly, pulmonary physiological responses and histopathology and bioassay studies should be done as well. Finally, species differences of the laboratory animals in pulmonary responses have to be considered.

B. Animal Exposure Chambers

Various animal exposure chambers have been constructed for evaluating the toxicological effects of the products of combustion (Dressler et al., 1975; Alarie and Anderson, 1979; Klimisch, 1980; Loke et al., 1981; Hilado, 1978; Drew, 1985). An analysis of the pyrolysis or combustion conditions, as well as the animal exposure conditions, must be considered in toxicological evaluation studies. Interlaboratory comparison of toxicological inhalation experiments may be difficult with different exposure chambers. Certain guidelines have been published by the Fire Toxicology Committee of National Academy of Sciences for building smoke exposure chambers (Fire Toxicology, 1977). Criteria include: (1) there should be a single smoke exposure chamber, with the animal exposure area and the furnace both housed in this single chamber; (2) test animals in the exposure chamber should be shielded from heat and hot gases; (3) the temperature in the exposure chamber should be controllable; (4) there should be adequate mixing of gaseous products in the chamber; (5) the chamber should be free from air leaks; (6) there should be a pressure relief safety valve so the exposure chamber can be ventilated in the event of a pressure build-up; (7) the exposure chamber should be easy to clean; (8) the furnace should generate a uniform temperature but have the capability of generating a wide range of temperatures to sustain either pyrolysis or combustion by varying access of air to the furnace area; (9) the test material should be weighed before and after burning; (10) the oxygen concentration in the exposure chamber should not decrease below 16%; and (11) the temperature should not exceed 35°C in the animal exposure area. The National Bureau of Standards developed a small-scale exposure chamber in 1980 for assessing toxicity of combustion products, and among seven laboratories evaluating this chamber there were reproducible results (Levin et al., 1983a). In this chamber, the autoignition temperature of the test material can be determined and the furnace can control the temperature enabling either a flaming or a nonflaming mode of the material to develop. The temperature in the animal exposure area has not exceeded 35°C during a 30 minute exposure period, and chemical measurements of carbon monoxide, carbon dioxide and oxygen in the exposure chamber area have been monitored during experiments.

Biological assays of the blood carboxyhemoglobin levels of experimental animals have also been done. The furnace for this exposure chamber is critical for the characterization of toxic gases from combustion products. It has been indicated that the most toxic conditions may be generated at temperatures which approximate the autoignition point of the test material. The autoignition temperature is defined as the lowest furnace temperature which ignites the test material spontaneously within 30 minutes. In the nonflaming mode, as the temperature increases and reaches the autoignition temperature, more of the material is decomposed and more toxic products are generated. In contrast, in the flaming mode there is more complete combustion with the production of two end products, carbon dioxide and water (Levin et al., 1985a). It is essential that a progressive, incremental rise in temperature occurs in the nonflaming mode when evaluating the toxicity or LC_{50} of products of combustion. Finally, it should be noted that screening tests with the specially designed exposure chamber evaluate only a segment of the complex combustion conditions in a real fire environment, and may not be applicable in human fire victims. More research is required of the full scale fire situation (Lowry et al., 1985) rather than excessive fine tuning of bench scale tests (Levin et al., 1985a).

IX. Diagnosis of Acute Smoke Inhalation

A. Clinical Evaluation

Fire victims with acute smoke inhalation may arrive at the emergency room with only a nonproductive cough, eye irritation, and mild shortness of breath, or they may be cyanotic, comatose, and hypotensive requiring immediate intubation and mechanical ventilation. Burns may be evident on the face and other parts of the body, and the patient's clothing may smell of smoke. Facial burns and thermal inhalation injury may be seen in patients with a sore throat, hoarseness, and stridor. Headache, dizziness, cough with carbonaceous sputum production, dyspnea, and chest pain may be present. The mental status of the victims should be assessed since arterial hypoxemia, severe carbon monoxide intoxication, drug abuse or alcohol intoxication all can alter the level of consciousness. A description of the fire environment may be helpful with special reference to the kinds of materials (e.g., plastics, polyurethane foam, etc.) that were burned. Fire victims are exposed to an extremely hot and heated environment in a fire, or to cold temperatures if the victim is rescued and left in a cold icy environment. Upon physical examination, the patient may be conscious but in respiratory distress with an increased respiratory rate. There may be soot in the oral pharynx besides edema of the supraglottic and laryngeal areas in fire victims with thermal inhalation injury. Stridor in the neck region and wheezes in the lungs may be present.

Fiberoptic bronchoscopy has been used to evaluate the upper and lower airways in acute inhalation injury patients with severe burns. At bronchoscopy there are extramucosal and mucosal abnormalities of the upper and lower respiratory tract. Carbonaceous material and secretions may be seen, while mucosal changes consist of edema, blister formation, hemorrhage, ulceration, and ischemia of the supraglottic and glottic areas. There may be significant swelling of the epiglottic and aryepiglottic folds and the ventricular folds (Hunt et al., 1975). As pointed out by Shirani et al. (Chap. 7), in certain patients rigid bronchoscopy may be required to remove large pieces of sloughed bronchial mucosa. (Beal et al., 1968). Indirect laryngoscopy may be used to evaluate the upper airways in some patients. Pulmonary function tests utilizing maximal expiratory flow-volume curve studies may reveal upper and lower airway obstruction (Landa et al., 1972; Wanner and Cutchavaree, 1973).

The chest roentgenogram is an insensitive indicator of inhalation lung injury (Putman et al., 1977), and may be normal initially in patients with tracheobronchitis and arterial hypoxemia. Focal and patchy pulmonary infiltrates may occur as late as 24 to 36 hours after smoke inhalation, while a diffuse alveolar filling pattern may occur as late as 96 hours after admission. Fire victims who have jumped from a high building to escape a fire may have a pneumothorax and/or a hemothorax, a pulmonary contusion, as well as rib or other bone fractures evident on chest roentgenogram. Radionuclide imaging studies with ventilation and perfusion lung scans have been used in the assessment of inhalation lung injury (Putman et al., 1977; Moylan et al., 1972) and ammonia inhalation (Taplin et al., 1976). The ventilation/perfusion lung scan may be abnormal in patients with chronic obstructive pulmonary disease. Using multiple inert gas analysis in human victims of acute smoke inhalation with surface burns and in laboratory animals exposed to wood smoke, it was found that the early alterations of ventilation ($\dot{V}$) and perfusion ($\dot{Q}$) resulted from increased high $\dot{V}_{alveolar}/\dot{Q}$ units and increased dead-space ventilation. Late alterations were due to increased perfusion of low $\dot{V}_{alveolar}/\dot{Q}$ units. True intrapulmonary shunt was not present. These $\dot{V}/\dot{Q}$ alterations may suggest early regional pulmonary vasospasm followed by regional bronchial obstruction and alveolar collapse secondary to bronchospasm, bronchial edema, or partial obstruction by cellular debris (Robinson et al., 1981).

Fire victims with a history of ischemic heart disease who complain of chest pain but no significant dyspnea should be hospitalized for observation to exclude acute myocardial ischemia, especially if the blood carboxyhemoglobin level is elevated. Acute myocardial infarction has been demonstrated in patients with an elevated carboxyhemoglobin and pre-existing coronary artery disease (Landa et al., 1972).

In laboratory studies, arterial blood gas analysis has revealed a near normal arterial oxygen tension (P_aO_2) and a metabolic acidosis with increased serum lactate (Buehler et al., 1975; Landa et al., 1972). Anticoagulated whole blood should be obtained to determine the blood carboxyhemoglobin (COHb) level. The COHb level is valuable in assessing the severity of acute smoke inhalation. Hemoglobin and methemoglobin are other parameters that can be measured when the blood carboxyhemoglobin level is obtained using the CO-Oximeter analyzer. Patients with elevation in COHb may have a normal P_aO_2 and a normal *calculated* oxygen saturation (Eckfeldt, 1978). However, the *measured* arterial oxygen saturation and arterial oxygen content will both be decreased. In a patient who has arterial hypoxemia, as well as a reduced measured oxygen saturation, the lung inhalation injury may be more severe than in an individual who has a reduction in measured arterial oxygen saturation and a normal P_aO_2. Falsely elevated values of blood hemoglobin and carboxyhemoglobin can occur in patients with markedly increased levels of triglycerides and chylomicrons (Hodgkin and Chan, 1975).

Augmented ventilation and oxygen therapy decrease the half life of carboxyhemoglobin. Accordingly, after oxygen therapy has been given to fire victims by the emergency medical team, the COHb level in blood determined at the hospital will be lower than at the scene of the fire prior to transporting the patient to the hospital.

Other blood levels obtained in fire victims include cyanide, benzene and ethanol. In 32% of autopsied fire victims in Baltimore City, Maryland, there was an increase in blood alcohol levels (Levine and Radford, 1977). Whether drug abuse screening needs to be performed in selected fire victims remains to be elucidated. The diagnosis of cyanide poisoning may be difficult, and should be suspected in the minority of acutely ill fire victims with both carbon monoxide poisoning and an unexplained severe anion gap metabolic acidosis (Crapo, 1981). Blood samples for cyanide and thiocyanate levels should be obtained in such cases. Also, a minority of patients with acute smoke inhalation present with severe dyspnea, refractory hypoxemia, a diffuse lung infiltrate on chest roentgenogram, and a clinical picture suggestive of the diagnosis of the adult respiratory distress syndrome.

The diagnosis of acute smoke inhalation with or without thermal upper airway injury can be made on the basis of history, clinical findings and laboratory examination. Although fiberoptic bronchoscopy offers a high diagnostic yield in the evaluation of thermal and smoke inhalation injury, it should not be performed routinely on all patients with acute smoke inhalation, except perhaps in selected specialized burn centers.

X. Management of Acute Smoke Inhalation Victims

The therapy of acute smoke inhalation includes oxygen, bronchodilators, chest physiotherapy, corticosteroids, antibiotics, endotracheal intubation, tracheostomy, and mechanical ventilation. Each of these treatment modalities will be reviewed. However, the management of surface burns will not be discussed.

A. Oxygen

Maintaining adequate oxygenation is critical in patient management. The initial arterial blood gas and carboxyhemoglobin values will determine the need for oxygen therapy. When there are clinical findings of respiratory distress, cough with carbonaceous sputum, or central nervous system dysfunction, 100% oxygen by face mask should be administered immediately, even before arterial blood gas and carboxyhemoglobin results are available. The half-life of carboxyhemoglobin is decreased to approximately 80 minutes by breathing 100% oxygen and can be decreased even further with hyperbaric oxygen. At 2.5 atmospheres of oxygen, the COHb level will decrease to 20% in about 50 minutes (Winter and Miller, 1976).

Prognosis of carbon monoxide poisoning depends upon the COHb level and blood pH. In a study by Larkin et al. (1976), 5 patients with an average COHb level of 48% and a pH of less than 7.4 (mean, 7.26) died. In contrast, 10 patients in this report with a pH greater than 7.4 and an average COHb level of 29% recovered. Both groups were treated with high flow oxygen therapy. The authors suggest than an initial uncompensated metabolic acidosis indicates a poor prognosis, and perhaps more aggressive treatment with either endotracheal intubation and mechanical ventilation or hyperbaric oxygen may benefit those patients with a high COHb blood level and a severe hypoxic insult to avoid death or severe neurological sequelae. In a subsequent study of three fire victims with an average COHb saturation of 51% and an average pH of 6.89, all three had full neurological recovery in spite of the presence of severe metabolic acidosis and COHb poisoning (Strohl et al., 1980). In the latter study, one patient received sodium bicarbonate and methylprednisolone and was emergently intubated and mechanically ventilated with 100% oxygen. The other two were electively intubated and mechanically ventilated with 100% oxygen. Therefore, it was concluded that severe metabolic acidosis may not be a poor prognostic factor provided early intubation and mechanical ventilation with 100% oxygen are accomplished.

In severe carbon monoxide intoxication (COHb level > 40%), the application of hyperbaric oxygen is recommended. At three atmospheres pressure of oxygen, there is a 50% clearance of carbon monoxide from the blood within 25 minutes (Dinman, 1974). Hyperbaric oxygen therapy has been recommended as the most efficacious mode of oxygen administration to decrease the morbidity and mortality from carbon monoxide poisoning and to reduce the neurological sequelae of headache, irritability, personality changes, confusion and loss of memory (Myers et al., 1985b; Norkool and Kirkpatrick, 1985; Brandon, 1984). In severe carbon monoxide poisoning, our treatment of choice is early elective intubation and mechanical ventilation with 100% oxygen. Alternatively, hyperbaric oxygen therapy should be given when this form of oxygen delivery is available.

In mild to moderate carbon monoxide poisoning without severe metabolic acidosis and significant neurological dysfunction, 100% oxygen should be administered by face mask and the COHb monitored serially. Caution is required when giving 100% oxygen to patients with severe chronic obstructive pulmonary disease and carbon dioxide retention since these individuals may become apneic. Patients with severe arterial hypoxemia, metabolic acidosis and severe carbon monoxide poisoning, as well as those who are comatose or have acute upper airway obstruction, require prompt endotracheal intubation and mechanical ventilation with 100% oxygen.

B. Bronchodilators

When wheezing is detected or there is a history of obstructive airway disease (e.g., asthma), bronchodilator therapy can be administered by the oral, inhaled, or intravenous route. Beta$_2$ agonists can be given by inhalation or nebulization, and racemic epinephrine aerosol inhalation may benefit patients with upper airway obstruction who do not require endotracheal intubation. Aminophylline should be administered in an initial intravenous bolus of 5.6 mg/kg over 20-30 min followed by a continuous intravenous infusion of 0.4-0.5 mg/kg/hr. Theophylline blood levels should be monitored to ensure therapeutic blood levels of 10-20 μg/ml and to guide adjustment of the aminophylline infusion. Chest physiotherapy in conjunction with beta$_2$ agonist aerosol therapy may be of value in patients with significant sputum production.

C. Antibiotics

Fever, purulent sputum production, leukocytosis, and infiltrates on the chest roentgenogram herald the onset of pulmonary infection and pneumonia. Clinical assessment of patients together with sputum findings should guide the use of antibiotic therapy. Penicillin, ampicillin, or a cephalosporin may be used depending on the findings on the sputum gram stain and culture. In a prospective study using aerosolized gentamicin to control infection in burn patients, there was no significant difference in morbidity and mortality between treated and control groups (Levine et al., 1978). The predominant organisms recovered from blood in both treated and control groups were *Pseudomonas aeruginosa* and *Klebsiella pneumoniae.* Pseudomonas organisms were present on sputum culture in 75% of both control and treated groups. In fire victims with inhalation injury and significant surface burns (average burn area 55%), the Brooke Army Medical Center burn team does not recommend prophylactic aerosol therapy with gentamicin. Moreover, even though there are abnormalities in the chemotactic, bactericidal and phagocytic functions of the pulmonary alveolar macrophage in acute smoke inhalation victims, the use of prophylactic antibiotic therapy for victims of smoke inhalation is not recommended.

D. Corticosteroids

In a prospective trial of dexamethasone versus placebo therapy in inhalation injury patients with a significant body surface area burn of more than 50%, parenteral dexamethasone (20 mg daily for three days) did not decrease pulmonary complications or mortality (Levine et al., 1978). In a double-blind study of methylprednisolone (30 mg/kg/day IV bolus for two days) versus saline placebo in 33 unselected burn patients with inhalation injury, the corticosteroid-treated group had a mortality rate four times that of the placebo group. Infections in the corticosteroid treated group were almost three times those of the placebo group (Moylan, 1979). Thus, the use of corticosteroids to treat patients with inhalation injury and surface burns is not recommended. Corticosteroids have been used to treat patients with pulmonary thermal and acrid smoke injury, and have been recommended during the acute phase of pulmonary injury (Beal et al., 1968).

In animal studies of acute smoke inhalation to white pine smoke without surface burn, both methylprednisolone and dexamethasone (but not hydrocortisone) reduced mortality in rats (Dressler et al., 1976). Moreover, methylprednisolone (10 mg twice daily for two days) was found to be effective in reducing mortality in these animals when given 1 hour after smoke inhalation. In another animal study, rabbits were exposed to acrolein vapor for 15 minutes, and 30 minutes later the animals were divided into three treatment groups: (1) saline placebo intramuscularly at 12 hr intervals, (2) 100 mg of methylprednisolone intramuscularly at 12 hr intervals, and (3) a single 100 mg dose of methylprednisolone intramuscularly followed by doses of saline at 12 hr intervals (Beeley et al., 1986). The animals were evaluated over a 72 hr period. In this study, there was a significantly lower mortality in the corticosteroid-treated groups than in the nontreated group.

In two hotel fires in Las Vegas, Nevada, victims were triaged in a random fashion to one of four local hospitals. In two of these institutions, corticosteroids (equivalent dosage equal to 10 mg dexamethasone every 6 hr for 48 hr) were given to 141 fire victims while 84 received no corticosteroids. Ventilatory insufficiency and pneumonia were present in 1% of both broups, and there were no deaths in either group. The authors concluded that corticosteroid therapy has little beneficial effect upon pulmonary-related morbidity and mortality following isolated smoke inhalation injury (Robinson et al., 1982). It should be noted that the COHb levels in the steroid- and nonsteroid-treated groups were 14% and 12%, respectively. Thus, with mild smoke inhalation corticosteroid therapy is apparently not indicated.

There may be a dichotomy between circulating and intrapulmonary inflammatory cell populations. For example, although systemic corticosteroid-treated guinea pigs showed a marked reduction in the percentage of T lymphocytes in the peripheral blood, no significant decrease in the percentage of T lymphocytes in the bronchoalveolar cell population was noted (Domby and Whitcomb, 1978). Therefore, significant differences could exist for other cell populations as well It has been shown that there is an inflammatory response in the lungs determined with bronchoalveolar lavage after smoke inhalation. The effectiveness of corticosteroids in blocking this response is uncertain. Moreover, the effectiveness of acutely inhaled corticosteroids in ameliorating inflammatory responses directly in the lungs of inhalation victims remains to be studied. In patients with smoke inhalation, systemic corticosteroid therapy has been recommended to be given early in one large dose (Mellins and Park, 1975). Moreover, possible long-term beneficial effects of corticosteroid treatment have been observed in patients with chlorine gas inhalation (Chester et al., 1977). This treatment has also been recommended in patients with smoke bomb inhalation lung injury (Matarese and Matthews, 1986).

Although there are no controlled studies in humans, we recommend a trial of corticosteroids (about 2 mg/kg/day of methylprednisolone equivalent) for 24-48 hr in acute smoke inhalation victims without thermal cutaneous burns but with evidence of upper airway obstruction, respiratory insufficiency, and/or severe bronchospasm. Recently, ibuprofen has been shown to prevent synthetic smoke-induced pulmonary edema in laboratory animals (Shinozawa et al., 1986), but this agent has not been studied systematically in humans with inhalation lung injury.

E. Specific Therapy of Smoke Inhalation

In case of smoke inhalation associated with chemical plants or in which hydrogen cyanide is suspected, specific antidotes (available as the Lilly Cyanide Antidote Kit) with inhaled amyl nitrite perles, 10% sodium nitrite, and 25% sodium thiosulfate solutions are required. In adults, the amyl nitrite perles can be cracked and are inhaled for 30 seconds per minute, sodium nitrite and sodium thiosulfate are available as 10 ml and 50 ml ampules, respectively, and are given slowly by the intravenous route (Hall and Rumack, 1986).

XI. Late Complications of Smoke Inhalation

Residual lung damage in the form of chronic obstructive pulmonary disease or bronchiectasis may be a sequela of smoke inhalation (Loke et al., 1980; Putman et al., 1977; Panke and McLeod, 1985). Tracheal stenosis may also be a late complication. Evaluation of patients with or without abnormal lung function but with respiratory complaints can be performed utilizing serial lung function tests, methacholine challenge test (Chan-Yeung and Lam, 1986), or clinical exercise testing.

Finally, fire prevention is still the best policy to prevent smoke inhalation, and automatic sprinklers and smoke detectors are recommended in residential and commercial buildings (Council on Scientific Affairs, 1987).

References

Abrams, C. S. (1984). Chronic effects of fire fighting on pulmonary function. MD Thesis, Yale University School of Medicine, New Haven.

Adams, C., Moisan, T., Chandrasekhar, A. J., and Warpeha, R. (1979). Endobronchial polyposis secondary to thermal inhalation injury. *Chest* **75**: 643-645.

Adelson, L., and Kaufman, J. (1971). Fatal chlorine poisoning: report of two cases with clinicopathologic correlation. *Am. J. Clin. Pathol.* **56**:430-442.

Alarie, Y. (1985). The toxicity of smoke from polymeric materials during thermal decomposition. *Ann. Rev. Pharmacol. Toxicol.* **25**:325-347.

Alarie, Y. C., and Anderson, R. C. (1979). Toxicologic and acute lethal hazard evaluation of thermal decomposition products of synthetic and natural polymers. *Toxicol. Appl. Pharmacol.* **51**:341-362.

Anderson, E. W., Andelman, R. J., Strauch, J. M., Fortuin, N. J., and Knelson, J. H. (1973). Effect of low-level carbon monoxide exposure on onset and duration of angina pectoris. A study in ten patients with ischemic heart disease. *Ann. Intern. Med.* **79**:46-50.

Anderson, R. F., Allensworth, D. C., and Degroot, W. J. (1967). Myocardial toxicity from carbon monoxide poisoning. *Ann. Intern. Med.* **67**:1172-1182.

Aronow, W. S., and Isbell, M. W. (1973). Carbon monoxide effect on exercise induced angina pectoris. *Ann. Intern. Med.* **79**:392-395.

Aronow, W. S., Ferlinz, J., and Glauser, F. (1977). Effect of carbon monoxide on exercise performance in chronic obstructive pulmonary disease. *Am. J. Med.* **63**:904-908.

Arora, N. S., and Aldrich, T. K. (1980). Bronchiolitis obliterans from a burning automobile. *South Med. J.* **73**:507-510.

Astrup, P. (1972). Some physiological and pathological effects of moderate carbon monoxide exposure. *Br. Med. J.* **4**:447-452.

Ayres, S. M., Giannelli, Jr., S., and Mueller, H. (1970). Myocardial and systemic responses to carboxyhemoglobin. *Ann. N.Y. Acad. Sci.* **174**:268-293.

Ayres, S. M., Giannelli, Jr., S., and Mueller, H. (1973). Carboxyhemoglobin and the access to oxygen. *Arch. Environ. Health* **26**:8-15.

Barnard, R. J., and Anthony, D. F. (1980). Effect of health maintenance programs on Los Angeles City Firefighters. *J. Occup. Med.* **22**:667-669.

Barnard, R. J., and Duncan, H. W. (1975). Heart rate and ECG responses of fire fighters. *J. Occup. Med.* **17**:247-250.

Barnard, R. J., Gardner, G. W., Diaco, N. V., and Kattus, A. A. (1975). Near-maximal ECG stress testing and coronary artery disease risk factor analysis in Los Angeles Fire Fighters. *J. Occup. Med.* **17**:693-695.

Barnard, R. J., and Weber, J. S. (1979). Carbon monoxide: A hazard to fire fighters. *Arch. Environ. Health* **34**:255-257.

Beal, D. D., Lambeth, J. T., and Conner, G. H. (1968). Follow-up studies on patients treated with steroids following pulmonary thermal and acrid smoke injury. *Laryngoscope* **78**:396-403.

Beard, R. R., and Grandstaff, N. (1970). Carbon monoxide exposure and cerebral function. *Ann. N.Y. Acad. Sci.* **174**:385-395.

Beck, B. D., Gerson, B., Feldman, H. A., and Brain, J. D. (1983). Lactate dehydrogenase isoenzymes in hamster lung lavage fluid after lung injury. *Toxicol. Appl. Pharmacol.* **71**:59-71.

Beeley, J. M., Crow, J., Jones, J. G., Minty, B., Lynch, R. D., and Pryce, D. P. (1986). Mortality and lung histopathology after inhalation lung injury. The effect of corticosteroids. *Am. Rev. Respir. Dis.* **133**:191-196.

Birky, M. M. (1976). Philosophy of testing for assessment of toxicological aspects of fire exposure. *J. Combust. Toxicol.* **3**:5-21.

Blank, M. L., Dalbey, W., Nettesheim, P., Price, J., Creasia, D., and Snyder, F. (1978). Sequential changes in phospholipid composition and synthesis in lungs exposed to nitrogen dioxide. *Am. Rev. Respir. Dis.* **117**:273-280.

Brandon, S. (1984). Late sequelae of carbon monoxide poisoning. *Lancet* **2**: 637.

Breysse, P. A. (1981). The health cost of tight homes. *JAMA* **245**:267-268.

Brody, J. S., and Coburn, R. F. (1969). Carbon monoxide-induced arterial hypoxemia. *Science* **164**:1297-1298.

Buehler, J. H., Berns, A. S., Webster, J. R., Addington, W. W., and Cugell, D. W. (1975). Lactic acidosis from carboxyhemoglobinemia after smoke inhalation. *Ann. Intern. Med.* **82**:803-805.

Cahalane, M., and Demling, R. H. (1984). Early respiratory abnormalities from smoke inhalation. *JAMA* **251**:771-773.

Caplan, Y. H., Thompson, B. C., Levine, B., and Masemore, W. (1986). Accidental poisonings involving carbon monoxide, heating systems, and confined spaces. *J. Forensic Sci.* **31**:117-121.

Chan-Yeung, M., and Lam, S. (1986). Occupational asthma. *Am. Rev. Respir. Dis.* **133**:686-703.

Charan, N. B., Myers, C. G., Lakshminarayan, S., and Spencer, T. M. (1979). Pulmonary injuries associated with acute sulfur dioxide inhalation. *Am. Rev. Respir. Dis.* **119**:555-560.

Chester, E. H., Kaimal, P. J., Payne, Jr., C. B., and Kohn, P. M. (1977). Pulmonary injury following exposure to chlorine gas. Possible beneficial effects of steroid treatment. *Chest* **72**:247-250.

Chiodi, H., Dill, D. B., Consolazio, F., and Horvath, S. M. (1941). Respiratory and circulatory responses to acute carbon monoxide poisoning. *Am. J. Physiol.* **134**:683-693.

Chu, C. S. (1981). New concepts of pulmonary burn injury. *J. Trauma* **21**: 958-961.

Clark, C. J., Campbell, D., and Reid, W. H. (1981). Blood carboxyhaemoglobin and cyanide levels in fire survivors. *Lancet* **1**:1332-1335.

Coleman, D. L. (1981). Smoke inhalation. Medical Staff Conference. University of California, San Francisco. *West. J. Med.* **135**:300-309.

Colice, G. L., Munster, A. M., and Haponik, E. F. (1986). Tracheal stenosis complicating cutaneous burns: an underestimated problem. *Am. Rev. Respir. Dis.* **134**:1315-1318.

Collison, H. A., Rodkey, F. L., and O'Neal, J. D. (1968). Determination of carbon monoxide in blood by gas chromatography. *Clin. Chem.* **14**:162-171.

Committee on Fire Toxicology (1986). Fire and Smoke: Understanding the hazards. National Research Council, Board on environmental studies and toxicology, National Academy Press, Washington, D.C.

Conner, E. H., DuBois, A. B., Comroe, Jr., J. H. (1962). Acute chemical injury of the airway and lungs. Experience with six cases. *Anesthesiology* **23**: 538-547.

Cornish, H. H., and Abar, E. L. (1969). Toxicity of pyrolysis products of vinyl plastics. *Arch. Environ. Health* **19**:15-21.

Costa, D. L., Kutzman, R. S., Lehmann, J. R., and Drew, R. T. (1986). Altered lung function and structure in the rat after subchronic exposure to acrolein. *Am. Rev. Respir. Dis.* **133**:286-291.

Council on Scientific Affairs, American Medical Association (1987). Preventing death and injury from fires with automatic sprinklers and smoke detectors. *JAMA* **257**:1618-1620.

Crapo, R. O. (1981). Smoke-inhalation injuries. *JAMA* **246**:1694-1696.

Czaja, A. J., McAlhany, J. C., and Pruitt, B. A. Jr. (1974). Acute gastroduodenal disease after thermal injury. An endoscopic evaluation of incidence and natural history. *N. Engl. J. Med.* **291**:925-929.

Demarest, G. B., Hudson, L. D., and Altman, L. C. (1979). Impaired alveolar macrophage chemotaxis in patients with acute smoke inhalation. *Am. Rev. Respir. Dis.* **119**:279-286.

Demling, R. H. (1985). Burns. *N. Engl. J. Med.* **313**:1389-1398.

Demling, R. H. (1983). Improved survival after massive burns. *J. Trauma* **23**: 179-184.

Dilley, J. V., Martin, S. B., McKee, R., and Pryor, G. (1979). A smoke toxicity methodology. *J. Combust. Toxicol.* **6**:20-29.

Dinman, B. D. (1974). The management of acute carbon monoxide intoxication. *J. Occup. Med.* **16**:662-664.

DiVincenti, F. C., Pruitt, Jr., B. A., and Reckler, J. M. (1971). Inhalation injuries. *J. Trauma* **11**:109-117.

Domby, W. R., and Whitcomb, M. E. (1978). The effects of corticosteroid administration on the bronchoalveolar cells obtained from guinea pigs by lung lavage. *Am. Rev. Respir. Dis.* **117**:893-896.

Douglas, D. B., Douglas, R. B., Oakes, D., and Scott, G. (1985). Pulmonary function of London Firemen. *Br. J. Ind. Med.* **42**:55-58.

Dressler, D. P., Skornik, W. A., Bloom, S. B., and Dougherty, J. D. (1975). Smoke toxicity of common aircraft carpets. *Aviat. Space Environ. Med.* **46**:1141-1143.

Dressler, D. P., Skornik, W. A., and Kupersmith, S. (1976). Corticosteroid treatment of experimental smoke inhalation. *Ann. Surg.* **183**:46-52.

Drew, R. T. (1985). The design and operation of systems for inhalation exposure of animals. In *Toxicology of Inhaled Materials.* Edited by H. P. Witschi and J. D. Brain. Springer-Verlag, Berlin, Heidelberg, pp. 3-22.

Dyer, R. F., and Esch, V. H. (1976). Polyvinyl chloride toxicity in fires: hydrogen chloride toxicity in fire fighters. *JAMA* **235**:393-397.

Eckfeldt, J. H. (1978). Diagnosis of carbon monoxide poisoning. *JAMA* **240**:1140-1141.

Eckholm, E. (1986). Radon: Threat is real, but scientists argue over its severity. *The New York Times,* September 2, p. C1.

Epler, G. R., Colby, T. V., McLoud, T. C., Carrington, C. B., and Gaensler, E. A. (1985). Bronchiolitis obliterans organizing pneumonia. *N. Engl. J. Med.* **312**:152-158.

Evanoff, B. A., and Rosenstock, L. (1986). Reproductive hazards in the workplace: A case study of women fire fighters. *Am. J. Indust. Med.* **9**:503-515.

Fein, A., Leff, A., and Hopewell, P. C. (1980). Pathophysiology and management of the complications resulting from fire and the inhaled products of combustion: Reveiw of the literature. *Crit. Care Med.* **8**:94-98.

Fein, A., Grossman, R. F., Jones, J. G., Hoeffel, J., and McKay, D. (1980a). Carbon monoxide effect on alveolar epithelial permeability. *Chest* **78**:726-731.

Feuer, E., and Rosenman, K. (1986). Mortality in police and firefighters in New Jersey. *Am. J. Indust. Med.* **9**:517-527.

Ferguson, J. S., Schaper, M., Stock, M. F., Weyel, D. A., and Alarie, Y. (1986). Sensory and pulmonary irritation with exposure to methyl isocynate. *Toxicol. Appl. Pharmacol.* **82**:329-335.

Fick, Jr., R. B., Paul, E. S., Merrill, W. W., Reynolds, H. Y., and Loke, J. S. O. (1984). Alterations in the antibacterial properties of rabbit pulmonary macrophages exposed to wood smoke. *Am. Rev. Respir. Dis.* **129**:76-81.

Finley, T. N., and Ladman, A. J. (1972). Low yield of pulmonary surfactant in cigarette smokers. *N. Engl. J. Med.* **286**:223-227.

Fire Toxicology: Methods for evaluation of toxicity of pyrolysis and combustion products. (1977). Report No. 2, National Academy of Science, Washington, D.C.

Fisher, J., and Rubin, K. P. (1982). Occult carbon monoxide poisoning. *Arch. Intern. Med.* **142**:1270-1271.

Fleming, G. M., Chester, E. H., and Montenegro, H. D. (1979). Dysfunction of small airways following pulmonary injury due to nitrogen dioxide. *Chest* **75**:720-721.

Freedman, A. L. (1975). Hypercarboxyhemoglobinemia from inhalation of cigar smoke. *Ann. Intern. Med.* **82**:537.

Frost, J. K., Gupta, P. K., Erozan, Y. S., Carter, D., Hollander, D. H., Levin, M. L., and Ball, Jr., W. C. (1973). Pulmonary cytologic alterations in toxic environmental inhalation. *Hum. Pathol.* **4**:521-536.

Genovesi, M. G., Tashkin, D. P., Chopra, S., Morgan, M., and McElroy, C. (1977). Transient hypoxemia in firemen following inhalation of smoke. *Chest* **71**: 441-444.

Glassroth, J., Adams, G. D., and Schnoll, S. (1987). The impact of substance abuse on the respiratory system. *Chest* **91**:596-602.

Gold, A., Burgess, W. A., and Clougherty, E. V. (1978). Exposure of fire fighters to toxic air contaminants. *Am. Indust. Hyg. Assoc. J.* **39**:534-539.

Goldfrank, L. R., Lewin, N. A., Kirstein, R. H., and Weisman, R. S. (1986). Carbon monoxide. In *Goldfrank's Toxicologic Emergencies,* 3rd Edition. Appleton Century-Crofts/Norwalk, Connecticut, Chap. 64, pp. 662-668.

Gosink, B. B., Friedman, P. J., and Liebow, A. A. (1973). Bronchiolitis obliterans: Roentgenologic-pathologic correlation. *Am. J. Roentgenol. Radium Ther. Nucl. Med.* **117**:816-832.

Grace, T. W., and Platt, F. W. (1981). Subacute carbon monoxide poisoning. Another great imitator. *JAMA* **246**:1698-1700.

Graham, D. L., Laman, D., Theodore, J., and Robin, E. D. (1977). Acute cyanide poisoning complicated by lactic acidosis and pulmonary edema. *Arch. Intern. Med.* **137**:1051-1055.

Halebian, P. H., Madden, M. R., Finklestein, J. L., Corder, V. J., and Shires, G. T. (1986). Improved burn center survival of patients with toxic epidermal necrolysis managed without corticosteroids. *Ann. Surg.* **204**:503-512.

Halebian, P., Yurt, R., Petito, C., and Shires, G. T. (1985). Diabetes insipidus after carbon monoxide poisoning and smoke inhalation. *J. Trauma* **25**: 662-663.

Hall, A. H., and Rumack, B. H. (1986). Clinical toxicology of cyanide. *Ann. Emer. Med.* **15**:1067-1074.

Haponik, E. F., Meyers, D. A., Munster, A. M., Smith, P. L., Britt, E. J., Wise, R. A., and Bleecker, E. R. (1987). Acute upper airway injury in burn patients. Serial changes of flow-volume curves and nasopharyngoscopy. *Am. Rev. Respir. Dis.* **135**:360-366.

Hartnett, L. (1986). Environmental contamination. In *Goldfrank's Toxicologic Emergencies,* 3rd edition. Appleton Century-Crofts/Norwalk, CT, Chap. 69, pp. 729-738.

Hartzell, G. E., Packham, S. C., and Switzer, W. G. (1983). Toxic products from fires. *Am. Ind. Indust. Assoc. J.* **44**:248-255.

Head, J. M. (1980). Inhalation injury in burns. *Am. J. Surg.* **139**:508-512.

Hebbel, R. P., Eaton, J. W., Modler, S., and Jacob, H. S. (1978). Extreme but asymptomatic carboxyhemoglobinemia and chronic lung disease. *JAMA* **239**:2584-2856.

Henderson, R. F., Rebar, A. H., DeNicola, D. B., Henderson, T. R., and Damon, E. G. (1981). The use of pulmonary washings as a probe to detect lung injury. *Chest* **80(S)**:12S-15S.

Henderson, R. F., Rebar, A. H., Pickrell, J. A., and Newton, G. J. (1979). Early damage indicators in the lung III. Biochemical and cytological response of the lung to inhaled metal salts. *Toxicol. Appl. Pharmacol.* **50**:123-136.

Henderson, Y., and Haggard, H. W. (1943). Chemical Asphyxiants. In *Noxious Gases and the Principles of Respiration Influencing Their Action.* Reinhold Publishing Co., New York, pp. 159-176.

Herndon, D. N., Traber, D. L., Niehaus, G. D., Linares, H. A., and Traber, L. D. (1984). The pathophysiology of smoke inhalation injury in a sheep model. *J. Trauma* **24**:1044-1051.

Hilado, C. J. (1978). The practical use of the USF (University of San Francisco) toxicity screening test method. *J. Combust. Toxicol.* **5**:331-338.

Hilado, C. J., and Huttlinger, P. A. (1981). Comparison of time to death, survival time and LT_{50}. *J. Combust. Toxicol.* **8**:33-36.

Himmelstein, J. S., and Frumkin, H. (1985). The right to know about toxic exposures. Implications for physicians. *N. Engl. J. Med.* **312**:687-690.

Hirsch, C. S., Bost, R. O., Gerber, S. R., Cowan, M. E., Adelson, L., and Sunshine, I. (1977). Carboxyhemoglobin concentrations in flash fire victims. Report of six simultaneous fire fatalities without elevated carboxyhemoglobin. *Am. J. Clin. Pathol.* **68**:317-320.

Hocking, W. G., and Golde, D. W. (1979). The pulmonary-alveolar macrophage. *N. Engl. J. Med.* **301**:580-587, 639-645.

Hodgkin, J. E., and Chan, D. M. (1975). Diabetic ketoacidosis presenting as carbon monoxide poisoning. *JAMA* **231**:1164-1165.

Hogg, J. C. (1985). Response of the lung to inhaled particles. *Med. J. Aust.* **142**:675-678.

Holmberg, B., and Lundberg, P. (1985). Benzene: standards, occurrence and exposures. *Am. J. Indust. Med.* 7:375-383.

Horovitz, J. H. (1981). Diagnostic tools for use in smoke inhalation. *J. Trauma* 21:717-719.

Hunninghake, G., Gadek, J. E., Kawanami, O., Ferrans, V. J., and Crystal, R. G. (1979). Inflammatory and immune processes in the human lung in health and disease: evaluation by bronchoalveolar lavage. *Am. J. Pathol.* 97: 149-206.

Hunt, J. L., Agee, R. N., and Pruitt, Jr., B. A. (1975). Fiberoptic bronchoscopy in acute inhalation injury. *J. Trauma* 15:641-648.

Jones, R. N., Hughes, J. M., Glindmeyer, H., and Weill, H. (1986). Lung function after acute chlorine exposure. *Am. Rev. Respir. Dis.* 134:1190-1195.

Kamat, S. R., Mahashur, A. A., Tiwari, A. K. B., Potdar, P. V., Gaur, M., Kolhatkar, V. P., Vaidya, P., Parmar, D., Rupwate, R., Chatterjee, T. S., Jain, K., Kelkar, M. D., and Kinare, S. G. (1985). Early observations on pulmonary changes and clinical morbidity due to the isocyanate gas leak at Bhopal. *J. Postgrad. Med. (India)* 31:63-72.

Karter, M. J., Jr. (1986). Fire loss in the United States during 1985. *Fire J.* 80: 26-65.

Kelly, J. S., and Sophocleus, G. J. (1978). Retinal hemorrhage in subacute carbon monoxide poisoning. *JAMA* 239:1515-1517.

Kimmerle, M. G. (1974). Aspects and methodology for the evaluation of toxicological parameters during fire exposure. *JFF/Combust. Toxicol.* 1:4-51.

Kirkpatrick, J. N. (1987). Occult carbon monoxide poisoning. *West. J. Med.* 146:52-56.

Kirkpatrick, M. B., and Bass. J. B. (1979). Severe obstructive lung disease after smoke inhalation. *Chest* 76:108-110.

Kishitani, K. (1971). Study on injurious properties of combustive products of building materials at the initial stage of fire. *J. Faculty Eng.* (University Tokyo) (B) 31:1-35.

Kizer, K. W. (1984). Toxic inhalations. *Emer. Med. Clin. North Am.* 2:649-666.

Klimisch, H. J., Hollander, H. W. M., and Thyssen, J. (1980). Comparative measurements of the toxicity to laboratory animals of products of thermal decomposition generated by the method of DIN 53.436. *J. Combust. Toxicol.* 7:209-230.

Kuller, L. H., Radford, E. P., Swift, D., Perper, J. A., and Fisher, R. (1975). Carbon monoxide and heart attacks. *Arch. Environ. Health* 30:477-482.

Landa, J., Avery, W. G., and Sachner, M. A. (1972). Some physiologic observations in smoke inhalation. *Chest* 61:62-64

Larkin, J. M., Brahos, G. J., and Moylan, J. A. (1976). Treatment of carbon monoxide poisoning: prognostic factors. *J. Trauma* **16**:111-114.

Lawther, P. J. (1975). Carbon monoxide. *Br. Med. Bull.* **31**:256-260.

Lawther, P. J., and Commins, B. T. (1970). Cigarette smoking and exposure to carbon monoxide. *Ann. N.Y. Acad. Sci.* **174**:135-147.

Leaderer, B. P. (1982). Air pollutant emissions from kerosene space heaters. *Science* **218**:1113-1115.

Lee-Jones, M., Bennett, M. A., and Sherwell, J. M. (1970). Cyanide self-poisoning. *Br. Med. J.* **4**:780-781.

Lefcoe, N. M., and Wonnacott, T. H. (1974). Chronic respiratory disease in four occupational groups. *Arch. Environ. Health* **29**:143-146.

Levin, B. C., Paabo, M., and Birky, M. M. (1983a). An interlaboratory evaluation of the 1980 version of the National Bureau of Standards Test Method for assessing the acute inhalation toxicity of combustion products. NBSIR 83-2678. U.S. Department of Commerce, National Bureau of Standards, National Engineering Laboratory, Center for Fire Research, Washington, D.C., pp. 1-82.

Levin, B. C., Paabo, M., Fultz, M. L., Bailey, C., Yin, W., and Harris, S. E. (1983b). An acute inhalation toxicological evaluation of combustion products from fire retarded and non-fire retarded flexible polyurethane foam and polyester. NBSIR 83-2791. U.S. Department of Commerce, National Bureau of Standards, National Engineering Laboratory, Center for Fire Research, Washington, D.C., pp. 1-62.

Levin, B. C., Babrauskas, V., Braun, E., Gurman, J., and Paabo, M. (1985a). An exploration of combustion limitations and alternatives to the NBS toxicity test method. NBSIR 85-3274. U.S. Department of Commerce, National Bureau of Standards, National Engineering Laboratory, Center for Fire Research, Gaithersburg, MD 20899.

Levin, B. C., Paabo, M., Fultz, M. L., and Bailey, C. S. (1985b). Generation of hydrogen cyanide from flexible polyurethane foam decomposed under different combustion conditions. *Fire Mater.* **9**(3):125-134.

Levine, B. A., Petroff, P. A., Slade, C. L., Pruitt, Jr., B. A. (1978). Prospective trials of dexamethasone and aerosolized gentamicin in the treatment of inhalation injury in the burned patient. *J. Trauma* **18**:188-193.

Levine, M. S., and Radford, E. P. (1977). Fire victims: medical outcomes and demographic characteristics. *Am. J. Public Health* **67**:1077-1080.

Levine, M. S., and Radford, E. P. (1978). Occupational exposures to cyanide in Baltimore fire fighters. *J. Occup. Med.* **20**:53-56.

Loke, J., Farmer, W. C., Matthay, R. A., Virgulto, J. A., and Bouhuys, A. (1976). Carboxyhemoglobin levels in fire fighters. *Lung* **154**:35-39.

Loke, J., Farmer, W., Matthay, R. A., Putman, C. E., and Walker-Smith, G. J.

(1980). Acute and chronic effects of fire fighting on pulmonary function. *Chest* **77**:369-373.

Loke, J., and Matthay, R. A. (1981). Managing victims of smoke inhalation. *J. Respir. Dis.* **2**:87-98.

Loke, J., Paul, E., and Virgulto, J. (1981). Smoke exposure chamber and bronchoalveolar lavage as a method for the evaluation of toxicity of pyrolysis and combustion products in laboratory animals. *J. Combust. Toxicol.* **8**: 37-44.

Loke, J., Paul, E., Virgulto, J., and Matthay, R. (1981a). Smoke inhalation in humans and laboratory animals. Proc. Third Calif. Conf. Fire Toxicity, SRI International, Menlo Park, CA, Vol. 3:96-98.

Loke, J., Paul, E., Virgulto, J. A., and Walker-Smith, G. J. (1984). Rabbit lung after acute smoke inhalation. Cellular responses and scanning electron microscopy. *Arch. Surg.* **119**:956-959.

Lowry, W. T., Juarez, L., Petty, C. S., and Roberts, B. (1985a). Studies of toxic gas production during actual structural fires in the Dallas area. *J. Forensic Sci.* **30**:59-72.

Lowry, W. T., Peterson, J., Petty, C. S., and Badgett, J. L. (1985b). Free radical production from controlled low-energy fires: toxicity considerations. *J. Forensic Sci.* **30**:73-85.

MacFarland, H. N., and Leong, K. J. (1962). Hazards from the thermodecomposition of plastics. *Arch. Environ. Health* **4**:39-45.

Mallory, T. B., and Brickley, W. J. (1943). Pathology: with special reference to the pulmonary lesions. *Ann. Surg.* **117**:865-884.

Martin, F. M., and Witschi, H. P. (1985). Cadmium-induced lung injury: cell kinetics and long-term effects. *Toxicol. Appl. Pharmacol.* **80**:215-227.

Mastromatteo, E. (1959a). Mortality in city firemen. I. A review. *AMA Arch. Ind. Health* **20**:1-7.

Mastromatteo, E. (1959b). Mortality in city firemen II. A study of mortality in firemen of a city fire department. *AMA Arch. Ind. Health* **20**:227-233.

Matarese, S. L., and Matthews, J. I. (1986). Zinc chloride (smoke bomb) inhalational lung injury. *Chest* **89**:308-309.

McAlhany, J. C., Jr., Czaja, A. J., and Pruitt, B. A., Jr. (1976). Antacid control of complications from acute gastroduodenal disease after burns. *J. Trauma* **16**:645-647.

Meier, B. (1986). Bhopal gas-leak victims likely to face life-long health problems, U.S. Finds. *The Wall Street Journal*, February 4, p. 8.

Mellins, R. B., and Park, S. (1975). Respiratory complications of smoke inhalation in victims of fires. *J. Pediatr.* **87**:1-7.

Mierley, M. C., and Baker, S. P. (1983). Fatal house fires in an urban population. *JAMA* **249**:1466-1468.

Milroy, W. C. (1984). Management of irradiated and contaminated casualty victims. *Emer. Med. Clin. North Am.* 2:667-686.

Mohler, S. R. (1975). Air crash survival: Injuries and evacuation toxic hazards. *Aviat. Space Environ. Med.* 46:86-88.

Moritz, A. R., Henriques, Jr., F. C., and McLean, R. (1945). The effects of inhaled heat on the air passages and lungs. *Am. J. Pathol.* 21:311-331.

Moylan, J. A. (1979). Diagnostic techniques and steroids. *J. Trauma* 19 (suppl.):917.

Moylan, J. A., Wilmore, D. W., Mouton, D. E., and Pruitt, B. A. (1972). Early diagnosis of inhalation injury using [133] Xenon lung scan. *Ann. Surg.* 176: 477-484.

Mullin, L. S., Wood, C. K., and Krivanek, N. D. (1983). Guinea pig respiratory response to isocyanates. *Toxicol. Appl. Pharmacol.* 71:113-122.

Murphy, D. M. F., Fairman, R. P., Lapp, N. L., and Morgan, W. K. C. (1976). Severe airway disease due to inhalation of fumes from cleansing agents. *Chest* 69:372-376.

Musk, A. W., Peters, J. M., and Wegman, D. H. (1977a). Lung function in fire fighter, I. A three year follow-up of active subjects. *Am. J. Public Health* 67:626-629.

Musk, A. W., Peters, J. M., and Wegman, D. H. (1977b). Lung function in fire fighters, II. A five year follow-up of retirees. *Am. J. Public Health* 67: 630-633.

Musk, A. W., Monson, R. R., Peters, J. M., and Peters, R. K. (1978). Mortality among Boston firefighters 1915-1975. *Br. J. Indust. Med.* 35:104-108.

Musk, A. W., Peters, J. M., Bernstein, L., Rubin, C., and Monroe, C. B. (1982). Pulmonary function in firefighters: A six-year follow-up in the Boston Fire Department. *Am. J. Indust. Med.* 3:3-9.

Myers, R. A. M., Snyder, S. K., and Majerus, T. C. (1985a). Cutaneous blisters and carbon monoxide poisoning. *Ann. Emer. Med.* 14:603-606.

Myers, R. A. M., Snyder, S. K., and Emhoff, T. A. (1985b). Subacute sequelae of carbon monoxide poisoning. *Ann. Emer. Med.* 14:1163-1167.

Neilan, B. A., Taddeini, L., and Strate, R. G. (1977). T lymphocyte rosette formation after major burns. *JAMA* 238:493-496.

Nemery, B., Dinsdale, D., Sparrow, S., and Ray, D. (1985). Effects of methyl isocyanate on the respiratory tract of rats. *Br. J. Indust. Med.* 42:799-805.

Nichols, B. H. (1930). The clinical effects of the inhalation of nitrogen dioxide. *Am. J. Roentgenol.* 23:516-520.

Niederman, M. S., Abrams, C., Virgulto, J. A., Snyder, P., Wiedemann, H. P., Matthay, R. A., and Loke, J. (1983). Increase in bronchial reactivity of fire fighters with normal lung function. *Am. Rev. Respir. Dis.* **127**(4) (Suppl.):173 (Abstr.).

Niederman, M. S., Paul, E., Virgulto, J., Walker Smith, G. J., and Loke, J. (1981). In vitro tracheal repair after in vivo smoke inhalation in rabbits. Proc. Third Calif. Conf. Fire Toxicity, SRI International, Menlo Park, CA, Vol. 3:97-98.

Nieman, G. F., Clark, Jr., W. R., Wax, S. D., and Webb, W. R. (1980). The effect of smoke inhalation on pulmonary surfactant. *Ann. Surg.* **191**:171-181.

Norkool, D. M., and Kirkpatrick, J. N. (1985). Treatment of acute carbon monoxide poisoning with hyperbaric oxygen: a review of 115 cases. *Ann. Emer. Med.* **14**:1168-1171.

O'Flaherty, E. J., and Thomas, W. C. (1982). The cardiotoxicity of hydrogen cyanide as a component of polymer pyrolysis smoke. *Toxicol. Appl. Pharmacol.* **63**:373-381.

Olsen, J. H., and Asnaes, S. (1986). Formaldehyde and the risk of squamous cell carcinoma of the sinonasal cavities. *Br. J. Indust. Med.* **43**:769-774.

Panke, T. W., and McLeod, Jr., C. G. (1985). Respiratory system. In *Pathology of Thermal Injury: A Practical Approach.* Grune and Stratton, Inc., Orlando, Florida, Chap. 10, pp. 126-148.

Petajan, J. H., Voorhees, K. J., Packham, S. C., Baldwin, R. C., Einhorn, I. N., Grunnet, M. L., Dinger, B. G., and Birky, M. M. (1975). Extreme toxicity from combustion products of a fire-retarded polyurethane foam. *Sicence* **187**:742-744.

Peters, J. M., Theriault, G. P., Fine, L. J., and Wegman, D. H. (1974). Chronic effect of fire fighting on pulmonary function. *N. Engl. J. Med.* **291**:1320-1322.

Phillips, A. W., Tanner, J. W., and Cope, O. (1963). Brun therapy: IV. Respiratory tract damage (an account of the clinical, x-ray and postmortem findings) and the meaning of restlessness. *Ann. Surg.* **158**:799-811.

Pierson, D. J. (1976). Respiratory complications in the burned patient: pathophysiology and management. *Resp. Care* **21**:123-133.

Pitt, B. R., Radford, E. P., Gurtner, G. H., and Traystman, R. J. (1979). Interaction of carbon monoxide and cyanide on cerebral circulation and metabolism. *Arch. Environ. Health* **34**:354-359.

Planas, M., Wachtel, T., Frank, H., and Henderson, L. W. (1982). Characterization of acute renal failure in the burned patient. *Arch. Intern. Med.* **142**:2087-2091.

Pruitt, Jr., B. A. (1987). Burn treatment for the unburned. *JAMA* **257**:2207-2208.

Pruitt, Jr., B. A., and McManus, A. T. (1984). Opportunistic infections in severely burned patients. *Am. J. Med.* **76**:146-154.

Purser, D. A., and Berrill, K. R. (1983). Effects of carbon monoxide on behavior in monkeys in relation to human fire hazard. *Arch. Environ. Health* **38**:308-315.

Purser, D. A., Grimshaw, P., and Berrill, K. R. (1984). Intoxication by cyanide in fires: a study in monkeys using polyacrylonitrile. *Arch. Environ. Health* **39**:394-400.

Putman, C. E., Loke, J., Matthay, R. A., and Ravin, C. E. (1977). Radiographic manifestations of acute smoke inhalation. *Am. J. Roentgenol.* **129**:865-870.

Radford, E. P., and Levine, M. S. (1976). Occupational exposures to carbon monoxide in Baltimore fire fighters. *J. Occup. Med.* **18**:628-632.

Radford, E. P., and Renard, K. G. S. C. (1984). Lung cancer in Swedish iron miners exposed to low doses of radon daughters. *N. Engl. J. Med.* **310**: 1485-1494.

Rall, D. P. (1984). Toxic agent and radiation control: meeting the 1990 objectives for the nation. Public Health Reports. *J. US Public Health Service* **99**:532-538.

Ranieri, A., Jr., Jatlow, P., and Seligson, D. (1974). New method for rapid determination of carboxyhemoglobin by use of double-wave length spectrophotometry. *Clin. Chem.* **20**:278-281.

Rapaport, F. T., Backvaroff, R. J., Grullon, J., Kunz, H., Gill, III, T. J. (1982). Genetics of natural resistance to thermal injury. *Ann. Surg.* **195**:294-304.

Ratner, D., and Eshel, E. (1986). Aerial pesticide spraying: an environmental hazard. *JAMA* **256**:2516-2517.

Rees, P. J., Chilvers, C., and Clark, T. J. H. (1980). Evaluation of methods used to estimate inhaled dose of carbon monoxide. *Thorax* **35**:47-51.

Reisz, G. R., and Gammon, R. S. (1986). Toxic pneumonitis from mixing household cleaners. *Chest* **89**:40-52.

Richardson, P. S. (1982). Protective mechanisms of the respiratory tract. In *The Lung and Its Environment.* Edited by G. Bonsignore and G. Cumming. Plenum Press, New York, pp. 27-34.

Robinson, N. B., Hudson, L. D., Riem, M., Miller, E., Willoughby, J., Ravenholt, O., Carrico, C. J., and Heimbach, D. M. (1982). Steroid therapy following isolated smoke inhalation injury. *J. Trauma* **22**:876-879.

Robinson, N. B., Hudson, L. D., Robertson, H. T., Thorning, D. R., Carrico, C. J., and Heimbach, D. M. (1981). Ventilation and perfusion alterations after smoke inhalation injury. *Surgery* **90**:352-361.

Rooney, S. A. (1985). The surfactant system of the lung. In *Toxicology of In-*

haled Materials. Edited by H. P. Witschi and J. D. Brain. Springer-Verlag, Berlin-Heidelberg, pp. 471-502.

Rosenthal, T., Baum, G. L., Frand, U., and Molho, M. (1978). Poisoning caused by inhalation of hydrogen chloride, phosphorus oxychloride, phosphorus pentachloride, oxalyl chloride and oxalic acid. *Chest* **73**:623-626.

Saenger, E. L. (1986). Radiation accidents. *Ann. Emer. Med.* **15**:1061-1066.

Said, S. I. (1978). Environmental injury of the lung: role of humoral mediators. *Fed. Proc.* **37**:2504-2507.

Salmon, A. G., Muir, M. K., and Andersson, N. (1985). Acute toxicity of methyl isocyanate: a preliminary study of the dose response for eye and other effects. *Br. J. Indust. Med.* **42**:795-798.

Scharf, S. M., Thames, M. D., and Sargent, R. K. (1974). Transmural myocardial infarction after exposure to carbon monoxide in coronary artery disease. *N. Engl. J. Med.* **291**:85-86.

Schottenfeld, D. (1984). Chronic disease in the workplace and environment: cancer. *Arch. Environ. Health* **39**:150-157.

Sheppard, D., Distefano, S., Morse, L., and Becker, C. (1986). Acute effects of routine firefighting on lung function. *Am. J. Indust. Med.* **9**:333-340.

Sheps, D. S., Adams, Jr., K. F., Bromberg, P. A., Goldstein, G. M., O'Neil, J. J., Horstman, D., and Koch, G. (1987). Lack of effect of low levels of carboxyhemoglobin on cardiovascular function in patients with ischemic heart disease. *Arch. Environ. Health* **42**:108-116.

Shinozawa, Y., Hales, C., Jung, W., and Burke, J. (1986). Ibuprofen prevents synthetic smoke-induced pulmonary edema. *Am. Rev. Respir. Dis.* **134**: 1145-1148.

Shirani, K. Z., Pruitt, B. A., Jr., and Mason, A. D., Jr. (1987). The influence of inhalation injury and pneumonia on burn mortality. *Ann. Surg.* **205**: 82-87.

Sidor, R., Peterson, N. H., and Burgess, W. A. (1973). A carbon monoxide-oxygen sampler for evaluation of fire fighter exposures. *Am. Indust. Hyg. Assoc. J.* **34**(6):264-274.

Sidor, R., and Peters, J. M. (1974). Fire fighting and pulmonary function. *Am. Rev. Respir. Dis.* **109**:249-254.

Small, K. A., Radford, E. P., Frazier, J. M., Rodkey, F. L., and Collison, H. A. (1971). A rapid method for simultaneous measurement of carboxy-and methemoglobin in blood. *J. Appl. Physiol.* **31**:154-160.

Smith, J. R., and Landaw, S. A. (1978). Smokers' polycythemia. *N. Engl. J. Med.* **298**:6-10.

Smith, J. S., and Brandon, S. (1973). Morbidity from acute carbon monoxide poisoning at three year follow-up. *Br. Med. J.* **1**:318-321.

Sorenson, W. R. (1976). Polyvinyl chloride in fires. *JAMA* **236**:1449.

Sparrow, D., Bosse, R., Rosner, B., and Weiss, S. T. (1982). The effect of occupational exposure on pulmonary function. A longitudinal evaluation of fire fighters and nonfire fighters. *Am. Rev. Respir. Dis.* **125**:319-322.

Spebar, M. J., and Pruitt, B. A., Jr. (1981). Candidiasis in the burned patients. **21**:237-239.

Steenland, K. (1986). Lung cancer and diesel exhaust: a review. *Am. J. Indust. Med.* **10**:177-189.

Stewart, R. (1974). Cyanide poisoning. **7**:561-564.

Stewart, R. D., and Hake, C. L. (1976). Paint-remover hazard. *JAMA* **235**:398-401.

Stewart, R. D., Stewart, R. S., Stamm, W., and Seelen, R. P. (1976). Rapid estimation of carboxyhemoglobin level in fire fighters. *JAMA* **235**:390-392.

Stewart, R. D. (1975). The effect of carbon monoxide on humans. *Ann. Rev. Pharmacol.* **15**:409-423.

Stone, W. R. (1974). Safe use and hazards of coal and wood stoves. *Fire J.* May, pp. 87-92.

Strohl, K. P., Feldman, N. T., Saunders, N. A., and O'Connor, N. (1980). Carbon monoxide poisoning in fire victims: a reappraisal of prognosis. *J. Trauma* **20**:78-80.

Sturgess, J. M. (1985). Mucociliary clearance and mucus secretion in the lung. In *Toxicology of Inhaled Materials.* Edited by H. P. Witschi and J. D. Brain. Springer-Verlag, Berlin, Heidelberg, pp. 319-367.

Symington, I. S., Anderson, R. A., Oliver, J. S., Thomson, I., Harland, W. A., and Kerr, J. W. (1978). Cyanide exposure in fires. *Lancet* **2**:91-92.

Taplin, G. V., Chopra, S., Yanda, R. L., and Elam, D. (1976). Radionuclide lung-imaging procedures in the assessment of injury due to ammonia inhalation. *Chest* **69**:582-586.

Tashkin, D. P., Genovesi, M. G., Chopra, S., Coulson, A., and Simmons, M. (1977). Respiratory status of Los Angeles firemen: one month follow-up after inhalation of dense smoke. *Chest* **71**:445-449.

Terrill, J. B., Montgomery, R. R., and Reinhardt, C. F. (1978). Toxic gases from fires. *Science* **200**:1343-1347.

Thomas, W. C., and O'Flaherty, E. J. (1982). The cardiotoxicity of carbon monoxide as a component of polymer pyrolysis smoke. *Toxicol. Appl. Pharmacol.* **63**:363-372.

Thompson, P. B., Herndon, D. N., Traber, D. L., and Abston, S. (1986). Effect on mortality of inhalation injury. *J. Trauma* **26**:163-165.

Trunkey, D. D. (1978). Inhalation injury. *Surg. Clin. North Am.* **58**:1133-1140.

Unger, K. M., Snow, R. M., Mestas, J. M., and Miller, W. C. (1980). Smoke inhalation in firemen. *Thorax* **35**:838-842.

Upton, A. C. (1986). The place of laboratory animal testing in occupational and preventive medicine. *Am. J. Indust. Med.* **9**:69-71.

U.S. National Air Pollution Control Administration: Air quality criteria for carbon monoxide. (1970). U.S. Government Printing Office, Washington, D.C. AP-62:8-52.

Vena, J. E., and Fiedler, R. C. (1987). Mortality of a municipal-worker cohort: IV. Fire fighters. *Am. J. Indust. Med.* **11**:671-684.

Viadana, E., Bross, I. D. J., and Houten, L. (1976). Cancer experience of men exposed to inhalation of chemicals or to combustion products. *J. Occup. Med.* **18**:787-792.

Vogel, S. N., Sultan, T. R., and TenEyck, R. P. (1981). Cyanide poisoning. *Clin. Toxicol.* **18**:367-383.

Walker, H. L., McLeod, Jr., C. G., and McManus, W. F. (1981). Experimental inhalation injury in the goat. *J. Trauma* **21**:962-964.

Wanner, A., and Cutchavaree, A. (1973). Early recognition of upper airways obstruction following smoke inhalation. *Am. Rev. Respir. Dis.* **108**:1421-1423.

Webster, J. R., McCabe, M. M., and Karp, M. (1967). Recognition and management of smoke inhalation. **201**:287-290.

Wegman, D. H., Musk, A. W., Main, D. M., and Pagnotto, L. D. (1982). Accelerated loss of FEV_1 in polyurethane production workers: a four-year prospective study. *Am. J. Indust. Med.* **3**:209-215.

Wexler, J., Whittenberger, J. L., and Dumke, P. R. (1947). The effect of cyanide on the electrocardiogram of man. *Am. Heart J.* **34**:163-173.

Whitener, D. R., Whitener, L. M., Robertson, K. J., Baxter, C. R., and Pierce, A. K. (1980). Pulmonary function measurements in patients with thermal injury and smoke inhalation. *Am. Rev. Respir. Dis.* **122**:731-739.

Widdicombe, J. (1982). Defense mechanisms of the upper airways. In *The Lung in Its Environment.* Edited by G. Bonsignore and G. Cumming. Plenum Press, New York, pp. 121-130.

Wiedemann, H. P., Mahler, D. A., Loke, J., Virgulto, J. A., Snyder, P., and Matthay, R. A. (1986). Acute effects of passive smoking on lung function and airway reactivity in asthmatic subjects. *Chest* **89**:180-185.

Williams, D. O., Vanecko, R. M., and Glassroth, J. (1983). Endobronchial polyposis following smoke inhalation. *Chest* **84**:774-776.

Winter, P. M., and Miller, J. N. (1976). Carbon monoxide poisoning. *JAMA* **236**:1502-1504.

Winternitz, M. C. (1920). *Pathology of War Gas Poisoning.* Yale University Press, New Haven.

Witschi, H. (1976). Proliferation of Type II alveolar cells: a review of common responses in toxic lung injury. *Toxicology* **5**:267-277.

Woods, J. S. (1979). Epidemiologic considerations in the design of toxicologic studies: an approach to risk assessment in humans. *Fed. Proc.* **38**:1891-1896.

Young, I., Jackson, J., and West, S. (1980). Chronic respiratory disease and respiratory function in a group of fire fighters. *Med. J. Aust.* **1**:654-658.

Zaidi, S. H. (1986). Bhopal and after. *Am. J. Indust. Med.* **9**:215-216.

Zapp, Jr., J. A. (1962). Toxic and health effects of plastics and resins. *Arch. Environ. Health* **4**:125-136.

Zawacki, B. E., Jung, R. C., Joyce, J., and Rincon, E. (1977). Smoke, burns, and the natural history of inhalation injury in fire victims: a correlation of experimental and clinical data. *Ann. Surg.* **185**:100-110.

Zikria, B. A., Ferrer, J. M., and Floch, H. F. (1972). The chemical factors contributing to pulmonary damage in "smoke poisoning." *Surgery* **71**:704-709.

Zikria, B. A., Budd, D. C., Floch, F., and Ferrer, J. M. (1975). What is clinical smoke poisoning? *Ann. Surg.* **181**:151-156.

Zikria, B. A., Sturner, W. Q., Astarjian, N. K., Fox, C. L., Jr., and Ferrer, J. M., Jr. (1968). Respiratory tract damage in burns: pathophysiology and therapy. *Ann. NY Acad. Sci.* **150**:618-626.

AUTHOR INDEX

Italic numbers give page on which the complete reference is listed.

SUBJECT INDEX

A

Absorption
  gaseous and microparticulate, 134
  routes of administration, 136
Acetaldehyde, 466
Acrolein, 466-467
Acquired immune deficiency syndrome, 351, 353, 396
Acute brain syndrome, 376, 377
Acute gastrointestinal disease, 470
Acute hypertensive crises, 391
Acute inhalation injury in burn patients
  bronchoscopy, 250-252
  complications, 264-267
  diagnostic tests, 249-253
  differential diagnosis, 253
  parenchymal injury, 261
  pneumonia, 265-267
  pulmonary effects, 246-247
  pulmonary function tests, 235
  pulmonary insufficiency, 259-261
  respiratory tract injury, 256-257
  [133]Xenon lung scan, 250-253
Acute myocardial infarction, 384
Acute respiratory distress syndrome (ARDS), 188, 195, 198

Acute smoke inhalation, diagnosis, 482
Aerosols, 126
  environmental levels, 126
  propellants, 394, 395
Air flow velocity, 129
Air pollution, 49, 126
  ambient, 427-429
Airborne chemicals, 67
Airway, 49
  deposition, 130
  equivalent aerodynamic diameter, 130-131
  hyperreactivity, 478
  intubation in burn patients
    complications, 265
    indications, 257-258
  monodisperse, 130
  polydisperse, 130
Albumin, 216
  [99m]Tc macroaggregated, 196
Aldehydes, 466-467
Alkaline phosphatase, 226
Aluminum, 154-155
  absorption and excretion, 154
  Shaver's disease, 154
  Threshold limit value, 154
  toxicity, 154
Alveolar macrophages, 219-221
Aminotiols, 307
Amotivational syndrome, 367
Amyl nitrite, 307, 395

For Product Safety Concerns and Information please contact our EU
representative GPSR@taylorandfrancis.com
Taylor & Francis Verlag GmbH, Kaufingerstraße 24, 80331 München, Germany

www.ingramcontent.com/pod-product-compliance
Ingram Content Group UK Ltd.
Pitfield, Milton Keynes, MK11 3LW, UK
UKHW021426080625
459435UK00011B/180